Linear Algebra

and its Applications

Linear Algebra

and its Applications

Ganesh A MSc MPhil PhD PGDCA MISTE

Associate Professor
Department of Mathematics
The Oxford College of Engineering
Bangalore 560068 Karnataka

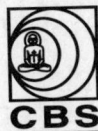

CBS Publishers & Distributors Pvt Ltd

New Delhi • Bengaluru • Chennai • Kochi • Kolkata • Mumbai
Bhopal • Bhubaneswar • Hyderabad • Jharkhand • Nagpur • Patna • Pune • Uttarakhand • Dhaka (Bangladesh)

Linear Algebra
and its Applications

ISBN: 978-81-239-2408-3

Copyright © Author and Publisher

First Edition: 2014
Reprint: 2019

Published by Satish Kumar Jain and produced by Varun Jain for
CBS Publishers & Distributors Pvt Ltd
4819/XI Prahlad Street, 24 Ansari Road, Daryaganj, New Delhi 110 002, India.
Ph: 23289259, 23266861, 23266867   Website: www.cbspd.com
Fax: 011-23243014   e-mail: delhi@cbspd.com; cbspubs@airtelmail.in.
Corporate Office: 204 FIE, Industrial Area, Patparganj, Delhi 110 092
Ph: 4934 4934   Fax: 4934 4935   e-mail: publishing@cbspd.com; publicity@cbspd.com

Branches

- **Bengaluru:** Seema House 2975, 17th Cross, K.R. Road,
  Banasankari 2nd Stage, Bengaluru 560 070, Karnataka
  Ph: +91-80-26771678/79   Fax: +91-80-26771680   e-mail: bangalore@cbspd.com
- **Chennai:** 7, Subbaraya Street, Shenoy Nagar, Chennai 600 030, Tamil Nadu
  Ph: +91-44-26680620, 26681266   Fax: +91-44-42032115   e-mail: chennai@cbspd.com
- **Kochi:** 42/1325, 1326, Power House Road, Opp KSEB, Power House,
  Ernakulam 682 018, Kochi, Kerala
  Ph: +91-484-4059061-65   Fax: +91-484-4059065   e-mail: kochi@cbspd.com
- **Kolkata:** 6/B, Ground Floor, Rameswar Shaw Road, Kolkata-700 014, West Bengal
  Ph: +91-33-22891126, 22891127, 22891128   e-mail: kolkata@cbspd.com
- **Mumbai:** 83-C, Dr E Moses Road, Worli, Mumbai-400018, Maharashtra
  Ph: +91-22-24902340/41   Fax: +91-22-24902342   e-mail: mumbai@cbspd.com

Representatives

• Bhopal	0-8319310552	• Bhubaneswar	0-9911037372	• Hyderabad	0-9885175004
• Jharkhand	0-9811541605	• Nagpur	0-9421945513	• Patna	0-9334159340
• Pune	0-9623451994	• Uttarakhand	0-9716462459	• Dhaka (Bangladesh)	01912-003485

Printed at: Swastik Packaging, Patparganj Industrial Area, Delhi, India

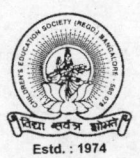

CHILDREN'S EDUCATION SOCIETY (Regd.)
Administrative Office :
1st Phase, J.P. Nagar, Bangalore - 560 078
✆ : 080 - 3041 0501 - 502   Fax : 080 - 2654 8658

THE OXFORD COLLEGE OF ENGINEERING
(Recognised by Govt. of Karnataka, Affiliated to Visveswaraiah Technological University, Belgaum & Approved by A.I.C.T.E., New Delhi & Accredited by National Board of Accreditation)
Bommanahalli, Hosur Road, Bangalore - 560 068
✆ : 080 - 3021 9601 - 602   Fax : 080 - 2573 0551 / 3021 9629
E-mail : engprincipal@theoxford.edu   Web : www.theoxford.edu

Estd. : 1974

Foreword

I am happy to present to the reader this book on *Linear Algebra and its Applications,* which is conceptualized and written by Dr A Ganesh, Associate Professor, Department of Mathematics, The Oxford College of Engineering, Bangalore. It mainly caters to the needs of postgraduate students and it can also be used as a reference book by undergraduate students as well as 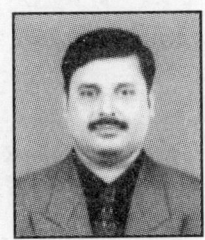 research students. A sound knowledge of linear algebra is very important for engineers and scientists.

It is pleasant to find that the book does not presume any knowledge of matrices on the part of the reader. The book begins with topics that explain matrix operations of addition, subtraction, scalar multiplication, and matrix multiplication. Next, it explores the notations of inverse, determinant, consistent and inconsistent systems. The book also provides an introduction to Markov chains, curve fitting, Eigenpairs, and some of the challenges encountered when matrices are used to solve real world problems.

This book is the outcome of the passionate work by Dr A Ganesh, who is already well known in student community and academic circles as a prolific author of popular textbooks in the field of mathematics. I am confident that this book will be very well received by the students. I am proud of his accomplishments and wish him all the best for the success of this book and in all his future endeavours.

Dr Nagaraj R
Principal
The Oxford College of Engineering
Bommanahalli, Hosur Road
Bangalore 560 068

to

_____

my dear parents,
Shiridi Sai Baba,
my loving son G. Monish Sri Sai,
my nephew Bhavesh L.
and
my wife Mamatha Ganesh

Aim and Motivation

This module aims to provide students with further knowledge in calculus and linear algebra essential for studies in engineering courses at the university level. Topics in the modules include multiple integrals, partial derivatives and their geometric significance and applications, sequences, infinite series and power series, matrices, determinants, systems of linear equations, eigenvalue and eigenvectors.

The teaching of linear algebra has always been a challenge for teachers of mathematics because it is extremely important that students become introduced into complex and abstract mathematical system of linear algebra and learn concepts which can be successfully applied later in other mathematical topics. It is necessary that teachers better understand how students learn and recognize and allow that the appropriate content, methods and context could be different in different environments.

The traditional approach that "only talking is teaching" is not acceptable anymore and it is not sufficient because it completely ignores the cognitive level and degree of development of each individual student. The role of teacher is to assist students in this construction process to acquire knowledge, but it is quite clear that simply talking and showing, no matter how qualitative it may be, probably will not significantly improve their learning of such abstract topics. It is recommended that students acquire knowledge by themselves.

As mathematicians, we are aware of the significant interconnections of different ideas and concepts, which are difficult to recognize and understand. We should not forget that understanding of these kinds of interconnections develops through active and hard exploration of mathematical topics through permanent discovering of new inter-connections and relations.

Thus, the primary role of a teacher is to try to motivate students to take active part during the class concerning important and difficult concepts, either through individual opinions or through group discussions. Even when the lectures have been supported by powerful technology, it is possible that students are still passive observers and we know that passive students are rarely successful in qualitative learning.

It is not easy to suggest teaching methods, especially in comparison to traditional lectures, which would be effective and would actively engage students and generate stimulating learning. Some very interesting questions for teachers considering linear algebra are:

1. What is optimal to teach at the first course and what should be the student's previous knowledge?
2. Which degree of abstraction should the teaching aim at?
3. Which facts should be used in the proofs?
4. How much time should be spent on each lesson topics?
5. What is the measure of qualitative understanding of basic principles and conceptual learning in linear algebra?
6. Whether, when, and how to use technology?

There are several different roles that technology can play in instructions. It may vary eliminating computations in realistic applications of providing environments for active exploration of the properties of mathematical structures and objects or getting a variety of experience using different software tools. Sometimes teachers can use adequate software tools for some topics to facilitate calculation of some examples and then they can direct the discussion to analyzing results.

Some teachers have lectures in electronic form for all the topics in their linear algebra courses. They hold lectures in computer laboratories and students work on these lessons individually or in groups, while the teacher is present and assist as much as necessary, which is an effective collaborative learning method.

Classroom voting through multiple choice questions or true/false questions is a powerful technique which can easily be incorporated into a traditional class. These techniques prevent students to be passive listeners and require their active participation creating a more effective learning environment. The students vote on the correct answer for the following type of questions: "Who thinks that this idea will be correct? Who does not?" either by raising up a hand or using an electronic clicker device, and then teacher can guide or direct the class through a discussion towards the concepts involved. The discussions are usually very live and typically result in correct responses from a large majority of the students. It is a practice that some of the students who understand correctly, explain their answers.

Self-evaluation and self-regulation are very meaningful parameters of a student's work. Also, students learn best in a non-stressful environment in psychological, emotional and physical sense. However, some research suggests that a natural environment, such as computer environment, is best for older, highly-motivated students. The natural environment allow students to have a choice in selecting tasks and activities whenever possible, or allow them to participate in group work, group discussions, especially in cooperative learning, which successfully increases motivation of students.

Conclusion

The essence of teaching is to help students to learn the material that they need and want to learn since different students want to learn different material in different ways, we should expect to change the way of our teaching. The integration of theoretical mathematics is natural in linear algebra, so that students can use their experience with linear algebra as a starting point for seeking similar integration in other mathematical areas and understanding of mathematics. Students have learned new techniques and have been able to model and evaluate a situation that was challenging, interesting and real. Technology brings to students and teachers the opportunity to individualize learning, generate illustrative examples, follow interesting topics to the desired depth, choose their own problems and appropriate tools for solving them. Information technologies have transformed the workplace for teaching-learning of mathematics, but not yet the curriculum of mathematics. Methodologically various teaching-learning models, which involve mathematical software, need to be developed in future.

Preface

Our original purpose in writing this book is to provide a text for the undergraduate and postgraduate linear algebra course.

Linear Algebra and its Applications is an introductory text for undergraduate and postgraduate students throughout the country. The organization of this text is motivated by what our experience tells us are the essential concepts that students should master in one-semester undergraduate linear algebra course. The centerpiece of our philosophy regarding the presentation of the material is that each topic should be fully developed before the reader moves onto the next. In addition, there should be a natural connection between the topics. We take great care to meet both of these objectives. As a result, the reader is prepared for each new unit and there is no need to repeat a concept in a subsequent chapter when it is utilized.

On the other hand, we have been keenly aware of the backgrounds which the students may possess and, in particular, of the fact that the students have very experience with abstract mathematical reasoning.

Throughout the book we have included a great variety of examples of the important concepts which occur. The study of such examples is of fundamental importance and tends to minimize the number of students who can repeat definition, theorem, and proof in logical order without grasping the meaning of the abstract concepts. This book also contains a wide variety of graded exercises ranging from routine applications to ones which will extend to the very best students.

The chapters deals with systems of linear equations and their solutions by means of elementary row operations on matrices, vector spaces, subspaces, basis and dimensions, linear transformations, their representation by matrices as well as isomorphism, linear functional and dual spaces, inner products, Jordan canonical forms, diagonalizable, eigenvalues and eigenvectors, Jordan form, quadratic forms, etc.

To motivate the definition of an abstract vector space and the suitable concept of linear independence, we use addition and scalar multiplication of vectors in Euclidean space. This approach equips students with the necessary skills and problem solving strategies in an abstract setting that allows for a greater understanding and appreciation for the numerous applications of the subject.

Ganesh A

Applications

Over the last few decades, the applications of linear algebra have mushroomed increasing not only in their numbers but also in the diversity of fields to which they apply. Much of this growth is fueled by the power of modern computers and the availability of computer algebra systems used to carry out computations for problems involving large matrices. This impressive power has made linear algebra more relevant than ever. Recently, a consortium of mathematics educators has placed its importance, relative to applications, second only to calculus. Increasingly, universities are offering courses in linear algebra that are specifically geared towards its applications. Whether the intended audience is engineering, economics, science or mathematics students, the abstract theory is essential for understanding how linear algebra is applied.

In this text, we show how linear systems can be used to solve problems related to chemistry, engineering, economics, nutrition and urban planning. However, many types of applications involve the more sophisticated concepts that we develop in the text. These applications require the theoretical notions beyond the basic ideas of the chapter and are presented at the end of a chapter as soon as the required background material is completed. Naturally, we had to limit the number of applications considered. The topics chosen will interest the reader and lead to further inquiry.

Specifically, the role of linear algebra in computer graphics, the connection between differential equations and linear algebra and the problem of finding approximate solutions to inconsistent linear systems have been considered. One of the most familiar applications here is the problem of finding the equation of a line which best fits a set of data points. Finally, we consider the singular value decomposition of a matrix and its application to data compression.

Technology

Computations are an integral part of any introductory course in mathematics and certainly in linear algebra also. To gain mastery of the techniques, we encourage the students to solve as many problems as possible by hand. We also encourage the students to make appropriate use of the available technologies designed to facilitate, or to completely carry out, some of the more tedious computations. For example, it is quite reasonable to use a computer algebra system, such as MAPLE or MATLAB to row reduce a large matrix. Our approach to linear algebra with applications is to assume that some form of technology will be used, but leave the choice to the individual instructor and the student. We do not think that it is necessary to include discussions or exercises that use particular software. The degree to which it is used is left to the discretion of the instructor. From our own experience, we have found that scientific notebookTM, which offers a front end for LATEX along with menu access to the computer algebra system MuPad, allows the students to gain experience using technology to carry out computations while learning to write clear mathematics. Another option is to use LATEX for writing mathematics and a computer algebra system to perform computations.

Another aspect of technology in linear algebra has to do with the accuracy and efficiency of computations. Some applications, like those related to internet search engines, involve very large matrices which require extensive processing. Moreover, the accuracy of the results can be affected by computer round off error. For example, using the characteristic equation to find the eigenvalues of a large matrix is not feasible. Overcoming problems of this kind is extremely important. The field of study known as numerical linear algebra is an area of vibrant research for both software engineers and applied mathematicians who are concerned with developing practical solutions. In our text, the fundamental concepts of linear algebra are introduced using simple examples. However, students should be made aware of the computational difficulties that arise when extending these ideas beyond the small matrices used in the illustrations.

Acknowledgements

First and foremost, I thank Almighty for showering his grace for the endeavour possible.

It gives me great pleasure to present this book *Linear Algebra and its Applications* throughout the country. My indebtedness remains to those who contributed to this first edition.

I am ever indebted to Dr G Balasubramaniam, Associate Professor, Department of Mathematics, Govt. Arts College (Men), Krishnagiri, for his excellent constructive guidance, continued interest and utmost motivation throughout the period of my work.

I wish to place my heartly and sincere thanks to my respectable Professor Dr Nityananda Pradhan, National Institute of Mental Health and Neurosciences (NIMHANS), Bangalore-29, for his constant encouragement, wealthy advice and administrative support.

I would like to thank The Oxford College of Engineering Chairman Mr S Narasaraju Garu, Executive Director Mr SNLV Narasimha Raju Garu, Principal Dr R Nagaraj and Head of the Department Dr. Mallikarjun K and the faculty members of the mathematics department for their valuable suggestions and encouragement.

My special thanks to well-wishers Dr KS Basavarajappa, Prof and Head, Department of Mathematics, Bapuji College of Engineering, Davanagiri, Karnataka, Prof KV Narayana, Vivekananda Degree College, Bangalore, Mr D Srinivas Murthy, Balasubramani, Telugu Pandit, Prof Chandran M, Department of Mathematics, The Oxford College of Engineering, Bangalore.

My sincere thanks to my family members for their prayers, affection and moral support throughout the period.

In addition, I would like to thank my students and colleagues whose perceptive comments led to this edition and the staff of CBS Publishers for their patience in dealing with me.

Ganesh A

Contents

1

Preliminary Concepts

1.1 INTRODUCTION

This chapter provides a brief review of all basic concepts, definitions, theorems, etc. which will be used in the subsequent chapters. Various theorems and results have been stated only without giving their proofs as the same may be looked up in any standard textbook on Algebra. It has been assumed that the reader is familiar with the elementary set theory.

1.2 OUTLINE

Here is a listing and brief description of the material in this set of notes.

Systems of Equation and Matrices

Systems of equations In this section, we will introduce most of the basic topics that we will need in order to solve systems of equations including augmented matrices and row operations.

Solving systems of equations Here we will look at the Gaussian elimination and Gauss-Jordan method of solving systems of equations.

Matrices We will introduce many of the basic ideas and properties involved in the study of matrices.

Matrix arithmetic and operations In this section, we will take a look at matrix addition, subtraction and multiplication and also take a quick look at the transpose and trace of a matrix.

Properties of matrix arithmetic We will take a more in-depth look at many of the properties of matrix arithmetic and the transpose.

Inverse and elementary matrices Here we will define the inverse and take a look at some of its properties and also introduce the idea of elementary matrices.

Finding inverse matrices In this section, we will develop a method for finding inverse matrices.

Special matrices We will introduce diagonal, triangular and symmetric matrices in this section.

LU-decompositions In this section, we will introduce the LU-decomposition, a way of "factoring" certain kinds of matrices.

1

Systems revisited Here we will revisit solving systems of equations. We will take a look at how inverse matrices and *LU*-decompositions can help with the solution process. We will also take a look at a couple of other ideas in the solution of systems of equations.

Determinants

The determinant function We will give the formal definition of the determinant in this section. We will also give formulae for computing determinants of 2×2 and 3×3 matrices.

Properties of determinants Here we will take a look at quite a few properties of the determinant function including formulae for determinants of triangular matrices.

The method of cofactors In this section, we will take a look at the first of two methods for computing determinants of general matrices.

Using row reduction to find determinants Here we will take a look at the second method for computing determinants in general.

Cramer's rule We will take a look at yet another method for solving systems. This method will involve the use of determinants.

Euclidean *n*-Space

Vectors In this section, we will introduce vectors in 2-space and 3-space as well as some of the important ideas about them.

Dot product and cross product Here we will look at the dot product and the cross product, two important products of vectors. We will also take a look at an application of the dot product.

Euclidean n-space We will introduce the idea of Euclidean *n*-space in this section and extend many of the ideas of the previous two sections.

Linear transformations In this section, we will introduce the topic of linear transformations and look at many of their properties.

Examples of linear transformations We will take a look at quite a few examples of linear transformations in this section.

Vector Spaces

Vector spaces In this section, we will formally define vectors and vector spaces.

Subspaces Here we will be looking at vector spaces that live inside of other vector spaces.

Span The concept of the span of a set of vectors will be investigated in this section.

Linear independence Here we will take a look at what it means for a set of vectors to be linearly independent or linearly dependent.

Basis and dimension We will be looking at the idea of a set of basis vectors and the dimension of a vector space.

Change of basis In this section, we will see how to change the set of basis vectors for a vector space.

Fundamental subspaces Here we will take a look at some of the fundamental subspaces of a matrix, including the row space, column space and null space.

Inner product spaces We will be looking at a special kind of vector spaces as well as define the inner product.

Orthonormal basis In this section, we will develop and use the Gram-Schmidt process for constructing an orthogonal/orthonormal basis for an inner product space.

Least squares In this section, we will take a look at an application of some of the ideas that we will be discussing in this chapter.

R-decomposition Here we will take a look at the QR-decomposition for a matrix and how it can be used in the least squares process.

Orthogonal matrices In this section, will take a look at a special kind of matrix, i.e. the orthogonal matrix.

Eigenvalues and Eigenvectors

Review of determinants In this section, we will do a quick review of determinants.

Eigenvalues and eigenvectors Here, we will take a look at the main section of this chapter. We will be looking at the concept of eigenvalues and eigenvectors.

Diagonalization We will be looking at diagonalizable matrices in this section.

1.3 CARTESIAN PRODUCT OF SETS AND RELATIONS

Cartesian Product of Sets

Let A and B be any two non-empty sets. The set of all ordered pairs (a, b) such that $a \in A$ and $b \in B$ is called the cartesian product of the sets A and B and is denoted by $A \times B$, that is,

$$A \times B = \{(a, b) : a \in A \text{ and } b \in B\}$$

If $A = \phi$ or $B = \phi$, then we define $A \times B = \phi$

Relation

Let A and B be two sets. A relation R from set A to set B is a subset of $A \times B$.

If R is a relation from a non-void set A to a non-void set B and if $(a, b) \in R$, then we write $a \, R \, b$ which is read as 'a is related to b by the relation R'. If $(a, b) \notin R$, then $(a, b) \in R^1$.

A relation from a set A to itself is called a relation on set A.

Inverse of a relation Let A and B be two sets and let R be a relation from a set A to a set B. Then the inverse of R denoted by R^{-1} is a relation from B to A and is defined by

$$R^{-1} = \{(b, a) : b \in B, a \in A\}$$

Clearly, $(a,b) \in R \Leftrightarrow (b,a) \in R^{-1}$

Identity relation The relation I_A on a set is identity relation if every element of A is related to itself only, that is

$$I_A = \{(a,a) : a \in A\}$$

Reflexive relation A relation R on set A is said to be reflexive if every element of A is related to itself.

Thus, R is reflexive on set A iff $(a, a) \in R$ for all $a \in A$.

Symmetric relation A relation R on set A is said to be a symmetric relation iff $(a,b) \in R \Rightarrow (b,a) \in R$ for all $a,b \in A$.

Transitive relation A relation R on a set A is said to be a transitive relation iff

$$(a,b) \in R \text{ and } (b,c) \in R \Rightarrow (a,c) \in R \text{ for all } a, b, c \in A.$$

Equivalence relation A relation R on a set A is said to be an equivalence relation iff R is :

(i) Reflexive, i.e. $(a, a) \in R$ for all $a \in A$.

(ii) Symmetric, i.e. $(a, b) \in R \Rightarrow (b, a) \in R$ for all $a, b \in A$.

If R is an equivalence relation on a non-empty set A and $a \in A$, then the set of all those elements of A which are related to a by the relation R is called the equivalence class determined by a and is denoted by $[a]$.

Thus, $[a] = \{x \in A : (x,a) \in R\}$

For any $a, b \in A$

(i) if $b \in [a]$, then $[b] = [a]$

(ii) $[a] = [b]$ iff $(a, b) \in R$

(iii) either $[a] = [b]$ or $[a] \cap [b] = \phi$

1.4 FUNCTIONS

Function as a Set of Ordered Pairs

Let A and B be two non-empty sets. A relation f from A to B, i.e. a subset of $A \times B$ is called a function (or a mapping or a map) from A to B if

(i) for each $a \in A$ there exists $b \in B$ such that $(a, b) \in f$

(ii) $(a, b) \in f$, then b is called the image of a under f

Function as a Correspondence

Let A and B be two non-empty sets. A function 'f' from set A to set B is a rule relating elements of set A to elements of set B such that

(i) all elements of set A are associated to elements in set B.

(ii) an element of set A is associated to a unique element in set B.

Terms such as 'map' (for "mapping"), "correspondence" are used as synonyms for "function".

If f is a function from a set A to a set B, then we write $f : A \rightarrow B$ or $A \xrightarrow{f} B$, which is read as 'f' is a function from A to B or f maps A to B. If an element $a \in A$ is associated to an element $b \in B$, then b is called "the f image of a" or "image of a under function" or "the value of the function f at a". Also, a is called the pre-image of b under the function f and we write $b = f(a)$ or $f^{-1}(b) = a$.

The set A is known as the domain of f and the set B is known as the co-domain of f. The set of all f-images of elements of A is known as the range of f or image set of A under f and is denoted by $f(A)$.

Thus, $\qquad f(A) = \{ f(x) : x \in A \} = $ range of f.

The set of all functions or mappings from a set X to a set A is denoted by A^X.

Remark: A rule relating all elements of set A to elements of set B is a function or a well-defined rule iff

$$x = y \Rightarrow f(x) = f(y) \text{ for all } x, y \in A$$

Injective Map

A function $f : A \rightarrow B$ is said to be an injective map or a one-one function if distinct elements in A have distinct images in B.

Thus, f is injective if and only if

$$x \neq y \Rightarrow f(x) \neq f(y) \text{ for all } x, y \in A$$

$$\Leftrightarrow \qquad f(x) = f(y) \Rightarrow x = y \text{ for all } x, y \in A$$

If $f : A \rightarrow B$ is not a one-one function, then it is said to be a many-one function, that is, a function $f : A \to B$ is said to be a many-one function if two or more elements of set A have the same image in B.

Surjective Map

A function $f : A \to B$ is said to be an onto function or a surjective map if every element of B is the f image of some element of A, i.e. if $f(A) = B$ or range of f is the co-domain of f or $l_m(f) = B$.

$f : A \to B$ is said to be a bijective map if it is injective as well as surjective.

Bijective Map

A function $f : A \to B$ is said to be a bijective map if it is injective as well as surjective.

In other words, a function $f : A \to B$ is a bijective map or a bijection if

(i) it is injective, i.e. $f(x) = f(y) \Rightarrow x = y$ for all $x, y \in A$

(ii) it is surjective, i.e. for all $y \in A$ there exists $x \in A$ such that $f(x) = y$

Permutation

Let A be a non-empty set. A bijective map from A to itself is called a permutation on A.

If A is a finite set equal to $\{a_1, a_2, ..., a_n\}$, then a permutation f on A is written in two row notation as follows.

$$f = \begin{pmatrix} a_1 & a_2 & a_3 & \cdots & a_n \\ f(a_1) & f(a_2) & f(a_3) & \cdots & f(a_n) \end{pmatrix}$$

Inverse of a Function

Let $f : A \to B$ be a bijection. Then a function $g : B \to A$ which associate each element $y \in B$ to a unique element $x \in A$ such that $f(x) = y$ is called the inverse of f and is denoted by f^{-1}.

Thus, if $f : A \to B$ is bijection, then $f^{-1} : B \to A$ is such that

$$f(x) = y \Leftrightarrow f^{-1}(y) = x$$

If f has an inverse, then f is said to be invertible. The inverse of an invertible function is unique.

Clearly f is invertible iff f is a bijection.

Composition of Functions

Let $f : A \to B$ and $g : C \to D$ be two functions such that $B \subset C$ or range $f \subset C$, then the composite h of f and g, denoted by *gof*, is the

mapping $h : A \to D$ defined by
$$h(x) = g\big(f(x)\big) \text{ for each } x \in A.$$

The composition of functions is not necessarily commutative, i.e. $gof \neq fog$. But it is always associative, i.e. for any three functions f, g, h, we have

$(fog)oh = fo(goh)$ provided that fog and goh are defined.

Also, if $f : A \to B$, then
$$foI_B = f = I_A of$$

where I_A and I_B are identity functions on A and B respectively.

If f and g are both invertible functions such that gof is defined, then gof is also invertible and $(gof)^{-1} = f^{-1}og^{-1}$.

Following are some useful results on composition of functions:

(i) If $f : A \to B$ and $g : B \to A$ are two functions such that $gof = I_A$, then f is an injection and g is a surjection.

(ii) If $f : A \to B$ and $g : B \to A$ are two functions such that $fog = I_B$, then f is a surjection and g is an injection.

(iii) If $f : A \to B$ and $g : B \to C$ be two functions, then

    (a) g of $A \to C$ is onto $\Rightarrow g : B \to C$ is onto

    (b) g of $A \to C$ is one-one $\Rightarrow f : A \to B$ is one-one

    (c) g of $A \to C$ is onto and $g : B \to C$ is one-one $\Rightarrow f : A \to B$ is onto

    (d) g of $A \to C$ is one and $f : A \to B$ is onto $\Rightarrow g : B \to C$ is one-one

List: Let n denote the set of first n natural numbers, i.e. $N = \{1, 2, ..., n\}$. Then a function $f : n \to A$ is called a list of elements in A and is written $(f_1, f_2, f_3, ..., f_n)$.

We use the notation n to denote the list $(1, 2, 3, ..., n)$.

1.5 BINARY OPERATIONS

Binary Operations: Let S be a non-empty set. A function $f : S \times S \to S$ is called a binary operation (or a binary composition) on this set S.

Thus, a binary operation f on a set S associates each ordered pair (a, b) in S. We shall use the notation of fb instead of $f(a, b)$ for a binary operation f on a set S. Generally, binary operations are denoted by the symbols like $*$, $\circ$, $\odot$, $\oplus$, etc. Thus, if $*$ is a binary operation on a set S, then image of an element $(a, b) \in S \times S$ is written as $a * b$ (instead of the usual notation $*(a, b)$).

Addition $(+)$ and multiplication $(\cdot)$ are binary operations on N but subtraction and division are not binary operations on N. Subtraction is a binary operation on each of sets Z, Q, R and C.

Commutative binary operation A binary operation $*$ on a set S is said to be commutative if

$$a * b = b * a \text{ for all } a, b \in S$$

Addition on R is commutative but subtraction is not commutative.

Associative binary operation A binary operation $*$ on a set S is said to be associative if

$$(a * b) * c = a * (b * c) \text{ for all } a, b, c \in S$$

Distributivity Let S be a non-void set and $*$ and $\odot$ be two binary operations on S. The binary operation $*$ is said to be

(i) left distributive over $\odot$ $(b \odot c) * a = (b * a) \odot (c * a)$

(ii) Right distributive over $\odot$ $a * (b \odot c) = (a * b) \odot (a * c)$ for all $a, b, c \in S$

The binary operation $*$ is said to be distributive over $\odot$ if it is both left as well as right distributive.

Closure property Let $*$ be a binary operation on a set S. A subset T of S is said to be closed under $*$ if $a * b \in T$ for all $a, b \in T$.

Clearly, S is closed under $*$ by the definition.

Restriction of a binary operation Let S and T be two sets such that $T \subset S$. A binary operation $*$ on T is said to be the restriction of a binary operation $\odot$ on S if $a * b \in T$ for all $a, b \in T$, that is, $*$ and $\odot$ are equal on T. If $*$ is restriction of $\odot$ on S, then we also say that the binary operation $*$ is induced by $\odot$ on S.

Usually, we use the same symbol for the binary operation $\odot$ and its restriction $*$ on T.

Addition on Z is restriction of addition on R. Similarly, multiplication on R is restriction of multiplication on C.

Left identity Let $*$ be a binary operation on a set S. An element $e_1 \in S$ is called a left identity if

$$e_1 * a = a \text{ for all } a \in S$$

Right identity Let $*$ be a binary operation on a set S. An element $e_2 \in S$ is called a right identity if

$$a * e_2 = a \text{ for all } a \in S$$

Identity element Let $*$ be a binary operation on a set S. An element $e \in S$ is called identity element if it is both a left identity and a right identity, i.e. $e * a = a = a * e$ for all $a \in S$

The identity element for a binary operation $*$ on a set S, if it exists, is unique.

Left inverse Let $*$ be a binary operation on a set S and $e \in S$ be the identity element for $*$ on S. An element b is a left inverse of $a \in S$ if

$$b * a = e$$

Right inverse Let $*$ be a binary operation on a set S and $e \in S$ be the identity element for $*$ on S. An element c is a right inverse of $a \in S$ if

$$a * c = e$$

Inverse of an element Let $*$ be a binary operation on a set S and $e \in S$ be the identity element for $*$ on S. An element x is an inverse of an element $a \in S$ if x is both left inverse as well as right inverse of a, i.e.

$$x * a = e = a * x$$

The inverse of a is usually denoted by a^{-1}. For additive binary operation on a set S, the inverse of a is denoted by $-a$.

An element $a \in S$ is said to be invertible, if it possesses its inverse. The inverse of an invertible element is unique. The identity element is always invertible and is inverse of itself.

Algebraic Structure

A non-empty set S equipped with one or more binary operations on it is called an algebraic structure.

1.6 GROUPS

Semigroup An algebraic structure $(G, *)$ consisting of a non-void set G and a binary operation $*$ defined on G is called a semigroup if it satisfies the following axiom.

SG-1 Associativity The binary operation $*$ is associative on G

i.e. $\qquad (a * b) * c = a * (b * c)$ for all $a, b, c \in G$

The algebraic structures $(N, +), (Q, +)\ (R, +), (C, +)\ (Z, +), (Q, +)$, etc. are semigroups.

Let $P(S)$ be the power set of a set S. Then, $(P(S), \cup)$ and $(P(S), \cap)$ are semigroups.

Monoid: An algebraic structure $(G, *)$ consisting of a non-void set G and a binary operation $*$ defined on G is called a monoid if it satisfies the following axioms.

M-1 Associativity The binary operation $*$ is associative on G

i.e. $\qquad (a * b) * c = a * (b * c)$ for all $a, b, c \in G$.

M-2 Existence of identity There exists a unique element $e \in G$ such that
$$a * e = a = e * a \text{ for all } a \in G.$$

The algebraic structures $(N, \times)$, $(Z, +)$, $(Q, \times)$ are monoids but $(N, +)$ is not a monoid.

Group: An algebraic structure $(G, *)$ consisting of a non-void set G and a binary operation $*$ defined on G is called a group if it satisfies the following axioms:

G-1 Associativity The binary operation $*$ is associative on G,

i.e. $\qquad (a * b) * c = a * (b * c) \text{ for all } a, b, c \in G$

G-2 Existence of Identity There exists an element $e \in G$ such that
$$a * e = a = e * a \text{ for all } a \in G$$

G-3 Existence of Inverse For each $a \in G$ there exists an element $a' \in G$ such that
$$a * a' = e = a' * a$$

The element a' is called the inverse of a and is denoted by a^{-1}.

The algebraic structures $(Z, +)$, $(Q, +)$, $(R, +)$, $(C, +)$ and $(Q, \times)$ are groups.

When it is not necessary to indicate the binary operation $*$, the group $(G, *)$ is simply referred to as the group G. If the binary operation on a group G is addition, it is usually called an additive group, its identity element is called zero, written as 0, and the inverse of a is called the negative of a, written as $-a$. When the binary operation on a group G is multiplication, then G is called a multiplicative group and $a \times b$ is written as ab. The identity element is usually denoted by 1 and the inverse of an element a is written as $\dfrac{1}{a}$.

Abelian Group

A group $(G, *)$ is called an abelian group if $*$ is commutative on G,

i.e. $a * b = b * a$ for all $a, b \in G$.

$(Z, +), (Q, \times), (R, +), (C, +)$, etc. are abelian groups.

Following are some useful properties of groups.

(i) The identity element in a group $(G, *)$ is unique.

(ii) The inverse of every element of a group $(G, *)$ is unique.

(iii) The inverse of identity element in a group is the identity element itself.

(iv) In a group $(G, *)$, $(a * b)^{-1} = b^{-1} * a^{-1}$ for all $a, b \in G$.

(v) Let $(G, *)$ be a group. Then for all $a, b, c \in G$

$a * b = a * c \Rightarrow b = c$ (Left cancellation law)

and $b * a = c * a \Rightarrow b = c$ (Right cancellation law)

(vi) In a group $(G, *)$, $(a^{-1})^{-1} = a$, $a \in G$

(vii) Let $(G, *)$ be a group. Then for any $a, b \in G$, the equation $a * x = b$ and $y * a = b$ have unique solutions in G.

Cyclic Group

A group $(G, *)$ is said to be cyclic, if there exists an element $a \in G$ such that every element of G is expressible as some integral power of a.

The element $a \in G$ is called the generator of G and we write $G = |a|$.

For example, $(Z, +)$ is a cyclic group generated by 1.

Following are some useful properties of a cyclic group:

(i) Every cyclic group is abelian but an abelian group need not be cyclic.

(ii) If a is generator of a cyclic group, then a^{-1} is also a generator of G.

(iii) The order of a cyclic group is the same as the order of its generator.

(iv) Every infinite cyclic group has two and only two generators.

Subgroup

Let $(G, *)$ be a group and H be a non-void subset of G such that

(i) H is closed for the binary operation $*$ on G

(ii) H itself is group for the composition induced by that of G, i.e. H itself is a group under the restriction of $*$ on H. Then, we say that $(H, *)$ is the subgroup of $(G, *)$.

Trivially $\{e\}$ and G itself are subgroups of G.

For the sake of convenience, we simply say that H is a subgroup of G if $(H, *)$ is a subgroup of $(G, *)$.

Cosets: Let H be a subgroup of a group G and let $a \in G$. Then the sets

$$aH = \{ah : h \in H\} \text{ and } Ha = \{ha : h \in H\}$$

are known as left and right cosets respectively of H in G.

Obviously, $aH \subset G$ and $Ha \subset G$ for all $a \in G$.

If the binary operation on G is addition, then

$$a + H = \{a + h : h \in H\} \text{ and } \{h + a : h \in H\}$$

are respectively the left and right cosets of H in G.

Any two right (left) cosets of a subgroup H of group G are identical or disjoint.

If H is a subgroup of a group G and $a, b \in G$, then

$$Ha = Hb \Leftrightarrow ab^{-1} \in H$$

If H is a subgroup of a group G and $a, b \in G$, then

$$H + a = H + b \Leftrightarrow a - b \in H$$

Normal Subgroup

A subgroup N of a group G is said to be a normal subgroup of G if $xax^{-1} \in N$ for all $x \in G$ and all $a \in N$

$$\Rightarrow \qquad\qquad xNx^{-1} \subset N \text{ for all } x \in G$$

A subgroup N of a group G is a normal subgroup of G iff $xN = Nx$ for all $x \in G$.

This means that there is no distinction between left and right cosets of a normal subgroup of a group.

If N is a normal subgroup of a group G, then $NaNb = Nab$ for all $a, b \in G$

Quotient Group

Let N be a normal subgroup of a group G. Then the set $\dfrac{G}{N} = \{Nx : x \in G\}$ of

all cosets of N in G is a group under the multiplication of cosets as a binary operation, i.e.

$$Na\,Nb = Nab \text{ for all } a, b \in G$$

This group is known as the quotient group or factor group of G by N.

1.7 RINGS AND FIELDS

Ring An algebraic structure $(R, +)$ consisting of a non-empty set R and two binary operations '+' and '×' on R is called a ring if the following axioms are satisfied.

Axiom-1: $(R, +)$ is an abelian group

Axiom-2: $(R, \cdot)$ is a semigroup

Axiom-3: '$\cdot$' is distributive over '+', i.e. for all $a, b \in G$

(i) $a \cdot (b + c) = a \cdot b + a \cdot c$

(ii) $(b + c) \cdot a = b \cdot a + c \cdot a$

Clearly, $(Z, +, \times)$, $(Q, +, \times)$ and $(R, +, \times)$ are rings.

Ring with unity A ring $(R, +, \cdot)$ is said to be a ring with unity if R has the identity element for multiplicative binary operation.

The identity element for multiplicative binary operation is denoted by 1.

Commutative ring A ring $(R, +, \cdot)$ is said to be a commutative ring if its multiactive binary operation is commutative,

i.e. $a \cdot b = b \cdot a$ for all $a, b \in R$

Following are some useful results in a ring $(R, +, \cdot)$:

(i) $a + 0 = 0 + a = 0$ for all $a \in R$, where 0 is the zero element, i.e. additive identity in R.

(ii) $a(-b) = -(ab) = (-a)b$ for all $a, b \in R$

(iii) $(-a)(-b) = ab$ for all $a, b \in R$

(iv) $a(b - c) = ab - ac$ for all $a, b, c \in R$

(v) $(b - c)a = ba - ca$ for all $a, b, c \in R$

Let $(R, +, \cdot)$ be a ring and n be a positive integer, then we define

$$na = a + a + a + \ldots + a \text{ (up to } n\text{-terms)}$$

Also, we define $0a = 0$, where 0 on the left-hand side is integer 0 and 0 on the right-hand side is the zero element (additive identity) of the ring.

Characteristic of a ring Let $(R, +, \cdot)$ be a ring with zero element 0. If there exists a positive integer n such that $na = 0$,

i.e. $a + a + a + \ldots + a$ (n times) $= 0$ (zero of the ring) for all $a \in R$. Then, we say that the ring is of finite characteristic. If n is the smallest positive integer such that $na = 0$ for all $a \in R$, then n is called the characteristic of ring R.

If there exists no positive integer n, such that $na = 0$ for all $a \in R$, then R is said to be of characteristic zero or infinite.

The ring $(Z, +, \times)$ is of characteristic zero, whereas $(Z_6, +_6, \times_6)$ is of characteristic 6.

Subring A non-void subset S of a ring $(R, +, \times)$ is a subring of R iff

(i) S is closed with respect to the binary operations of addition and multiplication on R

(ii) S itself is a ring for the induced binary operations.

The necessary and sufficient conditions for a non-void subset S of a ring R to be a subring of R are (i) $a - b \in S$ and (ii) $ab \in S$.

Field An algebraic structure $(F, +, \cdot)$ consisting of a non-void set F and two binary operations '+' and '$\cdot$' on F is called a field if the following axioms are satisfied.

Axiom-1: $(F, +)$ is an abelian group

Axiom-2: $(F, \cdot)$ is an abelian group

Axiom-3: '$\cdot$' is distributive over '+', i.e. for all $a, b, c \in G$

(i) $a \cdot (b + c) = a \cdot b + a \cdot c$

(ii) $(b + c) \cdot a = b \cdot a + c \cdot a$

A commutative ring with unity is a field, if its every non-zero element has multiplicative inverse.

$(Q,+,\times),(R,+,\times)$ and $(E,+,\times)$ are fields.

Subfield A non-void subset K of a field $(F,+,\cdot)$ is a subfield of F iff

(i) K is closed under the binary operations on F.

(ii) K itself is a field for the induced binary operations.

The necessary and sufficient conditions for a non-void subset K of a field F to be a subfield of F are

(i) $ab = ba$ for all $a,b \in K$

(ii) $ab^{-1} \in K$ for all $a \ne b \in K$

1.8 MATRICES

Matrix A matrix over a field F or simply a matrix A (when F is implicit) is a rectangular arrangement of scalars.

If there are mn scalars $a_{ij} \in F$, where $i \in m$ and $j \in n$, then the following arrangement of these mn scalars is a matrix.

$$A = \begin{bmatrix} a_{11} & a_{12} & \cdots & a_{1j} & \cdots & a_{1n} \\ a_{21} & a_{22} & \cdots & a_{2j} & \cdots & a_{2n} \\ \vdots & \vdots & & \vdots & & \vdots \\ a_{i1} & a_{i2} & \cdots & a_{ij} & \cdots & a_{in} \\ \vdots & \vdots & & \vdots & & \vdots \\ a_{m1} & a_{m2} & \cdots & a_{in} & \cdots & a_{mn} \end{bmatrix}$$

The element a_{ij} is called the ij-element or ij-entry which appears in ith row and jth column. Such a matrix is usually denoted by $A = [a_{ij}]_{m \times n}$ or simply $A = [a_{ij}]$.

A matrix with m rows and n columns is called an m by n matrix, written as $m \times n$.

The rows of matrix A (given above) are m horizontal lists of scalars as

$$(a_{11},a_{12},a_{13},\ldots,a_{1n}),\ (a_{21},a_{22},a_{23},\ldots,a_{2n}),\ (a_{m1},a_{m2},a_{m3},\ldots,a_{mn})$$

If we denote these rows by $A_1, A_2, A_3, \ldots, A_m$ respectively, then matrix A can also be written as a vertical list as given below.

$$A = \begin{bmatrix} A_1 \\ A_2 \\ \vdots \\ A_m \end{bmatrix}$$

The columns of matrix A are n vertical lists of scalars

$$\begin{bmatrix} a_{11} \\ a_{21} \\ \vdots \\ a_{n1} \end{bmatrix}, \begin{bmatrix} a_{12} \\ a_{22} \\ \vdots \\ a_{n2} \end{bmatrix} \cdots \begin{bmatrix} a_{1n} \\ a_{2n} \\ \vdots \\ a_{mn} \end{bmatrix}$$

These columns are generally denoted by $A^1, A^2,..., A^n$ and the matrix A can be written as list of n columns as given below.

$$A = (A^1, A^2,..., A^n)$$

Matrix as a mapping Let F be a field and m, n be positive integers. A mapping $A : m \times n \to F$ associating each ordered pair $(i, j) \in m \times n$ to the scalar $a_{ij} \in F$ is called an $m \times n$ matrix.

Clearly, a_{ij} is the image of $(i, j) \in m \times n$ under mapping A, i.e. $A(i, j) = a$ and is called the *ij-entry* or *ij-element* of matrix A. In such a case, the matrix A is also written as $A = [a_{ij}]$.

Column matrix A matrix with only one column is called a column matrix or a column vector.

As discussed above, a matrix A can be written as a row vector of its columns $A^1, A^2,..., A^n$ and a column vector of its rows $A_1, A_2,..., A_m$.

Square matrix An $n \times n$ matrix A is called a square matrix of order n.

If $A = [a_{ij}]$ is a square matrix of order n, then the elements $a_{11}, a_{22},..., a_{nn}$ are called the diagonal elements and the line along which they lie is called the principal diagonal or leading diagonal of the matrix. The diagonal elements are also written as $a_{ii}, i \in n$.

Diagonal matrix A square matrix $A = [a_{ij}]$ is called a diagonal matrix if all the elements except those in the leading diagonal are zero, i.e. $a_{ij} = 0$ for all $i \neq j$.

A diagonal matrix of order $n \times n$, having $d_1, d_2,..., d_n$ as diagonal elements is denoted by diag $(d_1, d_2,..., d_n)$.

For example, the diagonal matrix

$$A = \begin{bmatrix} 1 & 0 & 0 \\ 0 & 2 & 0 \\ 0 & 0 & 3 \end{bmatrix}$$

is written as diag $(1, 2, 3)$.

Scalar matrix A square matrix $A = \begin{bmatrix} a_{ij} \end{bmatrix}$ is called a scalar matrix if

(i) $a_{ij} = 0$ for all $i \neq j$

(ii) $a_{ii} = c$ for all i, where $c \neq 0$.

Identity matrix A square matrix $A = \begin{bmatrix} a_{ij} \end{bmatrix}_{n \times n}$ is called an identity matrix if

(i) $a_{ij} = 0$ for all $i \neq j$ and (ii) $a_{ii} = 1$ for all $i \in n$

An identity matrix of order $n \times n$ is generally denoted by I_n.

Null matrix A matrix whose all elements are zero is called a null matrix or a zero matrix.

Upper triangular matrix A square matrix $A = \begin{bmatrix} a_{ij} \end{bmatrix}_{n \times n}$ is called an upper triangular matrix if $a_{ij} = 0$ for all $i \neq j$.

All elements below the leading diagonal of an upper triangular matrix are zero.

Lower triangular matrix A square matrix $A = \begin{bmatrix} a_{ij} \end{bmatrix}_{n \times n}$ is a lower triangular matrix if $a_{ij} = 0$ for all $i < j$.

All elements above the leading diagonal of a lower triangular matrix are zero.

A triangular matrix $A = \begin{bmatrix} a_{ij} \end{bmatrix}$ is called strictly triangular iff $a_n = 0$ for all $i \in n$.

Echelon matrix A matrix is called an echelon matrix or is said to be in echelon form if A is either the null matrix or satisfies the following conditions.

(i) All zero rows, if any, are at the bottom of the matrix. Here zero row means a row whose all entries are zeros.

(ii) The number of zeros before the first non-zero element in a row is less than the number of such zeros in the next row.

That is, $A = \begin{bmatrix} a_{ij} \end{bmatrix}$ is an echelon matrix if there exist non-zero entries.

$$a_{j_1}, a_{j_2}, \ldots, a_{jr} \text{ where } j_1 < j_2 < \ldots < j_r$$

with the property that

$$a_{ij} = 0 \text{ for } \begin{cases} i \leq r \text{ and } j < j_i \\ i > r \text{ and } j < j_i \end{cases}$$

The elements a_{1j}, a_{2j}, a_{3j}, which are the leading non-zero elements in their respective rows are called the pivots of the echelon matrix.

The matrix A given by

$$A = \begin{bmatrix} 0 & ③ & 2 & 1 \\ 0 & 0 & ② & 5 \\ 0 & 0 & 0 & 0 \end{bmatrix}$$

is an echelon matrix whose pivots have been encircled.

Clearly, each pivot is to the right of the one above.

The following matrix is also an echelon matrix whose pivots have been encircled.

$$\begin{bmatrix} ③ & 4 & 2 & 0 & -1 & -2 & 3 \\ 0 & 0 & ⑤ & 1 & -2 & 3 & 0 \\ 0 & 0 & 0 & 0 & 0 & ⑦ & 3 \\ 0 & 0 & 0 & 0 & 0 & 0 & 0 \end{bmatrix}$$

Matrix in Row Canonical Form

A matrix A is said to be in row canonical form if it is an echelon matrix satisfying the following additional conditions.

(i) Each pivot is equal to 1.

(ii) Each pivot is the only non-zero entry of its column.

It should be noted that in echelon matrix there must be zeros below the pivots but in a matrix in row canonical form each pivot must be equal to 1 and there must also be zeros above the pivots.

The null matrix O and the identity matrix I (of any order) are examples of matrices in row canonical form.

The matrix A given by

$$A = \begin{bmatrix} 0 & ① & 2 & 0 & 0 & 4 \\ 0 & 0 & 0 & ① & 0 & 2 \\ 0 & 0 & 0 & 0 & ① & 3 \end{bmatrix}$$

is in row canonical form but the matrix B given on next page

$$B = \begin{bmatrix} \textcircled{-1} & 2 & 3 & 0 & 5 & -46 \\ 0 & 0 & \textcircled{1} & -2 & 3 & 0 \\ 0 & 0 & 0 & 0 & \textcircled{6} & 5 \\ 0 & 0 & 0 & 0 & 0 & 0 \end{bmatrix}$$

is not in row canonical form.

Equality of Matrices

Two matrices $A = \begin{bmatrix} a_{ij} \end{bmatrix}_{m \times n}$ and $B = \begin{bmatrix} b_{ij} \end{bmatrix}_{r \times s}$ are equal if (i) $m = r$ (ii) $n = s$ and (iii) $a_{ij} = b_{ij}$ for all i, j.

Scalar Multiplication

Let $A = \begin{bmatrix} a_{ij} \end{bmatrix}$ be an $m \times n$ matrix and k be a scalar. Then the matrix obtained by multiplying every element of A by k is called the scalar multiple of A by k and it is denoted by kA, that is,

$$kA = \begin{bmatrix} ka_{ij} \end{bmatrix}_{m \times n}$$

The negative of an $m \times n$ matrix $A = [a_{ij}]$, written as $-A$ is defined to be the $m \times n$ matrix given by $-A = [-a_{ij}]$ for all $i \in m, j \in n$.

Addition of Matrices

Let $A = [a_{ij}]$ and $B = [b_{ij}]$ be two $m \times n$ matrices over a field F. Then their sum $A + B$ is also an $m \times n$ matrix over F such that

$$(A + B)_{ij} = a_{ij} + b_{ij} \text{ for all } i \in m, \ j \in n$$

Let F be a field and m, n be positive integers. Then $F^{m \times n}$ denotes the set of all $m \times n$ matrices over field F. It is evident from the above definition that addition of matrices is a binary operation which possesses the following properties.

(i) Matrix addition on $F^{m \times n}$ is commutative,
   i.e. $A + B = B + A$ for all $A, B \in F^{m \times n}$

(ii) Matrix addition on $F^{m \times n}$ is associative,
   i.e. $(A + B) + C = A + (B + C)$ for all $A, B, C \in F^{m \times n}$

(iii) Null matrix O is the additive identity,
   i.e. $A + O = A = O + A$ for all $A \in F^{m \times n}$

(iv) For every matrix $A \in F^{m \times n}$, there exists $-A \in F^{m \times n}$ such that
   $A + (-A) = O = (-A) + A$

It follows from the above properties that $(F^{m \times n}, +)$ is an abelian group. Let A, B, $C \in F$ and λ, μ are scalars. Then we also have the following results:

(i) $\lambda(A + B) = \lambda A + \lambda B$

(ii) $(\lambda + \mu)A = \lambda A + \mu A$

(iii) $(\lambda\mu)A = \lambda(\mu A) = \mu(\lambda A)$

(iv) $1A = A$.

Multiplication of Matrices

If $A = [a_1, a_2, ..., a_n]$ is a row matrix and $B = \begin{bmatrix} b_1 \\ b_2 \\ \vdots \\ b_n \end{bmatrix}$ is a column matrix, then

their product AB is defined to be the scalar (or 1×1 matrix) obtained by multiplying corresponding entries and adding, that is,

$$AB = [a_1, a_2, ..., a_n]\begin{bmatrix} b_1 \\ b_2 \\ \vdots \\ b_n \end{bmatrix} = a_1 b_1 + a_2 b_2 + ... + a_n b_n = \sum_{r=1}^{n} a_r b_r$$

Note that the product AB is not defined when A and B have different number of elements. Let us now generalize the above definition for arbitrary matrices.

Let $A = [a_{ij}]$ and $B = [b_{ij}]$ be the two matrices over a field F such that the number of columns of A is equal to the number of rows of B; say A is $m \times p$ matrix and B is $p \times n$ matrix. Then, the product AB is $m \times n$ matrix whose ij-entry is obtained by multiplying ith row of A by the jth column of B, that is,

$$(AB)_{ij} = [a_1, a_2, ..., a_n]\begin{bmatrix} b_1 \\ b_2 \\ \vdots \\ b_n \end{bmatrix} = \sum_{r=1}^{n} a_{ir} b_{rj}$$

The multiplication of matrices is not commutative. However, matrix multiplication satisfies the following properties.

Theorem: Let A, B and C be the three matrices over a field F such that various products and sums are defined. Then

(i) $(AB)C = A(BC)$

(ii) $A(B+C) = AB + AC$

(iii) $(B+C)A = BA + CA$

(iv) $k(AB) = (kA)B = A(kB)$, where $k \in F$

(v) $A_{m \times n} O_{n \times p} = O_{m \times p}$ and $O_{p \times m} A_{m \times n} = O_{p \times n}$

Here A is an $m \times n$ matrix.

Positive Integral Powers of a Square Matrix

For any square matrix A, we define (i) $A^1 = A$ and (ii) $A^{n+1} = A^n A$, where $n \in N$.

It is evident from the above definition that:

$$A^2 = AA, \ A^3 = A^2 A = AAA \text{ etc.}$$

Also

(i) $A^m A^n = A^{m+n}$ and (ii) $(A^m)^n = A^{mn}$ for all $m, n \in N$.

Matrix Polynomial

Let $f(x) = a_0 x^n + a_1 x^{n-1} + \dots + a_{n-1} x + a_n$ be a polynomial over a field F and A be a square matrix over F. Then

$$f(A) = a_0 A^n + a_1 A^{n-1} + \dots + a_{n-1} A + a_n I$$

is called a matrix polynomial.

Let F be a field and n be a positive integer. Then the product of two $n \times n$ matrices over F is an $n \times n$ matrix over F. So the set $F^{n \times n}$ of all $n \times n$ matrices over F is closed under multiplication of matrices. The foregoing discussion suggests that $(F^{n \times n}, +, \times)$ is a non-commutative ring with unity if $n > 1$.

Transpose of a Matrix

Let $A = [a_{ij}]$ be an $m \times n$ matrix over a field F. Then the transpose of A denoted by A^T or A' is an $n \times m$ matrix such that

$$\left(A^T\right)_{ij} = a_{ji} \text{ for all } i \in m, j \in n.$$

Clearly, A^T is obtained from A by interchanging rows and columns of A.

Following are the basic properties of the transpose operation.

Let A and B be the two matrices over a field F and λ be a scalar in F. Then whenever the sum and product are defined

(i) $\left(A^T\right)^T = A$ (ii) $(A+B)^T = A^T + B^T$ (iii) $(\lambda A)^T = \lambda A^T$

(iv) $(AB)^T = B^T A^T$

Symmetric Matrix

A square matrix $A = [a_{ij}]$ over a field F is said to be a symmetric matrix if

$$a_{ij} = a_{ji} \text{ for all } i, j \in n$$

$$\Leftrightarrow \qquad A = A^T$$

Skew-Hermitian Matrix

A matrix A over the field C of all complex numbers is a skew-hermitian matrix if its conjugate transpose is equal to $-A$, i.e. $A^{-T} = -A$ or $A^* = -A$.

The diagonal elements of a skew-hermitian matrix are purely imaginary.

Unitary matrix A square matrix A over C is a unity matrix if $A^* A = 1 = AA^*$.

If A is the square matrix over C, then A is a normal matrix if $AA^* = A^* A$.

Clearly, this definition reduces to the definition of a normal matrix over R if C is replaced by R.

The conjugate transpose of a square matrix satisfies the following properties.

(i) $\left(A^*\right)^* = A$ (ii) $(\lambda A)^* = \bar{\lambda} A^*, \lambda \in C$ (iii) $(A+B)^* = A^* + B^*$

(iv) $(AB)^* = B^* A^*$ (v) $\left(A^*\right)^{-1} = \left(A^{-1}\right)^*$

Inverse of a Matrix

A square matrix B is said to be the inverse of a square matrix A if $AB = BA = 1$.

If the inverse of a square matrix A exists, then it is unique and we say that A is invertible. The inverse of A is denoted by A^{-1}.

Following are the properties of inverse of a matrix.

(i) If A is an invertible matrix, then $\left(A^{-1}\right)^{-1} = A$.

(ii) A square matrix is invertible if it is non-singular.

(iii) Let A and B be invertible matrices, then AB is invertible and
$$(AB)^{-1} = B^{-1} A^{-1}$$

(iv) Let A, B, C be square matrices of the same order and if A is an invertible matrix, then
$$AB = AC \Rightarrow B = C \text{ and } BA = CA \Rightarrow B = C$$

(v) If A is an invertible matrix, then A^T is also invertible and
$$\left(A^T\right)^{-1} = \left(A^{-1}\right)^T$$

(vi) The inverse of an invertible symmetric matrix is symmetric matrix.

(vii) The set $F^{n \times n}$ of all invertible matrices over a field F is a non-abelian group under multiplication of matrices.

1.9 DETERMINANTS

Determinants: Every square matrix over a field F can be associated to a scalar in F which is known as its determinant.

The determinant of A is denoted by $|A|$.

If $A = \begin{bmatrix} a_{11} & a_{12} \\ a_{21} & a_{22} \end{bmatrix}$ is a square matrix over a field F, then

$$|A| = \begin{vmatrix} a_{11} & a_{12} \\ a_{21} & a_{22} \end{vmatrix} = a_{11}a_{22} - a_{12}a_{21}$$

If $A = \begin{bmatrix} a_{11} & a_{12} & a_{13} \\ a_{21} & a_{22} & a_{23} \\ a_{31} & a_{32} & a_{33} \end{bmatrix}$ is a square matrix over a field F, then

$$|A| = \begin{vmatrix} a_{11} & a_{12} & a_{13} \\ a_{21} & a_{22} & a_{23} \\ a_{31} & a_{32} & a_{33} \end{vmatrix}$$

$$= a_{11} \begin{vmatrix} a_{22} & a_{23} \\ a_{32} & a_{33} \end{vmatrix} - a_{12} \begin{vmatrix} a_{21} & a_{23} \\ a_{31} & a_{33} \end{vmatrix} + a_{13} \begin{vmatrix} a_{21} & a_{22} \\ a_{31} & a_{32} \end{vmatrix}$$

$$= a_{11}(a_{22}a_{33} - a_{23}a_{32}) - a_{12}(a_{33}a_{21} - a_{23}a_{31}) + a_{13}(a_{21}a_{32} - a_{22}a_{31})$$

$$= a_{11}a_{22}a_{33} - a_{12}a_{23}a_{31} + a_{13}a_{32}a_{21} - a_{11}a_{23}a_{32} - a_{12}a_{21}a_{33} - a_{13}a_{22}a_{31}$$

Singular Matrix

A matrix A over a field F is called a singular matrix if $|A| = 0$. Otherwise, it is a non-singular matrix.

Minor

Let $A = \begin{bmatrix} a_{ij} \end{bmatrix}$ be a square matrix of order n. Then the minor M_{ij} of a_{ij} in A is the determinant of the square submatrix of order $(n - 1)$ obtained by leaving ith row and jth column of A.

Cofactor: Let $A = \begin{bmatrix} a_{ij} \end{bmatrix}$ be a square matrix of order n. Then the cofactor C_{ij} of a_{ij} in A is equal to $(-1)^{i+j}$ times the determinant of the submatrix of order $(n-1)$ obtained by leaving ith row and jth column of A.

Also,

(i) $\displaystyle\sum_{i=1}^{n} a_{ij}C_{ij} = |A|$ and $\displaystyle\sum_{j=1}^{n} a_{ij}C_{ij} = |A|$

(ii) $\displaystyle\sum_{i=1}^{n} a_{ij}C_{ij} = 0$ and $\displaystyle\sum_{j=1}^{n} a_{ij}C_{ij} = 0$

Adjoint of a Square Matrix

Let $A = \left[a_{ij} \right]$ be a square matrix of order n and let C_{ij} be a cofactor of a_{ij} in A. Then the transpose of the matrix of cofactor of elements of A is called the adjoint of A and is denoted by adj A, that is,

$$\text{adj}A = \left[C_{ij} \right]^{T} \text{ for all } i, \ j \in n$$

Following are some useful properties of adjoint of a matrix.

(i) For any square matrix A of order n

$A(\text{adj}A) = |A| I_n = (\text{adj}A)A$

(ii) For any square matrices A and B of order n

$\text{adj}AB = \text{adj}B \ \text{adj}A$

(iii) If A is an invertible matrix, then $\text{adj}A^{T} = (\text{adj}A)^{T}$

(iv) If A is an invertible matrix of order n, then

$\text{adj}(\text{adj}A) = |A|^{n-2} A$

(v) If A is a non-singular matrix, then $A^{-1} = \dfrac{1}{|A|}(\text{adj}A)$

1.10 SYSTEMS OF LINEAR EQUATIONS

A system of m linear equations in n unknowns $x_1, x_2, \ldots, x_n$ can be put in the standard form as follows:

$$a_{11}x_1 + a_{12}x_2 + \ldots + a_{1n}x_n = b_1$$
$$a_{21}x_1 + a_{22}x_2 + \ldots + a_{2n}x_n = b_2$$
$$\ldots \quad \ldots \quad \ldots \quad \ldots \quad \ldots$$
$$\ldots \quad \ldots \quad \ldots \quad \ldots \quad \ldots$$
$$a_{m1}x_1 + a_{m2}x_2 + \ldots + a_{mn}x_n = b_m$$

where a_{ij} and b_{ij} are constants.

This system of equations is known as $m \times n$ (read as m by n) system and can be written in the matrix form as follows :

$$\begin{bmatrix} a_{11} & a_{12} & \cdots & a_{1n} \\ a_{21} & a_{22} & \cdots & a_{2n} \\ \vdots & \vdots & & \vdots \\ a_{m1} & a_{m2} & \cdots & a_{mn} \end{bmatrix} \begin{bmatrix} x_1 \\ x_2 \\ \vdots \\ x_n \end{bmatrix} = \begin{bmatrix} b_1 \\ b_2 \\ \vdots \\ b_m \end{bmatrix}$$

Or $AX = B$, where $A = \begin{bmatrix} a_{11} & a_{12} & \cdots & a_{1n} \\ a_{21} & a_{22} & \cdots & a_{2n} \\ \vdots & \vdots & & \vdots \\ a_{m1} & a_{m2} & \cdots & a_{mn} \end{bmatrix}_{m \times n}$, $X = \begin{bmatrix} x_1 \\ x_2 \\ \vdots \\ x_n \end{bmatrix}_{n \times 1}$ and

$$B = \begin{bmatrix} b_1 \\ b_2 \\ \vdots \\ b_m \end{bmatrix}_{m \times 1}$$

The matrix $A = \begin{bmatrix} a_{ij} \end{bmatrix}_{m \times n}$ is called the coefficient matrix and the matrix

$$\begin{bmatrix} a_{11} & a_{12} & \cdots & a_{1n} & b_1 \\ a_{21} & a_{22} & \cdots & a_{2n} & b_2 \\ \cdots & \cdots & \cdots & \cdots & \cdots \\ \cdots & \cdots & \cdots & \cdots & \cdots \\ a_{m1} & a_{m2} & \cdots & a_{mn} & b_m \end{bmatrix}$$

is called the **augmented matrix** and is generally denoted by $[A : B]$.

A system of equations $AX = B$ is called a homogeneous system if $B = 0$. Otherwise, the system is said to be non-homogeneous.

A solution of the system of equations $AX = B$ is a list of the values for the unknowns which satisfy each equation of the system. Equivalently, a vector $U \in F^n$ is a solution of the system of equations $AX = B$.

If $AX = B$ is a system of n equations with n unknowns such that $|A| = 0$, then the system has unique solution given by $X = A^{-1}B$.

If $|A| \neq 0$, then the system of equations is either inconsistent or it has infinitely many solutions.

A homogeneous system of equations $AX = 0$ is always consistent and has trivial solution only if $|A| \neq 0$. If $|A| = 0$, then $AX = 0$ has non-trivial solutions also.

1.10.1 Systems of Equations in Triangular Form

Consider the following system of linear equations:

$$3x_1 - 2x_2 + 4x_3 - 3x_4 = 8$$
$$5x_2 - 2x_3 + 3x_4 = 7$$
$$7x_3 - 2x_4 = 3$$
$$3x_4 = 6$$

We observe that the system is square and the first unknown x_1 is the leading unknown in the first equation, the second unkonwn x_2 is the leading unknown in the second equation and so on. Such a system is said to be in triangular form.

Thus, a square system of linear equations is said to be in triangular form if each leading unknown is directly to the right of the leading unknown in the preceding equation.

Clearly, a triangular system always has a unique solution which may be obtained by back substitution.

1.10.2 Systems of Equations in Echelon Form

A system of simultaneous linear equations is said to be in echelon form if the leading unknown in each equation other than the first is to the right of the leading unknown in the preceding equation.

Consider the following system of equations in echelon form

$$3x_1 - 5x_2 + 3x_3 + 3x_4 - x_5 = 13$$
$$x_3 - 5x_4 + 2x_5 = 7$$
$$2x_4 - 7x_5 = 9$$

Clearly, x_1, x_3 and x_4 are the leading unknowns in this system.

These unknowns are called **pivot** variables and the other unknowns x_2 and x_5 are called **free variables.**

The solution set of a system of m simultaneous linear equations in n unknowns in echelon form is described into the following theorem.

Theorem: Let there be a system of simultaneous linear equations in n unknowns in echelon form, then

(i) The system has a unique solution if $m = n$, i.e. the system is in triangular form.

(ii) The system has an infinite number of solutions, if $m < n$, i.e. there are more variables than the number of equations.

Remark: If the echelon system of simultaneous linear equations contains more variables than equations, then each of the remaining $n - m$ free variables may take any value. So, the system has infinitely many solutions. The general solution of such a system may be obtained in either of the following two equivalent ways.

(i) Arbitrarily assign values to the $n - m$ free variables and solve uniquely for the m pivot variables to obtain a solution of the system.

(ii) Find the values of m pivot variables in terms of $(n - m)$ free variables to obtain the general solution of the system.

1.11 RANK OF A MATRIX

The rank of a matrix is defined in many different ways. But all the definitions lead to the same number.

Rank of a Matrix

The rank of a matrix is the order of the highest order non-singular square submatrix.

It is evident from the above definition that a positive integer r is rank of an $m \times n$ matrix if

(i) Every square submatrix of order $(r + 1)$ or more is singular.

(ii) There exists at least one square submatrix of order r which is non-singular.

The rank of a matrix A is written as rank (A).

Clearly, the rank of the identity matrix I_n is n.

If A is an $m \times n$ matrix, then rank $(A) \leq \min (m, n)$.

The rank of a matrix in echelon form is equal to the number of non-zero rows of the matrix or the number of pivots.

Theorem 1: The system of linear equations $AX = B$ is consistent iff the rank of the augmented matrix $[A : B]$ is equal to the rank of the coefficient matrix A.

Theorem 2: Let $AX = B$ be a system of m simultaneous linear equations in n unknowns such that $m \geq n$.

(i) If $r(A) = r([A : B]) = n$, the system has a unique solution.

(ii) If $r(A) = r([A : B]) = r > n$, the system is consistent and has infinite number of solutions.

In fact, in this case $(n - r)$ variables are free variables.

(iii) If $r(A) \neq r([A : B])$, the system is inconsistent, i.e. it has no solution.

2

Linear Equations

2.1 INTRODUCTION

Any straight line in the xy-plane can be represented algebraically by an equation of the form $a_1x + a_2y = b$, where a_1, a_2 and b are real constants and a_1 and a_2 both are not zero. An equation of the form is called a **"linear equation"** in the variables x and y. Generally, we define a linear equation in the n variables x_1, x_2,..., x_n to be one that can be expressed in the form

$$a_1x_1 + a_2x_2 + ... + a_nx_n = b$$

where a_1, a_2,..., a_n and b are real constants.

The variables in a linear equation are sometimes called *unknowns*.

Examples

$\Rightarrow \quad x + 3y = 7, \quad y = \dfrac{1}{2}x + 3z + 1, \quad x_1 - 2x_2 - 3x_3 + x_4 = 7$

are linear (the power should be one and no product involved).

$\Rightarrow x + 3\sqrt{y} = 5, 3x + 2y - z + xz = 4, y = \sin x$ are not linear (trigonometric and logarithmic equations are not linear)

2.2 FiELDS

Suppose F is a non-empty set with two binary operations called addition and multiplication denoted by '+' and '·' respectively, i.e. $\forall\, a + b \in F$ and $a \cdot b \in F$, then the algebraic structure $(F, +, \cdot)$ is called a field if the following postulates are satisfied.

F_1 : Addition is commutative, i.e. $a + b = b + a \,\,\forall\, a \cdot b \in F$

F_2 : Addition is associative $(a + b) + c = a + (b + c) \,\,\forall\, a, b, c \in F$

F_3 : If there exist an element denoted by 0 called zero in F, then $a + 0 = a \,\,\forall\, a \in F$

F_4 : To each element a in F there exist an element $- a$ in F such that $a + (-a) = 0$

F_5 : Multiplication is commutative, i.e. $a \cdot b = b \cdot a \,\,\forall\, a, b \in F$

F_6 : Multiplication is associative, i.e. $a \cdot (b \cdot c) = (a \cdot b) \cdot c \,\,\forall\, a, b, c \in F$

F_7 : If there exist a non-zero element denoted by 1 called one in F, then $a \cdot 1 = a \,\,\forall\, a \in F$

F_8: To every non-zero element a in F there corresponds an element a^{-1} (or $1/a$) in F such that $aa^{-1} = 1$.

F_9: Multiplication is distributive w.r.t addition in F, i.e. $a \cdot (b + c) = a \cdot b + a \cdot c \ \forall \, a, b, c$

Note: $0 \rightarrow$ zero element of field.

$1 \rightarrow$ identity element for multiplication $F \rightarrow$ unity

In field, each non-zero element has its unity.

2.3 FINDING A SOLUTION SET

Finding a solution set of (a) $4x - 2y = 1$ (b) $x_1 - 4x_2 + 7x_3 = 5$

Solution: (a) We can assign an arbitrary value to x and solve for y.

For example: $t = 3 \Rightarrow x = 3$

$$y = 2(3) - \frac{1}{2} = 6 - \frac{1}{2} = \frac{12-1}{2} = \frac{11}{2}$$

$$y = \frac{11}{2} \text{ and}$$

$$t = -\frac{1}{2} \text{ i.e. } x = -\frac{1}{2} \Rightarrow y = 2\left(-\frac{1}{2}\right) - \frac{1}{2} = -1 - \frac{1}{2}$$

$$= \frac{-2-1}{2} = -\frac{3}{2} \Rightarrow y = -\frac{3}{2}$$

Alternative approach: Assign of the arbitrary value 't'

i.e. $y = t, x = \frac{1}{2}t + \frac{1}{4}$

$$t = \frac{11}{2} \Rightarrow y = \frac{11}{2}, \ x = \frac{1}{2}\frac{11}{2} + \frac{1}{4} = \frac{11}{4} + \frac{1}{4} = \frac{12}{4} = 3$$

$$x = 3$$

$$t = -\frac{3}{2}, \text{ i.e. } y = -\frac{3}{2}, \ x = \frac{1}{2}\left(-\frac{3}{2}\right) + \frac{1}{4} = -\frac{3}{4} + \frac{1}{4} = -\frac{2}{4} = -\frac{1}{2}$$

All the sets of solutions should be the real numbers / values.

(b) To find the solution set of (b), we can assign arbitrary values to any two variables and solve for the third variable.

In particular, if we assign arbitrary values s and t to x_2 and x_3 respectively and solve for x_1, we obtain

$$x_1 = 5 + 4s - 7t, \quad x_2 = s, \quad x_3 = t$$

For example, $x_2 = 2, x_3 = 3$

$$x_1 = 5 + 4(2) - 7(3) = 5 + 8 - 21 = -8$$

$$x_1 = 8, \quad x_2 = 2$$

$$7x_3 = 5 - x_1 + 4x_2, \quad x_3 = \frac{5 - 8 + 8}{7} = \frac{5}{7}$$

$$x_1 = 8, \quad x_3 = 3$$

$$-4x_2 = 5 - 7x_3 - x_1 \implies x_2 = \frac{1}{4}(7x_3 + x_1 - 5)$$

$$= \frac{1}{4}(21 + 8 - 5)$$

$$= \frac{1}{4}(24) = 6$$

Sets of solutions are different.

2.4 SYSTEMS OF LINEAR EQUATIONS

Every system of linear equations has either no solution, exactly one solution or infinitely many solutions.

An arbitrary system of m linear equations in n unknowns can be written as

$$a_{11}x_1 + a_{12}x_2 + \ldots + a_{1n}x_n = b_1$$
$$a_{21}x_1 + a_{22}x_2 + \ldots + a_{2n}x_n = b_2$$
$$\vdots \qquad \vdots \qquad \qquad \vdots \qquad \vdots$$
$$a_{m1}x_1 + a_{m2}x_2 + \ldots + a_{mn}x_n = b_m$$

where $x_1, x_2, \ldots, x_n$ are the unknowns and a's and b's are constants.

Example: A general system of 3 linear equations in 3 unknowns can be written as

$$a_{11}x_1 + a_{12}x_2 + a_{13}x_3 = b_1$$
$$a_{21}x_1 + a_{22}x_2 + a_{23}x_3 = b_2$$
$$a_{31}x_1 + a_{32}x_2 + a_{33}x_3 = b_3$$

This system of equations can be written in the matrix form as

$$\begin{bmatrix} a_{11} & a_{12} & a_{13} \\ a_{21} & a_{22} & a_{23} \\ a_{31} & a_{32} & a_{33} \end{bmatrix} \begin{bmatrix} x_1 \\ x_2 \\ x_3 \end{bmatrix} = \begin{bmatrix} b_1 \\ b_2 \\ b_3 \end{bmatrix} \qquad \ldots(1)$$

$$AX = B$$

Equations (1) is called a solution of the system (or) non-homogeneous equation.

If $b_1 = b_2 = b_3 = ... = b_n = 0$, we say that the system is *homogeneous*.

Every homogeneous system of linear equations is consistent, since all such systems have $x_1 = 0$, $x_2 = 0$,..., $x_n = 0$ as a solution.

This solution is called the trivial solution. If there are other solutions, they are called non-trivial solutions.

Example: In the special case of a homogeneous system of two equations in two unknowns as say

$$a_1 x + b_1 y = 0 \qquad (a_1, b_1 \neq 0)$$
$$a_2 x + b_2 y = 0 \qquad (a_2, b_2 \neq 0)$$

Augmented Matrix

A system of m linear equations in n unknowns can be written only in the rectangular array of numbers.

$$\begin{bmatrix} a_{11} & a_{12} & \cdots & a_{1n} & b_1 \\ a_{21} & a_{22} & \cdots & a_{2n} & b_2 \\ \vdots & \vdots & \vdots & \vdots & \vdots \\ a_{m1} & a_{m2} & \cdots & a_{mn} & b_m \end{bmatrix}$$

This is called the augmented matrix for the system.

Elementary Row Operations

From the system of equations (1) $AX = B$

$$A = \begin{bmatrix} a_{11} & a_{12} & \cdots & a_{1n} \\ a_{21} & a_{22} & \cdots & a_{2n} \\ a_{m1} & a_{m2} & \cdots & a_{mn} \end{bmatrix}, \quad X = \begin{bmatrix} x_1 \\ x_2 \\ \vdots \\ x_n \end{bmatrix} \quad \text{and} \quad B = \begin{bmatrix} b_1 \\ b_2 \\ \vdots \\ b_m \end{bmatrix}$$

WORKED EXAMPLES

Example 1: Solve the system of equations.

$$x + y + 2z = 9$$
$$2x + 4y - 3z = 1$$
$$3x + 6y - 5z = 0$$

Solution:
$$[A:B] = \begin{bmatrix} 1 & 1 & 2 & :9 \\ 2 & 4 & -3 & :1 \\ 3 & 6 & -5 & :0 \end{bmatrix}$$

$R_2 \to R_2 - 2R_1, \quad R_3 \to R_3 - 3R_1$

$$= \begin{bmatrix} 1 & 1 & 2 & : & 9 \\ 0 & 2 & -7 & : & -17 \\ 0 & 3 & -11 & : & -27 \end{bmatrix}$$

$R_2 \rightarrow R_2/2$

$$= \begin{bmatrix} 1 & 1 & 2: & 9 \\ 0 & 1 & \dfrac{-7}{2}: & \dfrac{-17}{2} \\ 0 & 3 & -11: & -27 \end{bmatrix}$$

$R_3 \rightarrow R_3 - 3R_2$

$$= \begin{bmatrix} 1 & 1 & 2 & : & 9 \\ 0 & 1 & \dfrac{-7}{2} & : & \dfrac{-17}{2} \\ 0 & 0 & \dfrac{-1}{2} & : & \dfrac{-3}{2} \end{bmatrix}$$

$R_3 \rightarrow -2R_3$

$$= \begin{bmatrix} 1 & 1 & 2 & : & 9 \\ 0 & 1 & \dfrac{-7}{2} & : & \dfrac{-17}{2} \\ 0 & 0 & 1 & : & 3 \end{bmatrix}$$

$R_1 \rightarrow R_1 - R_2$

$$= \begin{bmatrix} 1 & 0 & \dfrac{11}{2} & : & \dfrac{35}{2} \\ 0 & 1 & \dfrac{-7}{2} & : & \dfrac{-17}{2} \\ 0 & 0 & 1 & : & 3 \end{bmatrix}$$

$R_1 \rightarrow R_1 - \dfrac{11}{2} R_3, \quad R_2 \rightarrow R_2 + \dfrac{7}{2} R_3$

$$= \begin{bmatrix} 1 & 0 & 0 & 1 \\ 0 & 1 & 0 & 2 \\ 0 & 0 & 1 & 3 \end{bmatrix}$$

$x = 1, y = 2, z = 3$

Example 2: Suppose F is the field of rational numbers and

$$A = \begin{bmatrix} 2 & -1 & 3 & 2 \\ 1 & 4 & 0 & -1 \\ 2 & 6 & -1 & 5 \end{bmatrix}$$

Solution: We shall perform a finite sequence of elementary row operations on A.

$$A = \begin{bmatrix} 2 & -1 & 3 & 2 \\ 1 & 4 & 0 & -1 \\ 2 & 6 & -1 & 5 \end{bmatrix} \quad R_1 \leftrightarrow R_2$$

$$\simeq \begin{bmatrix} 1 & 4 & 0 & -1 \\ 2 & -1 & 3 & 2 \\ 2 & 6 & -1 & 5 \end{bmatrix}$$

$R_2 \to R_2 - 2R_1, \quad R_3 \to R_3 - 2R_1$

$$\simeq \begin{bmatrix} 1 & 4 & 0 & -1 \\ 0 & -9 & 3 & 4 \\ 0 & -2 & -1 & 7 \end{bmatrix} \quad R_3 \to R_3 / -2$$

$$\simeq \begin{bmatrix} 1 & 4 & 0 & -1 \\ 0 & -9 & 3 & 4 \\ 0 & 1 & \dfrac{1}{2} & \dfrac{-7}{2} \end{bmatrix}$$

$R_1 \to R_1 - 4R_3, \quad R_2 \to R_2 + 9R_3$

$$\simeq \begin{bmatrix} 1 & 0 & -2 & 13 \\ 0 & 0 & \dfrac{15}{2} & \dfrac{-55}{2} \\ 0 & 1 & \dfrac{1}{2} & \dfrac{-7}{2} \end{bmatrix}$$

$R_2 \to 2R_2$

$$\simeq \begin{bmatrix} 1 & 0 & -2 & 13 \\ 0 & 0 & 15 & -55 \\ 0 & 1 & \dfrac{1}{2} & \dfrac{-7}{2} \end{bmatrix}$$

$R_2 \to R_2 / 5$

$$\simeq \begin{bmatrix} 1 & 0 & -2 & 13 \\ 0 & 0 & 3 & -11 \\ 0 & 1 & \dfrac{1}{2} & \dfrac{-7}{2} \end{bmatrix}$$

$R_2 \to R_2/3$

$$\simeq \begin{bmatrix} 1 & 0 & -2 & 13 \\ 0 & 0 & 1 & \dfrac{-11}{3} \\ 0 & 1 & \dfrac{1}{2} & \dfrac{-7}{2} \end{bmatrix}$$

$R_1 \to R_1 + 2R_2, \quad R_3 \to R_3 - \dfrac{1}{2}R_2$

$$\simeq \begin{bmatrix} 1 & 0 & 0 & \dfrac{17}{3} \\ 0 & 0 & 1 & \dfrac{-11}{3} \\ 0 & 1 & 0 & \dfrac{-5}{3} \end{bmatrix}$$

$$x_1 + \frac{17}{3}x_4 = 0$$

$$x_3 - \frac{11}{3}x_4 = 0$$

$$x_2 - \frac{5}{3}x_4 = 0$$

Example 3: Suppose F is the field of complex numbers and

$$A = \begin{bmatrix} -1 & i \\ -i & 3 \\ 1 & 2 \end{bmatrix}$$

Solution: $R_1 \to R_1 + R_3, \quad R_2 \to R_2 + iR_3$

$$\simeq \begin{bmatrix} 0 & 2+i \\ 0 & 3+2i \\ 1 & 2 \end{bmatrix}$$

$R_1 \to R_1/(2+i)$

$$\simeq \begin{bmatrix} 0 & 1 \\ 0 & 3+2i \\ 1 & 2 \end{bmatrix}$$

$R_2 \rightarrow R_2 - (3 + 2i) R_1$

$R_3 \rightarrow R_3 - 2R_1$

$$\simeq \begin{bmatrix} 0 & 1 \\ 0 & 0 \\ 1 & 0 \end{bmatrix}$$

Thus the system of equations

$$-x_1 + ix_2 = 0$$
$$-ix_1 + 3x_2 = 0$$
$$x_1 + 2x_2 = 0$$

has only the solution $\quad x_1 = x_2 = 0$

Example 4: If $\quad A = \begin{bmatrix} 3 & -1 & 2 \\ 2 & 1 & 1 \\ 1 & -3 & 0 \end{bmatrix}$,

find all solutions of $A X = 0$ by row-reducing A.

Solution: $\quad R_1 \leftrightarrow R_3$

$$A = \begin{bmatrix} 1 & -3 & 0 \\ 2 & 1 & 1 \\ 3 & -1 & 2 \end{bmatrix}$$

$R_2 \rightarrow R_2 - 2R_1$, $R_3 \rightarrow R_3 - 3R_1$

$$\simeq \begin{bmatrix} 1 & -3 & 0 \\ 0 & 7 & 1 \\ 0 & 8 & 2 \end{bmatrix}$$

$R_2 \rightarrow R_2 / 7$, $R_3 \rightarrow R_3 / 2$

$$\simeq \begin{bmatrix} 1 & -3 & 0 \\ 0 & 1 & \dfrac{1}{7} \\ 0 & 4 & 1 \end{bmatrix}$$

$R_1 \rightarrow R_1 + 3R_2$, $R_3 \rightarrow R_3 - 4R_2$

$$\simeq \begin{bmatrix} 1 & 0 & \dfrac{3}{7} \\ 0 & 1 & \dfrac{1}{7} \\ 0 & 0 & \dfrac{3}{7} \end{bmatrix}$$

$$R_3 \rightarrow \frac{7}{3} R_3$$

$$\simeq \begin{bmatrix} 1 & 0 & \dfrac{3}{7} \\ 0 & 1 & \dfrac{1}{7} \\ 0 & 0 & 1 \end{bmatrix}$$

$$R_1 \rightarrow R_1 - \frac{3}{7} R_3$$

$$R_2 \rightarrow R_2 - \frac{1}{7} R_3$$

$$\simeq \begin{bmatrix} 1 & 0 & 0 \\ 0 & 1 & 0 \\ 0 & 0 & 1 \end{bmatrix}$$

2.5 OPERATIONS ON MATRICES

So far, we have used matrices to abbreviate the work in solving systems of linear equations. For other applications, however, it is desirable to develop an "algebra of matrices" in which matrices can be added, subtracted and multiplied in a useful way.

Equal Matrices

Two matrices are said to be equal if they have the same size and their corresponding entries are equal.

In matrix notation, if $A = [a_{ij}]$ and $B = [b_{ij}]$ have the same size, then $A = B$ iff $(A)_{ij} = (B)_{ij}$ or equivalently, $a_{ij} = b_{ij}, \forall\ i = 1,2,\ldots,m,\ j = 1,2,\ldots,n$.

Example:

Consider the matrices

$$A = \begin{bmatrix} 2 & 1 \\ 3 & x \end{bmatrix}, \quad B = \begin{bmatrix} 2 & 1 \\ 3 & 5 \end{bmatrix}, \quad C = \begin{bmatrix} 2 & 1 & 0 \\ 2 & 4 & 0 \end{bmatrix}$$

If $x = 5$, then $A = B$ but for all other values of x the matrices A and B are not equal. There is no value of x for which $A = C$ since A and C have different sizes.

2.5.1 Sum and Difference of the Matrices

If A and B are matrices of the same size, then the sum $A + B$ is the matrix obtained by adding the entries of B to the corresponding entries of A and the difference $A - B$ is the matrix obtained by subtracting the entries of B from the corresponding entries of A.

Matrices of different sizes cannot be added or subtracted.

In matrix notation, if $A = [a_{ij}]$ and $B = [b_{ij}]$ have the same size, then

$$A + B = [a_{ij} + b_{ij}]$$

$$A - B = [a_{ij} - b_{ij}]$$

Example:

Consider the matrices

$$A = \begin{bmatrix} 2 & 1 & 0 & 3 \\ -1 & 0 & 2 & 4 \\ 4 & -2 & 7 & 0 \end{bmatrix}, \ B = \begin{bmatrix} -4 & 3 & 5 & 1 \\ 2 & 2 & 0 & -1 \\ 3 & 2 & -4 & 5 \end{bmatrix} \text{ and } C = \begin{bmatrix} 1 & 1 \\ 2 & 2 \end{bmatrix}$$

$$A + B = \begin{bmatrix} -2 & 4 & 5 & 4 \\ 1 & 2 & 2 & 3 \\ 7 & 0 & 3 & 5 \end{bmatrix} \text{ and } A - B = \begin{bmatrix} 6 & -2 & -5 & 2 \\ -3 & -2 & 2 & 5 \\ 1 & -4 & 11 & -5 \end{bmatrix}$$

The expressions $A + C$, $B + C$, $A - C$ and $B - C$ are undefined.

2.5.2 Scalar Multiple of Matrix

If A is any matrix and c is any scalar, then the product cA is the matrix obtained by multiplying each entry of the matrix A by c. The matrix cA is said to be a scalar multiple of A.

In matrix notation, if $A = [a_{ij}]$, then

$$(cA)_{ij} = c(A)_{ij} = ca_{ij}$$

Example:

For the matrices

$$A = \begin{bmatrix} 2 & 3 & 4 \\ 1 & 3 & 1 \end{bmatrix}, \ B = \begin{bmatrix} 0 & 2 & 7 \\ -1 & 3 & -5 \end{bmatrix} \text{ and } C = \begin{bmatrix} 9 & -6 & 3 \\ 3 & 0 & 12 \end{bmatrix}$$

We have

$$2A = \begin{bmatrix} 4 & 6 & 8 \\ 2 & 6 & 2 \end{bmatrix}, \ (-1)B = \begin{bmatrix} 0 & -2 & -7 \\ 1 & -3 & 5 \end{bmatrix} \text{ and } \frac{1}{3}C = \begin{bmatrix} 3 & -2 & 1 \\ 1 & 0 & 4 \end{bmatrix}$$

If $A_1, A_2,..., A_n$ are matrices of the same size and $c_1, c_2,...,c_n$ are scalars, then an expression of the form

$$c_1 A_1 + c_2 A_2 +...+ c_n A_n$$

is called "linear combination" of $A_1, A_2,...,A_n$ with coefficients $c_1, c_2,...,c_n$. For example, if A, B and C are the matrices in the above examples, then

$$2A - B + \frac{1}{3}C = 2A + (-1)B + \frac{1}{3}C$$

$$= \begin{bmatrix} 4 & 6 & 8 \\ 2 & 6 & 2 \end{bmatrix} + \begin{bmatrix} 0 & -2 & -7 \\ 1 & -3 & 5 \end{bmatrix} + \begin{bmatrix} 3 & -2 & 1 \\ 1 & 0 & 4 \end{bmatrix}$$

$$= \begin{bmatrix} 7 & 2 & 2 \\ 4 & 3 & 11 \end{bmatrix}$$

is the linear combination of A, B and C with scalar coefficients 2, -1 and $\frac{1}{3}$.

Matrix Multiplication

If A is an $m \times r$ matrix and B is an $r \times n$ matrix, the product AB is the $m \times n$ matrix.

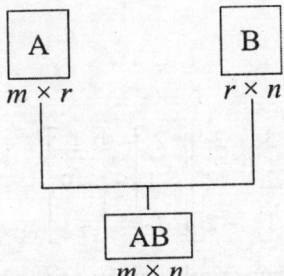

Example:

$$A = \begin{bmatrix} 1 & 2 & 4 \\ 2 & 6 & 0 \end{bmatrix}_{2\times3} \quad \text{and} \quad B = \begin{bmatrix} 4 & 1 & 4 & 3 \\ 0 & -1 & 3 & 1 \\ 2 & 7 & 5 & 2 \end{bmatrix}_{3\times4}$$

$$AB = 2 \times 4$$

$$AB = \begin{bmatrix} 12 & 27 & 30 & 13 \\ 8 & -4 & 26 & 12 \end{bmatrix}$$

2.6 MATRIX PRODUCT AS LINEAR COMBINATIONS

Row and column matrices provide an alternative way of thinking about matrix multiplication.

Example:

$$A = \begin{bmatrix} a_{11} & a_{12} & \cdots & a_{1n} \\ a_{21} & a_{22} & \cdots & a_{2n} \\ \vdots & \vdots & & \vdots \\ a_{m1} & a_{m2} & \cdots & a_{mn} \end{bmatrix} \quad \text{and} \quad X = \begin{bmatrix} x_1 \\ x_2 \\ \vdots \\ x_n \end{bmatrix}$$

Then,

$$AX = \begin{bmatrix} a_{11}x_1 + a_{12}x_2 + a_{13}x_3 + \ldots + a_{1n}x_n \\ a_{21}x_1 + a_{22}x_2 + a_{23}x_3 + \ldots + a_{2n}x_n \\ \vdots \qquad \vdots \qquad\qquad \vdots \\ a_{m1}x_1 + a_{m2}x_2 + a_{m3}x_3 + \ldots + a_{mn}x_n \end{bmatrix}$$

$$AX = x_1 \begin{bmatrix} a_{11} \\ a_{21} \\ \vdots \\ a_{m1} \end{bmatrix} + x_2 \begin{bmatrix} a_{12} \\ a_{22} \\ \vdots \\ a_{m2} \end{bmatrix} + \ldots + x_n \begin{bmatrix} a_{1n} \\ a_{2n} \\ \vdots \\ a_{mn} \end{bmatrix}$$

The product AX of a matrix A with a column matrix X is a linear combination of the column matrices of A with the coefficients coming from the matrix X.

Example 1:

The matrix product

$$\begin{bmatrix} -1 & 3 & 2 \\ 1 & 2 & -3 \\ 2 & 1 & -2 \end{bmatrix} \begin{bmatrix} 2 \\ -1 \\ 3 \end{bmatrix} = \begin{bmatrix} 1 \\ -9 \\ -3 \end{bmatrix}$$

can be written as the linear combination of the column matrices.

$$2\begin{bmatrix} -1 \\ 1 \\ 2 \end{bmatrix} - 1\begin{bmatrix} 3 \\ 2 \\ 1 \end{bmatrix} + 3\begin{bmatrix} 2 \\ -3 \\ -2 \end{bmatrix} = \begin{bmatrix} 1 \\ -9 \\ -3 \end{bmatrix}$$

The matrix product

$$\begin{bmatrix} 1 & -9 & -3 \end{bmatrix}_{1\times 3} \begin{bmatrix} -1 & 3 & 2 \\ 1 & 2 & -3 \\ 2 & 1 & -2 \end{bmatrix}_{3\times 3} = \begin{bmatrix} -16 & -18 & 35 \end{bmatrix}$$

can be written as the linear combination of row matrices.

$$1\begin{bmatrix} -1 & 3 & 2 \end{bmatrix} - 9\begin{bmatrix} 1 & 2 & -3 \end{bmatrix} - 3\begin{bmatrix} 2 & 1 & -2 \end{bmatrix} = \begin{bmatrix} -16 & -18 & 35 \end{bmatrix}$$

Example 2:

Columns of a product AB as linear combinations

$$AB = \begin{bmatrix} 1 & 2 & 4 \\ 2 & 6 & 0 \end{bmatrix} \begin{bmatrix} 4 & 1 & 4 & 3 \\ 0 & -1 & 3 & 1 \\ 2 & 7 & 5 & 2 \end{bmatrix} = \begin{bmatrix} 12 & 27 & 30 & 13 \\ 8 & -4 & 26 & 12 \end{bmatrix}$$

The column matrices of AB can be expressed as linear combinations of the column matrices of A as follows

$$4\begin{bmatrix}1\\2\end{bmatrix}+0\begin{bmatrix}2\\6\end{bmatrix}+2\begin{bmatrix}4\\0\end{bmatrix}=\begin{bmatrix}12\\8\end{bmatrix}$$

$$1\begin{bmatrix}1\\2\end{bmatrix}-1\begin{bmatrix}2\\6\end{bmatrix}+7\begin{bmatrix}4\\0\end{bmatrix}=\begin{bmatrix}27\\-4\end{bmatrix}$$

$$4\begin{bmatrix}1\\2\end{bmatrix}+3\begin{bmatrix}2\\6\end{bmatrix}+5\begin{bmatrix}4\\0\end{bmatrix}=\begin{bmatrix}30\\26\end{bmatrix}$$

$$3\begin{bmatrix}1\\2\end{bmatrix}+1\begin{bmatrix}2\\6\end{bmatrix}+2\begin{bmatrix}4\\0\end{bmatrix}=\begin{bmatrix}13\\12\end{bmatrix}$$

2.7 MATRIX FORM OF A LINEAR SYSTEM

Matrix multiplication has an important application to systems of linear equations. Consider any system of m linear equations in n unknowns.

$$a_{11}x_1 + a_{12}x_2 + \ldots + a_{1n}x_n = b_1$$
$$a_{21}x_1 + a_{22}x_2 + \ldots + a_{2n}x_n = b_2$$
$$\vdots \qquad \vdots \qquad \qquad \vdots \qquad \vdots$$
$$a_{m1}x_1 + a_{m2}x_2 + \ldots + a_{mn}x_n = b_n$$

$$\begin{bmatrix} a_{11} & a_{12} & \cdots & a_{1n} \\ a_{21} & a_{22} & \cdots & a_{2n} \\ \vdots & \vdots & & \vdots \\ a_{m1} & a_{m2} & \cdots & a_{mn} \end{bmatrix}\begin{bmatrix} x_1 \\ x_2 \\ \vdots \\ x_n \end{bmatrix}=\begin{bmatrix} b_1 \\ b_2 \\ \vdots \\ b_n \end{bmatrix}$$

$$AX = B$$

The matrix A in this equation is called the coefficient matrix of the system. The augmented matrix for the system is obtained by adjoining B to A as the last column, then the augmented matrix is

$$\left[A\,|\,B\right]=\begin{bmatrix} a_{11} & a_{12} & \cdots & a_{1n} & b_1 \\ a_{21} & a_{22} & \cdots & a_{2n} & b_2 \\ \vdots & \vdots & & \vdots & \vdots \\ a_{m1} & a_{m2} & \cdots & a_{mn} & b_n \end{bmatrix}$$

Transpose of a Matrix

If A is any $m \times n$ matrix, then the transpose of A, denoted by A^T is defined to be the $n \times m$ matrix that results from interchanging the rows and columns of A, i.e. the first column of A^T is the first row of A, etc.

Example 1:

$$A = \begin{bmatrix} a_{11} & a_{12} & a_{13} & a_{14} \\ a_{21} & a_{22} & a_{23} & a_{24} \\ a_{31} & a_{32} & a_{33} & a_{34} \end{bmatrix} \text{ and } A^T = \begin{bmatrix} a_{11} & a_{21} & a_{31} \\ a_{12} & a_{22} & a_{32} \\ a_{13} & a_{23} & a_{33} \\ a_{14} & a_{24} & a_{34} \end{bmatrix}$$

Example 2:

$$B = \begin{bmatrix} 2 & 3 \\ 1 & 4 \\ 5 & 6 \end{bmatrix} \text{ and } B^T = \begin{bmatrix} 2 & 1 & 5 \\ 3 & 4 & 6 \end{bmatrix}$$

Example 3:

$$= \begin{bmatrix} 0 & 0 & -2 & 0 & 7 & 12 \\ 2 & 4 & -10 & 6 & 12 & 28 \\ 2 & 4 & -5 & 6 & -5 & -1 \end{bmatrix}$$

$R_2 \rightarrow R_2/2$

$$= \begin{bmatrix} 0 & 0 & -2 & 0 & 7 & 12 \\ 1 & 2 & -5 & 3 & 6 & 14 \\ 2 & 4 & -5 & 6 & -5 & -1 \end{bmatrix}$$

$R_1 \leftrightarrow R_2$

$$= \begin{bmatrix} 1 & 2 & -5 & 3 & 6 & 14 \\ 0 & 0 & -2 & 0 & 7 & 12 \\ 2 & 4 & -5 & 6 & -5 & -1 \end{bmatrix}$$

$R_3 \rightarrow R_3 - 2R_1$

$$= \begin{bmatrix} 1 & 2 & -5 & 3 & 6 & 14 \\ 0 & 0 & -2 & 0 & 7 & 12 \\ 0 & 0 & 5 & 0 & -17 & -29 \end{bmatrix}$$

$R_2 \rightarrow R_2/2$

$$= \begin{bmatrix} 1 & 2 & -5 & 3 & 6 & 14 \\ 0 & 0 & -1 & 0 & \dfrac{7}{2} & 6 \\ 0 & 0 & 5 & 0 & -17 & -29 \end{bmatrix}$$

$R_3 \rightarrow R_3 + 5R_2$

$$= \begin{bmatrix} 1 & 2 & -5 & 3 & 6 & 14 \\ 0 & 0 & -1 & 0 & \dfrac{7}{2} & 6 \\ 0 & 0 & 0 & 0 & \dfrac{1}{2} & 1 \end{bmatrix}$$

$R_3 \rightarrow R_3 / 2$

$$= \begin{bmatrix} 1 & 2 & -5 & 3 & 6 & 14 \\ 0 & 0 & -1 & 0 & \dfrac{7}{2} & 6 \\ 0 & 0 & 0 & 0 & 1 & 2 \end{bmatrix}$$

$R_1 \rightarrow R_1 - 5R_2$

2.8 ROW-REDUCED ECHELON MATRICES

Definition: An $m \times r$ matrix R is called a row-reduced echelon matrix if:

1. A row does not consist entirely of zeros, then the non-zero numbers in the row is a 1. We call this as leading 1.
2. There is any row that consists entirely of zeros, they are grouped together at the bottom of the matrix.
3. Each column that contains a leading 1 has zero everywhere else.

Example: The following matrices are in reduced row-echelon form

$$\begin{bmatrix} 1 & 0 & 0 & 4 \\ 0 & 1 & 0 & 7 \\ 0 & 0 & 1 & -1 \end{bmatrix}, \begin{bmatrix} 1 & 0 & 0 \\ 0 & 1 & 0 \\ 0 & 0 & 1 \end{bmatrix}, \begin{bmatrix} 0 & 1 & -2 & 0 & 1 \\ 0 & 0 & 0 & 1 & 3 \\ 0 & 0 & 0 & 0 & 0 \\ 0 & 0 & 0 & 0 & 0 \end{bmatrix}, \begin{bmatrix} 0 & 0 \\ 0 & 0 \end{bmatrix}$$

Solutions of Four Linear Systems

Suppose that the augmented matrices for a system of linear equations has been reduced by row operations to the given reduced row-echelon form.

Example 1: Solve the system

(a) $\begin{bmatrix} 1 & 0 & 0 & 5 \\ 0 & 1 & 0 & -2 \\ 0 & 0 & 1 & 4 \end{bmatrix}$

Solution: The corresponding system of equations is
$$x_1 = 5, \, x_2 = -2, \, x_3 = 4$$

(b)
$$\begin{bmatrix} 1 & 0 & 0 & 4 & -1 \\ 0 & 1 & 0 & 2 & 6 \\ 0 & 0 & 1 & 3 & 2 \end{bmatrix}$$

Solution: The system of equations is
$$x_1 + 4x_4 = -1$$
$$x_2 + 2x_4 = 6$$
$$x_3 + 3x_4 = 2$$

Since x_1, x_2 and x_3 correspond to leading 1's in the augmented matrix, we call these terms as leading variables. The non-leading variables (x_4) are called "free variables".

$$x_1 = -1 - 4x_4$$
$$x_2 = 6 - 2x_4$$
$$x_3 = 2 - 3x_4$$

For free variables $x_4 = t$
$$x_1 = -1 - 4t, \quad x_2 = 6 - 2t, \quad x_3 = 2 - 3t, \quad x_4 = t$$
Then there are many solutions.

(c)
$$\begin{bmatrix} 1 & 6 & 0 & 0 & 4 & -2 \\ 0 & 0 & 1 & 0 & 3 & 1 \\ 0 & 0 & 0 & 1 & 5 & 2 \\ 0 & 0 & 0 & 0 & 0 & 0 \end{bmatrix}$$

Solution: The row of zeros leads to equation
$$0x_1 + 0x_2 + 0x_3 + 4x_4 + 0x_5 = 0$$
Then we can omit this equation and write the corresponding system as
$$x_1 + 6x_2 + 4x_5 = -2$$
$$x_3 + 3x_5 = 1$$
$$x_4 + 5x_5 = 2$$

x_5 is free variable
$$x_5 = t$$
$$x_2 = s$$
There are infinitely many solutions.
Therefore, the general solution is
$$x_1 = -2 - 6s - 4t, \quad x_2 = s, x_3 = 1 - 3t, \quad x_4 = 2 - 5t, \quad x_5 = t$$

(d)
$$\begin{bmatrix} 1 & 0 & 0 & 0 \\ 0 & 1 & 2 & 0 \\ 0 & 0 & 0 & 1 \end{bmatrix}$$

Solution: The least equation in the corresponding system of equations
$$0x_1 + 0x_2 + 0x_3 = 1$$
Since this equation cannot be satisfied, there is no solution of the system.
Let F be the field of rational numbers and

$$A = \begin{bmatrix} 1 & -2 & 1 \\ 2 & 1 & 1 \\ 0 & 5 & -1 \end{bmatrix}$$

To solve the system $AX = Y$ for some $y_1, y_2, y_3, \ldots$, let us perform a sequence of row operations on the augmented matrix A' which row-reduced A:

$$= \begin{bmatrix} 1 & -2 & 1 & y_1 \\ 2 & 1 & 1 & y_2 \\ 0 & 5 & -1 & y_3 \end{bmatrix}$$

$R_2 \rightarrow R_2 - 2R_1$

$$= \begin{bmatrix} 1 & -2 & 1 & y_1 \\ 0 & 5 & -1 & y_2 - 2y_1 \\ 0 & 5 & -1 & y_3 \end{bmatrix}$$

$R_3 \rightarrow R_3 - R_2$

$$= \begin{bmatrix} 1 & -2 & 1 & y_1 \\ 0 & 5 & -1 & y_2 - 2y_1 \\ 0 & 0 & 0 & y_3 - y_2 + 2y_1 \end{bmatrix}$$

$R_2 \rightarrow R_2 / 5$

$$= \begin{bmatrix} 1 & -2 & 1 & y_1 \\ 0 & 1 & \dfrac{-1}{5} & \dfrac{1}{5}(y_2 - 2y_1) \\ 0 & 0 & 0 & y_3 - y_2 + 2y_1 \end{bmatrix}$$

$R_1 \rightarrow R_1 + 2R_2$

$$= \begin{bmatrix} 1 & 0 & \dfrac{3}{5} & \dfrac{1}{5}(y_1 + 2y_2) \\ 0 & 1 & \dfrac{-1}{5} & \dfrac{1}{5}(y_2 - 2y_1) \\ 0 & 0 & 0 & y_3 - y_2 + 2y_1 \end{bmatrix}$$

The condition that the system $AX = Y$ has a solution is then
$$2y_1 - y_2 + y_3 = 0$$

$$x_1 = \frac{-3}{5}x_3 + \frac{1}{5}(y_1 + 2y_2)$$

$$x_2 = +\frac{1}{5}x_3 + \frac{1}{5}(y_2 - 2y_1)$$

x_3 is transverse

$$x_3 = k$$

$$x_1 = \frac{-3}{5}k + \frac{1}{5}(y_1 + 2y_2)$$

$$x_2 = \frac{1}{5}k + \frac{1}{5}(y_2 - 2y_1)$$

$y_1,...,y_n$ are in F.
$x_1, x_2,...$ are real numbers.

Example 2: Reducing the following matrices to reduced row-echelon form:

$$\begin{bmatrix} 0 & 0 & -2 & 0 & 7 & 12 \\ 2 & 4 & -10 & 6 & 12 & 28 \\ 2 & 4 & -5 & 6 & -5 & -1 \end{bmatrix}$$

Solution:
Step 1:

$$= \begin{bmatrix} 0 & 0 & -2 & 0 & 7 & 12 \\ 2 & 4 & -10 & 6 & 12 & 28 \\ 2 & 4 & -5 & 6 & -5 & -1 \end{bmatrix}$$

↖ Leftmost non-zero column
Step 2:
$R_1 \leftrightarrow R_2$

$$= \begin{bmatrix} 2 & 4 & -10 & 6 & 12 & 28 \\ 0 & 0 & -2 & 0 & 7 & 12 \\ 2 & 4 & -5 & 6 & -5 & -1 \end{bmatrix}$$

Step 3:
$R_1 \rightarrow R_1/2$

$$= \begin{bmatrix} 1 & 2 & -5 & 3 & 6 & 14 \\ 0 & 0 & -2 & 0 & 7 & 12 \\ 2 & 4 & -5 & 6 & -5 & -1 \end{bmatrix}$$

Step 4:

$R_3 \to R_3 - 2R_1$

$$= \begin{bmatrix} 1 & 2 & -5 & 3 & 6 & 14 \\ 0 & 0 & -2 & 0 & 7 & 12 \\ 0 & 0 & 5 & 0 & -17 & -29 \end{bmatrix}$$

↖ Leftmost non-zero column in the sub-matrix

$R_2 \to R_2 / -2$

$$= \begin{bmatrix} 1 & 2 & -5 & 3 & 6 & 14 \\ 0 & 0 & 1 & 0 & \dfrac{-7}{2} & -6 \\ 0 & 0 & 5 & 0 & -17 & -29 \end{bmatrix}$$

$R_3 \to R_3 - 5R_2$

$$= \begin{bmatrix} 1 & 2 & -5 & 3 & 6 & 14 \\ 0 & 0 & 1 & 0 & \dfrac{-7}{2} & -6 \\ 0 & 0 & 0 & 0 & \dfrac{1}{2} & 1 \end{bmatrix}$$

↖ Non-zero column matrix in the new sub-matrix

$R_3 \to 2R_3$

$$= \begin{bmatrix} 1 & 2 & -5 & 3 & 6 & 14 \\ 0 & 0 & 1 & 0 & \dfrac{-7}{2} & -6 \\ 0 & 0 & 0 & 0 & 1 & 2 \end{bmatrix}$$

Step 5:

$R_2 \to R_2 + \dfrac{7}{2} R_3$

$$= \begin{bmatrix} 1 & 2 & -5 & 3 & 6 & 14 \\ 0 & 0 & 1 & 0 & 0 & 1 \\ 0 & 0 & 0 & 0 & 1 & 2 \end{bmatrix}$$

$R_1 \rightarrow R_1 + 5R_2$

$$= \begin{bmatrix} 1 & 2 & 0 & 3 & 6 & 19 \\ 0 & 0 & 1 & 0 & 0 & 1 \\ 0 & 0 & 0 & 0 & 1 & 2 \end{bmatrix}$$

$R_1 \rightarrow R_1 - 6R_3$

$$= \begin{bmatrix} 1 & 2 & 0 & 3 & 0 & 7 \\ 0 & 0 & 1 & 0 & 0 & 1 \\ 0 & 0 & 0 & 0 & 1 & 2 \end{bmatrix}$$

$$x_1 + 2x_2 + 3x_4 = 7$$
$$x_3 = 1$$
$$x_5 = 2$$
$$x_1 + 2x_2 + 3x_4 = 7$$
$$x_1 = -(2x_2 + 3x_4) + 7$$
$$x_2 = t, \, x_4 = s$$
$$x_1 = -(2t + 3s) + 7$$

Example 3: Solve by Gauss-Jordan elimination:
$$x_1 + 3x_2 - 2x_3 + 2x_5 = 0$$
$$2x_1 + 6x_2 - 5x_3 - 2x_4 + 4x_5 - 3x_6 = -1$$
$$5x_3 + 10x_4 + 15x_6 = 5$$
$$2x_1 + 6x_2 + 8x_4 + 4x_5 + 18x_6 = 6$$

Solution:

The augmented matrix for the system is

$$= \begin{bmatrix} 1 & 3 & -2 & 0 & 2 & 0 & 0 \\ 2 & 6 & -5 & -2 & 4 & -3 & -1 \\ 0 & 0 & 5 & 10 & 0 & 15 & 5 \\ 2 & 6 & 0 & 8 & 4 & 18 & 6 \end{bmatrix}$$

$R_2 \rightarrow R_2 - 2R_1$
$R_4 \rightarrow R_4 - 2R_1, \quad R_3 \rightarrow R_3 / 5$

$$= \begin{bmatrix} 1 & 3 & -2 & 0 & 2 & 0 & 0 \\ 0 & 0 & -1 & -2 & 0 & -3 & -1 \\ 0 & 0 & 1 & 2 & 0 & 3 & 1 \\ 0 & 0 & 4 & 8 & 0 & 18 & 6 \end{bmatrix}$$

$R_3 \to R_3 + R_2$, $R_4 \to R_4 + 4R_2$

$$= \begin{bmatrix} 1 & 3 & -2 & 0 & 2 & 0 & 0 \\ 0 & 0 & -1 & -2 & 0 & -3 & -1 \\ 0 & 0 & 0 & 0 & 0 & 0 & 0 \\ 0 & 0 & 0 & 0 & 0 & 6 & 2 \end{bmatrix}$$

$R_4 \to R_4/6$

$$= \begin{bmatrix} 1 & 3 & -2 & 0 & 2 & 0 & 0 \\ 0 & 0 & -1 & -2 & 0 & -3 & -1 \\ 0 & 0 & 0 & 0 & 0 & 0 & 0 \\ 0 & 0 & 0 & 0 & 0 & 1 & \dfrac{1}{3} \end{bmatrix}$$

$R_2 \to (-)R_2$, $R_3 \leftrightarrow R_4$

$$= \begin{bmatrix} 1 & 3 & -2 & 0 & 2 & 0 & 0 \\ 0 & 0 & +1 & +2 & 0 & +3 & +1 \\ 0 & 0 & 0 & 0 & 0 & 1 & \dfrac{1}{3} \\ 0 & 0 & 0 & 0 & 0 & 0 & 0 \end{bmatrix}$$

$R_2 \to R_2 - 3R_3$

$$= \begin{bmatrix} 1 & 3 & -2 & 0 & 2 & 0 & 0 \\ 0 & 0 & 1 & 2 & 0 & 0 & 0 \\ 0 & 0 & 0 & 0 & 0 & 1 & \dfrac{1}{3} \\ 0 & 0 & 0 & 0 & 0 & 0 & 0 \end{bmatrix}$$

$$x_1 + 3x_2 - 2x_3 + 2x_5 = 0$$
$$x_3 + 2x_4 = 0$$
$$x_6 = \frac{1}{3}$$

We have discarded the equation
$$0x_1 + 0x_2 + 0x_3 + 0x_4 + 0x_5 + 0x_6 = 0$$
We solve the leading variables
$$x_1 = -3x_2 + 2x_3 - 2x_5$$
$$x_3 = -2x_4$$
$$x_6 = \frac{1}{3}$$

Assign the free variables x_2, x_4 and x_5 arbitrary values as r, s and t respectively.

Therefore the general solution,
$$x_1 = -3r - 4 - 2t$$

$$x_3 = -2s, \ x_4 = s, \ x_5 = t, \ x_6 = \frac{1}{3}$$

Example 4: Solve
$$x + y + 2z = 9$$
$$2x + 4y - 3z = 1$$
$$3x + 6y - 5z = 0$$

Solution:

Any matrix

$$= \begin{bmatrix} 1 & 1 & 2 & : & 9 \\ 2 & 4 & -3 & : & 1 \\ 3 & 6 & -5 & : & 0 \end{bmatrix}$$

to the row-echelon form,
$$R_2 \rightarrow R_2 - 2R_1 , \quad R_3 \rightarrow R_3 - 3R_1$$

$$= \begin{bmatrix} 1 & 1 & 2 & 9 \\ 0 & 2 & -7 & -17 \\ 0 & +3 & -11 & -27 \end{bmatrix}$$

$R_2 \rightarrow R_2 / 2$

$$= \begin{bmatrix} 1 & 1 & 2 & 9 \\ 0 & 1 & \dfrac{-7}{2} & \dfrac{-17}{2} \\ 0 & +3 & -11 & -27 \end{bmatrix}$$

$R_3 \rightarrow R_3 - 3R_2$

$$= \begin{bmatrix} 1 & 1 & 2 & 9 \\ 0 & 1 & \dfrac{-7}{2} & \dfrac{-17}{2} \\ 0 & 0 & \dfrac{-1}{2} & \dfrac{-3}{2} \end{bmatrix}$$

$R_3 \rightarrow -2R_3$

$$= \begin{bmatrix} 1 & 1 & 2 & 9 \\ 0 & 1 & \dfrac{-7}{2} & \dfrac{-17}{2} \\ 0 & 0 & 1 & 3 \end{bmatrix}$$

$$x + y + 2z = 9$$

$$y - \frac{7}{2}z = \frac{-17}{2}$$

$$z = 3 \quad \therefore \quad x = 1, \ y = 2, \ z = 3$$

Example 5: (a) $A = \begin{bmatrix} 1 & -1 & 1 \\ 2 & 0 & 1 \\ 3 & 0 & 1 \end{bmatrix}$ and $B = \begin{bmatrix} 2 & -2 \\ 1 & 3 \\ 4 & 4 \end{bmatrix}$

Verify that $A(AB) = A^2 B$

(b) $A = \begin{bmatrix} 2 & -1 & 1 \\ 1 & 2 & 1 \end{bmatrix}$, $B = \begin{bmatrix} 3 \\ 1 \\ -1 \end{bmatrix}$ and $C = \begin{bmatrix} 1 & -1 \end{bmatrix}$

Compute ABC and CAB.

2.9 INVERTIBLE MATRICES

Definition: If A is a square matrix and if a matrix B of the same order can be found such that $AB = BA = I$, then A is said to be invertible and B is called an inverse of A $[B = A^{-1}]$.

Example 1: The matrix $B = \begin{bmatrix} 3 & 5 \\ 1 & 2 \end{bmatrix}$ is an inverse of $A = \begin{bmatrix} 2 & -5 \\ -1 & 3 \end{bmatrix}$.

Since $\quad AB = \begin{bmatrix} 2 & -5 \\ -1 & 3 \end{bmatrix}\begin{bmatrix} 3 & 5 \\ 1 & 2 \end{bmatrix} = \begin{bmatrix} 1 & 0 \\ 0 & 1 \end{bmatrix} = I$

and $\quad BA = \begin{bmatrix} 3 & 5 \\ 1 & 2 \end{bmatrix}\begin{bmatrix} 2 & -5 \\ -1 & 3 \end{bmatrix} = \begin{bmatrix} 1 & 0 \\ 0 & 1 \end{bmatrix} = I$

$$x_1 y_1 = 64, \ 25x_1 = 64, \ x_1 = \frac{64}{25}$$

Example 2:

The matrix $A = \begin{bmatrix} 1 & 4 & 0 \\ 2 & 5 & 0 \\ 3 & 6 & 0 \end{bmatrix}$ is singular.

Let $B = \begin{bmatrix} b_{11} & b_{12} & b_{13} \\ b_{21} & b_{22} & b_{23} \\ b_{31} & b_{32} & b_{33} \end{bmatrix}$ be any 3×3 matrix.

The third column of BA is

$$\begin{bmatrix} b_{11} & b_{12} & b_{13} \\ b_{21} & b_{22} & b_{23} \\ b_{31} & b_{32} & b_{33} \end{bmatrix} \begin{bmatrix} 0 \\ 0 \\ 0 \end{bmatrix} = \begin{bmatrix} 0 \\ 0 \\ 0 \end{bmatrix}$$

Thus $BA \neq I = \begin{bmatrix} 1 & 0 & 0 \\ 0 & 1 & 0 \\ 0 & 0 & 1 \end{bmatrix}$

Theorem 1: If B and C are both inverses of the matrix A, then $B = C$.

Proof: Since B is an inverse of A,
we have $BA = I$

Multiplying both sides on the right by C

$\quad\quad (BA)\,C = IC = C$

But $\quad (BA)\,C = B\,(AC) = BI = B$

So that $\quad C = B$

Theorem 2: If A and B are invertible matrix of the same order, then AB is invertible and $(AB)^{-1} = B^{-1}\,A^{-1}$
i.e. prove that $(AB)\,B^{-1}\,A^{-1} = (B^{-1}\,A^{-1})\,AB = I$

Proof: If we can show that

$$(AB)\,(B^{-1}\,A^{-1}) = (B^{-1}\,A^{-1})\,AB = I$$

then the matrix AB is invertible and that $(AB)^{-1} = B^{-1}\,A^{-1}$

But $(AB)\,(B^{-1}\,A^{-1}) = A\,(BB^{-1})\,A^{-1} = A\,I\,A^{-1} = I$

A similar argument shows that $(B^{-1}\,A^{-1})\,AB = I$

Theorem 3: If A is an invertible matrix, then A^T is also invertible and
$$(A^{-1})^{-1} = (A^{-1})^T \qquad\qquad \text{...(2)}$$

Proof: We can prove the invariability of A^T and obtain equation (2) by showing that

$$A^T\,(A^{-1})^T = (A^{-1})^T\,A^T = I$$
$$(AA^{-1})^T = (A^{-1}\,A)^T = I^T = I$$
$$(A^{-1})^T\,A^T = (AA^{-1})^T = I^T = I$$

which completes the proof.

Example: Suppose F is the field of rational numbers and $A = \begin{bmatrix} 2 & -1 \\ 1 & 3 \end{bmatrix}$
(let us find the inverse of the form $AX = Y$)

Solution:
$$\approx \begin{bmatrix} 2 & -1 & y_1 \\ 1 & 3 & y_2 \end{bmatrix}$$

$R_1 \leftrightarrow R_2$

$$\approx \begin{bmatrix} 1 & 3 & y_2 \\ 2 & -1 & y_1 \end{bmatrix}$$

$R_2 \rightarrow R_2 - 2R_1$

$$\approx \begin{bmatrix} 1 & 3 & y_2 \\ 0 & -7 & y_1 - 2y_2 \end{bmatrix}$$

$R_3 \rightarrow R_3 / 7$

$$\approx \begin{bmatrix} 1 & 3 & y_2 \\ 0 & 1 & \frac{1}{7}(2y_2 - y_1) \end{bmatrix}$$

$R_1 \rightarrow R_1 - 3R_2$

$$= \begin{bmatrix} 1 & 0 & \frac{1}{7}(y_2 + 3y_1) \\ 0 & 1 & \frac{1}{7}(2y_2 - y_1) \end{bmatrix}$$

from which it is clear that A is invertible and

$$A^{-1} = \begin{bmatrix} \dfrac{3}{7} & \dfrac{1}{7} \\ \dfrac{-1}{7} & \dfrac{2}{7} \end{bmatrix}$$

$(y_1, y_2, ...$ are the arbitrary scalars)

Elementary Matrices and a Method for Finding A^{-1}.

Definition: A $n \times n$ matrix is called an elementary matrix if it can be obtained from $n \times n$ identity matrix by performing a single elementary row operations.

Example 1: Elementary matrices and row operations.

Four elementary matrices and the operation to produce them.

$$\begin{bmatrix} 1 & 0 \\ 0 & -3 \end{bmatrix}, \begin{bmatrix} 1 & 0 & 0 & 0 \\ 0 & 0 & 0 & 1 \\ 0 & 0 & 1 & 0 \\ 0 & 1 & 0 & 0 \end{bmatrix}, \begin{bmatrix} 1 & 0 & 3 \\ 0 & 1 & 0 \\ 0 & 0 & 1 \end{bmatrix} \text{ and } \begin{bmatrix} 1 & 0 & 0 \\ 0 & 1 & 0 \\ 0 & 0 & 1 \end{bmatrix}$$

Example 2: Using row operations to find A^{-1}.

(a) Find the inverse of $A = \begin{bmatrix} 1 & 2 & 3 \\ 2 & 5 & 3 \\ 1 & 0 & 8 \end{bmatrix}$

Solution:

$$A/I \simeq \begin{bmatrix} 1 & 2 & 3 & | & 1 & 0 & 0 \\ 2 & 5 & 3 & | & 0 & 1 & 0 \\ 1 & 0 & 8 & | & 0 & 0 & 1 \end{bmatrix}$$

$R_2 \rightarrow R_2 - 2R_1$, $R_3 \rightarrow R_3 - R_1$

$$\simeq \begin{bmatrix} 1 & 2 & 3 & | & 1 & 0 & 0 \\ 0 & 1 & -3 & | & -2 & 1 & 0 \\ 0 & -2 & 5 & | & -1 & 0 & 1 \end{bmatrix}$$

$R_1 \rightarrow R_1 - 2R_2$, $R_3 \rightarrow R_3 + 2R_2$

$$= \begin{bmatrix} 1 & 0 & 9 & 5 & -2 & 0 \\ 0 & 1 & -3 & -2 & 1 & 0 \\ 0 & 0 & -1 & -5 & 2 & 1 \end{bmatrix}$$

$$= \begin{bmatrix} 1 & 0 & 9 & 5 & -2 & 0 \\ 0 & 1 & -3 & -2 & 1 & 0 \\ 0 & 0 & 1 & 5 & -2 & -1 \end{bmatrix}$$

$R_1 \rightarrow R_1 - 9R_3$, $R_2 \rightarrow R_2 + 3R_3$

$$= \begin{bmatrix} 1 & 0 & 0 & -40 & 16 & +9 \\ 0 & 1 & 0 & 13 & -5 & -3 \\ 0 & 0 & 1 & 5 & -2 & -1 \end{bmatrix}$$

$\therefore$ $\qquad A^{-1} = \begin{bmatrix} -40 & 16 & 9 \\ 13 & -5 & -3 \\ 5 & -2 & -1 \end{bmatrix} \rightarrow$ invertible

(b) Find the inverse of $A = \begin{bmatrix} 1 & \dfrac{1}{2} & \dfrac{1}{3} \\ \dfrac{1}{2} & \dfrac{1}{3} & \dfrac{1}{4} \\ \dfrac{1}{3} & \dfrac{1}{4} & \dfrac{1}{5} \end{bmatrix}$

Solution:

$$= \begin{bmatrix} 1 & \dfrac{1}{2} & \dfrac{1}{3} & 1 & 0 & 0 \\[2ex] \dfrac{1}{2} & \dfrac{1}{3} & \dfrac{1}{4} & 0 & 1 & 0 \\[2ex] \dfrac{1}{3} & \dfrac{1}{4} & \dfrac{1}{5} & 0 & 0 & 1 \end{bmatrix}$$

$R_2 \to R_2 - \dfrac{1}{2}R_1$, $R_3 \to R_3 - \dfrac{1}{3}R_1$

$$= \begin{bmatrix} 1 & \dfrac{1}{2} & \dfrac{1}{3} & 1 & 0 & 0 \\[2ex] 0 & \dfrac{1}{12} & \dfrac{1}{12} & \dfrac{-1}{2} & 1 & 0 \\[2ex] 0 & \dfrac{1}{12} & \dfrac{4}{45} & \dfrac{-1}{3} & 0 & 1 \end{bmatrix}$$

$R_2 \to 12R_2$

$$= \begin{bmatrix} 1 & \dfrac{1}{2} & \dfrac{1}{3} & 1 & 0 & 0 \\[2ex] 0 & 1 & 1 & -6 & 12 & 0 \\[2ex] 0 & \dfrac{1}{12} & \dfrac{4}{45} & \dfrac{-1}{3} & 0 & 1 \end{bmatrix}$$

$R_1 \to R_1 - \dfrac{1}{2}R_2$, $R_3 \to R_3 - \dfrac{1}{12}R_2$

$$= \begin{bmatrix} 1 & 0 & \dfrac{-1}{6} & 4 & -6 & 0 \\[2ex] 0 & 1 & 1 & -6 & 12 & 0 \\[2ex] 0 & 0 & \dfrac{1}{180} & \dfrac{1}{6} & -1 & 1 \end{bmatrix}$$

$R_3 \to 18R_3$

$$= \begin{bmatrix} 1 & 0 & \dfrac{-1}{6} & 4 & -6 & 0 \\[2ex] 0 & 1 & 1 & -6 & 12 & 0 \\[2ex] 0 & 0 & 1 & 30 & -180 & 180 \end{bmatrix}$$

$$R_1 \rightarrow R_1 + \frac{1}{6} R_3 , \quad R_2 \rightarrow R_2 - R_3$$

$$\begin{bmatrix} 1 & 0 & 0 & 9 & -36 & -30 \\ 0 & 1 & 0 & -36 & 192 & -180 \\ 0 & 0 & 1 & 30 & -180 & 180 \end{bmatrix}$$

$$A^{-1} = \begin{bmatrix} 9 & -36 & 36 \\ -36 & -192 & -180 \\ 30 & -180 & 180 \end{bmatrix}$$

Example 3: For each of the two matrices

$$\begin{bmatrix} 2 & 5 & -1 \\ 4 & -1 & 2 \\ 6 & 4 & 1 \end{bmatrix} \quad \text{and} \quad \begin{bmatrix} 1 & -1 & 2 \\ 3 & 2 & 4 \\ 0 & 1 & -2 \end{bmatrix}$$

use elementary row operations to discover whether it is invertible and find the inverse.

Example 4: Show that a matrix is not invertible.

Consider the matrix

$$A = \begin{bmatrix} 1 & 6 & 4 \\ 2 & 4 & -1 \\ -1 & 2 & 5 \end{bmatrix}$$

Solution:

$$= \begin{bmatrix} 1 & 6 & 4 & 1 & 0 & 0 \\ 2 & 4 & -1 & 0 & 1 & 0 \\ -1 & 2 & 5 & 0 & 0 & 1 \end{bmatrix}$$

$$R_2 \rightarrow R_2 - 2R_1 , \quad R_3 \rightarrow R_3 + R_1$$

$$= \begin{bmatrix} 1 & 6 & 4 & 1 & 0 & 0 \\ 0 & -8 & -9 & -2 & 1 & 0 \\ 0 & 8 & 9 & 1 & 0 & 1 \end{bmatrix}$$

$$R_3 \rightarrow R_3 + R_2$$

$$= \begin{bmatrix} 1 & 6 & 4 & 1 & 0 & 0 \\ 0 & -8 & -9 & -2 & 1 & 0 \\ 0 & 0 & 0 & -1 & 1 & 1 \end{bmatrix}$$

Since we have obtained a row of zeros on the left side, A is not invertible.

Example 5: Show that a matrix is not invertible:

$$A = \begin{bmatrix} 1 & 6 & 4 \\ 2 & 4 & -1 \\ -1 & 2 & 5 \end{bmatrix}$$

Solution:

$$= \begin{bmatrix} 1 & 6 & 4 \\ 2 & 5 & -1 \\ -1 & 2 & 5 \end{bmatrix} \begin{matrix} 1 & 0 & 0 \\ 0 & 1 & 0 \\ 0 & 0 & 1 \end{matrix}$$

$R_2 \rightarrow R_2 - 2R_1$, $R_3 \rightarrow R_3 + R_1$

$$= \begin{bmatrix} 1 & 6 & 4 \\ 0 & -7 & -7 \\ 0 & 8 & 9 \end{bmatrix} \begin{matrix} 1 & 0 & 0 \\ -2 & 1 & 0 \\ 1 & 0 & 0 \end{matrix}$$

$R_2 \rightarrow R_2 / -7$

$$= \begin{bmatrix} 1 & 6 & 4 \\ 0 & 1 & 1 \\ 0 & 8 & 9 \end{bmatrix} \begin{matrix} 1 & 0 & 0 \\ \dfrac{2}{7} & \dfrac{-1}{7} & 0 \\ 1 & 0 & 0 \end{matrix}$$

$R_1 \rightarrow R_1 - 6R_2$, $R_3 \rightarrow R_3 - 8R_2$

$$= \begin{bmatrix} 1 & 0 & -2 \\ 0 & 1 & 1 \\ 0 & 0 & -1 \end{bmatrix} \begin{matrix} \dfrac{-5}{7} & \dfrac{6}{7} & 0 \\ \dfrac{2}{7} & \dfrac{-1}{7} & 0 \\ \dfrac{-9}{7} & \dfrac{8}{7} & 0 \end{matrix}$$

$$\begin{bmatrix} 1 & 0 & 0 \\ x_1 & 1 & 0 \\ x_2 & x_3 & 1 \end{bmatrix} \begin{bmatrix} y_1 & y_2 & y_3 \\ 0 & y_4 & y_5 \\ 0 & 0 & y_6 \end{bmatrix} = \begin{bmatrix} 25 & 5 & 1 \\ 64 & 8 & 1 \\ 144 & 12 & 1 \end{bmatrix}$$

$$y_1 = 25, \quad y_2 = 0, \quad y_3 = 1 \text{ and } x_1 = \frac{64}{25}$$

Example 6: Show that a matrix is not invertible.

$$A = \begin{bmatrix} 1 & 6 & 4 \\ 2 & 4 & -1 \\ -1 & 2 & 5 \end{bmatrix} = \begin{bmatrix} 1 & 6 & 4 \\ 0 & -8 & -9 \\ 0 & 0 & 0 \end{bmatrix} \begin{bmatrix} 1 & 0 & 0 \\ -2 & 1 & 0 \\ -1 & 1 & 1 \end{bmatrix} \rightarrow \text{Not invertible}$$

LU-Decomposition/Factorization

LU-decomposition or triangular decomposition or triangular factorization is a different approach in which the coefficient matrix A is factored into the product of a lower triangular matrix (L) and a upper triangular matrix (U),

i.e. $$A = LU$$

Since a matrix that is either upper triangular or lower triangular is called "triangles", so *LU*-decomposition is also referred to as triangular factorization. *LU* method can be easily adopted to solve a system with new RHS.

2.10 SOLUTION OF LINEAR SYSTEM BY *LU*-DECOMPOSITION

A non-singular matrix A is said to have a triangular factorization or *LU*-decomposition of A if it can be expressed as the product of a lower triangular matrix (L) and an upper triangular matrix (U).

i.e. $A = LU$

For $n = 3$, we have

$[A]_{3 \times 3} = [L]_{3 \times 3} [U]_{3 \times 3}$

$$\begin{bmatrix} a_{11} & a_{12} & a_{13} \\ a_{21} & a_{22} & a_{23} \\ a_{31} & a_{32} & a_{33} \end{bmatrix} = \begin{bmatrix} 1 & 0 & 0 \\ l_{21} & 1 & 0 \\ l_{31} & l_{32} & 1 \end{bmatrix} \begin{bmatrix} u_{11} & u_{12} & u_{13} \\ 0 & u_{22} & u_{23} \\ 0 & 0 & u_{33} \end{bmatrix}$$

The condition of non-singularity of A implies that $U_{kk} \neq 0$ for all k. Now consider the system of equations

$AX = B$

(or) $LUX = B$

Put $Y = UX$, then $LY = B$ and $UX = Y$

First row: $LY = B$ for Y using forward substitution and then solve $UX = Y$ for X using back substitution. Here X is required solution vector.

LU-decomposition is also known as Do little's method.

Note that *LU*-decomposition is not unique.

Any matrix A with all non-zero diagonal elements (i.e. $a_{ii} \neq 0$ for $i = 1$ to n) can be factored in a number of ways.

Example 1: $\begin{bmatrix} 2 & -1 & -1 \\ 0 & -4 & 2 \\ 6 & -3 & 1 \end{bmatrix}$

Solution: $A = LU$

$$\begin{bmatrix} 2 & -1 & -1 \\ 0 & -4 & 2 \\ 6 & -3 & 1 \end{bmatrix} = \begin{bmatrix} 1 & 0 & 0 \\ x_1 & 1 & 0 \\ x_2 & x_3 & 1 \end{bmatrix} \begin{bmatrix} y_1 & y_2 & y_3 \\ 0 & y_4 & y_5 \\ 0 & 0 & y_6 \end{bmatrix}$$

First row: $y_1 = 2, y_2 = -1, y_3 = -1$

Second row: $x_1 y_1 = 0 \Rightarrow x_1 = 0$

$\qquad x_1 y_2 + y_4 = -4 \Rightarrow (-1) + y_4 = -4 \Rightarrow y_4 = -4$

$\qquad x_1 y_3 + y_5 = 2 \Rightarrow y_5 = 2$

Third row: $x_2 y_1 = 6 \Rightarrow 2x_2 = +6 \Rightarrow x_2 = 3$

$\qquad x_2 y_2 + x_3 y_4 = -3 \Rightarrow (3)(-1) + x_3(-4) = -3 \Rightarrow x_3 = 0$

$x_2 y_3 + x_3 y_5 + y_6 = 1 \Rightarrow (3)(-1) + (0) + y_6 = 1 \Rightarrow y_6 = 4$

$$A = \begin{bmatrix} 2 & -1 & -1 \\ 0 & -4 & 2 \\ 6 & -3 & 1 \end{bmatrix} = \begin{bmatrix} 1 & 0 & 0 \\ 0 & 1 & 0 \\ 3 & 0 & 1 \end{bmatrix} \begin{bmatrix} 2 & -1 & -1 \\ 0 & -4 & 2 \\ 0 & 0 & 4 \end{bmatrix} = LU$$

Verify that $LU = A$ (multiply LU)

Example 2: $\begin{bmatrix} 8 & 2 & 9 \\ 4 & 9 & 4 \\ 6 & 7 & 9 \end{bmatrix}$

Solution: Reader should do the problem.

Example 3: Express the matrix $A = \begin{bmatrix} 1 & 3 & 6 \\ 2 & 8 & 16 \\ 5 & 21 & 45 \end{bmatrix}$ as the product of LU of

lower triangular (L) and an upper triangular matrices (U).

where $\qquad L = \begin{bmatrix} 1 & 0 & 0 \\ l_{21} & 1 & 0 \\ l_{31} & l_{32} & 1 \end{bmatrix}$ and $U = \begin{bmatrix} u_{11} & u_{12} & u_{13} \\ 0 & u_{22} & u_{23} \\ 0 & 0 & u_{33} \end{bmatrix}$

By writing $UX = Y$ and $LY = B$,
solve the system of equations

$$x + 3y + 6z = 17$$
$$2x + 8y + 16z = 42$$
$$5x + 21y + 45z = 91$$

Solution:

$$\begin{bmatrix} 1 & 3 & 6 \\ 2 & 8 & 16 \\ 5 & 21 & 45 \end{bmatrix} \begin{bmatrix} x_1 \\ x_2 \\ x_3 \end{bmatrix} = \begin{bmatrix} 17 \\ 42 \\ 91 \end{bmatrix}$$

$$\quad A \qquad\quad X \qquad B$$

Step 1:

$$A = L\,U$$

$$\begin{bmatrix} 1 & 3 & 6 \\ 2 & 8 & 16 \\ 5 & 21 & 45 \end{bmatrix} = \begin{bmatrix} 1 & 0 & 0 \\ x_1 & 1 & 0 \\ x_2 & x_3 & 1 \end{bmatrix} \begin{bmatrix} y_1 & y_2 & y_3 \\ 0 & y_4 & y_5 \\ 0 & 0 & y_6 \end{bmatrix}$$

First row: $y_1 = 1$, $y_2 = 3$, $y_3 = 6$

Second row: $x_1 y_1 = 2 \Rightarrow x_1 = 2$

$x_1 y_2 + y_4 = 8 \Rightarrow (2)(3) + y_4 = 8 \Rightarrow y_4 = 2$

$x_1 y_3 + y_5 = 16 \Rightarrow (2)(6) + y_5 = 16 \Rightarrow y_5 = 4$

Third row: $x_2 y_1 = 5$, $y_2 = 3$, $x_2 = 5$

$x_2 y_2 + x_3 y_4 = 21 \Rightarrow (5)(3) + x_3 (2) = 21 \Rightarrow 2x_3 = 6$, $x_3 = 3$

$x_2 y_3 + x_3 y_5 + y_6 = 45 \Rightarrow y_6 = 3$

Replacing $x_1, x_2, \ldots$

$$\begin{bmatrix} 1 & 3 & 6 \\ 2 & 8 & 16 \\ 5 & 21 & 45 \end{bmatrix} = \begin{bmatrix} 1 & 0 & 0 \\ 2 & 1 & 0 \\ 5 & 3 & 1 \end{bmatrix} \begin{bmatrix} 1 & 3 & 6 \\ 0 & 2 & 4 \\ 0 & 0 & 3 \end{bmatrix}$$

$$LU = A$$

The product of LU is equal to A.

Step 2: $L\,Y = B$

$$\begin{bmatrix} 1 & 0 & 0 \\ 2 & 1 & 0 \\ 5 & 3 & 1 \end{bmatrix} \begin{bmatrix} y_1 \\ y_2 \\ y_3 \end{bmatrix} = \begin{bmatrix} 17 \\ 42 \\ 91 \end{bmatrix}$$

$$y_1 = 17, \; 2y_1 + y_2 = 42 \Rightarrow y_2 = 8$$

$$5y_1 + 3y_2 + y_3 = 91 \Rightarrow y_3 = -18$$

Step 3: $UX = Y$

$$\begin{bmatrix} 1 & 3 & 6 \\ 0 & 2 & 4 \\ 0 & 0 & 3 \end{bmatrix} \begin{bmatrix} x_1 \\ x_2 \\ x_3 \end{bmatrix} = \begin{bmatrix} 17 \\ 8 \\ -18 \end{bmatrix}$$

$$x_1 + 3x_2 + 6x_3 = 17, \; 2x_2 + 4x_3 = 8, \; 3x_3 = -18$$

$$x_1 = 5 \qquad x_2 = 16 \qquad x_3 = -6$$

$\therefore$ The solution is $x = 5, \; y = 16, \; z = -6$.

Example 4: Solve $AX = B$ by LU-decomposition using Gauss elimination where

$$A = \begin{bmatrix} 2 & 4 & -6 \\ 1 & 5 & 3 \\ 1 & 3 & 2 \end{bmatrix} \text{ and (a) } B^T = (-4, 10, 5) \quad \text{(b) } B^T = (20, 49, 32)$$

Example 5: Solve the system of equations

$$3x_1 - 6x_2 - 3x_3 = -3$$
$$2x_1 + 6x_3 = -22$$
$$-4x_1 + 7x_2 + 4x_3 = 3$$

Solution:

$$A = \begin{bmatrix} 3 & -6 & -3 \\ 2 & 0 & 6 \\ -4 & 7 & 4 \end{bmatrix} \text{ and } B = \begin{bmatrix} -3 \\ -22 \\ 3 \end{bmatrix}$$

Consider $A = LU$

$$\begin{bmatrix} 3 & -6 & -3 \\ 2 & 0 & 6 \\ -4 & 7 & 4 \end{bmatrix} = \begin{bmatrix} 1 & 0 & 0 \\ \dfrac{2}{3} & 1 & 0 \\ \dfrac{-4}{3} & \dfrac{-1}{4} & 1 \end{bmatrix} \begin{bmatrix} 3 & -6 & -3 \\ 0 & 4 & 8 \\ 0 & 0 & 2 \end{bmatrix}$$

$\Rightarrow$ $\qquad\qquad\qquad\qquad LY = B$

$$\begin{bmatrix} 1 & 0 & 0 \\ \dfrac{2}{3} & 1 & 0 \\ \dfrac{-4}{3} & \dfrac{-1}{4} & 1 \end{bmatrix} \begin{bmatrix} y_1 \\ y_2 \\ y_3 \end{bmatrix} = \begin{bmatrix} -3 \\ -22 \\ 3 \end{bmatrix} \quad y_1 = -3,\ y_2 = -20,\ y_3 = -6$$

$$\Rightarrow \qquad\qquad UX = Y$$

$$\begin{bmatrix} 3 & -6 & 3 \\ 0 & 4 & 8 \\ 0 & 0 & 2 \end{bmatrix} \begin{bmatrix} x_1 \\ x_2 \\ x_3 \end{bmatrix} = \begin{bmatrix} -3 \\ -20 \\ -6 \end{bmatrix} \quad x_1 = -2,\ x_2 = 1,\ x_3 = -3$$

$$X^T = [-2 \quad 1 \quad -3]$$

Example 6: Solve the system of equations

$2x_1 - 2x_2 - 2x_3 = -4$

$\qquad -2x_2 + 2x_3 = -2$

$-x_1 + 5x_2 + 2x_3 = 6$

Solution: $x_1 = -1,\ x_2 = 1,\ x_3 = 0$

Example 7:
$$\begin{bmatrix} -1 & 0 & 1 & 0 \\ 2 & 3 & -2 & 6 \\ 0 & -1 & 2 & 0 \\ 0 & 0 & 1 & 5 \end{bmatrix} \begin{bmatrix} x_1 \\ x_2 \\ x_3 \\ x_4 \end{bmatrix} = \begin{bmatrix} 5 \\ -1 \\ 3 \\ 7 \end{bmatrix}$$

Solution: $A = LU$

$$\begin{bmatrix} -1 & 0 & 1 & 0 \\ 2 & 3 & -2 & 6 \\ 0 & -1 & 2 & 0 \\ 0 & 0 & 1 & 5 \end{bmatrix} = \begin{bmatrix} 1 & 0 & 0 & 0 \\ x_1 & 1 & 0 & 0 \\ x_2 & x_3 & 1 & 0 \\ x_4 & x_5 & x_6 & 1 \end{bmatrix} \begin{bmatrix} y_1 & y_2 & y_3 & y_4 \\ 0 & y_5 & y_6 & y_7 \\ 0 & 0 & y_8 & y_9 \\ 0 & 0 & 0 & y_{10} \end{bmatrix}$$

First row: $y_1 = -1,\ y_2 = 0,\ y_3 = 1,\ y_4 = 0$

Second row: $x_1 y_1 = 2 \Rightarrow x_1 (-1) = 2 \Rightarrow x_1 = -2$

$\qquad x_1 y_2 + y_5 = 3 \Rightarrow (-2)(0) + y_5 = 3 \Rightarrow y_5 = 3$

$\qquad x_1 y_3 + y_6 = -2 \Rightarrow (-2)(1) + y_6 = -2 \Rightarrow y_6 = 0$

$\qquad x_1 y_4 + y_7 = 6 \Rightarrow (-2)(0) + y_7 = 6 \Rightarrow y_7 = 6$

Third row: $x_2 y_1 = 0 \Rightarrow x_2 = 0$

$x_2 y_2 + x_3 y_5 = -1 \Rightarrow 0 + x_3 (3) = -1 \Rightarrow x_3 = \dfrac{-1}{3}$

$x_2 y_3 + x_3 y_6 + y_8 = 2 \Rightarrow (0) + \left(\dfrac{-1}{5}\right)(0) + y_8 = 2 \Rightarrow y_8 = 2$

$x_2 y_4 + x_3 y_7 + y_9 = 0 \Rightarrow 0 + \left(\dfrac{-1}{3}\right)(6) + y_9 = 0 \Rightarrow y_9 = 2$

Fourth row: $x_4 y_1 = 0 \Rightarrow x_4 = 0$

$x_4 y_2 + x_5 y_5 = 0 \Rightarrow 0 + x_5 (3) = 0 \Rightarrow x_5 = 0$

$x_4 y_3 + x_5 y_6 + x_6 y_8 = 1 \Rightarrow 0 + 0 + (2) x_6 = 1 \Rightarrow x_6 = \dfrac{1}{2}$

$x_4 y_4 + x_5 y_7 + x_6 y_9 + y_{10} = 5 \Rightarrow 0 + 0 + \left(\dfrac{1}{2}\right)\left(\dfrac{6}{7}\right) + y_{10} = 5$

$\dfrac{3}{7} + y_{10} = 5$

$y_{10} = 5 - \dfrac{3}{7} = \dfrac{35-3}{7} = 4 \Rightarrow y_{10} = 4$

$$\begin{bmatrix} -1 & 0 & 1 & 0 \\ 2 & 3 & -2 & 6 \\ 0 & -1 & 2 & 0 \\ 0 & 0 & 1 & 5 \end{bmatrix} = \begin{bmatrix} 1 & 0 & 0 & 0 \\ -2 & 1 & 0 & 0 \\ 0 & \dfrac{-1}{3} & 1 & 0 \\ 0 & 0 & \dfrac{1}{2} & 1 \end{bmatrix} \begin{bmatrix} -1 & 0 & 1 & 0 \\ 0 & 3 & 0 & 6 \\ 0 & 0 & 2 & 2 \\ 0 & 0 & 0 & 4 \end{bmatrix}$$

$L\,Y = B$

$$\begin{bmatrix} 1 & 0 & 1 & 0 \\ -2 & 1 & 0 & 0 \\ 0 & \dfrac{-1}{3} & 1 & 0 \\ 0 & 0 & \dfrac{1}{2} & 1 \end{bmatrix} \begin{bmatrix} y_1 \\ y_2 \\ y_3 \\ y_4 \end{bmatrix} = \begin{bmatrix} 5 \\ -1 \\ 3 \\ 7 \end{bmatrix}$$

$\dfrac{1}{2} y_3 + y_4 = 7$

$\dfrac{6}{2} + y_4 = 7 \Rightarrow y_4 = 4$

$y_1 = 5$

$$-2y_1 + y_2 = -1$$

$$-10 + y_2 = -1 \Rightarrow y_2 = 9$$

$$\frac{-1}{3} y_2 + y_3 = 3$$

$$\left(\frac{-1}{3}\right) + y_3 = 3 \Rightarrow y_3 = 6$$

$$UX = Y$$

$$\begin{bmatrix} -1 & 0 & 1 & 0 \\ 0 & 3 & 0 & 6 \\ 0 & 0 & 2 & 2 \\ 0 & 0 & 0 & 4 \end{bmatrix} \begin{bmatrix} x_1 \\ x_2 \\ x_3 \\ x_4 \end{bmatrix} = \begin{bmatrix} 5 \\ 9 \\ 6 \\ 4 \end{bmatrix}$$

$$4x_4 = 4 \Rightarrow x_4 = 1$$

$$2x_3 + 2x_4 = 6 \Rightarrow 2x_3 = 6 - 2 \Rightarrow x_3 = 2$$

$$3x_2 + 6x_4 = 9$$

$$3x_2 + 6 = 9 \Rightarrow 3x_2 = 3 \Rightarrow x_3 = 1$$

$$-x_1 + x_3 = 5 - x_1 + 2 = 5$$

$$-x_1 = 3 \Rightarrow x_1 = -3$$

Therefore

$$x_1 = -3, x_2 = 1, x_3 = 2, x_4 = 1$$

Verification

$$-x_1 + x_3 = 5$$

$$3 + 2 = 5$$

Solve the matrix $A = \begin{bmatrix} 3 & -0.1 & -0.2 \\ 0.1 & 7 & -0.3 \\ 0.3 & -0.2 & 10 \end{bmatrix}$

Solution:

$$f_{21} = \frac{a_{21}}{a_{11}} = \frac{0.1}{3} = 0.0333$$

$$R_1 \rightarrow R_1 (f_{21})$$

$$= \begin{bmatrix} 0.1 & -0.00333 & -0.00666 \\ 0.1 & 7 & -0.3 \\ 0.3 & -0.2 & 10 \end{bmatrix}$$

$R_2 \rightarrow R_2 - R_1$, $R_3 \rightarrow R_3 - 3R_1$

$$= \begin{bmatrix} 0.1 & -0.00333 & -0.00666 \\ 0 & 7.00333 & -0.29334 \\ 0 & -0.19001 & 10.01998 \end{bmatrix}$$

First row: $3x_1 - 0.1x_2 - 0.2x_3 = 0 \times \left(\dfrac{0.1}{3} \right)$

$$0.1x_1 + 7x_2 - 0.3x_3 = 0 \qquad \qquad \text{...(1)}$$
$$0.3x_1 - 0.2x_2 + 10x_3 = 0 \qquad \qquad \text{...(2)}$$
$$3x_1 - 0.1x_2 - 0.2x_3 = 0 \qquad \qquad \text{...(3)}$$

Second row: $\qquad \qquad 7.0033x_2 - 0.2x_3 = 0$

$$- 0.19001x_2 + 10.01998x_3 = 0$$

$\dfrac{a_{32}}{a_{22}} = \dfrac{-0.19001}{7.0033}$ and multiplied by (2) (0.02713)

$3x_1 - 0.1x_2 - 0.2\, x_3 = 0$
$- 0.19001x_2 + 0.0079583\, x_3 = 0$
$- 0.19001x_2 + 10.01998x_3 = 0$

LU-Decomposition to Find $(A^{-1})_{m \times n}$

Example 8: *LU*-decomposition of $\begin{bmatrix} 25 & 5 & 1 \\ 64 & 8 & 1 \\ 144 & 12 & 1 \end{bmatrix}$

Solution: $\underbrace{\begin{bmatrix} 25 & 5 & 1 \\ 64 & 8 & 1 \\ 144 & 12 & 1 \end{bmatrix}}_{A} = \underbrace{\begin{bmatrix} 1 & 0 & 0 \\ 2.56 & 1 & 0 \\ 5.76 & 3.5 & 1 \end{bmatrix}}_{L} \underbrace{\begin{bmatrix} 25 & 5 & 1 \\ 0 & -4.8 & -1.56 \\ 0 & 0 & 0.7 \end{bmatrix}}_{U}$

$$[B] = [A]^{-1} = \begin{bmatrix} b_{11} & b_{12} & b_{13} \\ b_{21} & b_{22} & b_{23} \\ b_{31} & b_{32} & b_{33} \end{bmatrix} \begin{bmatrix} 1 & 0 & 0 \\ 0 & 1 & 0 \\ 0 & 0 & 1 \end{bmatrix}$$

$$\begin{bmatrix} 1 & 0 & 0 \\ 0 & 1 & 0 \\ 0 & 0 & 1 \end{bmatrix}$$

$$\begin{bmatrix} 25 & 5 & 1 \\ 64 & 3 & 1 \\ 144 & 12 & 1 \end{bmatrix} \begin{bmatrix} b_{11} \\ b_{21} \\ b_{31} \end{bmatrix} = \begin{bmatrix} 1 \\ 0 \\ 0 \end{bmatrix}$$

$$[L][Z] = [C] \quad \Rightarrow \quad LY = B$$

$$[U][X] = [Z] \quad \Rightarrow \quad UX = Y$$

$$[L][Z] = \begin{bmatrix} 1 & 0 & 0 \\ 2.56 & 1 & 0 \\ 5.76 & 3.5 & 1 \end{bmatrix} \begin{bmatrix} z_1 \\ z_2 \\ z_3 \end{bmatrix} = \begin{bmatrix} 1 \\ 0 \\ 0 \end{bmatrix}$$

Example 9: Use LU-decomposition to find the inverse of

$$[A] = \begin{bmatrix} 25 & 5 & 1 \\ 64 & 8 & 1 \\ 144 & 12 & 1 \end{bmatrix}$$

Solution:

$$A = [L][U]$$

$$= \begin{bmatrix} 1 & 0 & 0 \\ 2.56 & 1 & 0 \\ 5.76 & 3.5 & 1 \end{bmatrix} \begin{bmatrix} 25 & 5 & 1 \\ 0 & -4.8 & -1.56 \\ 0 & 0 & 0.7 \end{bmatrix}$$

We can solve the 1st column of $[B] = [A]^{-1}$ by solving for

$$\begin{bmatrix} 25 & 5 & 1 \\ 64 & 8 & 1 \\ 144 & 12 & 1 \end{bmatrix} \begin{bmatrix} b_{11} \\ b_{21} \\ b_{31} \end{bmatrix} = \begin{bmatrix} 1 \\ 0 \\ 0 \end{bmatrix}$$

First solve: $[L][Z] = [C]$

i.e.

$$\begin{bmatrix} 1 & 0 & 0 \\ 2.56 & 1 & 0 \\ 5.76 & 3.5 & 1 \end{bmatrix} \begin{bmatrix} z_1 \\ z_2 \\ z_3 \end{bmatrix} = \begin{bmatrix} 1 \\ 0 \\ 0 \end{bmatrix}$$

For given $z_1 = 1$, $2.56z_1 + z_2 = 0$, $5.76z_1 + 3.5z_2 + z_3 = 0$,

forward substitution straight from the first equation gives

$$z_1 = 1, z_2 = -2.56, z_3 = 3.2$$

Hence $$[Z] = \begin{bmatrix} z_1 \\ z_2 \\ z_3 \end{bmatrix} = \begin{bmatrix} 1 \\ -2.56 \\ 3.2 \end{bmatrix}$$

Now solve $[U][X] = [Z]$

i.e.

$$\begin{bmatrix} 25 & 5 & 1 \\ 0 & -4.8 & -1.56 \\ 0 & 0 & 0.7 \end{bmatrix} \begin{bmatrix} b_{11} \\ b_{21} \\ b_{31} \end{bmatrix} = \begin{bmatrix} 1 \\ -2.56 \\ 3.2 \end{bmatrix}$$

$$25b_{11} + 5b_{21} + b_{31} = 1$$

$$-4.8b_{21} - 1.56b_{21} = -2.56$$

$$0.7b_{31} = 3.2$$

$$b_{31} = 4.571, \ b_{21} = -0.9524, \ b_{11} = 0.04762$$

Hence the 1st column of the inverse of $[A]$ is

$$\begin{bmatrix} b_{11} \\ b_{21} \\ b_{31} \end{bmatrix} = \begin{bmatrix} 0.04762 \\ -0.9524 \\ 4.571 \end{bmatrix}$$

Similarly by solving,

$$\begin{bmatrix} 25 & 5 & 1 \\ 64 & 8 & 1 \\ 144 & 12 & 1 \end{bmatrix} \begin{bmatrix} b_{12} \\ b_{22} \\ b_{32} \end{bmatrix} = \begin{bmatrix} 0 \\ 1 \\ 0 \end{bmatrix} \text{ gives } \begin{bmatrix} b_{12} \\ b_{22} \\ b_{32} \end{bmatrix} = \begin{bmatrix} -0.08333 \\ 1.417 \\ -5.000 \end{bmatrix}$$

and solving

$$\begin{bmatrix} 25 & 5 & 1 \\ 64 & 8 & 1 \\ 144 & 12 & 1 \end{bmatrix} \begin{bmatrix} b_{13} \\ b_{23} \\ b_{33} \end{bmatrix} = \begin{bmatrix} 0 \\ 1 \\ 0 \end{bmatrix} \text{ gives } \begin{bmatrix} b_{13} \\ b_{23} \\ b_{33} \end{bmatrix} = \begin{bmatrix} 0.03571 \\ -0.4643 \\ 1.429 \end{bmatrix}$$

$$[A]^{-1} = \begin{bmatrix} 0.04762 & -0.08333 & 0.03571 \\ -0.9524 & 1.417 & -0.4643 \\ 4.571 & -5.000 & 1.429 \end{bmatrix}$$

You can confirm the following equation

$$[A][A]^{-1} = I = [A]^{-1}[A]$$

Finding $[z_1 \ z_2 \ z_3]^T$

Forward Substitution

$$\begin{bmatrix} z_1 \\ z_2 \\ z_3 \end{bmatrix} = \begin{bmatrix} 1 \\ -2.56 \\ 3.2 \end{bmatrix}$$

$$UX = \begin{bmatrix} 25 & 5 & 1 \\ 0 & -4.8 & -1.56 \\ 0 & 0 & 0.7 \end{bmatrix} \begin{bmatrix} x_1 \\ x_2 \\ x_3 \end{bmatrix} = \begin{bmatrix} 1 \\ -2.56 \\ 3.2 \end{bmatrix}$$

Back substitute of decomposition

$$\begin{bmatrix} b_{11} \\ b_{21} \\ b_{31} \end{bmatrix} = \begin{bmatrix} x_1 \\ x_2 \\ x_3 \end{bmatrix} = \begin{bmatrix} 0.04762 \\ -0.9524 \\ 4.524 \end{bmatrix}$$

Second column:

$$\begin{bmatrix} 25 & 6 & 1 \\ 64 & 8 & 1 \\ 144 & 12 & 1 \end{bmatrix} \begin{bmatrix} b_{12} \\ b_{22} \\ b_{32} \end{bmatrix} = \begin{bmatrix} 0 \\ 1 \\ 0 \end{bmatrix}$$

Third column:

$$\begin{bmatrix} 25 & 6 & 1 \\ 64 & 8 & 1 \\ 144 & 12 & 1 \end{bmatrix} \begin{bmatrix} b_{12} \\ b_{23} \\ b_{32} \end{bmatrix} = \begin{bmatrix} 0 \\ 0 \\ 0 \end{bmatrix}$$

$$B = [A]^{-1} = \begin{bmatrix} 0.4762 & 0.08333 & 0.0357 \\ -0.9524 & 1.417 & -0.4643 \\ 4.571 & -5.000 & 1.429 \end{bmatrix}$$

$$A = \begin{bmatrix} 3 & -0.1 & -0.2 \\ 0.1 & 7 & -0.3 \\ 0.3 & -0.2 & 10 \end{bmatrix} = \overset{U}{\begin{bmatrix} 3 & -0.1 & -0.2 \\ 0 & 7.00333 & -0.29333 \\ 0 & 0 & 10.0120 \end{bmatrix}} \overset{L}{\begin{bmatrix} 1 & 0 & 0 \\ 0.03333 & 1 & 0 \\ 0.1000 & -0.0271300 & 1 \end{bmatrix}}$$

We can solve the 1st column if $[B] = [A]^{-1}$ by solving from

$$\begin{bmatrix} 3 & -0.1 & -0.2 \\ 0.1 & 7 & -0.3 \\ 0.3 & -0.2 & 10 \end{bmatrix} \begin{bmatrix} b_{11} \\ b_{21} \\ b_{31} \end{bmatrix} = \begin{bmatrix} 1 \\ 0 \\ 0 \end{bmatrix}$$

First solve $[L] = [Z] = [C]$

i.e.

$$\begin{bmatrix} 1 & 0 & 0 \\ 0.03333 & 1 & 0 \\ 0.1000 & -0.271300 & 1 \end{bmatrix} \begin{bmatrix} z_1 \\ z_2 \\ z_3 \end{bmatrix} = \begin{bmatrix} 1 \\ 0 \\ 0 \end{bmatrix} \Rightarrow z_1 = 1$$

$0.03333z_1 + z_2 = 0 \Rightarrow z_2 = -0.03333$

$0.1z_1 - 0.271300z_2 + z_3 = 0 \Rightarrow z_3 = -0.100904$

$$[Z] = \begin{bmatrix} z_1 \\ z_2 \\ z_3 \end{bmatrix} = \begin{bmatrix} 1 \\ -0.03333 \\ -0.100904 \end{bmatrix}$$

Now solve $[U] [X] = [Z]$

$$\begin{bmatrix} 3 & -0.1 & -0.2 \\ 0 & 7.00333 & -0.29333 \\ 0 & 0 & 10.0120 \end{bmatrix} \begin{bmatrix} x_1 \\ x_2 \\ x_3 \end{bmatrix} = \begin{bmatrix} z_1 \\ z_2 \\ z_3 \end{bmatrix} = \begin{bmatrix} 1 \\ -0.0333 \\ -0.100904 \end{bmatrix} = \begin{bmatrix} b_{11} \\ b_{21} \\ b_{31} \end{bmatrix}$$

$10.0120x_3 = -0.100904 \Rightarrow x_3 = -0.010078 = b_{31}$

$7.00333x_2 - 0.29333x_2 = -0.0333 \Rightarrow x_2 = -0.00518$

$3x_1 - 0.1x_2 - 0.2x_3 = 1 \Rightarrow x_1 = 0.33249$

Hence 1st column of the inverse of $[A]$

$$\begin{bmatrix} b_{11} \\ b_{21} \\ b_{31} \end{bmatrix} = \begin{bmatrix} 0.33249 \\ -0.00518 \\ -0.010078 \end{bmatrix}$$

Similarly $\begin{bmatrix} b_{11} \\ b_{22} \\ b_{32} \end{bmatrix} = \begin{bmatrix} 0.004944 \\ 0.142903 \\ 0.00271 \end{bmatrix}$ and $\begin{bmatrix} b_{13} \\ b_{23} \\ b_{33} \end{bmatrix} = \begin{bmatrix} 0.006798 \\ 0.004183 \\ 0.09986 \end{bmatrix}$

$$\therefore [A]^{-1} = \begin{bmatrix} 0.33249 & 0.004944 & 0.006798 \\ -0.00518 & 0.142903 & 0.004183 \\ 0.0108 & 0.00271 & 0.09988 \end{bmatrix}$$

$$= [A]\begin{bmatrix} A^{-1} \end{bmatrix} = I$$

EXERCISE

1. Solve: $\begin{bmatrix} 4 & 8 & 4 & 0 \\ 1 & 5 & 4 & -3 \\ 1 & 4 & 7 & 2 \\ 1 & 3 & 0 & -2 \end{bmatrix}\begin{bmatrix} x_1 \\ x_2 \\ x_3 \\ x_4 \end{bmatrix} = \begin{bmatrix} b_1 \\ b_2 \\ b_3 \\ b_4 \end{bmatrix}$

(a) $B^T = [8, -4, 10, -4]$

(b) $B^T = [28, 13, 23, 4]$

Ans. (a) $Y^T = [8, -6, 12, 2]$, $X^T = [3, -1, 1, 2]$

(b) $Y^T = [28, 6, 12, 1]$, $X^T = [3, 1, 2, 1]$

Hint:

$$L = \begin{bmatrix} 1 & 0 & 0 & 0 \\ \dfrac{1}{4} & 1 & 0 & 0 \\ \dfrac{1}{4} & \dfrac{2}{3} & 1 & 0 \\ \dfrac{1}{4} & \dfrac{1}{3} & -\dfrac{1}{2} & 1 \end{bmatrix}$$

$$U = \begin{bmatrix} 4 & 8 & 4 & 0 \\ 0 & 3 & 3 & -3 \\ 0 & 0 & 4 & 4 \\ 0 & 0 & 0 & 1 \end{bmatrix}$$

2. Solve:
$$\begin{bmatrix} 4 & 3 & -1 \\ -2 & -4 & 5 \\ 1 & 2 & 6 \end{bmatrix}$$

Ans.
$$L = \begin{bmatrix} 1 & 0 & 0 \\ -0.2 & 1 & 1 \\ -0.6 & 5.5 & 1 \end{bmatrix} \text{ and } U = \begin{bmatrix} -5 & 2 & -1 \\ 0 & 0.4 & 2.8 \\ 0 & 0 & -10 \end{bmatrix}$$

3. Solve:
$$\begin{bmatrix} 1 & 1 & 0 & 4 \\ 2 & -1 & 5 & 0 \\ 5 & 2 & 1 & 2 \\ -3 & 0 & 2 & 6 \end{bmatrix}$$

Ans.
$$L = \begin{bmatrix} 1 & 1 & 0 & 0 \\ 2 & 1 & 0 & 0 \\ 5 & 1 & 1 & 0 \\ -3 & -1 & -1.75 & 1 \end{bmatrix}$$

$$U = \begin{bmatrix} 1 & 1 & 0 & 4 \\ 0 & -3 & 5 & -8 \\ 0 & 0 & -4 & -10 \\ 0 & 0 & 0 & -7.5 \end{bmatrix}$$

2.11 APPLICATIONS OF LINEAR EQUATIONS I

Linear equations contains one or two variables. The word 'linear' comes from the fact that the graph of the equation is straight line. For example, $x + y = 10$ is a linear equation with two variables x and y. A variable as opposed to a constant can take different values depending on the equation.

Linear Equations in Everyday Life

People tend not to think in terms of equations and formulae in their daily lives. They use language to describe the situation. But words can be translated into the language of mathematics.

Take a very simple example:

1. A mother has to divide six apples among 3 children. Effortlessly she reaches the conclusion that each child gets two apples. What she has used is the mathematical function of division to reach the answer: $6/3 = 2$.
2. Converting hours to minutes: How many minutes are there in 4 hours? Let x = the number of hours and y = number of minutes.

By definition, there are 60 mins in one hour. So you can write a linear equation to describe this relationship: $y = 60x$. The number of minutes equal 60 times the number of hours.

For example: Let $x = 4$, then plug the number into the linear equation to get $y = 60 \times 4$, i.e. $y = 240$ mins.

Application to Traffic Flow

At rush hours, traffic congestion is encountered at the street intersections shown in the given figure. The city wishes to improve the traffic signals at these corners to improve the traffic flow. All streets are one-way and the directions are indicated by the arrows.

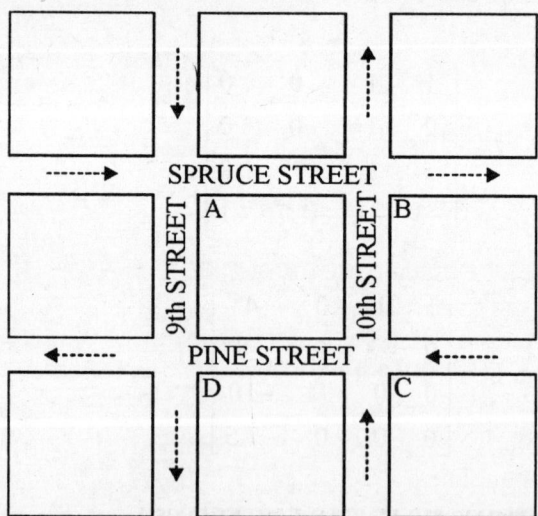

Data collection: The traffic engineers gathered the following information.

1. *Corner A*: 700 vehicles an hour come down spruce street to intersection *A*.

   300 vehicles an hour come down 9th street to intersection *A*.
2. *Corner B*: 200 vehicles an hour leave intersection *B* on spruce street.

900 vehicles an hour leave intersection B on 10th street.

3. *Corner C*: 400 vehicles an hour enter on pine street to intersection C. 300 vehicles an hour come down 10th street to intersection C.

4. *Corner D*: 200 vehicles an hour leave intersection D on pine street. 400 vehicles an hour leave intersection D on 9th street to intersection A.

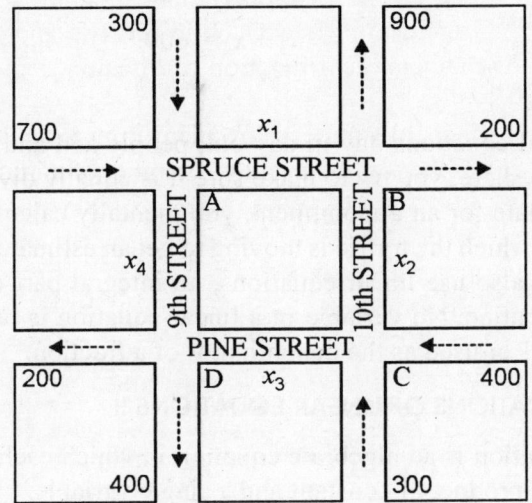

Let x_1 denote the number of vehicles leaving corner A on spruce street towards corner B.

Let x_2 denote the number of vehicles arriving to corner B on 10th street from corner C.

Let x_3 denote the number of vehicles leaving corner C on pine street towards corner D.

Let x_4 denote the number of vehicles arriving to corner D on 9th street from corner A.

Assumptions: We assume the following.

1. To speed the traffic flow every vehicle that arrives to a given corner must also leave. Hence at any corner, the number of cars arriving is equal to number of vehicles leaving.

2. All streets are one-way.

3. All variables $x_1, x_2, x_3,$ and x_4 are positive integers since they represent number of vehicles.

Equations: Using assumption 1 for each corner, we obtain the following equations:

At corner A: $x_1 + x_4 = 700 + 300$

At corner B: $x_1 + x_2 = 900 + 200$

At corner C: $x_2 + x_3 = 400 + 300$

At corner D: $x_3 + x_4 = 400 + 200$

These four equations form a system of linear equations that can be solved by using the Gauss-Jordan method

$$x_1 + x_4 = 1000$$
$$x_1 + x_2 = 1100$$
$$x_2 + x_3 = 700$$
$$x_3 + x_4 = 600.$$

Conclusions

Mathematical equations day in day out, people add and subtract. If you have a pie to share, you try to make sure it is equally divided. When you are running late for an appointment, you mentally calculate the distance and speed at which the traffic is moving to get an estimate of how late you will be. You also use linear equations, an integral part of arithmetic, in your daily routine. No variable in a linear equation is raised to a power greater than 1 or used as the denominator of a fraction.

2.12 APPLICATIONS OF LINEAR EQUATIONS II

A linear equation is an algebraic equation in which each term is either a constant or a product of constant and a single variable.

Linear equations can have one or more variables.

The equations having a one variable is called single variable linear equation.

Example: $3x + 2 = 17$

This equation contains a single unknown variable 'x'.

Similarly the equations having two variables is called two variables linear equation.

Example: $\left.\begin{array}{l} 3x + 2y = 1 \\ x - y = 2 \end{array}\right\} \rightarrow$ Non-homogeneous equations.

These two equations are called system of linear equations.

This system of linear equations is said to be **homogeneous** if and only if the RHS of the system of equations is zero. If it is not zero, then equations are called **non-homogeneous** equations.

i.e. $\left.\begin{array}{l} 3x + 2y = 0 \\ x - y = 0 \end{array}\right\} \rightarrow$ Homogeneous equations.

The values of the unknown variables are found by solving this system of linear equations.

$\therefore$ General form of a linear eq. is

$$a_1 x_1 + a_2 x_2 + \ldots + a_n x_n = b$$

2.12.1 Linear Equations in Mechanical Engineering Applications

Linear equations are used in so many mechanical applications. Here we will discuss about the **Spring Mass System.**

Spring Mass System

The spring mass system have numerous applications throughout the study of engineering. The linear equations can be used successfully in order to solve the problems associated with such systems.

   The figure below shows the spring mass system.

   It is composed of three masses suspended vertically by a series of springs.

   The left portion of the diagram indicates state of system before releases.

   However, after the masses are released, they are pulled downwards by force of gravity.

   The resulting displacement is measured with respect to local coordinates referenced to its initial position.

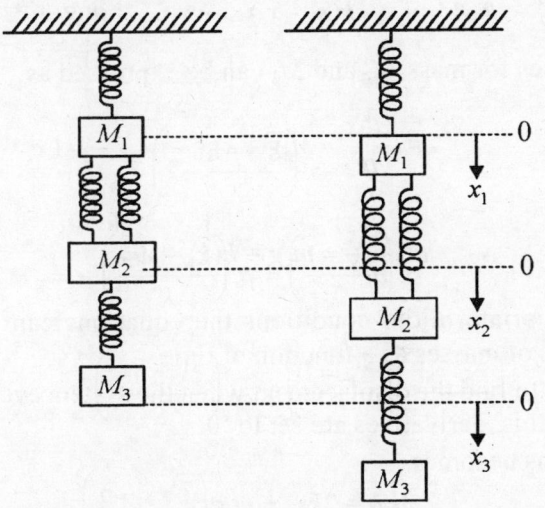

For each mass, Newton's second law of motion (i.e. $F = ma$) can be applied in conjuction with force to develop mathematical model of the system.

$$m\frac{d^2x}{dt^2} = F_D - F_U$$

In order to simplify the analysis, we will assume that all springs are identical.

$\therefore$ The free body diagram of M_1 is shown in the figure.

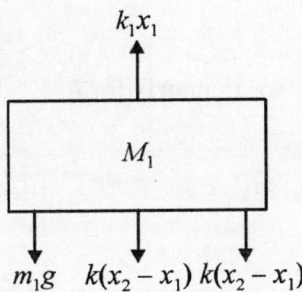

∴ Net force acting on mass m_1

$$m_1 \frac{d^2x}{dt^2} = m_1 g + 2k(x_2 - x_1) - kx_1 \qquad ...(1)$$

The solution for this equation cannot be obtained because the model includes a second dependent variable x_2. Consequently, free body diagrams must be developed for masses M_2 and M_3.

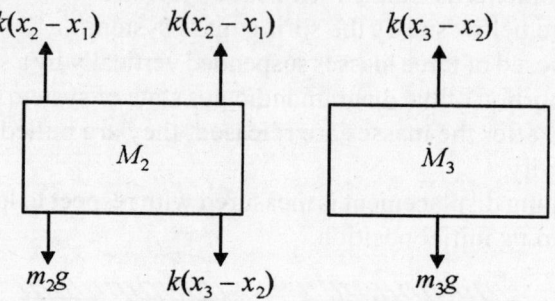

∴ Net forces for mass M_2 and M_3 can be expressed as

$$m_2 \frac{d^2x}{dt^2} = m_2 g + k(x_3 - x_2) - 2k(x_2 - x_1) \qquad ...(2)$$

$$m_3 \frac{d^2x}{dt^2} = m_3 g + k(x_3 - x_2) \qquad ...(3)$$

With appropriate initial conditions the equations can be solved for displacements of masses as a function of time.

∴ We have to find the displacement when the system eventually comes to rest. To do this, derivatives are set to '0'.

∴ Equations becomes

$$3kx_1 - 2kx_2 = m_1 g$$

$$-2kx_1 - 3kx_2 - kx_3 = m_2 g$$

$$-kx_2 + kx_3 = m_3 g$$

or in matrix form

$$[K][X] = [W]$$

or

$$[X] = [K]^{-1}[W]$$

∵

$$[K] = \begin{bmatrix} 3k & -2k & 0 \\ -2k & 3k & -k \\ 0 & -k & k \end{bmatrix}$$

$$[W] = g \begin{bmatrix} m_1 \\ m_2 \\ m_3 \end{bmatrix}$$

$$\begin{bmatrix} x_1 \\ x_2 \\ x_3 \end{bmatrix} = \begin{bmatrix} 3k & -2k & 0 \\ -2k & 3k & -k \\ 0 & -k & k \end{bmatrix} \begin{bmatrix} gm_1 \\ gm_2 \\ gm_3 \end{bmatrix}$$

Conclusion

Linear equations occur with a great regularity in applied mathematics. While there linear equations arise quite naturally, hence linear equations are particularly useful since many non-linear equations may be reduced to linear equations by assuming that quantities of interest vary to only a small extent from some background state.

3

Systems of Equations and Matrices

3.1 INTRODUCTION

We will start this chapter by looking at the application of matrices that almost every book on linear algebra starts off with, solving systems of linear equations. Looking at systems of equations will allow us to start getting used to the notation and some of the basic manipulations of matrices.

Once we have looked at solving systems of linear equations, we will move into the basic arithmetic of matrices and basic matrix properties. We will also take a look at a couple of other ideas about matrices that have some nice applications to the solution to systems of equations.

One word of warning about this chapter, and in fact about this complete set of notes for that matter, we will start out in the first section giving a lot of the details in the problems, but towards the end of this chapter and in the remaining chapters we will leave many of the details to you to check. We start off by giving lots of details to make sure you are comfortable working with matrices and the various operations involving them. However, we will eventually assume that you have become comfortable with the details and can check them on your own.

Here is a listing of the topics in this chapter.

Systems of equations In this section, we will introduce most of the basic topics that we will need in order to solve systems of equations including augmented matrices and row operations.

Solving systems of equations Here we will look at the Gaussian Elimination and Gauss-Jordan method of solving systems of equations.

Matrices We will introduce many of the basic ideas and properties involved in the study of matrices.

Matrix arithmetic and operations In this section, we will take a look at matrix addition, subtraction and multiplication. We will also take a quick look at the transpose and trace of a matrix.

Properties of matrix arithmetic We shall discuss in-depth at many of the properties of matrix arithmetic and the transpose.

Inverse matrices and elementary matrices Here we shall define the inverse and take a look at some of its properties and introduce the idea of elementary matrices.

Finding inverse matrices In this section, we will develop a method for finding inverse matrices.

Special matrices We will introduce diagonal, triangular and symmetric matrices in this section.

LU-decompositions In this section, we will introduce the *LU-*Decomposition as a way of "factoring" certain kinds of matrices.

Systems revisited Here we will revisit solving systems of equations. We will take a look at how inverse matrices and LU-Decompositions can help with the solution process. We will also take a look at a couple of other ideas in the solution of systems of equations.

Systems of Equations

Let us start this section with the definition of a linear equation. Here are a couple of examples of linear equations.

$$6x - 8y + 10z = 3 \qquad 7x_1 - \frac{5}{9}x_2 = -1$$

The most general linear equation is

$$a_1 x_1 + a_2 x_2 + \dots + a_n x_n = b \qquad \qquad \dots (1)$$

Here, there are n unknowns $x_1, x_2, \dots, x_n$ and $a_1, a_2, \dots, a_n, b$ are all known real numbers.

Next we need to take a look at the solution set of a single linear equation. A solution set (or often just solution) for equation (1) is a set of numbers $t_1, t_2, \dots, t_n$ so that if we set $x_1 = t_1, x_2 = t_2, \dots, x_n = t_n$, then equation (1) will be satisfied.

Recall the solution sets.

Example 1: Find the solution set for each of the following linear equations.

(a) $7x_1 - \frac{5}{9}x_2 = -1$

(b) $6x - 8y + 10z = 3$

Solution:

(a) $7x_1 - \frac{5}{9}x_2 = -1$

In this case, it will probably be slightly easier to solve for x_1.

$$7x_1 - \frac{5}{9}x_2 = -1 \quad \Rightarrow \quad 7x_1 = \frac{5}{9}x_2 - 1 \quad \Rightarrow \quad x_1 = \frac{5}{63}x_2 - \frac{1}{7}$$

Let $x_2 = t$, where t is any number.

The general solution set is as follows,

$$x_1 = \frac{5}{63}t - \frac{1}{7}, \quad x_2 = t$$

Choose any value of t and a pair of numbers x_1 and x_2 that will satisfy the equation.

$$t = 0: \quad x_1 = -\frac{1}{7}, x_2 = 0$$

$$t = 27: \quad x_1 = -\frac{5}{63}(27) - \frac{1}{7} = 2, x_2 = 27$$

We can easily check that these are in fact solutions to the equation

$$t = 0: \quad 7\left(-\frac{1}{7}\right) - \frac{5}{9}(0) = -1$$

$$t = 27: \quad 7(2) - \frac{5}{9}(27) = -1$$

(b) $6x - 8y + 10z = 3$

We will first solve the equation for one of the variables.

$$10z = 3 - 6x + 8y$$

$$z = \frac{3}{10} - \frac{3}{5}x + \frac{4}{5}y$$

In this case, we will need to know the values for both x and y in order to get a value for z. In this case, we will choose $x = t$ and $y = s$. Note that we choose different letters so that both x and y will have different values (although it is possible for them to have the same value).

The solution set to this linear equation is then

$$x = t, \quad y = s, \quad z = \frac{3}{10} - \frac{3}{5}t + \frac{4}{5}s$$

So if we choose any values for t and s, we can get number of solutions as follows.

$$x = 0, \quad y = -2, \quad z = \frac{3}{10} - \frac{3}{5}(0) + \frac{4}{5}(-2) = -\frac{13}{10}$$

$$x = -\frac{3}{2}, \quad y = 5, \quad z = \frac{3}{10} - \frac{3}{5}\left(-\frac{3}{2}\right) + \frac{4}{5}(5) = \frac{26}{5}$$

As with the first part if we take either set of three numbers to verify that the equation will be satisfied.

$$6\left(\frac{-3}{2}\right) - 8(5) + 10\left(\frac{26}{5}\right) = -9 - 40 + 52 = 3$$

The variables that we got to choose values for (x_2 in the first example and x and y in the second) are sometimes called free variables.

Here are some examples of systems of linear equations.

(1) $2x + 3y = 9$ (2) $4x_1 - 5x_2 + x_3 = 9$ (3) $6x_1 + x_2 = 9$

     $x - 2y = -13$ $-x_1 + 10x_3 = -2$ $-5x_1 - 3x_2 = 7$

                     $7x_1 - x_2 - 4x_3 = 5$ $3x_1 - 10x_2 = -4$

(4) $x_1 - x_2 + x_3 - x_4 + x_5 = 1$

     $3x_1 + 2x_2 - x_3 + 9x_4 = 0$

     $7x_1 + 10x_2 + 3x_3 + 6x_4 - 9x_5 = -7$

Theorem 1: Given a system of n equations and m unknowns there will be one of the three possibilities for solutions to the system.

1. There will be no solution.
2. There will be exactly one solution.
3. There will be infinitely many solutions.

Proof: If there is no solution to the system we call the system is inconsistent and if there is at least one solution to the system we call it consistent.

We are going to start with a simplified way of writing the system of equations. For this we will need the following general system of n equations and m unknowns.

$$a_{11}x_1 + a_{12}x_2 + \ldots + a_{1m}x_m = b_1$$
$$a_{21}x_1 + a_{22}x_2 + \ldots + a_{2m}x_m = b_2$$
$$\vdots$$
$$a_{n1}x_1 + a_{n2}x_2 + \ldots + a_{nm}x_m = b_n$$

In this system, the unknowns are $x_1, x_2, \ldots, x_m$ and the a_{ij}'s and b_{ij}'s are known numbers.

Any system of equations can be written as an augmented matrix. A matrix is just a rectangular array of numbers. Here is the augmented matrix for the general system.

$$\begin{bmatrix} a_{11} & a_{12} & \cdots & a_{1m} & b_1 \\ a_{21} & a_{22} & \cdots & a_{2m} & b_2 \\ \vdots & \vdots & & \vdots & \vdots \\ a_{n1} & a_{n2} & \cdots & a_{nm} & b_n \end{bmatrix}$$

Each row of the augmented matrix consists of the coefficients and constant on the right of the equal sign from a given equation in the system.

The first row is for the first equation, the second row is for the second equation, etc. Likewise each of the first m columns of the matrix consists of the coefficients from the unknowns. The first column contains the coefficients of x_1, the second column contains the coefficients of x_2, etc. The final column contains all the constants on the right of the equal sign. Note that the augmented part of the name arises because we take the b_i's onto the matrix and we have

$$\begin{bmatrix} a_{11} & a_{12} & \cdots & a_{1m} \\ a_{21} & a_{22} & \cdots & a_{2m} \\ \vdots & \vdots & & \vdots \\ a_{n1} & a_{n2} & \cdots & a_{nm} \end{bmatrix}$$

and we call this the coefficient matrix for the system.

Example 2: Write down the augmented matrix for the following system.

$$3x_1 - 10x_2 + 6x_3 - x_4 = 3$$
$$x_1 + 9x_3 - 5x_4 = -12$$
$$-4x_1 + x_2 - 9x_3 + 2x_4 = 7$$

Solution:

$$\begin{bmatrix} 3 & -10 & 6 & -1 & 3 \\ 1 & 0 & 9 & -5 & -12 \\ -4 & 1 & -9 & 2 & 7 \end{bmatrix}$$

Notice that the second equation did not contain x_2 and so we consider its coefficient to be zero.

Example 3: For the given augmented matrix write down the corresponding system of equations.

$$\begin{bmatrix} 4 & -1 & 1 \\ -5 & -8 & 4 \\ 9 & 2 & -2 \end{bmatrix}$$

Solution:

Since each row corresponds to an equation, we have three equations in the system. Here is the system that corresponds to this augmented matrix.

$$4x_1 - x_2 = 1$$
$$-5x_1 - 8x_2 = 4$$
$$9x_1 + 2x_2 = -2$$

Here are the three row operations, their equivalent equation operations as well as the notations that we will be using to denote each of them.

Row Operation	**Equation Operation**	**Notation**
Multiply row i by the constant c	Multiply equation i by the constant c	cR_i
Interchange rows i and j	Interchange equations i and j	$R_i \leftrightarrow R_j$
Add c times row i to row j	Add c times equation i to equation j	$R_j + cR_i$

Example 4: Perform each of the indicated row operations on given augmented matrix.

$$\begin{bmatrix} 2 & 4 & -1 & -3 \\ 6 & -1 & -4 & 10 \\ 7 & 1 & -1 & 5 \end{bmatrix}$$

(a) $-3R_1$ (b) $\frac{1}{2}R_2$ (c) $R_1 \leftrightarrow R_3$ (d) $R_2 + 5R_3$ (e) $R_1 - 3R_2$

Solution:

For reference purposes the system corresponding to the augmented matrix given for this problem is

$$2x_1 + 4x_2 - x_3 = -3$$
$$6x_1 - x_2 - 4x_3 = 10$$
$$7x_1 + x_2 - x_3 = 5$$

(a) $-3R_1$

$$\begin{bmatrix} -6 & -12 & -3 & -9 \\ 6 & -1 & -4 & 10 \\ 7 & 1 & -1 & 5 \end{bmatrix} \Leftrightarrow \begin{array}{l} -6x_1 - 12x_2 - 3x_3 = -9 \\ 6x_1 - x_2 - 4x_3 = 10 \\ 7x_1 + x_2 - x_3 = 5 \end{array}$$

(b) $\frac{1}{2}R_2$

This is similar to the first one. We will multiply each element of the second row by one-half or each coefficient of the second equation by one-half. Here are the results of this operation.

$$\begin{bmatrix} 2 & 4 & -1 & -3 \\ 3 & -\frac{1}{2} & -2 & 5 \\ 7 & 1 & -1 & 5 \end{bmatrix} \Leftrightarrow \begin{array}{l} 2x_1 + 4x_2 - x_3 = -3 \\ 3x_1 - \frac{1}{2}x_2 - 2x_3 = 5 \\ 7x_1 + x_2 - x_3 = 5 \end{array}$$

Note that often in cases like this we will say that we divided the second row by 2 instead of multiplied by one-half.

(c) $R_1 \leftrightarrow R_3$

In this case, we will just interchange the first and third rows or equations.

$$\begin{bmatrix} 7 & 1 & -1 & 5 \\ 6 & -1 & -4 & 10 \\ 2 & 4 & -1 & -3 \end{bmatrix} \Leftrightarrow \begin{array}{c} 7x_1 + x_2 - x_3 = 5 \\ 6x_1 - x_2 - 4x_3 = 10 \\ 2x_1 + 4x_2 - x_3 = -3 \end{array}$$

(d) $R_2 + 5R_3$

We now need to work an example of the third row operation. In this case, we will add 5 times the third row (equation) to the second row (equation).

Here are the individual computations for this operation.

1st entry: $6 + (5)(7) = 41$

2nd entry: $-1 + (5)(1) = 4$

3rd entry: $-4 + (5)(-1) = -9$

4th entry: $10 + (5)(5) = 35$

$41x_1 + 4x_2 - 9x_3 = 35$

$$\begin{bmatrix} 2 & 4 & -1 & -3 \\ 41 & 4 & -9 & 35 \\ 7 & 1 & -1 & 5 \end{bmatrix} \Leftrightarrow \begin{array}{c} 2x_1 + 4x_2 - x_3 = -3 \\ 41x_1 + 4x_2 - 9x_3 = 35 \\ 7x_1 + x_2 - x_3 = 5 \end{array}$$

(e) $R_1 - 3R_2$

In this part, we are going to subtract 3 times the second row (equation) from the first row (equation). Here are the results of this operation.

$$\begin{bmatrix} -16 & 7 & 11 & -33 \\ 6 & -1 & -4 & 10 \\ 7 & 1 & -1 & 5 \end{bmatrix} \Leftrightarrow \begin{array}{c} -16x_1 + 7x_2 + 11x_3 = -33 \\ 6x_1 - x_2 - 4x_3 = 10 \\ 7x_1 + x_2 - x_3 = 5 \end{array}$$

Solving Systems of Equations

In this section, we are going to look at linear algebra techniques to solve a system of linear equations.

A matrix (any matrix, not just an augmented matrix) is said to be in reduced row-echelon form if it satisfies all four of the following conditions.

1. If there are any rows of all zeros, then they are at the bottom of the matrix.

2. If a row does not consist of all zeros, then its first non-zero entry (i.e. the left most non-zero entry) is a 1. This 1 is called a leading 1.
3. In any two successive rows, neither of which consists of all zeros, the leading 1 of the lower row is to the right of the leading 1 of the higher row.
4. If a column contains a leading 1, then all the other entries of that column are zero.

A matrix (again any matrix) is said to be in row-echelon form if it satisfies items 1–3 of the reduced row-echelon form definition.

Notice from this definition that a matrix that is reduced to row-echelon form is also in row-echelon form while a matrix in row-echelon form may or may not be in reduced row-echelon form.

Example 1: The following matrices are all in row-echelon form.

$$\begin{bmatrix} 1 & -6 & 9 & 1 & 0 \\ 0 & 0 & 1 & -4 & -5 \\ 0 & 0 & 0 & 1 & 2 \end{bmatrix} \qquad \begin{bmatrix} 1 & 0 & 5 \\ 0 & 1 & 3 \\ 0 & 0 & 1 \end{bmatrix}$$

$$\begin{bmatrix} 1 & -8 & 10 & 9 & -3 \\ 0 & 1 & 13 & 9 & 12 \\ 0 & 0 & 0 & 1 & 1 \\ 0 & 0 & 0 & 0 & 0 \end{bmatrix}$$

Example 2: The following matrices are all in reduced row-echelon form.

$$\begin{bmatrix} 1 & 0 \\ 0 & 1 \end{bmatrix} \qquad \begin{bmatrix} 0 & 0 \\ 0 & 0 \end{bmatrix} \qquad \begin{bmatrix} 0 & 1 & 0 & -8 \\ 0 & 0 & 1 & 5 \\ 0 & 0 & 0 & 0 \end{bmatrix}$$

$$\begin{bmatrix} 1 & -7 & 10 \\ 0 & 0 & 0 \\ 0 & 0 & 0 \end{bmatrix} \qquad \begin{bmatrix} 1 & 9 & 0 & 0 & -2 \\ 0 & 0 & 1 & 0 & 16 \\ 0 & 0 & 0 & 1 & 1 \\ 0 & 0 & 0 & 0 & 0 \end{bmatrix}$$

Reducing the augmented matrix to reduced row-echelon form is called **Gauss-Jordan Elimination**.

If we stop at row-echelon form, we will have a little more work to do in order to get the solution but it is generally fairly simple arithmetic. Reducing the augmented matrix to row-echelon form and then stopping is called **Gaussian Elimination**.

Example 3: Use Gaussian elimination and Gauss-Jordan elimination to solve the following system of linear equations.

$$-2x_1 + x_2 - x_3 = 4$$
$$x_1 + 2x_2 + 3x_3 = 13$$
$$3x_1 + x_3 = -1$$

Solution: The augumented matrix for this system.

$$\simeq \begin{bmatrix} -2 & 1 & -1 & 4 \\ 1 & 2 & 3 & 13 \\ 3 & 0 & 1 & -1 \end{bmatrix}$$

$$\simeq \begin{bmatrix} -2 & 1 & -1 & 4 \\ 1 & 2 & 3 & 13 \\ 3 & 0 & 1 & -1 \end{bmatrix} \quad \begin{matrix} R_1 \leftrightarrow R_2 \\ \rightarrow \end{matrix} \quad \begin{bmatrix} 1 & 2 & 3 & 13 \\ -2 & 1 & -1 & 4 \\ 3 & 0 & 1 & -1 \end{bmatrix}$$

$$\simeq \begin{bmatrix} 1 & 2 & 3 & 13 \\ -2 & 1 & -1 & 4 \\ 3 & 0 & 1 & -1 \end{bmatrix} \quad \begin{matrix} R_2 + 2R_1 \\ R_3 - 3R_1 \\ \rightarrow \end{matrix} \quad \begin{bmatrix} 1 & 2 & 3 & 13 \\ 0 & 5 & 5 & 30 \\ 0 & -6 & -8 & -40 \end{bmatrix}$$

$$\simeq \begin{bmatrix} 1 & 2 & 3 & 13 \\ 0 & 5 & 5 & 30 \\ 0 & -6 & -8 & -40 \end{bmatrix} \quad \begin{matrix} \frac{1}{5}R_2 \\ \rightarrow \end{matrix} \quad \begin{bmatrix} 1 & 2 & 3 & 13 \\ 0 & 1 & 1 & 6 \\ 0 & -6 & -8 & -40 \end{bmatrix}$$

$$\simeq \begin{bmatrix} 1 & 2 & 3 & 13 \\ 0 & 1 & 1 & 6 \\ 0 & -6 & -8 & -40 \end{bmatrix} \quad \begin{matrix} R_3 + 6R_2 \\ \rightarrow \end{matrix} \quad \begin{bmatrix} 1 & 2 & 3 & 13 \\ 0 & 1 & 1 & 6 \\ 0 & 0 & -2 & -4 \end{bmatrix}$$

$$\simeq \begin{bmatrix} 1 & 2 & 3 & 13 \\ 0 & 1 & 1 & 6 \\ 0 & 0 & -2 & -4 \end{bmatrix} \quad \begin{matrix} -\frac{1}{2}R_3 \\ \rightarrow \end{matrix} \quad \begin{bmatrix} 1 & 2 & 3 & 13 \\ 0 & 1 & 1 & 6 \\ 0 & 0 & 1 & 2 \end{bmatrix}$$

Gaussian elimination on this matrix we will stop and go back to equations.

$$\simeq \begin{bmatrix} 1 & 2 & 3 & 13 \\ 0 & 1 & 1 & 6 \\ 0 & 0 & 1 & 2 \end{bmatrix} \quad \Rightarrow \quad \begin{matrix} x_1 + 2x_2 + 3x_3 = 13 \\ x_2 + x_3 = 6 \\ x_3 = 2 \end{matrix}$$

At this point solving is quite simple. In fact we can see from this that $x_3 = 2$. The second equation gives $x_2 = 4$. Finally, the first equation gives $x_1 = -1$. Summarizing up the solution to the system is

$$x_1 = -1, \quad x_2 = 4, \quad x_3 = 2$$

This substitution process is called back substitution.

$$\simeq \begin{bmatrix} 1 & 2 & 3 & 13 \\ 0 & 1 & 1 & 6 \\ 0 & 0 & 1 & 2 \end{bmatrix} \quad \begin{matrix} R_1 - 3R_3 \\ R_2 - R_3 \\ \rightarrow \end{matrix} \quad \begin{bmatrix} 1 & 2 & 0 & 7 \\ 0 & 1 & 0 & 4 \\ 0 & 0 & 1 & 2 \end{bmatrix}$$

$$\simeq \begin{bmatrix} 1 & 2 & 0 & 7 \\ 0 & 1 & 0 & 4 \\ 0 & 0 & 1 & 2 \end{bmatrix} \quad \begin{matrix} R_1 - 2R_2 \\ \rightarrow \end{matrix} \quad \begin{bmatrix} 1 & 0 & 0 & -1 \\ 0 & 1 & 0 & 4 \\ 0 & 0 & 1 & 2 \end{bmatrix}$$

In reduced row-echelon form all we need to do is to perform Gauss-Jordan elimination to go back to equations.

$$\simeq \begin{bmatrix} 1 & 0 & 0 & -1 \\ 0 & 1 & 0 & 4 \\ 0 & 0 & 1 & 2 \end{bmatrix} \quad \Rightarrow \quad \begin{matrix} x_1 = -1 \\ x_2 = 4 \\ x_3 = 2 \end{matrix}$$

We can see that one of the nice consequences to Gauss-Jordan elimination is when there is a single solution to the system. Note that it is the same solution as the one that we got by using Gaussian elimination as we should expect.

Example 4: Solve the following system of linear equations.

$$x_1 - 2x_2 + 3x_3 = -2$$
$$-x_1 + x_2 - 2x_3 = 3$$
$$2x_1 - x_2 + 3x_3 = 1$$

Solution:

The augmented matrix for this system

$$\simeq \begin{bmatrix} 1 & -2 & 3 & -2 \\ -1 & 1 & -2 & 3 \\ 2 & -1 & 3 & 1 \end{bmatrix}$$

and here is the work to put it into row-echelon form.

$$\simeq \begin{bmatrix} 1 & -2 & 3 & -2 \\ -1 & 1 & -2 & 3 \\ 2 & -1 & 3 & 1 \end{bmatrix} \quad \begin{matrix} R_2 + R_1 \\ R_3 - 2R_1 \\ \rightarrow \end{matrix} \quad \begin{bmatrix} 1 & -2 & 3 & -2 \\ 0 & -1 & 1 & 1 \\ 0 & 3 & -3 & 5 \end{bmatrix}$$

$$-R_2 \rightarrow \begin{bmatrix} 1 & -2 & 3 & -2 \\ 0 & 1 & -1 & -1 \\ 0 & 3 & -3 & 5 \end{bmatrix}$$

$$R_3 - 3R_2 \rightarrow \begin{bmatrix} 1 & -2 & 3 & -2 \\ 0 & 1 & -1 & -1 \\ 0 & 0 & 0 & 8 \end{bmatrix} \quad \frac{1}{8}R_3 \rightarrow \begin{bmatrix} 1 & -2 & 3 & -2 \\ 0 & 1 & -1 & -1 \\ 0 & 0 & 0 & 1 \end{bmatrix}$$

We are now in row-echelon form. Let us go back to equations and see what we have got.

$$x_1 - 2x_2 + 3x_3 = -2$$
$$x_2 - x_3 = -1$$
$$0 = 1$$

That last equation does not look correct, i.e. there is no solution to this system.

Example 5: Solve the following system of linear equations.

$$x_1 - 2x_2 + 3x_3 = -2$$
$$-x_1 + x_2 - 2x_3 = 3$$
$$2x_1 - x_2 + 3x_3 = -7$$

Solution:

The only difference between this system and the previous one is −7 in the third equation. In the previous example this was 1.

Here is the augmented matrix for this system.

$$\simeq \begin{bmatrix} 1 & -2 & 3 & -2 \\ -1 & 1 & -2 & 3 \\ 2 & -1 & 3 & -7 \end{bmatrix}$$

Now, since this is essentially the same augmented matrix as the previous example, the first few steps are identical. After taking the same steps as above, we get

$$\simeq \begin{bmatrix} 1 & -2 & 3 & -2 \\ 0 & 1 & -1 & -1 \\ 0 & 0 & 0 & 0 \end{bmatrix}$$

In this case, the last row converts to the equation $0 = 0$ and this is a perfectly acceptable equation.

At this point we shall stop and convert the first two rows of the matrix to equations and find a solution.

$$\simeq \begin{bmatrix} 1 & -2 & 3 & -2 \\ 0 & 1 & -1 & -1 \\ 0 & 0 & 0 & 0 \end{bmatrix} \quad \begin{matrix} R_1 + 2R_2 \\ \rightarrow \end{matrix} \quad \begin{bmatrix} 1 & 0 & 1 & -4 \\ 0 & 1 & -1 & -1 \\ 0 & 0 & 0 & 0 \end{bmatrix}$$

We are now in reduced row-echelon form

$$x_1 + x_3 = -4 \quad \Rightarrow \quad x_1 = -4 - x_3$$
$$x_2 - x_3 = -1 \quad \Rightarrow \quad x_2 = -1 + x_3$$

So, we can choose x_3 to be any value and hence it is a free variable, each choice of x_3 will give us a different solution to the system.

$$x_1 = -4 - t, \quad x_2 = -1 + t, \quad x_3 = t \text{ where } t \text{ is any number}$$

Therefore, we get infinitely many solutions, one for each possible value of t and since t can be any real number there are infinitely many choices for t.

Example 6: Solve the following system of linear equations.

$$3x_1 - 4x_2 = 10$$
$$-5x_1 + 8x_2 = -17$$
$$-3x_1 + 12x_2 = -12$$

Solution: The augmented matrix

$$\simeq \begin{bmatrix} 3 & -4 & 10 \\ -5 & 8 & -17 \\ -3 & 12 & -12 \end{bmatrix}$$

By reducing the matrix to row-echelon form

$$\simeq \begin{bmatrix} 3 & -4 & 10 \\ -5 & 8 & -17 \\ -3 & 12 & -12 \end{bmatrix} \quad \begin{matrix} \frac{1}{3}R_1 \\ \rightarrow \end{matrix} \quad \begin{bmatrix} 1 & -\dfrac{4}{3} & \dfrac{10}{3} \\ -5 & 8 & -17 \\ -3 & 12 & -12 \end{bmatrix}$$

$$\begin{matrix} R_2 + 5R_1 \\ R_3 + 3R_1 \\ \rightarrow \end{matrix} \quad \begin{bmatrix} 1 & -\dfrac{4}{3} & \dfrac{10}{3} \\ 0 & \dfrac{4}{3} & -\dfrac{1}{3} \\ 0 & 8 & -2 \end{bmatrix}$$

$$\frac{3}{4}R_2 \quad \begin{bmatrix} 1 & -\dfrac{4}{3} & \dfrac{10}{3} \\ 0 & 1 & -\dfrac{1}{4} \\ 0 & 8 & -2 \end{bmatrix} \quad R_3 - 8R_2 \quad \begin{bmatrix} 1 & -\dfrac{4}{3} & \dfrac{10}{3} \\ 0 & 1 & -\dfrac{1}{4} \\ 0 & 0 & 0 \end{bmatrix}$$

Here are the equations we get from the row-echelon form of the matrix and the back substituion.

$$x_1 - \frac{4}{3}x_2 = \frac{10}{3} \quad \Rightarrow \quad x_1 = \frac{10}{3} + \frac{4}{3}\left(-\frac{1}{4}\right) = 3$$

$$x_2 = -\frac{1}{4}$$

So the solution to this system is

$$x_1 = 3, \quad x_2 = -\frac{1}{4}$$

Example 7: Solve the following system of linear equations.

$$7x_1 + 2x_2 - 2x_3 - 4x_4 + 3x_5 = 8$$
$$-3x_1 - 3x_2 + 2x_4 + x_5 = -1$$
$$4x_1 - x_2 - 8x_3 + 20x_5 = 1$$

Solution: The augmented matrix for this system

$$\simeq \begin{bmatrix} 7 & 2 & -2 & -4 & 3 & 8 \\ -3 & -3 & 0 & 2 & 1 & -1 \\ 4 & -1 & -8 & 0 & 20 & 1 \end{bmatrix}$$

$$\simeq \begin{bmatrix} 7 & 2 & -2 & -4 & 3 & 8 \\ -3 & -3 & 0 & 2 & 1 & -1 \\ 4 & -1 & -8 & 0 & 20 & 1 \end{bmatrix} \quad \begin{array}{c} R_1 + 2R_2 \\ \rightarrow \end{array} \quad \begin{bmatrix} 1 & -4 & -2 & 0 & 5 & 6 \\ -3 & -3 & 0 & 2 & 1 & -1 \\ 4 & -1 & -8 & 0 & 20 & 1 \end{bmatrix}$$

$$\begin{array}{c} R_2 + 3R_1 \\ R_3 - 4R_1 \\ \rightarrow \end{array} \quad \begin{bmatrix} 1 & -4 & -2 & 0 & 5 & 6 \\ 0 & -15 & -6 & 2 & 16 & 17 \\ 0 & 15 & 0 & 0 & 0 & -23 \end{bmatrix}$$

$$R_2 \leftrightarrow R_3 \atop \rightarrow \quad \begin{bmatrix} 1 & -4 & -2 & 0 & 5 & 6 \\ 0 & 15 & 0 & 0 & 0 & -23 \\ 0 & -15 & -6 & 2 & 16 & 17 \end{bmatrix}$$

$$R_3 + R_2 \atop \rightarrow \quad \begin{bmatrix} 1 & -4 & -2 & 0 & 5 & 6 \\ 0 & 15 & 0 & 0 & 0 & -23 \\ 0 & 0 & -6 & 2 & 16 & -6 \end{bmatrix}$$

$$\begin{matrix} \dfrac{1}{15}R_2 \\[2mm] -\dfrac{1}{6}R_3 \\[2mm] \rightarrow \end{matrix} \quad \begin{bmatrix} 1 & -4 & -2 & 0 & 5 & 6 \\[2mm] 0 & 1 & 0 & 0 & 0 & -\dfrac{23}{15} \\[2mm] 0 & 0 & 1 & -\dfrac{1}{3} & -\dfrac{8}{3} & 1 \end{bmatrix}$$

$$\simeq \begin{bmatrix} 1 & -4 & -2 & 0 & 5 & 6 \\[2mm] 0 & 1 & 0 & 0 & 0 & -\dfrac{23}{15} \\[2mm] 0 & 0 & 1 & -\dfrac{1}{3} & -\dfrac{8}{3} & 1 \end{bmatrix} \quad \begin{matrix} R_1 + 2R_3 \\ \rightarrow \end{matrix}$$

$$\simeq \begin{bmatrix} 1 & -4 & 0 & -\dfrac{2}{3} & -\dfrac{1}{3} & 8 \\[2mm] 0 & 1 & 0 & 0 & 0 & -\dfrac{23}{15} \\[2mm] 0 & 0 & 1 & -\dfrac{1}{3} & -\dfrac{8}{3} & 1 \end{bmatrix}$$

$$\begin{matrix} R_1 + 4R_2 \\ \rightarrow \end{matrix} \quad \begin{bmatrix} 1 & 0 & 0 & -\dfrac{2}{3} & -\dfrac{1}{3} & \dfrac{28}{15} \\[2mm] 0 & 1 & 0 & 0 & 0 & -\dfrac{23}{15} \\[2mm] 0 & 0 & 1 & -\dfrac{1}{3} & -\dfrac{8}{3} & 1 \end{bmatrix}$$

We are now in reduced row-echelon form and so let us go back to equations

$$x_1 - \frac{2}{3}x_4 - \frac{1}{3}x_5 = \frac{28}{15} \quad \Rightarrow \quad x_1 = \frac{28}{15} + \frac{2}{3}x_4 + \frac{1}{3}x_5, \quad x_2 = -\frac{23}{15}$$

$$x_3 - \frac{1}{3}x_4 - \frac{8}{3}x_5 = 1 \quad \Rightarrow \quad x_3 = 1 + \frac{1}{3}x_4 + \frac{8}{3}x_5$$

We have got two free variables this time, x_4 and x_5. Here is the solution for this system.

$$x_1 = \frac{28}{15} + \frac{2}{3}t + \frac{1}{3}s, \quad x_2 = -\frac{23}{15}, \quad x_3 = 1 + \frac{1}{3}t + \frac{8}{3}s, \quad x_4 = t$$

$x_5 = s,$ s and t are any numbers.

3.2 HOMOGENEOUS SYSTEMS OF LINEAR EQUATIONS

A system of n linear equations in m unknowns in the form

$$a_{11}x_1 + a_{12}x_2 + \ldots + a_{1m}x_m = 0$$
$$a_{21}x_1 + a_{22}x_2 + \ldots + a_{2m}x_m = 0$$
$$\vdots$$
$$a_{n1}x_1 + a_{n2}x_2 + \ldots + a_{nm}x_m = 0$$

is called a homogeneous system. The one characteristic that defines a homogeneous system is the fact that all the equations are equal to zero unlike a general system in which each equation can be equal to a different (probably non-zero) number.

Hopefully, it is clear that if we take

$$x_1 = 0, \quad x_2 = 0, \quad x_3 = 0, \ldots, x_m = 0$$

we will have a solution to the homogeneous system of equations. The following theorems are for homogeneous systems.

Theorem 1: Given a homogeneous system of n equations and m unknowns, there will be one of two possibilities for solutions to the system.

1. There will be exactly one solution, $x_1 = 0, \ x_2 = 0, \ x_3 = 0, \ldots, x_m = 0$. This solution is called the trivial solution.
2. There will be infinitely many non-zero solutions in addition to the trivial solution.

Note that when we say non-zero solution in the above fact, we mean that at least one of the x_i's in the solution will not be zero. It is completely possible that some of them will still be zero but at least one will not be zero in a non-zero solution.

We assume that there are more unknowns than equations in a homogeneous system as the following theorem states.

Theorem 2: Given a homogeneous system of n linear equations in m unknowns and if $m > n$ (i.e. there are more unknowns than equations), there will be infinitely many solutions to the system.

Matrices

In the previous section, we used augmented matrices to denote a system of linear equations. In this section, we are looking at matrices in more generality. A matrix is nothing more than a rectangular array of numbers and each of the numbers in the matrix is called an entry. Here are some examples of matrices.

$$\approx \begin{bmatrix} 4 & 3 & 0 & 6 & -1 & 0 \\ 0 & 2 & -4 & -7 & 1 & 3 \\ -6 & 1 & 15 & \frac{1}{2} & -1 & 0 \end{bmatrix}, \quad \begin{bmatrix} 7 & 10 & -1 \\ 8 & 0 & -2 \\ 9 & 3 & 0 \end{bmatrix}, \quad \begin{bmatrix} 12 \\ -4 \\ 2 \\ -17 \end{bmatrix}$$

$$\begin{bmatrix} 3 & -1 & 12 & 0 & -9 \end{bmatrix}, \quad \begin{bmatrix} -2 \end{bmatrix}$$

The size of a matrix with n rows and m columns is denoted by $n \times m$. In denoting the size of a matrix we always list the number of rows first and the number of columns second.

Example 1: Give the size of each of the matrices above.

Solution:

$$\begin{bmatrix} 4 & 3 & 0 & 6 & -1 & 0 \\ 0 & 2 & -4 & -7 & 1 & 3 \\ -6 & 1 & 15 & \frac{1}{2} & -1 & 0 \end{bmatrix} \quad \Rightarrow \quad \text{size: } 3 \times 6$$

$$\begin{bmatrix} 7 & 10 & -1 \\ 8 & 0 & -2 \\ 9 & 3 & 0 \end{bmatrix} \quad \Rightarrow \quad \text{size: } 3 \times 3$$

In this matrix the number of rows is equal to the number of columns. Matrices that have the same number of rows as columns are called **square matrices**.

$$\begin{bmatrix} 12 \\ -4 \\ 2 \\ -17 \end{bmatrix} \quad \Rightarrow \quad \text{size: } 4 \times 1$$

This matrix has a single column and is often called a column matrix.

$$\begin{bmatrix} 3 & -1 & 12 & 0 & -9 \end{bmatrix} \Rightarrow \text{size: } 1 \times 5$$

This matrix has a single row and is often called a row matrix.

$$\begin{bmatrix} -2 \end{bmatrix} \Rightarrow \text{size: } 1 \times 1$$

Often when dealing with 1×1 matrices, we will drop the surrounding brackets and just write -2.

Example 2: Here are several partitions of a general 5×3 matrix.

(a) $A \doteq \begin{bmatrix} a_{11} & a_{12} & a_{13} \\ a_{21} & a_{22} & a_{23} \\ a_{31} & a_{32} & a_{33} \\ a_{41} & a_{42} & a_{43} \\ a_{51} & a_{52} & a_{53} \end{bmatrix} = \begin{bmatrix} A_{11} & A_{12} \\ A_{21} & A_{22} \end{bmatrix}$

In this case, we partitioned the matrix into four submatrices. Also notice that we simplified the matrix into a more compact form. The partitioned matrix can be thought of as a smaller matrix with four entries.

In this case A_{11} is a 2×1 submatrix of A, A_{12} is a 2×2 submatrix of A, A_{21} is a 3×1 submatrix of A and A_{22} is a 3×2 submatrix of A.

(b) $A = \begin{bmatrix} a_{11} & a_{12} & a_{13} \\ a_{21} & a_{22} & a_{23} \\ a_{31} & a_{32} & a_{33} \\ a_{41} & a_{42} & a_{43} \\ a_{51} & a_{52} & a_{53} \end{bmatrix} = \begin{bmatrix} c_1 & | & c_2 & | & c_3 \end{bmatrix}$

In this case, we partitioned A into three column matrices each representing one column in the original matrix. Again, note that we used the standard column matrix notation and subscripted each one with the location in the partitioned matrix. The c_i in the partitioned matrix are sometimes called the column matrices of A.

(c) $A = \begin{bmatrix} a_{11} & a_{12} & a_{13} \\ a_{21} & a_{22} & a_{23} \\ a_{31} & a_{32} & a_{33} \\ a_{41} & a_{42} & a_{43} \\ a_{51} & a_{52} & a_{53} \end{bmatrix} = \begin{bmatrix} r_1 \\ r_2 \\ r_3 \\ r_4 \\ r_5 \end{bmatrix}$

Just as we can partition a matrix into each of its columns as we did in the previous part, we can also partition a matrix into each of its rows. The r_i in the partitioned matrix are sometimes called the row matrices of A.

The first matrix is the zero matrix. The zero matrix is pretty much what the name implies. It is an $n \times m$ matrix whose all entries are zeros. The notation that we will use for the zero matrix is $0_{n \times m}$ for a general zero matrix or 0 for a zero column or row matrix.

$$0_{2 \times 4} = \begin{bmatrix} 0 & 0 & 0 & 0 \\ 0 & 0 & 0 & 0 \end{bmatrix} \qquad 0 = \begin{bmatrix} 0 & 0 & 0 & 0 \end{bmatrix} \qquad 0 = \begin{bmatrix} 0 \\ 0 \\ 0 \end{bmatrix}$$

If the size of a column or row zero matrix is important, we will sometimes subscript the size on those just to make it clear what the size is. Also, if the size of a full zero matrix is not important, we will drop the size from $0_{n \times m}$ and just denote it by 0.

The second special matrix we will look at in this section is the identity matrix. The identity matrix is a square $n \times n$ matrix usually denoted by I_n or just I if the size is unimportant or clear from the context of the problem. The entries on the main diagonal of the identity matrix are all ones and all the other entries in the identity matrix are zeros. Here are a couple of identity matrices.

$$I_2 = \begin{bmatrix} 1 & 0 \\ 0 & 1 \end{bmatrix} \qquad I_4 = \begin{bmatrix} 1 & 0 & 0 & 0 \\ 0 & 1 & 0 & 0 \\ 0 & 0 & 1 & 0 \\ 0 & 0 & 0 & 1 \end{bmatrix}$$

3.3 MATRIX ARITHMETIC AND OPERATIONS

Definition 1: If A and B are both $n \times m$ matrices, then we say that $A = B$ provided corresponding entries from each matrix are equal. Or, in other words, $A = B$ provided $a_{ij} = b_{ij}$, for all i and j.

Matrices of different sizes cannot be equal.

Example 1: Consider the following matrices.

$$A = \begin{bmatrix} -9 & 123 \\ 3 & -7 \end{bmatrix} \qquad B = \begin{bmatrix} -9 & b \\ 3 & -7 \end{bmatrix} \qquad C = \begin{bmatrix} -9 \\ 3 \end{bmatrix}$$

For these matrices, we have $A \neq C$ and $B \neq C$, since they have different sizes and so can not be equal. The fact that C is essentially the first column of both A and B is not important in determining equality in this case.

Next, $A = B$ provided we have $b = 123$. If $b \neq 123$, then we will have $A \neq B$.

Next we need to move onto addition and subtraction of two matrices.

Definition 2: If A and B are both $n \times m$ matrices, then $A \pm B$ is a new $n \times m$ matrix that is found by adding/subtracting corresponding entries from each matrix or in other words,

$$A \pm B = \left[a_{ij} \pm b_{ij} \right]$$

Matrices of different sizes cannot be added or subtracted.

Example 2: For the following matrices perform the indicated operation, if possible.

$$A = \begin{bmatrix} 2 & 0 & -3 & 2 \\ -1 & 8 & 10 & -5 \end{bmatrix} \qquad B = \begin{bmatrix} 0 & -4 & -7 & 2 \\ 12 & 3 & 7 & 9 \end{bmatrix} \qquad C = \begin{bmatrix} 2 & 0 & 2 \\ -4 & 9 & 5 \\ 6 & 0 & -6 \end{bmatrix}$$

(a) $A+B$ (b) $B-A$ (c) $A+C$

Solution:

(a) Both A and B are of the same sizes.

$$A + B = \begin{bmatrix} 2 & -4 & -10 & 4 \\ 11 & 11 & 17 & 4 \end{bmatrix}$$

(b) Again, A and B are of the same sizes. Just like the real number arithmetic, $B-A$ is different from $A-B$.

$$B - A = \begin{bmatrix} -2 & -4 & -4 & 0 \\ 13 & -5 & -3 & 14 \end{bmatrix}$$

(c) In this case, because A and C are of different sizes, the addition can not be done. Likewise, $A-C$, $C-A$, $B+C$, $C-B$ and $B-C$ can not be done for the same reason.

Definition 3: If A is any matrix and c is any number, then the product (or scalar multiple) cA is a new matrix of the same size as A and its entries are found by multiplying the original entries of A by c. In other words, $cA = \left[ca_{ij} \right]$ for all i and j.

Note that in the field of linear algebra, a number is often called a scalar and hence the name scalar multiple since we are multiplying a matrix by a scalar (number). From this point onwards we will generally call numbers as scalars.

If $A_1, A_2, ..., A_n$ are all matrices of the same sizes and $c_1, c_2, ..., c_n$ are scalars, then the linear combination of $A_1, A_2, ..., A_n$ with coefficients $c_1, c_2, ..., c_n$ is

$$c_1 A_1 + c_2 A_2 + ... + c_n A_n$$

Example 3: Given the matrices

$$A = \begin{bmatrix} 0 & 9 \\ 2 & -3 \\ -1 & 1 \end{bmatrix} \quad B = \begin{bmatrix} 8 & 1 \\ -7 & 0 \\ 4 & -1 \end{bmatrix} \quad C = \begin{bmatrix} 2 & 3 \\ -2 & 5 \\ 10 & -6 \end{bmatrix}$$

Compute $3A + 2B - \dfrac{1}{2}C$.

Solution:

Computing the scalar multiples and performing the addition and subtraction.

$$3A + 2B - \frac{1}{2}C = \begin{bmatrix} 0 & 27 \\ 6 & -9 \\ -3 & 3 \end{bmatrix} + \begin{bmatrix} 16 & 2 \\ -14 & 0 \\ 8 & -2 \end{bmatrix} - \begin{bmatrix} 1 & \dfrac{3}{2} \\ -1 & \dfrac{5}{2} \\ 5 & -3 \end{bmatrix} = \begin{bmatrix} 15 & \dfrac{55}{2} \\ -7 & -\dfrac{23}{2} \\ 0 & 4 \end{bmatrix}$$

Matrix Multiplication

Suppose we have the following two matrices,

$$A = \begin{bmatrix} a_1 & a_2 & \cdots & a_n \end{bmatrix} \text{ and } B = \begin{bmatrix} b_1 \\ b_2 \\ \vdots \\ b_n \end{bmatrix}$$

So A is a row matrix and B is a column matrix and they have the same number of entries. Then the product of A and B is defined to be,

$$AB = a_1 b_1 + a_2 b_2 + \ldots + a_n b_n$$

It is important to note that this product can only be done if A and B have the same number of entries. If they have a different number of entries, then this product is not defined.

Example 4: Compute AB, given that,

$$A = \begin{bmatrix} 4 & -10 & 3 \end{bmatrix} \quad B = \begin{bmatrix} -4 \\ 3 \\ 8 \end{bmatrix}$$

Solution: By using the definition

$$AB = (4)(-4) + (-10)(3) + (3)(8) = -22$$

Definition 4: If A is an $n \times p$ matrix and B is a $p \times m$ matrix, then the product (or matrix multiplication) is a new matrix with size $n \times m$ whose ij^{th} entry is found by multiplying row i of A with column j of B.

An easy way to check that a product is defined is to write down the two matrices in the order that we want to multiply them and underneath them write down the sizes as shown below.

$$\begin{array}{ccc} A & B & AB \\ n \times p & p \times m & n \times m \end{array}$$

If the two inner numbers are equal, then the product is defined and the size of the product will be given by the outside numbers.

Example 5: Compute AC and CA for the following two matrices, if possible.

$$A = \begin{bmatrix} 1 & -3 & 0 & 4 \\ -2 & 5 & -8 & 9 \end{bmatrix} \qquad C = \begin{bmatrix} 8 & 5 & 3 \\ -3 & 10 & 2 \\ 2 & 0 & -4 \\ -1 & -7 & 5 \end{bmatrix}$$

Solution: Let us first do AC. Here are the sizes for A and C.

$$\begin{array}{ccc} A & C & = AC \\ 2 \times 4 & 4 \times 3 & 2 \times 3 \end{array}$$

So the two inner numbers (4 and 4) are same and so the multiplication can be done and we can see that the new size of the matrix is 2×3.

For the first row and first column of AC, we shall multiply the first row of A by the first column of C as follows.

$$(1)(8) + (-3)(-3) + (0)(2) + (4)(-1) = 13$$

For the first row and second column of AC, we shall multiply the first row of A by the second column of C as follows.

$$(1)(5) + (-3)(10) + (0)(0) + (4)(-7) = -53$$

$$\begin{bmatrix} 1 & -3 & 0 & 4 \\ -2 & 5 & -8 & 9 \end{bmatrix} \begin{bmatrix} 8 & 5 & 3 \\ -3 & 10 & 2 \\ 2 & 0 & -4 \\ -1 & -7 & 5 \end{bmatrix} = \begin{bmatrix} 13 & -53 & \square \\ \square & \square & \square \end{bmatrix}$$

$$(1)(3) + (-3)(2) + (0)(-4) + (4)(5) = 17$$
$$(-2)(8) + (5)(-3) + (-8)(2) + (9)(-1) = -56$$
$$(-2)(5) + (5)(10) + (-8)(0) + (9)(-7) = -23$$
$$(-2)(3) + (5)(2) + (-8)(-4) + (9)(5) = 81$$

Here is the completed product.

$$\begin{bmatrix} 1 & -3 & 0 & 4 \\ -2 & 5 & -8 & 9 \end{bmatrix} \begin{bmatrix} 8 & 5 & 3 \\ -3 & 10 & 2 \\ 2 & 0 & -4 \\ -1 & -7 & 5 \end{bmatrix} = \begin{bmatrix} 13 & -53 & 17 \\ -56 & -23 & 81 \end{bmatrix}$$

Now let us do CA. Here are the sizes for this product.

$$\begin{array}{ccc} C & A & = CA \\ 4 \times 3 & 2 \times 4 & N/A \end{array}$$

In this case, the two inner numbers (3 and 2) are NOT same and so this product cannot be done.

Example 6: Compute BD and DB for the given matrices, if possible.

$$B = \begin{bmatrix} 3 & -1 & 7 \\ 10 & 1 & -8 \\ -5 & 2 & 4 \end{bmatrix} \qquad D = \begin{bmatrix} -1 & 4 & 9 \\ 6 & 2 & -1 \\ 7 & 4 & 7 \end{bmatrix}$$

Solution:
First, notice that both of these matrices are 3×3 matrices and so both BD and DB are defined.

Also note that in both cases the product will be a new 3×3 matrix.

$$BD = \begin{bmatrix} 3 & -1 & 7 \\ 10 & 1 & -8 \\ -5 & 2 & 4 \end{bmatrix} \begin{bmatrix} -1 & 4 & 9 \\ 6 & 2 & -1 \\ 7 & 4 & 7 \end{bmatrix} = \begin{bmatrix} 40 & 38 & 77 \\ -60 & 10 & 33 \\ 45 & 0 & -19 \end{bmatrix}$$

$$DB = \begin{bmatrix} -1 & 4 & 9 \\ 6 & 2 & -1 \\ 7 & 4 & 7 \end{bmatrix} \begin{bmatrix} 3 & -1 & 7 \\ 10 & 1 & -8 \\ -5 & 2 & 4 \end{bmatrix} = \begin{bmatrix} -8 & 23 & -3 \\ 43 & -6 & 22 \\ 26 & 11 & 45 \end{bmatrix}$$

Theorem 1: Assuming that A and B are appropriately sized so that AB is defined, then

1. The ith row of AB is given by the matrix product: [ith row of A]B.
2. The jth column of AB is given by the matrix product: A [jth column of B].

Example 7: Compute the second row and third column of AC given the following matrices.

$$A = \begin{bmatrix} 1 & -3 & 0 & 4 \\ -2 & 5 & -8 & 9 \end{bmatrix} \qquad C = \begin{bmatrix} 8 & 5 & 3 \\ -3 & 10 & 2 \\ 2 & 0 & -4 \\ -1 & -7 & 5 \end{bmatrix}$$

Solution: These are the matrices from Example 5 and so we can verify the results using this fact once we have done.

Let us find the second row first. So according to the fact this means we need to multiply the second row of A by C.

$$[-2 \quad 5 \quad -8 \quad 9] \begin{bmatrix} 8 & 5 & 3 \\ -3 & 10 & 2 \\ 2 & 0 & -4 \\ -1 & -7 & 5 \end{bmatrix} = [-56 \quad -23 \quad 81]$$

Second row of the product AC.

$$\text{Third column of } AC = \begin{bmatrix} 1 & -3 & 0 & 4 \\ -2 & 5 & -8 & 9 \end{bmatrix} \begin{bmatrix} 3 \\ 2 \\ -4 \\ 5 \end{bmatrix}$$

$$= \begin{bmatrix} 17 \\ 81 \end{bmatrix}$$

Let us start by assuming that we have got two matrices A (size $n \times p$) and B (size $p \times m$) so we know that the product AB is defined.

Now, the first new way of finding the product is to partition A into its row matrices as follows.

$$A = \begin{bmatrix} a_{11} & a_{12} & \cdots & a_{1p} \\ a_{21} & a_{22} & \cdots & a_{2p} \\ \vdots & \vdots & & \vdots \\ a_{n1} & a_{n2} & \cdots & a_{np} \end{bmatrix} = \begin{bmatrix} r_1 \\ r_2 \\ \vdots \\ r_n \end{bmatrix}$$

Now, we know that the ith row of AB is [ith row of A] B. Using this idea, the product AB can then be written as a new partitioned matrix as follows.

$$AB = \begin{bmatrix} r_1 \\ r_2 \\ \vdots \\ r_n \end{bmatrix} B = \begin{bmatrix} r_1 B \\ r_2 B \\ \vdots \\ r_n B \end{bmatrix}$$

For the second new way of finding the product, we will partition B into its column matrices as

$$B = \begin{bmatrix} b_{11} & b_{12} & \cdots & b_{1m} \\ b_{21} & b_{22} & \cdots & b_{2m} \\ \vdots & \vdots & & \vdots \\ b_{p1} & b_{p2} & \cdots & b_{pm} \end{bmatrix} = \begin{bmatrix} c_1 & c_2 & \cdots & c_m \end{bmatrix}$$

We can then use the fact that the jth column of AB is given by $A[\,j$th column of $B]$ and so the product AB can be written as a new partitioned matrix as follows.

$$AB = A \begin{bmatrix} c_1 & c_2 & \cdots & c_m \end{bmatrix} = \begin{bmatrix} Ac_1 & Ac_2 & \cdots & Ac_m \end{bmatrix}$$

Example 8: Use both the new methods for computing products to find AC for the following matrices.

$$A = \begin{bmatrix} 1 & -3 & 0 & 4 \\ -2 & 5 & -8 & 9 \end{bmatrix} \qquad C = \begin{bmatrix} 8 & 5 & 3 \\ -3 & 10 & 2 \\ 2 & 0 & -4 \\ -1 & -7 & 5 \end{bmatrix}$$

Solution:

First, let us use the row matrices of A. Here are the two row matrices of A.

$$r_1 = \begin{bmatrix} 1 & -3 & 0 & 4 \end{bmatrix} \qquad r_2 = \begin{bmatrix} -2 & 5 & -8 & 9 \end{bmatrix}$$

and product

$$r_1 C = \begin{bmatrix} 1 & -3 & 0 & 4 \end{bmatrix} \begin{bmatrix} 8 & 5 & 3 \\ -3 & 10 & 2 \\ 2 & 0 & -4 \\ -1 & -7 & 5 \end{bmatrix} = \begin{bmatrix} 13 & -53 & 17 \end{bmatrix}$$

$$r_2 C = \begin{bmatrix} -2 & 5 & -8 & 9 \end{bmatrix} \begin{bmatrix} 8 & 5 & 3 \\ -3 & 10 & 2 \\ 2 & 0 & -4 \\ -1 & -7 & 5 \end{bmatrix} = \begin{bmatrix} -56 & -23 & 81 \end{bmatrix}$$

Putting these together gives

$$AC = \begin{bmatrix} r_1 C \\ r_2 C \end{bmatrix} = \begin{bmatrix} 13 & -53 & 17 \\ -56 & -23 & 81 \end{bmatrix}$$

Now let us compute the product using columns. Here are the three column matrices for C.

$$c_1 = \begin{bmatrix} 8 \\ -3 \\ 2 \\ -1 \end{bmatrix} \qquad c_2 = \begin{bmatrix} 5 \\ 10 \\ 0 \\ -7 \end{bmatrix} \qquad c_3 = \begin{bmatrix} 3 \\ 2 \\ -4 \\ 5 \end{bmatrix}$$

Here are the columns of the product.

$$Ac_1 = \begin{bmatrix} 1 & -3 & 0 & 4 \\ -2 & 5 & -8 & 9 \end{bmatrix} \begin{bmatrix} 8 \\ -3 \\ 2 \\ -1 \end{bmatrix} = \begin{bmatrix} 13 \\ -56 \end{bmatrix}$$

$$Ac_2 = \begin{bmatrix} 1 & -3 & 0 & 4 \\ -2 & 5 & -8 & 9 \end{bmatrix} \begin{bmatrix} 5 \\ 10 \\ 0 \\ -7 \end{bmatrix} = \begin{bmatrix} -53 \\ -23 \end{bmatrix}$$

$$Ac_3 = \begin{bmatrix} 1 & -3 & 0 & 4 \\ -2 & 5 & -8 & 9 \end{bmatrix} \begin{bmatrix} 3 \\ 2 \\ -4 \\ 5 \end{bmatrix} = \begin{bmatrix} 17 \\ 81 \end{bmatrix}$$

Putting all these together as follows give the correct answer.

$$AB = \begin{bmatrix} Ac_1 & Ac_2 & Ac_3 \end{bmatrix} = \begin{bmatrix} 13 & -53 & 17 \\ -56 & -23 & 81 \end{bmatrix}$$

We can also write certain kinds of matrix product as a linear combination of column matrices. Consider A as $n \times p$ matrix and X as $p \times 1$ column matrix. We can easily compute this product directly as follows.

$$AX = \begin{bmatrix} a_{11} & a_{12} & \cdots & a_{1p} \\ a_{21} & a_{22} & \cdots & a_{2p} \\ \vdots & \vdots & & \vdots \\ a_{n1} & a_{n2} & \cdots & a_{np} \end{bmatrix} \begin{bmatrix} x_1 \\ x_2 \\ \vdots \\ x_p \end{bmatrix} = \begin{bmatrix} a_{11}x_1 + a_{12}x_2 + \ldots + a_{1p}x_p \\ a_{21}x_1 + a_{22}x_2 + \ldots + a_{2p}x_p \\ \vdots \\ a_{n1}x_1 + a_{n2}x_2 + \ldots + a_{np}x_p \end{bmatrix}_{n \times 1}$$

Now, using matrix addition, we can write the resultant $n \times 1$ matrix as follows.

$$\begin{bmatrix} a_{11}x_1 + a_{12}x_2 + \ldots + a_{1p}x_p \\ a_{21}x_1 + a_{22}x_2 + \ldots + a_{2p}x_p \\ \vdots \\ a_{n1}x_1 + a_{n2}x_2 + \ldots + a_{np}x_p \end{bmatrix} = \begin{bmatrix} a_{11}x_1 \\ a_{21}x_1 \\ \vdots \\ a_{n1}x_1 \end{bmatrix} + \begin{bmatrix} a_{12}x_2 \\ a_{22}x_2 \\ \vdots \\ a_{n2}x_2 \end{bmatrix} + \ldots + \begin{bmatrix} a_{1p}x_p \\ a_{2p}x_p \\ \vdots \\ a_{np}x_p \end{bmatrix}$$

Now, each of the p column matrices on the right above can also be rewritten as a scalar multiple as follows.

$$\begin{bmatrix} a_{11}x_1 \\ a_{21}x_1 \\ \vdots \\ a_{n1}x_1 \end{bmatrix} + \begin{bmatrix} a_{12}x_2 \\ a_{22}x_2 \\ \vdots \\ a_{n2}x_2 \end{bmatrix} + \ldots + \begin{bmatrix} a_{1p}x_p \\ a_{2p}x_p \\ \vdots \\ a_{np}x_p \end{bmatrix} = x_1 \begin{bmatrix} a_{11} \\ a_{21} \\ \vdots \\ a_{n1} \end{bmatrix} + x_2 \begin{bmatrix} a_{12} \\ a_{22} \\ \vdots \\ a_{n2} \end{bmatrix} + \ldots + x_p \begin{bmatrix} a_{1p} \\ a_{2p} \\ \vdots \\ a_{np} \end{bmatrix}$$

Finally, the column matrices that are multiplied by the x_i's are nothing more than the column matrices of A. So putting all this together gives us

$$AX = x_1 \begin{bmatrix} a_{11} \\ a_{21} \\ \vdots \\ a_{n1} \end{bmatrix} + x_2 \begin{bmatrix} a_{12} \\ a_{22} \\ \vdots \\ a_{n2} \end{bmatrix} + \ldots + x_p \begin{bmatrix} a_{1p} \\ a_{2p} \\ \vdots \\ a_{np} \end{bmatrix} = x_1 c_1 + x_2 c_2 + \ldots + x_p c_p$$

where $c_1, c_2, \ldots, c_p$ are the column matrices of A. Written in this manner we can see that Ax can be written as the linear combination of the column matrices of A, i.e. $c_1, c_2, \ldots, c_p$ with the entries of X, $x_1, x_2, \ldots, x_p$ as coefficients.

Example 9: Compute AX directly and as a linear combination for the following matrices.

$$A = \begin{bmatrix} 4 & 1 & 2 & -1 \\ -12 & 1 & 3 & 2 \\ 0 & -5 & -10 & 9 \end{bmatrix} \qquad X = \begin{bmatrix} 2 \\ -1 \\ 6 \\ 8 \end{bmatrix}$$

Solution:

The direct computation of the product gives

$$AX = \begin{bmatrix} 4 & 1 & 2 & -1 \\ -12 & 1 & 3 & 2 \\ 0 & -5 & -10 & 9 \end{bmatrix} \begin{bmatrix} 2 \\ -1 \\ 6 \\ 8 \end{bmatrix} = \begin{bmatrix} 11 \\ 9 \\ 17 \end{bmatrix}$$

Here is the linear combination method of computing the product.

$$AX = \begin{bmatrix} 4 & 1 & 2 & -1 \\ -12 & 1 & 3 & 2 \\ 0 & -5 & -10 & 9 \end{bmatrix} \begin{bmatrix} 2 \\ -1 \\ 6 \\ 8 \end{bmatrix}$$

$$= 2\begin{bmatrix} 4 \\ -12 \\ 0 \end{bmatrix} - 1\begin{bmatrix} 1 \\ 1 \\ -5 \end{bmatrix} + 6\begin{bmatrix} 2 \\ 3 \\ -10 \end{bmatrix} + 8\begin{bmatrix} -1 \\ 2 \\ 9 \end{bmatrix}$$

$$= \begin{bmatrix} 8 \\ -24 \\ 0 \end{bmatrix} - \begin{bmatrix} 1 \\ 1 \\ -5 \end{bmatrix} + \begin{bmatrix} 12 \\ 18 \\ -60 \end{bmatrix} + \begin{bmatrix} -8 \\ 16 \\ 72 \end{bmatrix}$$

$$= \begin{bmatrix} 11 \\ 9 \\ 17 \end{bmatrix}$$

3.4 NON-HOMOGENEOUS EQUATIONS

Let the system of equations be

$$a_{11}x_1 + a_{12}x_2 + \ldots + a_{1m}x_m = b_1$$
$$a_{21}x_1 + a_{22}x_2 + \ldots + a_{2m}x_m = b_2$$
$$\vdots$$
$$a_{n1}x_1 + a_{n2}x_2 + \ldots + a_{nm}x_m = b_n$$

Now, a set of equations can be written as a matrix of size $n \times 1$ as follows:

$$\begin{bmatrix} a_{11}x_1 + a_{12}x_2 + \ldots + a_{1m}x_m \\ a_{21}x_1 + a_{22}x_2 + \ldots + a_{2m}x_m \\ \vdots \\ a_{n1}x_1 + a_{n2}x_2 + \ldots + a_{nm}x_m \end{bmatrix} = \begin{bmatrix} b_1 \\ b_2 \\ \vdots \\ b_n \end{bmatrix}$$

In the above, we can see that the left side of it can be written as the following matrix product,

$$\begin{bmatrix} a_{11} & a_{12} & \cdots & a_{1m} \\ a_{21} & a_{22} & \cdots & a_{2m} \\ \vdots & \vdots & & \vdots \\ a_{n1} & a_{n2} & \cdots & a_{nm} \end{bmatrix} \begin{bmatrix} x_1 \\ x_2 \\ \vdots \\ x_m \end{bmatrix} = \begin{bmatrix} b_1 \\ b_2 \\ \vdots \\ b_n \end{bmatrix}$$

If the coefficient matrix is denoted by A, the column matrix containing the unknowns by X and the column matrix containing the b_i's by B, we can write the system in the following matrix form

$$AX = B$$

Definition 5: If A is an $n \times m$ matrix, then the transpose of A, denoted by A^T, is an $m \times n$ matrix that is obtained by interchanging the rows and columns of A. So the first row of A^T is the first column of A, the second row of A^T is the second column of A, etc. Likewise, the first column of A^T is the first row of A, the second column of A^T is the second row of A, etc.

The transpose is defined as follows,

$$A = \left[a_{ij} \right]_{n \times m} \quad \Rightarrow \quad A^T = \left[a_{ji} \right]_{m \times n} \quad \text{for all } i \text{ and } j$$

Notice the difference in the subscripts. Under this definition, the entry in the ith row and jth column of A will be in the jth row and ith column of A^T.

Definition 6: If A is a square matrix of size $n \times n$, then the trace of A, denoted by $\text{tr}(A)$, is the sum of the entries on main diagonal.

Or

$$\text{tr}(A) = a_{11} + a_{22} + \ldots + a_{nn}$$

If A is not square, then the trace is not defined.

Example 10: Determine the transpose (if it is defined) for each of the following matrices.

$$A = \begin{bmatrix} 4 & 10 & -7 & 0 \\ 5 & -1 & 3 & -2 \end{bmatrix} \qquad B = \begin{bmatrix} 3 & 2 & -6 \\ -9 & 1 & -7 \\ 5 & 0 & 12 \end{bmatrix} \qquad C = \begin{bmatrix} 9 \\ -1 \\ 8 \end{bmatrix}$$

$$D = [15] \qquad E = \begin{bmatrix} -12 & -7 \\ -7 & 10 \end{bmatrix}$$

Solution:

$$A^T = \begin{bmatrix} 4 & 5 \\ 10 & -1 \\ -7 & 3 \\ 0 & -2 \end{bmatrix} \quad \text{tr}(A): \text{Not defined since } A \text{ is not square.}$$

$$B^T = \begin{bmatrix} 3 & -9 & 5 \\ 2 & 1 & 0 \\ -6 & -7 & 12 \end{bmatrix} \quad \text{tr}(B) = 3 + 1 + 12 = 16$$

$$C^T = \begin{bmatrix} 9 & -1 & 8 \end{bmatrix} \quad \text{tr}(C): \text{Not defined since } C \text{ is not square.}$$

$$D^T = \begin{bmatrix} 15 \end{bmatrix} \quad \text{tr}(D) = 15$$

$$E^T = \begin{bmatrix} -12 & -7 \\ -7 & 10 \end{bmatrix} \quad \text{tr}(E) = -12 + 10 = -2$$

In the previous example note that $D^T = D$ and that $E^T = E$. In these cases, the matrix is called symmetric. So, in the previous example, D and E are symmetric while A, B and C are not symmetric.

3.5 PROPERTIES OF MATRIX ARITHMETIC

Properties

In the following set of properties, a and b are scalars and A, B and C are matrices. We will assume that the sizes of the matrices in each property are such that the operation in that property is defined.

1. $A + B = B + A$ Commutative law for addition

2. $A + (B + C) = (A + B) + C$ Associative law for addition

3. $A(BC) = (AB)C$ Associative law for multiplication

4. $A(B \pm C) = AB \pm AC$ Left distributive law

5. $(B \pm C)A = BA \pm CA$· Right distributive law

6. $a(B \pm C) = aB \pm aC$

7. $(a \pm b)C = aC \pm bC$

8. $(ab)C = a(bC)$

9. $a(BC) = (aB)C = B(aC)$

Example 1: Consider the following matrix

$$A = \begin{bmatrix} 10 & 0 \\ -3 & 8 \\ -1 & 11 \\ 7 & -4 \end{bmatrix}$$

Then,

$$I_4 A = \begin{bmatrix} 1 & 0 & 0 & 0 \\ 0 & 1 & 0 & 0 \\ 0 & 0 & 1 & 0 \\ 0 & 0 & 0 & 1 \end{bmatrix} \begin{bmatrix} 10 & 0 \\ -3 & 8 \\ -1 & 11 \\ 7 & -4 \end{bmatrix} = \begin{bmatrix} 10 & 0 \\ -3 & 8 \\ -1 & 11 \\ 7 & -4 \end{bmatrix}$$

$$A I_2 = \begin{bmatrix} 10 & 0 \\ -3 & 8 \\ -1 & 11 \\ 7 & -4 \end{bmatrix} \begin{bmatrix} 1 & 0 \\ 0 & 1 \end{bmatrix} = \begin{bmatrix} 10 & 0 \\ -3 & 8 \\ -1 & 11 \\ 7 & -4 \end{bmatrix}$$

Zero Matrix Properties

In the following properties, A is a matrix and 0 is the zero matrix sized appropriately for the indicated operation to be valid.

1. $A + 0 = 0 + A = A$
2. $A - A = 0$
3. $0 - A = -A$
4. $0A = 0$ and $A0 = 0$

We know that if $ab = ac$ and $a \neq 0$, then we must have $b = c$ (sometimes called the cancellation law). We also know that if $ab = 0$, then we have $a = 0$ or $b = 0$.

Example 2: Consider the following three matrices

$$A = \begin{bmatrix} -3 & 2 \\ -6 & 4 \end{bmatrix} \qquad B = \begin{bmatrix} -1 & 2 \\ 3 & -2 \end{bmatrix} \qquad C = \begin{bmatrix} 1 & 4 \\ 6 & 1 \end{bmatrix}$$

Verify that $AB = AC$

Clearly $A \neq 0$ and just as clearly $B \neq C$ and yet we do have $AB = AC$.

Example 3: Consider the following two matrices

$$A = \begin{bmatrix} 1 & 2 \\ 2 & 4 \end{bmatrix} \qquad B = \begin{bmatrix} -16 & 2 \\ 8 & -1 \end{bmatrix}$$

To verify that

$$AB = \begin{bmatrix} 0 & 0 \\ 0 & 0 \end{bmatrix}$$

So $AB = 0$ despite the fact that $A \neq 0$ and $B \neq 0$. So, in this case, this is zero factor.

Definition 1: If A is a square matrix, then

$$A^0 = 1 \qquad A^n = \underbrace{AA\ldots A}_{n\text{-times}}, n > 0$$

This is the standard integer exponent property.

3.6 PROPERTIES OF MATRIX EXPONENTS

If A is a square matrix and n and m are integers, then

$$A^n A^m = A^{n+m}, \qquad (A^n)^m = A^{nm}$$

$$p(x) = a_n x^n + a_{n-1} x^{n-1} + \ldots + a_1 x + a_0$$

and A is a square matrix, then

$$p(A) = a_n A^n + a_{n-1} A^{n-1} + \ldots + a_1 A + a_0 I$$

where the identity matrix on the constant term a_0 has the same size as A.

Example 4: Evaluate each of the following for the given matrix.

$$A = \begin{bmatrix} -7 & 3 \\ 5 & 1 \end{bmatrix}$$

(a) A^2

(b) A^3

(c) $p(A)$ where $p(x) = -6x^3 + 10x - 9$

Solution:

(a) Verify the multiplication

$$A^2 = \begin{bmatrix} -7 & 3 \\ 5 & 1 \end{bmatrix}\begin{bmatrix} -7 & 3 \\ 5 & 1 \end{bmatrix} = \begin{bmatrix} -538 & -18 \\ -30 & 16 \end{bmatrix}$$

(b) Verify the multiplication

$$A^3 = A^2 A = \begin{bmatrix} 64 & -18 \\ -30 & 16 \end{bmatrix}\begin{bmatrix} -7 & 3 \\ 5 & 1 \end{bmatrix} = \begin{bmatrix} -538 & 174 \\ 290 & -74 \end{bmatrix}$$

(c) $p(A) = -6A^3 + 10A - 9I$

$$= -6\begin{bmatrix} -538 & 174 \\ 290 & -74 \end{bmatrix} + 10\begin{bmatrix} -7 & 3 \\ 5 & 1 \end{bmatrix} - 9\begin{bmatrix} 1 & 0 \\ 0 & 1 \end{bmatrix}$$

$$= \begin{bmatrix} 3228 & -1044 \\ -1740 & 444 \end{bmatrix} + \begin{bmatrix} -70 & 30 \\ 50 & 10 \end{bmatrix} - \begin{bmatrix} 9 & 0 \\ 0 & 9 \end{bmatrix}$$

$$= \begin{bmatrix} 3149 & -1014 \\ -1690 & 445 \end{bmatrix}$$

Properties of the Transpose

If A and B are matrices such that the given operations are defined and c is any scalar, then

1. $(A^T)^T = A$
2. $(A \pm B)^T = A^T \pm B^T$
3. $(cA)^T = cA^T$
4. $(AB)^T = B^T A^T$

Proof of 4: We know that the entry in the ith row and jth column of AB is given by

$$(AB)_{ij} = a_{i1}b_{1j} + a_{i2}b_{2j} + a_{i3}b_{3j} + \ldots + a_{ip}b_{pj}$$

We also know that the entry in the ith row and jth column of $(AB)^T$ is found simply by interchanging the subscripts i and j and so it is

$$\left((AB)^T\right)_{ij} = (AB)_{ji} = a_{j1}b_{1i} + a_{j2}b_{2i} + a_{j3}b_{3i} + \ldots + a_{jp}b_{pi}$$

Now, let us denote the entries of A^T and B^T as $\overline{a}_{ij}$ and $\overline{b}_{ij}$ respectively. Again, based on the definition of the transpose, we know that

$$A^T = \left[\overline{a}_{ij}\right] = \left[a_{ji}\right] \qquad\qquad B^T = \left[\overline{b}_{ij}\right] = \left[b_{ji}\right]$$

and so from this we see that $\overline{a}_{ij} = a_{ji}$ and $\overline{b}_{ij} = b_{ji}$. Finally, the entry in the ith row and jth column of $B^T A^T$ is given by

$$\left(B^T A^T\right)_{ij} = \overline{b}_{i1}\overline{a}_{1j} + \overline{b}_{i2}\overline{a}_{2j} + \overline{b}_{i3}\overline{a}_{3j} + \ldots + \overline{b}_{ip}\overline{a}_{pj}$$

Now, plug in for $\overline{a}_{ij}$ and $\overline{b}_{ij}$ and we get that

$$(B^T A^T) = \overline{b}_{i1}\overline{a}_{1j} + \overline{b}_{i2}\overline{a}_{2j} + \overline{b}_{i3}\overline{a}_{3j} + \ldots + \overline{b}_{ip}\overline{a}_{pj}$$

$$= b_{1i}a_{j1} + b_{2i}a_{j2} + b_{3i}a_{j3} + \ldots + b_{pi}a_{jp}$$

$$= a_{j1}b_{1i} + a_{j2}b_{2i} + a_{j3}b_{3i} + \ldots + a_{jp}b_{pi} = \left((AB)^T\right)_{ij}$$

Note that property 4 can be naturally extended to more than two matrices. For example

$$(ABC)^T = C^T B^T A^T$$

Inverse Matrices and Elementary Matrices

Definition 1: If A is a square matrix and we can find another matrix of the same size, say B, such that

$$AB = BA = I$$

then we say A is invertible and B is an inverse of the matrix A.

If we cannot find such a matrix B, we call A, a singular matrix.

Also note that if A is invertible, then it will on occasions be called non-singular. We should also point out that B is invertible and that A is the inverse of B.

Theorem 1: Suppose that A is invertible and that both B and C are inverses of A. Then $B = C$ and we will denote the inverse as A^{-1}.

Proof: Since B is an inverse of A we know that $AB = I$. Now multiply both sides of this by C to get $C(AB) = CI = C$. However, by the associative law of matrix multiplication, we can also write $C(AB)$ as $C(AB) = (CA)B = IB = B$. Therefore, putting these two pieces together we see that $C = C(AB) = B$ or $C = B$.

So, the inverse for a matrix is unique.

Example 1: Given the matrix A, verify that the indicated matrix is in fact the inverse.

$$A = \begin{bmatrix} -4 & -2 \\ 5 & 5 \end{bmatrix} \qquad A^{-1} = \begin{bmatrix} -\dfrac{1}{2} & -\dfrac{1}{5} \\ \dfrac{1}{2} & \dfrac{2}{5} \end{bmatrix}$$

Solution:

To verify that we do, in fact, have the inverse, we will need to check that

$$AA^{-1} = A^{-1}A = I$$

To verify the multiplication

$$AA^{-1} = \begin{bmatrix} -4 & -2 \\ 5 & 5 \end{bmatrix} \begin{bmatrix} -\dfrac{1}{2} & -\dfrac{1}{5} \\ \dfrac{1}{2} & \dfrac{2}{5} \end{bmatrix} = \begin{bmatrix} 1 & 0 \\ 0 & 1 \end{bmatrix}$$

$$A^{-1}A = \begin{bmatrix} -\dfrac{1}{2} & -\dfrac{1}{5} \\ \dfrac{1}{2} & \dfrac{2}{5} \end{bmatrix} \begin{bmatrix} -4 & -2 \\ 5 & 5 \end{bmatrix} = \begin{bmatrix} 1 & 0 \\ 0 & 1 \end{bmatrix}$$

As the definition of an inverse matrix suggests, not every matrix will have an inverse. Here is an example of a matrix without an inverse.

Example 2: The matrix below does not have an inverse.

$$B = \begin{bmatrix} 3 & 9 & 2 \\ 0 & 0 & 0 \\ -4 & -5 & 1 \end{bmatrix}$$

If B has an inverse, then it must be a 3×3 matrix.

$$C = \begin{bmatrix} c_{11} & c_{12} & c_{13} \\ c_{21} & c_{22} & c_{23} \\ c_{31} & c_{32} & c_{33} \end{bmatrix}$$

The product BC

$$[2\text{nd row of } B]\, C = [0 \;\; 0 \;\; 0] \begin{bmatrix} c_{11} & c_{12} & c_{13} \\ c_{21} & c_{22} & c_{23} \\ c_{31} & c_{32} & c_{33} \end{bmatrix} = [0 \;\; 0 \;\; 0]$$

The second row of BC is $[0\; 0\; 0]$ but if C is to be the inverse of B the product BC must be the identity matrix and this means that the second row must in fact be $[0\; 1\; 0]$.

Now, C was a general 3×3 matrix and we have shown that the second row of BC is all zeros and hence the product will never be the identity matrix and so B cannot have an inverse and so it is a singular matrix.

Definition 2: If A is a square matrix and $n > 0$, then

$$A^{-n} = \left(A^{-1}\right)^n = \underbrace{A^{-1}A^{-1}\dots A^{-1}}_{n-\text{times}}$$

Example 3: Compute A^{-3} for the matrix

$$A = \begin{bmatrix} -4 & -2 \\ 5 & 5 \end{bmatrix}$$

Solution:
From Example 1, we know that the inverse of A is

$$A^{-1} = \begin{bmatrix} -\dfrac{1}{2} & -\dfrac{1}{5} \\ \dfrac{1}{2} & \dfrac{2}{5} \end{bmatrix}$$

So, this is easy to compute.

$$A^{-3} = \left(A^{-1}\right)^3 = \begin{bmatrix} -\dfrac{1}{2} & -\dfrac{1}{5} \\ \dfrac{1}{2} & \dfrac{2}{5} \end{bmatrix}\begin{bmatrix} -\dfrac{1}{2} & -\dfrac{1}{5} \\ \dfrac{1}{2} & \dfrac{2}{5} \end{bmatrix}\begin{bmatrix} -\dfrac{1}{2} & -\dfrac{1}{5} \\ \dfrac{1}{2} & \dfrac{2}{5} \end{bmatrix}$$

$$= \begin{bmatrix} \dfrac{3}{20} & \dfrac{1}{50} \\ -\dfrac{1}{20} & \dfrac{3}{50} \end{bmatrix}\begin{bmatrix} -\dfrac{1}{2} & -\dfrac{1}{5} \\ \dfrac{1}{2} & \dfrac{2}{5} \end{bmatrix}$$

$$= \begin{bmatrix} -\dfrac{13}{200} & -\dfrac{11}{500} \\ \dfrac{11}{200} & \dfrac{17}{500} \end{bmatrix}$$

Theorem 2: Suppose that A and B are invertible matrices of the same size. Then,

(a) AB is invertible and $(AB)^{-1} = B^{-1}A^{-1}$.

(b) A^{-1} is invertible and $(A^{-1})^{-1} = A$.

(c) For $n = 0, 1, 2,..., A^n$ is invertible and $(A^n)^{-1} = A^{-n} = (A^{-1})^n$

(d) If c is any non-zero scalar, then cA is invertible and $(cA)^{-1} = \dfrac{1}{c}\, A^{-1}$

(e) A^T is invertible and $(A^T)^{-1} = (A^{-1})^T$.

Proof:

We state that $(AB)^{-1} = B^{-1}A^{-1}$.

(a) We need to show that $(AB)(B^{-1}A^{-1}) = I$ and $(B^{-1}A^{-1})(AB) = I$.

$(AB)(B^{-1}A^{-1}) = A(BB^{-1})A^{-1} = AIA^{-1} = AA^{-1} = I$

$(B^{-1}A^{-1})(AB) = B^{-1}(A^{-1}A)B = B^{-1}IB = B^{-1}B = I$

So, we now know that AB is invertible and that $(AB)^{-1} = B^{-1}A^{-1}$.

(b) Now, we know from the fact that A is invertible such that
$$AA^{-1} = A^{-1}A = I$$
If we multiply A^{-1} by A on both sides, then we will get the identity matrix. To show that A^{-1} is invertible and that its inverse is A.

(c) The best way to prove this part is by a proof technique called induction. To show that $(A^n)(A^{-n}) = (A^{-n})(A^n) = I$, we shall see one of the inequalities

$$\left(A^n\right)\left(A^{-n}\right) = \left(\underbrace{AA...A}_{n-\text{times}}\right)\left(\underbrace{A^{-1}A^{-1}...A^{-1}}_{n-\text{times}}\right)$$

$$= \left(\underbrace{AA\ldots A}_{(n-1) \text{ times}} \right) \left(AA^{-1} \right) \left(\underbrace{A^{-1}A^{-1}\ldots A^{-1}}_{(n-1) \text{ times}} \right) \quad \text{but } AA^{-1} = I$$

$$= \left(\underbrace{AA\ldots A}_{(n-1) \text{ times}} \right) \left(\underbrace{A^{-1}A^{-1}\ldots A^{-1}}_{(n-1) \text{ times}} \right) \ldots, \text{ etc.}$$

$$= (AA)\,(A^{-1}A^{-1})$$

$$= A\,(AA^{-1})\,A^{-1} \quad \text{again } AA^{-1} = I$$

$$= AA^{-1} = I$$

Again, to verify that it is identical. After doing this product we can see that A^n is invertible and $(A^n)^{-1} = A^{-n} = (A^{-1})^n$.

(d) To prove this part we need to show that

$$(cA)\left(\frac{1}{c}A^{-1} \right) = \left(\frac{1}{c}A^{-1} \right)(cA) = I$$

$$(cA)\left(\frac{1}{c}A^{-1} \right) = \left(c.\frac{1}{c} \right)\left(AA^{-1} \right) = (1)(I) = I$$

We can see that cA is invertible and $(cA)^{-1} = \frac{1}{c}A^{-1}$.

(e) The part requires to show that $A^T (A^{-1}) = (A^{-1})\,A^T = I$. Now we need to verify $(CD)^T = D^T C^T$. Using this fact on $A^T (A^{-1})^T$ gives us

$$A^T (A^{-1}) = (A^{-1}A)^T = I^T = I$$

Note that we used the fact that $I^T = I$

$$(A^T)^{-1} = (A^{-1})^T$$

Note that the first part of this theorem can be easily extended to more than two matrices as follows

$$(ABC)^{-1} = C^{-1}B^{-1}A^{-1}$$

Theorem 3: Suppose that A is an invertible matrix and that B, C and D are matrices of the same size as A.

(a) If $AB = AC$, then $B = C$.

(b) If $AD = 0$, then $D = 0$.

Proof:

(a) Since we know that A is invertible, we know that A^{-1} exists so multiply on the left by A^{-1} to get

$$A^{-1}AB = A^{-1}AC$$

$$IB = IC$$
$$B = C$$

(b) Again we know that A^{-1} exists, so multiply on the left by A^{-1} to get

$$A^{-1}AD = A^{-1}0$$
$$ID = 0$$
$$D = 0$$

Definition 3: A square matrix is called an elementary matrix if it can be obtained by applying a single elementary row operation to the identify matrix of the same size.

Example 4: The following matrices are all elementary matrices. Also, given is the row operation on the appropriate sized identity matrix.

$$\begin{bmatrix} 9 & 0 \\ 0 & 9 \end{bmatrix} \qquad 9R_1 \text{ on } I_2$$

$$\begin{bmatrix} 0 & 0 & 0 & 1 \\ 0 & 1 & 0 & 0 \\ 0 & 0 & 1 & 0 \\ 1 & 0 & 0 & 0 \end{bmatrix} \qquad R_1 \leftrightarrow R_4 \text{ on } I_4$$

$$\begin{bmatrix} 1 & 0 & 0 & 0 \\ 0 & 1 & -7 & 0 \\ 0 & 0 & 1 & 0 \\ 0 & 0 & 0 & 1 \end{bmatrix} \qquad R_2 - 7R_3 \text{ on } I_4$$

$$\begin{bmatrix} 1 & 0 & 0 \\ 0 & 1 & 0 \\ 0 & 0 & 1 \end{bmatrix} \qquad 1.R_2 \text{ on } I_3$$

Theorem 4: Suppose E is an elementary matrix that was found by applying an elementary row operation to I_n. Then if A is an $n \times m$ matrix, EA is the matrix that will result by applying the same row operation to A.

Example 5: For the following matrix, perform the row operation $R_1 + 4R_2$ on it and then find the elementary matrix, E for this operation and verify that EA will give the same result.

$$A = \begin{bmatrix} 4 & 5 & -6 & 1 & -1 \\ -1 & 2 & -1 & 10 & 3 \\ 3 & 0 & 4 & -4 & 7 \end{bmatrix}$$

Solution:

Performing the row operation

$$\begin{bmatrix} 4 & 5 & -6 & 1 & -1 \\ -1 & 2 & -1 & 10 & 3 \\ 3 & 0 & 4 & -4 & 7 \end{bmatrix} \quad R_1 \rightarrow R_1 + 4R_2 \quad \begin{bmatrix} 0 & 13 & -10 & 41 & 11 \\ -1 & 2 & -1 & 10 & 3 \\ 3 & 0 & 4 & -4 & 7 \end{bmatrix}$$

Now, we can find E simply by applying the same operation to I_3 and so we have

$$E = \begin{bmatrix} 1 & 4 & 0 \\ 0 & 1 & 0 \\ 0 & 0 & 1 \end{bmatrix}$$

Verify that EA is the same matrix, then

$$EA = \begin{bmatrix} 1 & 4 & 0 \\ 0 & 1 & 0 \\ 0 & 0 & 1 \end{bmatrix} \begin{bmatrix} 4 & 5 & -6 & 1 & -1 \\ -1 & 2 & -1 & 10 & 3 \\ 3 & 0 & 4 & -4 & 7 \end{bmatrix} = \begin{bmatrix} 0 & 13 & -10 & 41 & 11 \\ -1 & 2 & -1 & 10 & 3 \\ 3 & 0 & 4 & -4 & 7 \end{bmatrix}$$

This is the same matrix as the theorem predicted.

Example 6: Give the operation that will take the elementary matrices from example 4 back to the original identity matrix.

$$\begin{bmatrix} 9 & 0 \\ 0 & 9 \end{bmatrix} \quad \begin{matrix} \frac{1}{9}R_1 \\ \rightarrow \end{matrix} \quad \begin{bmatrix} 1 & 0 \\ 0 & 1 \end{bmatrix}$$

$$\begin{bmatrix} 0 & 0 & 0 & 1 \\ 0 & 1 & 0 & 0 \\ 0 & 0 & 1 & 0 \\ 1 & 0 & 0 & 0 \end{bmatrix} \quad \begin{matrix} R_1 \leftrightarrow R_4 \\ \rightarrow \end{matrix} \quad \begin{bmatrix} 1 & 0 & 0 & 0 \\ 0 & 1 & 0 & 0 \\ 0 & 0 & 1 & 0 \\ 0 & 0 & 0 & 1 \end{bmatrix}$$

$$\begin{bmatrix} 1 & 0 & 0 & 0 \\ 0 & 1 & -7 & 0 \\ 0 & 0 & 1 & 0 \\ 0 & 0 & 0 & 1 \end{bmatrix} \quad \begin{matrix} R_2 + 7R_3 \\ \rightarrow \end{matrix} \quad \begin{bmatrix} 1 & 0 & 0 & 0 \\ 0 & 1 & 0 & 0 \\ 0 & 0 & 1 & 0 \\ 0 & 0 & 0 & 1 \end{bmatrix}$$

$$\begin{bmatrix} 1 & 0 & 0 \\ 0 & 1 & 0 \\ 0 & 0 & 1 \end{bmatrix} \xrightarrow{1.R_2} \begin{bmatrix} 1 & 0 & 0 \\ 0 & 1 & 0 \\ 0 & 0 & 1 \end{bmatrix}$$

These kinds of operations are called inverse operations and each row operation will have an inverse operation associated with it. The following table gives the inverse operation for each row operation.

Row operation	**Inverse operation**
Multiply row i by c	Multiply row i by $\dfrac{1}{c}$
Interchange rows i and j	Interchange rows j and i
Add c times row i to row j	Add $-c$ times row i to row j

For the inverse operation we can give the following theorem.

Theorem 5: Suppose that E is the elementary matrix associated with a particular row operation and that E_0 is the elementary matrix associated with the inverse operation. Then E is invertible and $E^{-1} = E_0$.

Proof: This is actually a simple proof. Let us start with $E_0 E$. We know from Theorem 4 that this is the same as the inverse operation to E but we also know that inverse operations will take an elementary matrix back to the original identity matrix. Therefore, we have

$$E_0 E = I$$

Likewise, if we look at EE_0 this will be the same as applying the original row operation to E_0. So we also have

$$EE_0 = I$$

Therefore, we proved that $EE_0 = E_0 E = I$ and so E is invertible and $E^{-1} = E_0$.

Example 7: Consider

$$A = \begin{bmatrix} 4 & 3 & -2 \\ -1 & 5 & 8 \end{bmatrix}$$

then

$$B = \begin{bmatrix} 4 & 3 & -2 \\ 14 & -1 & -22 \end{bmatrix}$$

is row equivalent to A because we reached B by first multiplying second row by (-2) and then adding 3 times row 1 onto row 2.

Here are the elementary matrices (and their inverses) for the operations on A.

$$-2R_2 \quad : \quad E_1 = \begin{bmatrix} 1 & 0 \\ 0 & -2 \end{bmatrix} \quad E_1^{-1} = \begin{bmatrix} 1 & 0 \\ 0 & -\dfrac{1}{2} \end{bmatrix}$$

$$R_2 + 3R_1 \quad : \quad E_2 = \begin{bmatrix} 1 & 0 \\ 3 & 1 \end{bmatrix} \quad E_2^{-1} = \begin{bmatrix} 1 & 0 \\ -3 & 1 \end{bmatrix}$$

Now, to reach B, Theorem 4 tells us that we need to multiply the left side of A by each of these in the same order as we applied the operations.

$$E_2 E_1 A = \begin{bmatrix} 1 & 0 \\ 3 & 1 \end{bmatrix} \begin{bmatrix} 1 & 0 \\ 0 & -2 \end{bmatrix} \begin{bmatrix} 4 & 3 & -2 \\ -1 & 5 & 8 \end{bmatrix}$$

$$= \begin{bmatrix} 1 & 0 \\ 3 & 1 \end{bmatrix} \begin{bmatrix} 4 & 3 & -2 \\ 2 & -10 & -16 \end{bmatrix}$$

$$= \begin{bmatrix} 4 & 3 & -2 \\ 14 & -1 & -22 \end{bmatrix} = B$$

Thus, we get B.

Now, since A and B are row equivalent this means that we should be able to get A from B by applying the inverse operations in the reverse order.

$$E_1^{-1} E_2^{-1} B = \begin{bmatrix} 1 & 0 \\ 0 & -\dfrac{1}{2} \end{bmatrix} \begin{bmatrix} 1 & 0 \\ -3 & 1 \end{bmatrix} \begin{bmatrix} 4 & 3 & -2 \\ 14 & -1 & -22 \end{bmatrix}$$

$$= \begin{bmatrix} 1 & 0 \\ 0 & -\dfrac{1}{2} \end{bmatrix} \begin{bmatrix} 4 & 3 & -2 \\ 2 & -10 & -16 \end{bmatrix}$$

$$= \begin{bmatrix} 4 & 3 & -2 \\ -1 & 5 & 8 \end{bmatrix} = A$$

3.7 FINDING INVERSE MATRICES

In the previous section, we introduced the idea of inverse matrices and elementary matrices. In this section, we need to devise a method for actually finding the inverse of a matrix and involve elementary matrices or at least the row operations that they represent.

Theorem 1: If A is an $n \times n$ matrix, then the following statements are equivalent.
  (a) A is invertible.
  (b) The only solution to the system $Ax = 0$ is the trivial solution.
  (c) A is row equivalent to I_n.
  (d) A is expressible as a product of elementary matrices.

Prove the following chain

$$(a) \Rightarrow (b), (b) \Rightarrow (c), (c) \Rightarrow (d), (d) \Rightarrow (a)$$

Proof:

$(a) \Rightarrow (b)$: We will assume that A is invertible and we need to show that this assumption also implies that $Ax = 0$ will have only the trivial solution. Since A is invertible, we know that A^{-1} exists. So start by assuming that x_0 is any solution to the system, then multiply (on the left) both sides by A^{-1} to get

$$A^{-1}Ax_0 = A^{-1}0, \quad Ix_0 = 0, \quad x_0 = 0$$

So $Ax = 0$ has only the trivial solution and we have managed to prove this implication.

$(b) \Rightarrow (c)$: Here we are assuming that $Ax = 0$ will have only the trivial solution and we need to show that A is row equivalent to I_n.

The augmented matrix for this system is

$$\begin{bmatrix} a_{11} & a_{12} & \cdots & a_{1n} & 0 \\ a_{21} & a_{22} & \cdots & a_{2n} & 0 \\ \vdots & \vdots & \ddots & \vdots & \vdots \\ a_{n1} & a_{n2} & \cdots & a_{nn} & 0 \end{bmatrix}$$

Now we know that the solution to this system must be

$$x_1 = 0, \, x_2 = 0, \, ..., \, x_n = 0$$

by assumption. Therefore, we also know the reduced row-echelon form of the augmented matrix. The reduced row-echelon form of this augmented matrix must be

$$\begin{bmatrix} 1 & 0 & \cdots & 0 & 0 \\ 0 & 1 & \cdots & 0 & 0 \\ \vdots & \vdots & \ddots & \vdots & \vdots \\ 0 & 0 & \cdots & 1 & 0 \end{bmatrix}$$

Now, the entries in the last column do not affect the values in the entries in the first n columns and so we take the same set of elementary row operations and apply them to A. So A is row equivalent to I_n. Since we can get to I_n by applying a finite set of row operations to A, therefore this implication has been proved.

$(c) \Rightarrow (d)$: In this case, we are going to assume that A is row equivalent to I_n and we need to show that A can be written as a product of elementary matrices.

So, since A is row equivalent to I_n, we know there is a finite set of elementary row operations that we can apply to A that will give us I_n. Suppose these row operations are represented by the elementary matrices $E_1, E_2, ..., E_k$. So, we will have the following

$$E_k ... E_2 E_1 A = I_n$$

Multiply by $E_k^{-1}, ..., E_2^{-1}, E_1^{-1}$ (in that order) to get,

$$A = E_1^{-1} E_2^{-1} ... E_k^{-1} I_n = E_1^{-1} E_2^{-1} ... E_k^{-1}$$

So, we see that A is a product of elementary matrices and this implication is proved.

$(\mathbf{d}) \Rightarrow (\mathbf{a})$: Here we will be assuming that A is a product of elementary matrices and we need to show that A is invertible. This is probably the easiest implication to prove.

First, A is a product of elementary matrices .

Theorem 2: Suppose that A is a square matrix, then
  (a) If B is a square matrix such that $BA = I$, then A is invertible and $A^{-1} = B$.
  (b) If B is a square matrix such that $AB = I$, then A is invertible and $A^{-1} = B$.

Proof:
  (a) This proof needs part (b) of Theorem 1. If we can show that $Ax = 0$ has only the trivial solution, then by Theorem 1 we will know that A is invertible. So, let x_0 be any solution to $Ax = 0$, then multiply both sides on the left by B.

$$Ax_0 = 0$$
$$BAx_0 = B0$$
$$Ix_0 = 0$$
$$x_0 = 0$$

So, this shows that any solution to $Ax = 0$ must be the trivial solution and so by Theorem 1, if one statement is true they all are true and so A is invertible. We know from the previous section that inverses are unique and because $BA = I$, we must then also have $A^{-1} = B$.

  (b) In this case, let x_0 be any solution to $Bx = 0$. Then multiplying both sides (on the left) of this by A, we can use a similar argument to that used in (a) to show that x_0 must be the trivial solution and so B is an invertible matrix and that in fact $B^{-1} = A$. Because B is invertible and its inverse is A, we know that

$$AB = BA = I$$

But this is exactly what it means for A to be invertible and that $A^{-1} = B$. So, this is done.

We recall from the last section that in order to show that a matrix B was the inverse of A, we need to show that $AB = BA = I$. In other words, we need to show that both of these products are the identity matrix.

Theorem 3: If A is an $n \times n$ matrix, then the following statements are equivalent.

(a) A is invertible.
(b) The only solution to the system $Ax = 0$ is the trivial solution.
(c) A is row equivalent to I_n.
(d) A is expressible as a product of elementary matrices.
(e) $Ax = B$ has exactly one solution for every $n \times 1$ matrix B.
(f) $Ax = B$ is consistent for every $n \times 1$ matrix B.

Prove the following implications

$$(a) \Rightarrow (e) \Rightarrow (f) \Rightarrow (a).$$

Proof: $(a) \Rightarrow (e)$: Assume that A is invertible and show that $Ax = B$ has exactly one solution for every $n \times 1$ matrix B. Since A is invertible, we know that A^{-1} exist

So $A^{-1}Ax = A^{-1}B$
$$Ix = A^{-1}B$$
$$x = A^{-1}B$$

So, if A is invertible, we show that the solution to the system will be $x = A^{-1}B$ and since matrix multiplication is unique, there is exactly one solution to the system.

$(e) \Rightarrow (f)$: This implication is trivial. Assuming that the system $Ax = B$ has exactly one solution for every $n \times 1$ matrix B but that also means that the system is consistent for every $n \times 1$ matrix B and so we are done with the proof of this implication.

$(f) \Rightarrow (a)$: Here assuming that $Ax = B$ is consistent for every $n \times 1$ matrix b and show that this implies A is invertible. So, if $Ax = B$ is consistent for every $n \times 1$ matrix B, it is consistent for the following n systems.

$$Ax = \begin{bmatrix} 1 \\ 0 \\ 0 \\ \vdots \\ 0 \end{bmatrix}_{n \times 1} \quad Ax = \begin{bmatrix} 0 \\ 1 \\ 0 \\ \vdots \\ 0 \end{bmatrix}_{n \times 1} \quad \cdots \quad Ax = \begin{bmatrix} 0 \\ 0 \\ 0 \\ \vdots \\ 1 \end{bmatrix}_{n \times 1}$$

Since, we know each of these systems have solutions, let $x_1, x_2, ..., x_n$ be those solutions and form a new matrix B, with these solutions as its columns. In other words,

$$B = [x_1 \mid x_2 \mid ... \mid x_n]$$

Now let us take a look at the product AB. We know from the matrix arithmetic section that the ith column of AB will be given by Ax_i, the product AB is

$$AB = [Ax_1 \mid Ax_2 \mid \cdots \mid Ax_n] = \begin{bmatrix} 1 & 0 & \cdots & 0 \\ 0 & 1 & \cdots & 0 \\ 0 & 0 & \cdots & 0 \\ \vdots & \vdots & & \vdots \\ 0 & 0 & \cdots & 1 \end{bmatrix} = I$$

So, we have shown that $AB = I$. By Theorem 2, this means that A must be invertible and so we are done with the proof.

Before proceeding, part (c) of this theorem is also telling us that if we reduce down A to reduced row-echelon form, then we have I_n. This can also be seen in the proof of the implication $(b) \Rightarrow (c)$ in Theorem 1.

Let us assume that A is in fact invertible and so all the statements in Theorem 3 are true. Now, go back to the proof of the implication $(c) \Rightarrow (d)$ of Theorem 1. In this proof, we saw that there were elementary matrices, $E_1, E_2, ..., E_k$, so that we get the following

$$E_k ... E_2 E_1 A = I_n$$

Since we know A is invertible, therefore we know that A^{-1} exists and so multiply (on the right) each side of this to get

$$E_k ... E_2 E_1 A A^{-1} = I_n A^{-1} \quad \Rightarrow \quad A^{-1} = E_k ... E_2 E_1 I_n$$

We need to find a series of row operations that will reduce A to I_n and then apply the same set of operations to I_n and the result will be A^{-1}.

Let us start by supposing that A is an invertible $n \times n$ matrix and then form the following new matrix

$$[A \mid I_n]$$

Note that all we did here was tack on I_n to the original matrix A. Now, if we apply a row operation to this, it will be equivalent to applying it simultaneously to both A and to I_n. So, all we need to do is to find a series of row operations that will reduce the "A" portion of this to I_n, making sure to apply the operations to the whole matrix. Once we have done this we would have

$$[I_n \mid A^{-1}]$$

provided A is, in fact, invertible of course. We will deal with singular matrices in a bit.

Let us take a look at a couple of examples.

Example 1: Determine the inverse of the following matrix given that it is invertible.

$$A = \begin{bmatrix} -4 & -2 \\ 5 & 5 \end{bmatrix}$$

Solution: Note that this is 2×2 matrix we looked at in Example 1 of the previous section. In that example, stated (and proved) that the inverse was

$$A^{-1} = \begin{bmatrix} -\dfrac{1}{2} & -\dfrac{1}{5} \\ \dfrac{1}{2} & \dfrac{2}{5} \end{bmatrix}$$

We can now show how we arrived at this for the inverse. We will first form the new matrix

$$\begin{bmatrix} -4 & -2 & | & 1 & 0 \\ 5 & 5 & | & 0 & 1 \end{bmatrix}$$

Next we will find row operations that will convert the first two columns into I_2 and the third and fourth columns should then contain A^{-1}.

$$\begin{bmatrix} -4 & -2 & | & 1 & 0 \\ 5 & 5 & | & 0 & 1 \end{bmatrix} \begin{array}{c} R_1 + R_2 \\ \rightarrow \end{array} \begin{bmatrix} 1 & 3 & | & 1 & 1 \\ 5 & 5 & | & 0 & 1 \end{bmatrix} \begin{array}{c} R_2 - 5R_1 \\ \rightarrow \end{array}$$

$$\begin{bmatrix} 1 & 3 & | & 1 & 1 \\ 0 & -10 & | & -5 & -4 \end{bmatrix}$$

$$\begin{array}{c} -\dfrac{1}{10}R_2 \\ \rightarrow \end{array} \begin{bmatrix} 1 & 3 & | & 1 & 1 \\ 0 & 1 & | & \dfrac{1}{2} & \dfrac{2}{5} \end{bmatrix} \begin{array}{c} R_1 - 3R_2 \\ \rightarrow \end{array} \begin{bmatrix} 1 & 0 & | & -\dfrac{1}{2} & -\dfrac{1}{5} \\ 0 & 1 & | & \dfrac{1}{2} & \dfrac{2}{5} \end{bmatrix}$$

So, the first two columns are in fact I_2 and in the third and fourth columns we have got the inverse

$$A^{-1} = \begin{bmatrix} -\dfrac{1}{2} & -\dfrac{1}{5} \\ \dfrac{1}{2} & \dfrac{2}{5} \end{bmatrix}$$

Example 2: Determine the inverse of the following matrix given that it is invertible.

$$A = \begin{bmatrix} 3 & 1 & 0 \\ -1 & 2 & 2 \\ 5 & 0 & -1 \end{bmatrix}$$

Solution:

First form the new matrix

$$\begin{bmatrix} 3 & 1 & 0 & | & 1 & 0 & 0 \\ -1 & 2 & 2 & | & 0 & 1 & 0 \\ 5 & 0 & -1 & | & 0 & 0 & 1 \end{bmatrix}$$

and we will use elementary row operations to reduce the first three columns to I_3 and then the last three columns will be the inverse of C.

$$= \begin{bmatrix} 3 & 1 & 0 & | & 1 & 0 & 0 \\ -1 & 2 & 2 & | & 0 & 1 & 0 \\ 5 & 0 & -1 & | & 0 & 0 & 1 \end{bmatrix} \begin{matrix} R_1 + 2R_2 \\ \rightarrow \end{matrix} \begin{bmatrix} 1 & 5 & 4 & | & 1 & 2 & 0 \\ -1 & 2 & 2 & | & 0 & 1 & 0 \\ 5 & 0 & -1 & | & 0 & 0 & 1 \end{bmatrix}$$

$$\begin{matrix} R_2 + R_1 \\ = R_3 - 5R_1 \\ \rightarrow \end{matrix} \begin{bmatrix} 1 & 5 & 4 & | & 1 & 2 & 0 \\ 0 & 7 & 6 & | & 1 & 3 & 0 \\ 0 & -25 & -21 & | & -5 & -10 & 1 \end{bmatrix}$$

$$\begin{matrix} = \dfrac{1}{7}R_2 \\ \rightarrow \end{matrix} \begin{bmatrix} 1 & 5 & 4 & | & 1 & 2 & 0 \\ 0 & 1 & \dfrac{6}{7} & | & \dfrac{1}{7} & \dfrac{3}{7} & 0 \\ 0 & -25 & -21 & | & -5 & -10 & 1 \end{bmatrix}$$

$$\begin{matrix} = R_3 + 25R_2 \\ \rightarrow \end{matrix} \begin{bmatrix} 1 & 5 & 4 & | & 1 & 2 & 0 \\ 0 & 1 & \dfrac{6}{7} & | & \dfrac{1}{7} & \dfrac{3}{7} & 0 \\ 0 & 0 & \dfrac{3}{7} & | & -\dfrac{10}{7} & \dfrac{5}{7} & 1 \end{bmatrix}$$

$$
= \frac{7}{3} R_3 \begin{bmatrix} 1 & 5 & 4 & | & 1 & 2 & 0 \\ 0 & 1 & \dfrac{6}{7} & | & \dfrac{1}{7} & \dfrac{3}{7} & 0 \\ 0 & 0 & 1 & | & -\dfrac{10}{3} & \dfrac{5}{3} & \dfrac{7}{3} \end{bmatrix}
$$

$$
\begin{aligned} R_2 - \dfrac{6}{7} R_3 \\ = R_1 - 4R_3 \\ \rightarrow \end{aligned} \begin{bmatrix} 1 & 5 & 0 & | & \dfrac{43}{3} & -\dfrac{14}{3} & -\dfrac{28}{3} \\ 0 & 1 & 0 & | & 3 & -1 & -2 \\ 0 & 0 & 1 & | & -\dfrac{10}{3} & \dfrac{5}{3} & \dfrac{7}{3} \end{bmatrix}
$$

$$
\begin{aligned} = R_1 - 5R_2 \\ \rightarrow \end{aligned} \begin{bmatrix} 1 & 0 & 0 & | & -\dfrac{2}{3} & \dfrac{1}{3} & \dfrac{2}{3} \\ 0 & 1 & 0 & | & 3 & -1 & -2 \\ 0 & 0 & 1 & | & -\dfrac{10}{3} & \dfrac{5}{3} & \dfrac{7}{3} \end{bmatrix}
$$

So, the first three columns reduced to I_3 and this means that the last three must be the inverse.

$$
C^{-1} = \begin{bmatrix} -\dfrac{2}{3} & \dfrac{1}{3} & \dfrac{2}{3} \\ 3 & 1 & -2 \\ -\dfrac{10}{3} & \dfrac{5}{3} & \dfrac{7}{3} \end{bmatrix}
$$

Verify that $CC^{-1} = C^{-1}C = I_3$.

Example 3: Show that the following matrix does not have an inverse, i.e. show that the matrix is singular.

$$
B = \begin{bmatrix} 3 & 3 & 6 \\ 0 & 1 & 2 \\ -2 & 0 & 0 \end{bmatrix}
$$

Solution: The problem statement says that the matrix is singular, that means we will need the new matrix

$$= \begin{bmatrix} 3 & 3 & 6 & | & 1 & 0 & 0 \\ 0 & 1 & 2 & | & 0 & 1 & 0 \\ -2 & 0 & 0 & | & 0 & 0 & 1 \end{bmatrix}$$

Now, let us get started on getting the first three columns reduced to I_3.

$$= \begin{bmatrix} 3 & 3 & 6 & | & 1 & 0 & 0 \\ 0 & 1 & 2 & | & 0 & 1 & 0 \\ -2 & 0 & 0 & | & 0 & 0 & 1 \end{bmatrix} \begin{matrix} R_1 + R_3 \\ \rightarrow \end{matrix} \begin{bmatrix} 1 & 3 & 6 & | & 1 & 0 & 1 \\ 0 & 1 & 2 & | & 0 & 1 & 0 \\ -2 & 0 & 0 & | & 0 & 0 & 1 \end{bmatrix}$$

$$\begin{matrix} R_3 + 2R_1 \\ \rightarrow \end{matrix} \begin{bmatrix} 1 & 3 & 6 & | & 1 & 0 & 1 \\ 0 & 1 & 2 & | & 0 & 1 & 0 \\ 0 & 6 & 12 & | & 2 & 0 & 3 \end{bmatrix} \begin{matrix} R_3 - 6R_2 \\ \rightarrow \end{matrix} \begin{bmatrix} 1 & 3 & 6 & | & 1 & 0 & 1 \\ 0 & 1 & 2 & | & 0 & 1 & 0 \\ 0 & 0 & 0 & | & 2 & -6 & 3 \end{bmatrix}$$

Theorem 4: The matrix $A = \begin{bmatrix} a & b \\ c & d \end{bmatrix}$

will be invertible if $ad - bc \neq 0$ and singular if $ad - bc = 0$. If the matrix is invertible, its inverse will be

$$A^{-1} = \frac{1}{ad - bc} \begin{bmatrix} d & -b \\ -c & a \end{bmatrix}$$

Example 4: Use the theorem to show that $A = \begin{bmatrix} -4 & -2 \\ 5 & 5 \end{bmatrix}$

is an invertible matrix and find its inverse.

Solution: First, we need

$$ad - bc = (-4)(5) - (5)(-2) = -10 \neq 0$$

So, the matrix is in fact invertible and here is the inverse

$$A^{-1} = \frac{1}{-10} \begin{bmatrix} 5 & 2 \\ -5 & -4 \end{bmatrix} = \begin{bmatrix} -\dfrac{1}{2} & -\dfrac{1}{5} \\ \dfrac{1}{2} & \dfrac{2}{5} \end{bmatrix}$$

Example 5: Determine if the following matrix is singular

$$B = \begin{bmatrix} -4 & -2 \\ 6 & 3 \end{bmatrix}$$

Solution:

Not much to do with this one

$$(-4)(3) - (-2)(6) = 0$$

So, by the theorem the matrix is singular.

3.8 SPECIAL MATRICES

Diagonal Matrix

The first one that we are going to look at is a diagonal matrix. A square matrix is called diagonal matrix if it has the following form.

$$D = \begin{bmatrix} d_1 & 0 & 0 & \cdots & 0 \\ 0 & d_2 & 0 & \cdots & 0 \\ 0 & 0 & d_3 & \cdots & 0 \\ \vdots & \vdots & \vdots & \ddots & \vdots \\ 0 & 0 & 0 & \cdots & d_n \end{bmatrix}_{n \times n}$$

In other words, a diagonal matrix is any matrix in which the only potentially non-zero entries are on the main diagonal. Any entry off the main diagonal must be zero and note that it is possible to have one or more of the main diagonal entries be zero.

Theorem 1: Suppose D is a diagonal matrix and $d_1, d_2, ..., d_n$ are the entries on the main diagonal. If one or more of the d_i's are zero, then the matrix is singular. On the other hand, if $d_i \neq 0$ for all i, then the matrix is invertible and the inverse is

$$D^{-1} = \begin{bmatrix} \dfrac{1}{d_1} & 0 & 0 & \cdots & 0 \\ 0 & \dfrac{1}{d_2} & 0 & \cdots & 0 \\ 0 & 0 & \dfrac{1}{d_3} & \cdots & 0 \\ \vdots & \vdots & \vdots & \ddots & \vdots \\ 0 & 0 & 0 & \cdots & \dfrac{1}{d_n} \end{bmatrix}$$

Triangular Matrix

The next kind of matrix will be triangular matrix. In fact, there are actually two kinds of triangular matrices. For an upper triangular matrix, the matrix must be square and all the entries below the main diagonal are zero and the main diagonal entries and the entries above it may or may not be zero. A lower triangular matrix is just the opposite. The matrix is still a square matrix and all the entries of a lower triangular matrix above the main diagonal are zero and the main diagonal entries and those below it may or may not be zero.

Here are the general forms of an upper and lower triangular matrix.

$$U = \begin{bmatrix} u_{11} & u_{12} & u_{13} & \cdots & u_{1n} \\ 0 & u_{22} & u_{23} & \cdots & u_{2n} \\ 0 & 0 & u_{33} & \cdots & u_{3n} \\ \vdots & \vdots & \vdots & \ddots & \vdots \\ 0 & 0 & 0 & \cdots & u_{nn} \end{bmatrix}_{n \times n} \qquad \text{Upper triangular}$$

$$L = \begin{bmatrix} l_{11} & 0 & 0 & \cdots & 0 \\ l_{21} & l_{22} & 0 & \cdots & 0 \\ l_{31} & l_{32} & l_{33} & \cdots & 0 \\ \vdots & \vdots & \vdots & \ddots & \vdots \\ l_{n1} & l_{n2} & l_{n3} & \cdots & l_{nn} \end{bmatrix}_{n \times n} \qquad \text{Lower triangular}$$

In these forms, the u_{ij} and l_{ij} may or may not be zero.

If the matrix is upper or lower triangular, we generally call it a triangular matrix.

Theorem 2: If A is a triangular matrix with main diagonal entries $a_{11}, a_{22}, ..., a_{nn}$, then if one or more of the a_{ii}'s are zero the matrix will be singular. On the other hand, if $a_{ii} \neq 0$ for all i, then the matrix is invertible.

Here is the outline of the proof.

Proof outline: First assume that $a_{ii} \neq 0$ for all i. In this case, we can divide each row by a_{ii} (since it is not zero) and that will put 1 in the main diagonal entry for each row. Now use the third row operation to eliminate all the non-zero entries above the main diagonal entry for an upper triangular matrix or below it for a lower triangular matrix. When done with these operations we have reduced A to the identity matrix.

In this case, A will not be row equivalent to the identity and so will be singular.

Theorem 3: If A and B are symmetric matrices of the same sizes and c is any scalar, then

(a) $A \pm B$ is symmetric.

(b) cA is symmetric.

(c) A^T is symmetric.

Note that the product of two symmetric matrices is probably not symmetric. Suppose both A and B are symmetric matrices of the same sizes, then

$$(AB)^T = B^T A^T = BA$$

Notice that, we used one of the properties of transpose we found earlier in the first step and the fact that A and B are symmetric in the last step. We have $(AB)^T = AB$ and the product will be symmetric. If A and B do commute, then the product will be symmetric.

Now, if A is any $n \times m$ matrix, then because A^T will have size $m \times n$, both AA^T and $A^T A$ will be defined and in fact will be square matrices where AA^T has size $n \times n$ and $A^T A$ has size $m \times m$.

Theorem 4:

(a) For any matrix A both AA^T and $A^T A$ are symmetric.

(b) If A is an invertible symmetric matrix, then A^{-1} is symmetric.

(c) If A is invertible, then AA^T and $A^T A$ are both invertible.

Proof:

(a) We will show that AA^T is symmetric and leave the other to you to verify. To show that AA^T is symmetric, we will need to show that $(AA^T)^T = AA^T$. This is actually quite simple if we recall the various properties of transpose matrices that we have

$$(AA^T)^T = (A^T)^T A^T = (A) A^T = AA^T$$

(b) In this case, to show that $(A^{-1})^T = A^{-1}$.

$$(A^{-1})^T = (A^T)^{-1} = (A)^{-1} = A^{-1}$$

(c) If A is invertible, then we also know that A^T is invertible and since the product of invertible matrices is invertible both AA^T and $A^T A$ are invertible.

Example 1: Given the following matrices, compute the indicated quantities.

$$A = \begin{bmatrix} 4 & -2 & 1 \\ 0 & 9 & -6 \\ 0 & 0 & -1 \end{bmatrix} \qquad B = \begin{bmatrix} -2 & 0 & 3 \\ 0 & 7 & -1 \\ 0 & 0 & 5 \end{bmatrix} \qquad C = \begin{bmatrix} 3 & 0 & 0 \\ 0 & 2 & 0 \\ 9 & 5 & 4 \end{bmatrix}$$

$$D = \begin{bmatrix} -2 & 0 & -4 & 1 \\ 1 & 0 & -1 & 6 \\ 8 & 2 & 1 & -1 \end{bmatrix} \qquad E = \begin{bmatrix} 1 & -2 & 0 \\ -2 & 3 & 1 \\ 0 & 1 & 0 \end{bmatrix}$$

(a) AB (b) C^{-1}

(c) $D^T D$ (d) E^{-1}

Solution:

(a) AB

$$A = \begin{bmatrix} -8 & -14 & 19 \\ 0 & 63 & -39 \\ 0 & 0 & -5 \end{bmatrix}$$

So, as suggested by Theorem 3, the product of upper triangular matrices is in fact an upper triangular matrix.

(b) C^{-1}

$$\begin{bmatrix} 3 & 0 & 0 & | & 1 & 0 & 0 \\ 0 & 2 & 0 & | & 0 & 1 & 0 \\ 9 & 5 & 4 & | & 0 & 0 & 1 \end{bmatrix} \begin{array}{c} \frac{1}{3}R_1 \\ \frac{1}{2}R_2 \\ \rightarrow \end{array} \begin{bmatrix} 1 & 0 & 0 & | & \frac{1}{3} & 0 & 0 \\ 0 & 1 & 0 & | & 0 & \frac{1}{2} & 0 \\ 9 & 5 & 4 & | & 0 & 0 & 1 \end{bmatrix}$$

$$\begin{array}{c} R_3 - 9R_1 \\ \rightarrow \end{array} \begin{bmatrix} 1 & 0 & 0 & | & \frac{1}{3} & 0 & 0 \\ 0 & 1 & 0 & | & 0 & \frac{1}{2} & 0 \\ 0 & 5 & 4 & | & -3 & 0 & 1 \end{bmatrix} \begin{array}{c} R_3 - 5R_2 \\ \rightarrow \end{array} \begin{bmatrix} 1 & 0 & 0 & | & \frac{1}{3} & 0 & 0 \\ 0 & 1 & 0 & | & 0 & \frac{1}{2} & 0 \\ 0 & 0 & 4 & | & -3 & -\frac{5}{2} & 1 \end{bmatrix}$$

$$\begin{array}{c} \frac{1}{4}R_3 \\ \rightarrow \end{array} \begin{bmatrix} 1 & 0 & 0 & | & \frac{1}{3} & 0 & 0 \\ 0 & 1 & 0 & | & 0 & \frac{1}{2} & 0 \\ 0 & 0 & 1 & | & -\frac{3}{4} & -\frac{5}{8} & \frac{1}{4} \end{bmatrix} \Rightarrow C^{-1} = \begin{bmatrix} \frac{1}{3} & 0 & 0 \\ 0 & \frac{1}{2} & 0 \\ -\frac{3}{4} & -\frac{5}{8} & \frac{1}{4} \end{bmatrix}$$

So, again as suggested by Theorem 3, the inverse of a lower triangular matrix is also a lower triangular matrix.

(c) $D^T D$

Hence the transpose and the product

$$D^T = \begin{bmatrix} -2 & 1 & 8 \\ 0 & 0 & 2 \\ -4 & -1 & 1 \\ 1 & 6 & -1 \end{bmatrix}$$

$$D^T D = \begin{bmatrix} -2 & 1 & 8 \\ 0 & 0 & 2 \\ -4 & -1 & 1 \\ 1 & 6 & -1 \end{bmatrix} \begin{bmatrix} -2 & 0 & -4 & 1 \\ 1 & 0 & -1 & 6 \\ 8 & 2 & 1 & -1 \end{bmatrix} = \begin{bmatrix} 69 & 16 & 15 & -4 \\ 16 & 4 & 2 & -2 \\ 15 & 2 & 18 & -11 \\ -4 & -2 & -11 & 38 \end{bmatrix}$$

So, as suggested by Theorem 4, this product is symmetric even though D was not symmetric.

(d) E^{-1}

Here is the work for finding E^{-1}.

$$E = \begin{bmatrix} 1 & -2 & 0 & | & 1 & 0 & 0 \\ -2 & 3 & 1 & | & 0 & 1 & 0 \\ 0 & 1 & 0 & | & 0 & 0 & 1 \end{bmatrix} \begin{array}{c} R_2 + 2R_1 \\ \rightarrow \end{array} \begin{bmatrix} 1 & -2 & 0 & | & 1 & 0 & 0 \\ 0 & -1 & 1 & | & 2 & 1 & 0 \\ 0 & 1 & 0 & | & 0 & 0 & 1 \end{bmatrix}$$

$$\begin{array}{c} R_2 \leftrightarrow R_3 \\ \rightarrow \end{array} \begin{bmatrix} 1 & -2 & 0 & | & 1 & 0 & 0 \\ 0 & 1 & 0 & | & 0 & 0 & 1 \\ 0 & -1 & 1 & | & 2 & 1 & 0 \end{bmatrix} \begin{array}{c} R_1 + 2R_2 \\ R_3 + R_2 \\ \rightarrow \end{array} \begin{bmatrix} 1 & 0 & 0 & | & 1 & 0 & 2 \\ 0 & 1 & 0 & | & 0 & 0 & 1 \\ 0 & 0 & 1 & | & 2 & 1 & 1 \end{bmatrix}$$

So, the inverse is

$$E^{-1} = \begin{bmatrix} 1 & 0 & 2 \\ 0 & 0 & 1 \\ 2 & 1 & 1 \end{bmatrix}$$

and as suggested by Theorem 5, the inverse is symmetric.

4

Vector Spaces

4.1 INTRODUCTION

The main idea of study in this chapter is that of a vector space. A vector space is nothing more than a collection of vectors that satisfies a set of axioms.

Here is a listing of the topics in this chapter.

Vector spaces In this section, we will formally define vectors and vector spaces.

Subspaces Here we will be looking at vector spaces that exist inside of other vector spaces.

Span The concept of the span of a set of vectors will be investigated in this section.

Linear independence Here we will take a look at what it means for a set of vectors to be linearly independent or linearly dependent.

Basis and dimension We will be looking at the idea of a set of basis vectors and the dimension of a vector space.

Change of basis In this section, we will see how to change the set of basis vectors for a vector space.

Fundamental subspaces Here we will take a look at some of the fundamental subspaces of a matrix, including the row space, column space and null space.

Inner product spaces We will be looking at a special kind of vector spaces in this section as well as define the inner product.

Orthonormal basis In this section, we will develop and use the Gram-Schmidt process for constructing an orthogonal/orthonormal basis for an inner product space.

Least squares In this section, we will take a look at an application of some of the ideas that we will discuss in this chapter.

QR-decomposition Here we will take a look at the *QR*-decomposition for a matrix and how it can be used in the least squares process.

Orthogonal matrices We will take a look at a special kind of matrix, the orthogonal matrix, in this section.

4.2 ESSENTIAL EXAMPLES

Before we dive into the axioms and proofs, we give some examples of vector spaces. Keep these examples in mind as you read the definitions which follows.

Example 1: $\mathbb{R}^n$

We define $\mathbb{R}^n$ to be the set of ordered n-tuples of real numbers,

i.e. $\qquad \mathbb{R}^n = \{(x_1, x_2, \ldots, x_n) : x_1, x_2, \ldots, x_n \in \mathbb{R}^n\}$

The elements of $\mathbb{R}^n$ are called vectors. Given a vector $x = (x_1, x_2, \ldots, x_n)$, the numbers $x_1, x_2, \ldots, x_n$ are called the components of x.

You are already quite familiar with $\mathbb{R}^n$ for normal values of n. For example, $\mathbb{R}^1 = \mathbb{R}$ may be interpreted as the number line and $\mathbb{R}^2$ as the cartesian plane. Furthermore, $\mathbb{R}^1 = \mathbb{R}$ may be interpreted as the number line and $\mathbb{R}^2$ as the cartesian plane. Furthermore, $\mathbb{R}^3$ can be interpreted as three-dimensional space, the components x^1, x^2 and x^3 correspond to the x, y and z coordinates of space.

We are interested in the algebraic properties of these sets, which can be abstracted away from a concrete geometric interpretation. Specifically, we shall focus on two operations:

(i) Addition: Given two vectors $x = (x_1, x_2, \ldots, x_n)$ and $y = (y_1, y_2, \ldots, y_n) \in \mathbb{R}^n$, we may add them componentwise to obtain a new vector $x + y \in \mathbb{R}^n$

$$x + y = (x_1 + y_1, x_2 + y_2, \ldots, x_n + y_n)$$

(ii) Scalar multiplication: Given a vector $x = (x_1, x_2, \ldots, x_n)$ and a real number $\lambda \in \mathbb{R}$ we may multiple x by λ componentwise to obtain a new vector $\lambda x \in \mathbb{R}^n$.

$$\lambda x = (\lambda x_1, \lambda x_2, \ldots, \lambda x_n).$$

The real number 1 is called a scalar, hence the terminology scalar multiplication. (You might try to guess the historical origin of this terminology by thinking about scalar multiplication geometrically in the case $n = 2$).

Example 2: Sequences

Let S denote the set of all sequences of real numbers.

$$S = \{(S_1, S_2, \ldots, S_n, \ldots)\}$$

We call the elements of S as vectors. The set S does not have the simple geometrical interpretations of $\mathbb{R}^n$, but it has many of the same algebraic properties. Specifically, we have the following operations on S.

(i) Addition: Given two vectors $S = (S_n)$, $t = (t_n) \in S$, we may add them term by term to obtain a new vector $S + t \in S$:

$$S + t = (S_1 + t_1, S_2 + t_2, \ldots, S_n + t_n)$$

(ii) Scalar multiplication: Given a vector $S = (S_n) \in S$ and a real number $\lambda \in \mathbb{R}$, we may multiply S and λ term by term to obtain a new vector $\lambda S \in S$

$$\lambda S = (\lambda S_1, \lambda S_2, \ldots, \lambda S_n, \ldots)$$

4.3 VECTOR SPACE AXIOMS

We give axioms for the common algebraic properties of these examples.

Definition 1: Let U be a set on which addition and scalar multiplication are defined (this means that if u and v are objects in U and c is a scalar, then we have defined $u + v$ and cu in some way). If the following axioms are true for all objects u, v and w in U and all scalars c and k, then U is called a **vector space** and the objects in U are called **vectors.**

(a) $u + v$ is in U–this is called **closed under addition**

(b) cu is in U–this is called **closed under scalar multiplication.**

(c) $u + v = v + u$

(d) $u + (v + w) = (u + v) + w$

(e) There is a special object in U, denoted by 0 and called the **zero vector** such that for all u in U we have $u + 0 = 0 + u = u$.

(f) For every u in U, there is another object in U, denoted by '$-u$' and called the **negative** of u such that $u - u = u + (-u) = 0$.

(g) $c\,(u + v) = cu + cv$

(h) $(c + k)\,u = cu + ku$

(i) $c\,(ku) = (ck)u$

(j) $1u = u$

Example 1: If n is any positive integer, then the set $U = R^n$ with the standard addition and scalar multiplication as defined in the Euclidean n-space section is a vector space.

Example 2: The set $U = R^3$ with the standard vector addition and scalar multiplication defined as

$$c\left(u_1,\ u_2,\ u_3\right) = \left(0,\ 0,\ cu_3\right)$$

is not a vector space.

There is a single axiom that fails in this case, to verify that the other should, in this case it is the last axiom (j) that fails as the following work shows.

$$1u = 1(u_1,\ u_2,\ u_3) = (0,\ 0,\ (1)u_3) = (0,\ 0,\ u_3) \neq (u_1,\ u_2,\ u_3) = u$$

Example 3: The set $U = R^2$ with the standard scalar multiplication and addition defined as,

$$(u_1, u_2)\ +\ (u_1, u_2) = (u_1 + 2u_1,\ u_2 + u_2)$$

is NOT a vector space.

To see that this is a vector space, consider the axiom (c).

$$u\ +\ v = (u_1,\ u_2)\ +\ (u_1,\ u_2) = (u_1 + 2u_1,\ u_2 + u_2)$$

Because only the first component of the second point listed gets multiplied by 2, we can see that $u + v \neq v + u$ and so this is not a vector space.

Theorem 1: Suppose that U is a vector space, u is a vector in U and c is any scalar. Then,

(a) $0u = 0$

(b) $(-1)u = -u$

Proof:

(a) Now, this can seem tricky, but each of these steps will come straight from a property of real numbers or one of the axioms above. We will start with $0u$ and use the fact that we can always write $0 = 0 + 0$ and then we will use axiom (h).

$$0u = (0 + 0)\ u = 0u + 0u$$

So, while just $0u$ is a vector, it is in the vector space and so we know from axiom (f) that it has a negative which we will denote by $-0u$. Add the negative to both sides and then use axiom (f) again to say that $0u + (-0u) = 0$

$$0u\ +\ (-0u) = 0u\ +\ 0u\ +\ (-0u)$$
$$0 = 0u\ +\ 0$$

Finally, use axiom (e) on the right side to get,

$$0 = 0u$$

and we proved (a).

(b) In this case, if we can show that $u + (-1)u = 0$, then from axiom (f) we will know that $(-1)u$ is the negative of u, or in other words that $(-1)u = -u$.

$$u + (-1)u = 1u + (-1)u$$

Next, use axiom (h) on the right side and then a property of real numbers.

$$u + (-1)u = [1 + (-1)]u$$
$$= 0u$$

Finally, use part (a) of this theorem on the right side and we get

$$u + (-1)u = 0$$

Definition 2: Suppose that U is a vector space and W is a subset of U. If, under the addition and scalar multiplication that is defined on U, W is also a vector space, then we call W is a subspace.

Suppose that W is a non-empty (i.e. at least one element in it) subset of the vector space U, then W will be a subspace if the following two conditions are true.

(a) If u and v are in W, then $u + v$ is also in W (i.e. W is closed under addition).

(b) If u is in W and c is any scalar, then cu is also in W (i.e. W is closed under scalar multiplication).

Where the definition of addition and scalar multiplication on W are the same as on U.

Example 1: Determine if the given set is a subspace of the given vector space.

(a) Let W be the set of all points (x, y), which is a subspace of R^2.

(b) Let W be the set of all points from R^3 of the form $(0, x_2, x_3)$. Is this a subspace of R^3?

(c) Let W be the set of all points from R^3 of the form $(1, x_2, x_3)$. Is this a subspace of R^3?

Solution:

In each of these cases, we need to show either that the set is closed under addition and scalar multiplication or it is not closed for at least one of those.

(a) Let W be the set of all points (x, y) from R^2 in which $x \geq 0$. Is this a subspace of R^2

This set is closed under addition because,

$$(x_1, y_1) + (x_2, y_2) = (x_1 + x_2, y_1 + y_2)$$

and since $x_1, x_2 \geq 0$ we also have $x_1 + x_2 \geq 0$ and so the resultant point is back in W.

However, this set is not closed under scalar multiplication. Let c be any negative scalar and further assume that $x > 0$, then

$$c(x, y) = (cx, cy)$$

Then, because $x > 0$ and $c < 0$, we must have $cx < 0$ and so the resultant point is not in W, because the first component is neither zero nor positive.

Therefore, W is not a subspace of U.

(b) Let W be the set of all points from R^3 of the form $(0, x_2, x_3)$. Is this a subspace of R^3?

This one is fairly simple to check. A point will be in W, if the first component is zero.

So, let $x = (0, x_2, x_3)$ and $y = (0, y_2, y_3)$ be any two points in W and let c be any scalar, then

$$x + y = (0, x_2, x_3) + (0, y_2, y_3) = (0, x_2 + y_2, x_3 + y_3)$$
$$cx = (0, cx_2, cx_3)$$

So, both $x + y$ and cx are in W and so W is closed under addition and scalar multiplication and so W is a subspace.

(c) Let W be the set of all points from R^3 of the form $(1, x_2, x_3)$. Is this a subspace of R^3?

This one is here just to keep us way from making any assumptions based on the previous part. This set is closed under neither addition nor scalar multiplication. In order to the points to be in W, in this case, the first component must be 1. However, if $x = (1, x_2, x_3)$ and $y = (1, y_2, y_3)$ be any two points in W and let c be any scalar other than 1, we get

$$x + y = (1, x_2, x_3) + (1, y_2, y_3) = (2, x_2 + y_2, x_3 + y_3)$$

$$cx = (c, cx_2, cx_3)$$

neither of which is in W and so W is not a subspace.

Example 2: Determine if the given set is a subspace of the given vector space.

(a) Let W be the set of diagonal matrices of size $n \times n$. Is this a subspace of M_{nn}?

(b) Let W be the set of matrices of the form $\begin{bmatrix} 0 & a_{12} \\ a_{21} & a_{22} \\ a_{31} & a_{32} \end{bmatrix}$. Is this subspace of M_{32}?

(c) Let W be the set of matrices of the form $\begin{bmatrix} 2 & a_{12} \\ 0 & a_{22} \end{bmatrix}$. Is this a subspace of M_{22}?

Solution:

(a) Let W be the set of diagonal matrices of size $n \times n$. Is this a subspace of M_{nn}?

Let u and v be any two $n \times n$ diagonal matrices and c be any scalar, then

$$u + v = \begin{bmatrix} u_1 & 0 & \cdots & 0 \\ 0 & u_2 & \cdots & 0 \\ \vdots & \vdots & \ddots & \vdots \\ 0 & 0 & \cdots & u_n \end{bmatrix} + \begin{bmatrix} v_1 & 0 & \cdots & 0 \\ 0 & v_2 & \cdots & 0 \\ \vdots & \vdots & \ddots & \vdots \\ 0 & 0 & \cdots & v_n \end{bmatrix}$$

$$= \begin{bmatrix} u_1 + v_1 & 0 & \cdots & 0 \\ 0 & u_2 + v_2 & \cdots & 0 \\ \vdots & \vdots & \ddots & \vdots \\ 0 & 0 & \cdots & u_n + v_n \end{bmatrix} \qquad cu = \begin{bmatrix} cu_1 & 0 & \cdots & 0 \\ 0 & cu_2 & \cdots & 0 \\ \vdots & \vdots & \ddots & \vdots \\ 0 & 0 & \cdots & cu_n \end{bmatrix}$$

Both $u + v$ and cu are also diagonal $n \times n$ matrices and so W is closed under addition and scalar multiplication and so is a subspace of M_{nn}.

(b) Let W be the set of matrices of the form $\begin{bmatrix} 0 & a_{12} \\ a_{21} & a_{22} \\ a_{31} & a_{32} \end{bmatrix}$. Is this a subspace of M_{32}?

Let u and v be any two matrices from W and c be any scalar, then

$$u + v = \begin{bmatrix} 0 & u_{12} \\ u_{21} & u_{22} \\ u_{31} & u_{32} \end{bmatrix} + \begin{bmatrix} 0 & v_{12} \\ v_{21} & v_{22} \\ v_{31} & v_{32} \end{bmatrix} = \begin{bmatrix} 0 & u_{12} + v_{12} \\ u_{21} + v_{21} & u_{22} + v_{22} \\ u_{31} + v_{31} & u_{32} + v_{32} \end{bmatrix}$$

$$cu = \begin{bmatrix} 0 & cu_{12} \\ cu_{21} & cu_{22} \\ cu_{31} & cu_{32} \end{bmatrix}$$

Both $u + v$ and cu are also in W and so W is closed under addition and scalar multiplication and hence is a subspace of M_{32}.

(c) Let W be the set of matrices of the form $\begin{bmatrix} 2 & a_{12} \\ 0 & a_{22} \end{bmatrix}$. Is this a subspace of M_{22}?

Let u and v be any two matrices from W, then

$$u + v = \begin{bmatrix} 2 & u_{12} \\ 0 & u_{22} \end{bmatrix} + \begin{bmatrix} 2 & v_{12} \\ 0 & v_{22} \end{bmatrix} = \begin{bmatrix} 4 & u_{12} + v_{12} \\ 0 & u_{22} + v_{22} \end{bmatrix}$$

So, $u + v$ is not in W since the entry in the first row and first column is not 2. Therefore, W is not closed under addition. You should also verify for yourself that W is not closed under scalar multiplication either.

In either case, W is not a subspace of M_{22}.

Example 3: Determine if the given set is a subspace of the given vector space.

(a) Let $C[a, b]$ be the set of all continuous functions on the interval $[a, b]$. Is this a subspace of $F[a, b]$, the set of all real valued functions on the interval $[a, b]$?

(b) Let P_n be the set of all polynomials of degree n or less. Is this a subspace of $F[a, b]$?

(c) Let W be the set of all polynomials of degree exactly n. Is this a subspace of $F[a, b]$?

(d) Let W be the set of all functions such that $f(6) = 10$. Is this a subspace of $F[a, b]$, where we have $a \le 6 \le b$?

Solution:

(a) Let $C[a, b]$ be the set of all continuous functions on the interval $[a, b]$. Is this a subspace of $F[a, b]$, the set of all real valued functions on the interval $[a, b]$.

So, $C[a, b]$ is a subspace of $F[a, b]$.

(b) Let P_n be the set of all polynomials of degree n or less. Is this a subspace of $F[a, b]$?

First recall that a polynomial is said to have degree n, if largest exponent of the variable in it is n. Let $u = a_n x^n + \ldots + a_1 x + a_0$ and $v = b_n x^n + \ldots + b_1 x + b_0$. Let c be any scalar. Then,

$$u + v = (a_n + b_n)x^n + \ldots + (a_1 + b_1)x + a_0 + b_0$$

$$cu = ca_n x^n + \ldots + ca_1 x + ca_0$$

In both cases, the degree of the new polynomial is not greater than n. Of course, in the case of scalar multiplication it will remain degree n, but with the sum, it is possible that some of the coefficients cancel out to zero and hence reduce the degree of the polynomial.

The point is that P_n is closed under addition and scalar multiplication and so will be a subspace of $F[a, b]$.

(c) Let W be the set of all polynomials of degree exactly n. Is this a subspace of $F[a, b]$?

In this case, W is not closed under addition. At $n = 2$ case to keep things simple (the same argument will work for other values of n), consider the following polynomials

$$u = ax^2 + bx + c \text{ and } v = ax^2 + dx + e$$

where a is not zero, we know this is true, because each polynomial must have degree 2. The other constants may or may not be zero. Both are polynomials of degree exactly 2 (since a is not zero) and if we add them we get

$$u + v = (b + d)x + c + e$$

So the sum had degree 1. Therefore, for $n = 2$, W is not closed under addition.

(d) Let W be the set of all functions such that $f(6) = 10$. Is this a subspace of $F[a, b]$, where we have $a \le 6 \le b$?

First notice that if we do not have $a \le 6 \le b$, so we will assume that $a \le 6 \le b$.

In this case, suppose that we have two elements from W, $f = f(x)$ and $g = g(x)$. This means that $f(6) = 10$ and $g(6) = 10$. In order to W to be a subspace we evaluate the sum and the scalar multiple at 6. The sum is

$$(f + g)(6) = f(6) + g(6) = 10 + 10 = 20 \ne 10$$

and so the sum will not be in W. Likewise, if c is any scalar, then

$$(cf)(6) = cf(6) = c(10) \ne 10$$

and so the scalar is not in W either.

Therefore, W is not closed under addition or scalar multiplication and so it is not a subspace.

First, we should just point out that the set of all continuous functions on the interval $[a, b]$ is a fairly important vector space in its own right to many areas of mathematical study.

Next, we saw that the set of all polynomials of degree less than or equal to n, P_n is a subspace of $F[a,b]$. However, that polynomials are continuous and so P_n can also be a subspace of $C[a,b]$ as well. In other words, subspaces can have subspaces in themselves.

Finally, here is something for you to think about. In the last part, we saw that the set of all functions for which $f(6) = 10$ was not a subspace of $F[a, b]$ with $a \le 6 \le b$. Let us take a more general look at this. For some fixed number k, let W be the set of all real valued functions for which $f(6) = k$.

Definition 3: Suppose A is an $n \times m$ matrix. The **null space** of A is the set of all x in R^m such that $Ax = 0$.

Example 4: Determine the null space of each of the following matrices.

(a) $A = \begin{bmatrix} 2 & 0 \\ -4 & 10 \end{bmatrix}$ (b) $B = \begin{bmatrix} 1 & -7 \\ -3 & 21 \end{bmatrix}$ (c) $O = \begin{bmatrix} 0 & 0 \\ 0 & 0 \end{bmatrix}$

Solution:

(a) $A = \begin{bmatrix} 2 & 0 \\ -4 & 10 \end{bmatrix}$

To find the null space of A, solve the following system of equations.

$$\begin{bmatrix} 2 & 0 \\ -4 & 10 \end{bmatrix} \begin{bmatrix} x_1 \\ x_2 \end{bmatrix} = \begin{bmatrix} 0 \\ 0 \end{bmatrix} \Rightarrow 2x_1 = 0$$

$$-4x_1 + 10x_2 = 0$$

We have given this in both matrix form and equation form. In equation form, it is easy to see that the only solution is $x_1 = x_2 = 0$. In terms of vectors from R^2, the solution consists of the single vector $\{0\}$ and hence the null space of A is $\{0\}$.

(b) $B = \begin{bmatrix} 1 & -7 \\ -3 & 21 \end{bmatrix}$

Here is the system that we need to solve for this part.

$$\begin{bmatrix} 1 & -7 \\ -3 & 21 \end{bmatrix} \begin{bmatrix} x_1 \\ x_2 \end{bmatrix} = \begin{bmatrix} 0 \\ 0 \end{bmatrix} \Rightarrow x_1 - 7x_2 = 0$$

$$-3x_1 + 21x_2 = 0$$

Now, we can see that these two equations are in fact the same equations and so we know there will be infinitely many solutions and that they will have the form

$x_1 = 7t$ and $x_2 = t$, where t is any real number.

Since the null space of B consists of all solutions to $Bx = 0$, therefore, the null space of B will consist of all the vectors $x = (x_1, x_2)$ from R^2 that are in the form

$x = (7t, t) = t(7, 1)$, where t is any real number.

In terms of equations, rather than vectors in R^2, let us note that the null space of B will be all of the points that are on the equation through the origin given by $x_1 - 7x_2 = 0$.

(c) $O = \begin{bmatrix} 0 & 0 \\ 0 & 0 \end{bmatrix}$

$$\begin{bmatrix} 0 & 0 \\ 0 & 0 \end{bmatrix} \begin{bmatrix} x_1 \\ x_2 \end{bmatrix} = \begin{bmatrix} 0 \\ 0 \end{bmatrix}$$

However, if you think about it, every vector x in R^2 will be a solution to this system since we are multiplying x by the zero matrix.

Hence the null space of O is all of R^2.

Definition 4: We say the vector w from the vector space U is a linear combination of the vectors $u_1, u_2,..., u_n$, all from U, if there are scalars $c_1, c_2,..., c_n$ so that w can be written as

$$w = c_1u_1 + c_2u_2 + ... + c_nu_n$$

So, we can see that the null space we were looking at above is in fact all the linear combinations of the vector $(7, 1)$. It may seem strange to talk about linear combinations of a single vector, such that it is really scalar multiplication.

When we were looking at Euclidean n-space, we introduced these things called the standard basis vectors. The standard basis vectors for R^n were defined as

$$e_1 = (1, 0, 0,...,0),\ e_2 = (0, 1, 0,...,0),...,\ e_n = (0, 0, 0,...,1)$$

We saw that we could take any vector $u = (u_1, u_2,...,u_n)$ from R^n and write it as

$$u = u_1 e_1 + u_2 e_2 + ... + u_n e_n$$

Or, in other words, we could write u as a linear combination of the standard basis vectors $e_1, e_2,..., e_n$.

Example 5: Determine if the vector is a linear combination of the two given vectors.

(a) Is $w = (-12, 20)$ a linear combination of $u_1 = (-1, 2)$ and $u_2 = (4, -6)$?

(b) Is $w = (4, 20)$ a linear combination of $u_1 = (2, 10)$ and $u_2 = (-3, -15)$?

(c) Is $w = (1, -4)$ a linear combination of $u_1 = (2, 10)$ and $u_2 = (-3, -15)$?

Solution:

(a) Is $w = (-12, 20)$ a linear combination of $u_1 = (-1, 2)$ and $u_2 = (4, -6)$?
Solve the following equation

$$w = c_1 u_1 + c_2 u_2$$
$$(-12, 20) = c_1(-1, 2) + c_2(4, -6)$$

Then set components equal to arrive at the following system of equations

$$-c_1 + 4c_2 = -12$$
$$2c_1 - 6c_2 = 20$$

The solution to this system is $c_1 = 4$ and $c_2 = -2$. Therefore, w is a linear combination of u_1 and u_2 and we can write $w = 4u_1 - 2u_2$.

(b) Is $w = (4, 20)$ a linear combination of $u_1 = (2, 10)$ and $u_2 = (-3, -15)$?

$$2c_1 - 3c_2 = 4$$
$$10c_1 - 15c_2 = 20$$

The solution to this system is

$$c_1 = 2 + \frac{3}{2}t,\quad c_2 = t$$

where t is any real number.

This means w is a linear combination of u_1 and u_2.

$$w = 2u_1 + (0)u_2 \text{ and } w = (0)u_1 - \frac{4}{3}u_2$$

$$w = 8u_1 + 4u_2 \text{ and } w = -u_1 - 2u_2$$

(c) Is $w = (1, -4)$ a linear combination of $u_1 = (2, 10)$ and $u_3 = (-3, -15)$?

$$2c_1 - 3c_2 = 1$$

$$10c_1 - 15c_2 = -4$$

This system does not have a solution and so w is not a linear combination of u_1 and u_2.

Definition 5: Let $S = \{u_1, u_2,...,u_n\}$ be a set of vectors in a vector space U and let W be the set of all linear combinations of the vectors $u_1, u_2,..., u_n$. The set W is the span of the vectors $u_1, u_2,...,u_n$ and is denoted by

$$W = \text{span}(S) \text{ or } W = \text{span } \{u_1, u_2,...,u_n\}$$

We also say that the vectors $u_1, u_2,...,u_n$ span W.

Theorem 1: Let $u_1, u_2,..., u_n$ be vectors in a vector space U and let their span be

$$W = \text{span } \{u_1, u_2,...,u_n\}, \text{ then}$$

(a) W is a subspace of U.

(b) W is the smallest subspace of U that contains all of the vectors $u_1, u_2,..., u_n$.

Proof:

(a) So we need to show that W is closed under addition and scalar multiplication. Let u and w be any two vectors from W. Now, since W is the set of all linear combinations of $u_1, u_2,..., u_n$, this means that both u and w must be a linear combination of these vectors. So, there are scalars $c_1, c_2,...,c_n$ and $k_1, k_2,...,k_n$ so that

$$u = c_1u_1 + c_2u_2 + ... + c_nu_n \text{ and } w = k_1u_1 + k_2u_2 + ... + k_nu_n$$

Now,

$$u + w = (c_1 + k_1)u_1 + (c_2 + k_2)u_2 + ... + (c_n + k_n)u_n$$

So the sum $u + w$ is a linear combination of the vectors $u_1, u_2,...,u_n$ and hence must be in W and so W is closed under addition.

Now, let k be any scalar

$$ku = (kc_1)u_1 + (kc_2)u_2 + ... + (kc_n)u_n$$

As we can see the scalar multiple ku is a linear combination of the vectors $u_1, u_2,..., u_n$ and hence must be in W and so W is closed under scalar multiplication.

Therefore, W must be a subspace.

(b) In these cases when we say that W is the smallest vector space that contains the set of vectors $u_1, u_2,...,u_n$ if W' is also a vector space that contains $u_1, u_2,...,u_n$, then

$$u_i = 0u_1 + 0u_2 + ... + 1u_i + ... + 0u_n$$

Now, let W be a vector space and consider any vector u from W. If we can show that u must also be in W', it will contain all the vectors in W. Now, u is in W and so must be a linear combination of $u_1, u_2,..., u_n$

$$u = c_1u_1 + c_2u_2 + ... + c_nu_n$$

Each of the terms in this sum, c_iu_i is a scalar multiple of a vector that is in W' and since W' is a vector space it must be closed under scalar multiplication and so each c_iu_i is in W'. But this means that u is the sum of a bunch of vectors that are in W' which is closed under addition and so this means that u must in fact be in W'.

Example 6: Describe the span of each of the following sets of vectors.

(a) $u_1 = (1,0,0)$ and $u_2 = (0,1,0)$.

(b) $u_1 = (1,0,1,0)$ and $u_2 = (0,1,0,-1)$

Solution:

(a) The span of this set of vectors, span $\{u_1, u_2\}$, is the set of all linear combinations and we can write down a general linear combination for these two vectors.

$$au_1 + bu_2 = (a, 0, 0) + (0, b, 0) = (a, b, 0)$$

So, it looks like span $\{u_1, u_2\}$ will be all of the vectors from R^3 that are in the form $(a, b, 0)$ for any choices of a and b.

(b) A general linear combination

$$au_1 + bu_2 = (a, 0, a, 0) + (0, b, 0, -b) = (a, b, a, -b)$$

So, span $\{u_1, u_2\}$ will be the vectors from R^4 of the form $(a, b, a, -b)$ for any choices of a and b.

Example 7: Describe the span of each of the following sets of "vectors".

(a) $u_1 = \begin{bmatrix} 1 & 0 \\ 0 & 0 \end{bmatrix}$ and $u_2 = \begin{bmatrix} 0 & 0 \\ 0 & 1 \end{bmatrix}$

(b) $u_1 = 1$, $u_2 = x$, and $u_3 = x^3$

Solution:

(a) Here is the general linear combination of these vectors.

$$au_1 + bu_2 = \begin{bmatrix} a & 0 \\ 0 & 0 \end{bmatrix} + \begin{bmatrix} 0 & 0 \\ 0 & b \end{bmatrix} = \begin{bmatrix} a & 0 \\ 0 & b \end{bmatrix}$$

Here the span$\{u_1, u_2\}$ will be all the diagonal matrices in M_{22}.

(b) A general linear combination in this case is

$$au_1 + bu_2 + cu_3 = a + bx + cx^3$$

In this case, span $\{u_1, u_2, u_3\}$ will be all the polynomials from P_3 that do not have a quadratic term.

4.4 LINEAR INDEPENDENCE

In the previous section, we saw several examples of writing a particular vector as a linear combination of other vectors. However, as we saw in Example 1(b) of that section there is sometimes more than one linear combination of the same set of vectors that can be used for a given vector.

Definition: Suppose $S = \{u_1, u_2,..., u_n\}$ is a non-empty set of vectors and form the vector equation

$$c_1u_1 + c_2u_2 + ... + c_nu_n = 0$$

This equation has at least one solution, namely $c_1 = 0$, $c_2 = 0,...,c_n = 0$. This solution is called the trivial solution.

If the trivial solution is the only solution to this equation, then the vectors in the set S are called linearly independent set. If there is another solution, then the vectors in the set S are called linearly dependent set.

Example 1: Determine whether each of the following sets of vectors are linearly independent or linearly dependent.

(a) $u_1 = (3, -1)$ and $u_2 = (-2, 2)$.

(b) $u_1 = (12, -8)$ and $u_2 = (-9, 6)$.

(c) $u_1 = (1, 0, 0)$, $u_2 = (0, 1, 0)$ and $u_3 = (0, 0, 1)$.

(d) $u_1 = (2, -2, 4)$, $u_2 = (3, -5, 4)$ and $u_3 = (0, 1, 1)$.

Solution:

The set up of the equation

$$c_1u_1 + c_2u_2 + ... + c_nu_n = 0$$

(a) $u_1 = (3, -1)$ and $u_2 = (-2, 2)$.

$c_1(3, -1) + c_2(-2, 2) = 0$

$(3c_1 - 2c_2, -c_1 + 2c_2) = (0, 0)$

Now, set each of the components equal to zero and arrive at the following system of equations.

$$3c_1 - 2c_2 = 0$$
$$-c_1 + 2c_2 = 0$$

Solving this system gives the following solution.

$$c_1 = 0, \quad c_2 = 0$$

The trivial solution is the only solution and so these two vectors are linearly independent.

(b) $u_1 = (12, -8)$ and $u_2 = (-9, 6)$.

Here is the vector equation we need to solve.

$$c_1(12, -8) + c_2(-9, 6) = 0$$

The system of equations that we need to solve

$$12c_1 - 9c_2 = 0$$

$$-8c_1 + 6c_2 = 0$$

and the solution to this system is

$$c_1 = \frac{3}{4}t \quad c_2 = t, \quad t \text{ is any real number}$$

We have got more than the trivial solution and so these vectors are linearly dependent.

(c) $u_1 = (1, 0, 0)$, $u_2 = (0, 1, 0)$ and $u_3 = (0, 0, 1)$.

We now have three vectors out of R^3. Here is the vector equation for this part.

$$c_1(1, 0, 0) + c_2(0, 1, 0) + c_3(0, 0, 1) = 0$$

The system of equations to solve for this part is

$$c_1 = 0$$

$$c_2 = 0$$

$$c_3 = 0$$

It is clear that the only solution will be the trivial solution and so these vectors are linearly independent.

(d) $u_1 = (2, -2, 4)$, $u_2 = (3, -5, 4)$ and $u_3 = (0, 1, 1)$.

Here is the vector equation for this final part.

$$c_1(2, -2, 4) + c_2(3, -5, 4) + c_3(0, 1, 1) = 0$$

The system of equations is

$$2c_1 + 3c_2 = 0$$

$$-2c_1 - 5c_2 + c_3 = 0$$

$$4c_1 + 4c_2 + c_3 = 0$$

The solution to this system is

$$c_1 = -\frac{3}{4}t \quad \text{and} \quad c_2 = \frac{1}{2}t$$

$c_3 = t$, where t is any real number.

So these vectors are linearly dependent.

Example 2: Determine whether the following sets of vectors are linearly independent or linearly dependent.

(a) $u_1 = (1, -3)$, $u_2 = (-2, 2)$ and $u_3 = (4, -1)$.

(b) $u_1 = (-2, 1)$, $u_2 = (-1, -3)$ and $u_3 = (4, -2)$.

(c) $u_1 = (1, 1, -1, 2)$, $u_2 = (2, -2, 0, 2)$ and $u_3 = (2, -8, 3, -1)$.

(d) $u_1 = (1, -2, 3, -4)$, $u_2 = (-1, 3, 4, 2)$ and $u_3 = (1, 1, -2, -2)$.

Solution:

(a) $u_1 = (1, -3)$, $u_2 = (-2, 2)$ and $u_3 = (4, -1)$.

Here is the vector equation we need to solve.

$$c_1(1, -3) + c_2(-2, 2) + c_3(4, -1) = 0$$
$$(c_1 - 2c_2 + 4c_3, -3c_1 + 2c_2 - c_3) = (0, 0)$$

This system of equations is

$$c_1 - 2c_2 + 4c_3 = 0$$
$$-3c_1 + 2c_2 - c_3 = 0$$

and this has the solution

$$c_1 = \frac{3}{2}t, \; c_2 = \frac{11}{4}t, \; c_3 = t, \text{ where } t \text{ is any real number.}$$

Therefore, these vectors are linearly dependent.

(b) $u_1 = (-2, 1)$, $u_2 = (-1, -3)$ and $u_3 = (4, -2)$.

Here is the vector equation

$$c_1(-2, 1) + c_2(-1, -3) + c_3(4, -2) = 0$$

The system of equations is

$$-2c_1 - c_2 + 4c_3 = 0$$
$$c_1 - 3c_2 - 2c_3 = 0$$

Here is the solution.

$c_1 = 2t$, $c_2 = 0$, $c_3 = t$, where t is any real number.

In this case one of the scalars is zero. There is nothing wrong with this as u_1 and u_3 are linearly dependent.

(c) $u_1 = (1, 1, -1, 2)$, $u_2 = (2, -2, 0, 2)$ and $u_3 = (2, -8, 3, -1)$.

Here is the vector equation for this part.

$$c_1(1, 1, -1, 2) + c_2(2, -2, 0, 2) + c_3(2, -8, 3, -1) = 0$$

The system of equations

$$c_1 + 2c_2 + 2c_3 = 0$$
$$c_1 - 2c_2 - 8c_3 = 0$$
$$-c_1 + 3c_3 = 0$$
$$2c_1 + 2c_2 - c_3 = 0$$

The solution to this system is

$$c_1 = 3t, \quad c_2 = -\frac{5}{2}t, \quad c_3 = t, \text{ where } t \text{ is any real number.}$$

So these three vectors are linearly dependent.

(d) $u_1 = (1, -2, 3, -4)$, $u_2 = (-1, 3, 4, 2)$ and $u_3 = (1, 1, -2, -2)$.

The vector equation

$$c_1(1, -2, 3, -4) + c_2(-1, 3, 4, 2) + c_3(1, 1, -2, -2) = 0$$

The system of equations is

$$c_1 - c_2 + c_3 = 0$$
$$-2c_1 + 3c_2 + c_3 = 0$$
$$3c_1 + 4c_2 - 2c_3 = 0$$
$$-4c_1 + 2c_2 - 2c_3 = 0$$

This system has only the trivial solution and so these three vectors are linearly independent.

Theorem 1: A finite set of vectors that contains the zero vector will be linearly dependent.

Proof: Let $S = \{0, u_1, u_2,..., u_n\}$ be any set of vectors that contains the zero vector as shown. We can then set up the following equation

$$1(0) + 0u_1 + 0u_2 + ... + 0u_n = 0$$

We have a non-trivial solution to this equation and so the set of vectors is linearly dependent.

Theorem 2: Suppose that $S = \{v_1, v_2,..., v_k\}$ is a set of vectors in R^n. If $k > n$, then the set of vectors is linearly dependent.

Example 3: Determine if the following sets of vectors are linearly independent or linearly dependent.

(a) $v_1 = \begin{bmatrix} 1 & 0 & 0 \\ 0 & 0 & 0 \end{bmatrix}, v_2 = \begin{bmatrix} 0 & 0 & 1 \\ 0 & 0 & 0 \end{bmatrix}$ and $v_3 = \begin{bmatrix} 0 & 0 & 0 \\ 0 & 1 & 0 \end{bmatrix}$

(b) $v_1 = \begin{bmatrix} 1 & 2 \\ 0 & -1 \end{bmatrix}$ and $v_2 = \begin{bmatrix} 4 & 1 \\ 0 & -3 \end{bmatrix}$

(c) $v_1 = \begin{bmatrix} 8 & -2 \\ 10 & 0 \end{bmatrix}$ and $v_2 = \begin{bmatrix} -12 & 3 \\ -15 & 0 \end{bmatrix}$

Solution:

(a) $v_1 = \begin{bmatrix} 1 & 0 & 0 \\ 0 & 0 & 0 \end{bmatrix}, v_2 = \begin{bmatrix} 0 & 0 & 1 \\ 0 & 0 & 0 \end{bmatrix}$ and $v_3 = \begin{bmatrix} 0 & 0 & 0 \\ 0 & 1 & 0 \end{bmatrix}$

The vector equation

$$c_1 v_1 + c_2 v_2 + c_3 v_3 = 0$$

$$c_1 \begin{bmatrix} 1 & 0 & 0 \\ 0 & 0 & 0 \end{bmatrix} + c_2 \begin{bmatrix} 0 & 0 & 1 \\ 0 & 0 & 0 \end{bmatrix} + c_3 \begin{bmatrix} 0 & 0 & 0 \\ 0 & 1 & 0 \end{bmatrix} = \begin{bmatrix} 0 & 0 & 0 \\ 0 & 0 & 0 \end{bmatrix}$$

$$\begin{bmatrix} c_1 & 0 & c_2 \\ 0 & c_3 & 0 \end{bmatrix} = \begin{bmatrix} 0 & 0 & 0 \\ 0 & 0 & 0 \end{bmatrix} \Rightarrow \begin{array}{l} c_1 = 0 \\ c_2 = 0 \\ c_3 = 0 \end{array}$$

As the solution is trivial,

$\therefore$ These vector are linearly independent.

(b) $v_1 = \begin{bmatrix} 1 & 2 \\ 0 & -1 \end{bmatrix}$ and $v_2 = \begin{bmatrix} 4 & 1 \\ 0 & -3 \end{bmatrix}$

Here is the vector equation

$$c_1 \begin{bmatrix} 1 & 2 \\ 0 & -1 \end{bmatrix} + c_2 \begin{bmatrix} 4 & 1 \\ 0 & -3 \end{bmatrix} = \begin{bmatrix} 0 & 0 \\ 0 & 0 \end{bmatrix}$$

The system of equations

$$c_1 + 4c_2 = 0$$
$$2c_1 + c_2 = 0$$
$$-c_1 - 3c_2 = 0$$

$\therefore$ The solution to the system is

$$c_1 = 0 \text{ and } c_2 = 0$$

So these vectors are linearly independent.

(c) $v_1 = \begin{bmatrix} 8 & -2 \\ 10 & 0 \end{bmatrix}$ and $v_2 = \begin{bmatrix} -12 & 3 \\ -15 & 0 \end{bmatrix}$

Here is the vector equation

$$c_1 \begin{bmatrix} 8 & -2 \\ 10 & 0 \end{bmatrix} + c_2 \begin{bmatrix} -12 & 3 \\ -15 & 0 \end{bmatrix} = \begin{bmatrix} 0 & 0 \\ 0 & 0 \end{bmatrix}$$

and the system of equations is

$$8c_1 - 12c_2 = 0$$
$$-2c_1 + 3c_2 = 0$$
$$10c_1 - 15c_2 = 0$$

The solution to this system is

$$c_1 = \frac{3}{2}t, \ c_2 = t, \text{ where } t \text{ is any real number.}$$

$\therefore$ It is linearly dependent.

4.5 BASIS AND DIMENSION

In this section, we are going to take a look at an important idea in the study of vector spaces.

Definition: Suppose $S = \{u_1, u_2,...,u_n\}$ is a set of vectors from the vector space U. Then S is called a basis (plural is bases) for U if both of the following conditions hold.

(a) Span $(S) = U$, i.e. S spans the vector space U.

(b) S is a linearly independent set of vectors.

Let us take a look at some examples.

Example 1: Determine if each of the sets of vectors will be a basis for R^3.

(a) $u_1 = (1, -1, 1)$, $u_2 = (0, 1, 2)$ and $u_3 = (3, 0, -1)$.

(b) $u_1 = (1, 0, 0)$, $u_2 = (0, 1, 0)$ and $u_3 = (0, 0, 1)$.

(c) $u_1 = (1, 1, 0)$, $u_2 = (-1, 0, 0)$.

(d) $u_1 = (1, -1, 1)$, $u_2 = (-1, 2, -2)$ and $u_3 = (-1, 4, -4)$.

Solution:

(a) $u_1 = (1, -1, 1)$, $u_2 = (0, 1, 2)$ and $u_3 = (3, 0, -1)$.

We need to determine the scalars c_1, c_2 and c_3, so that a general vector $u = (u_1, u_2, u_3)$ from R^3 can be expressed as a linear combination for these three vectors.

$$c_1(1, -1, 1) + c_2(0, 1, 2) + c_3 (3, 0, -1) = (u_1, u_2, u_3)$$

$$\begin{bmatrix} 1 & 0 & 3 \\ -1 & 1 & 0 \\ 1 & 2 & -1 \end{bmatrix} \begin{bmatrix} c_1 \\ c_2 \\ c_3 \end{bmatrix} = \begin{bmatrix} u_1 \\ u_2 \\ u_3 \end{bmatrix}$$

Verify that det $(A) = 0$ and so these three vectors do not span R^3. To determine this, we need to solve the following equation.

$$c_1(1, -1, 1) + c_2(0, 1, 2) + c_3(3, 0, -1) = 0 = (0, 0, 0)$$

If this system has only the trivial solution the vectors will be linearly independent and if it has solutions other than the trivial solution, then the vectors will be linearly dependent.

$$\begin{bmatrix} 1 & 0 & 3 \\ -1 & 1 & 0 \\ 1 & 2 & -1 \end{bmatrix} \begin{bmatrix} c_1 \\ c_2 \\ c_3 \end{bmatrix} = \begin{bmatrix} 0 \\ 0 \\ 0 \end{bmatrix}$$

So, here is the determinant of the coefficient matrix.

$$A = \begin{vmatrix} 1 & 0 & 3 \\ -1 & 1 & 0 \\ 1 & 2 & -1 \end{vmatrix} \Rightarrow \det(A) = -10 \neq 0$$

So, these vectors will form a basis for R^3.

(b) $u_1 = (1, 0, 0)$, $u_2 = (0, 1, 0)$ and $u_3 = (0, 0, 1)$.

Likewise, in Example 1(c) from the section on linear independence, we saw that these vectors are linearly independent.

(c) $u_1 = (1, 1, 0)$ and $u_2 = (-1, 0, 0)$

The method is similar to part (a) here because the coefficient matrix would not be square, two vectors will span R^3, then for each $u = (u_1, u_2, u_3)$ in R^3, there must be scalars c_1 and c_2 to satisfy the above equation.

Therefore, these two vectors do not span R^3 and hence cannot be a basis for R^3.

(d) $u_1 = (1, -1, 1)$, $u_2 = (-1, 2, -2)$ and $u_3 = (-1, 4, -4)$

The general equation is

$$c_1(1, -1, 1) + c_2(-1, 2, -2) + c_3(-1, 4, -4) = (u_1, u_2, u_3)$$

and the matrix form of this is

$$\begin{bmatrix} 1 & -1 & -1 \\ -1 & 2 & 4 \\ 1 & -2 & -4 \end{bmatrix} \begin{bmatrix} c_1 \\ c_2 \\ c_3 \end{bmatrix} = \begin{bmatrix} 0 \\ 0 \\ 0 \end{bmatrix}$$

Verify that $\det(A) = 0$ and so these three vectors do not span R^3 and are not linearly independent, either of which will mean that these three u vectors are not a basis for R^3.

$$e_1 = (1, 0, 0, ..., 0)$$
$$e_2 = (0, 1, 0, ..., 0), ..., \ e_n = (0, 0, 0, ..., 1)$$

will span R^n as we saw in the section on span and it is fairly simple to show that these vectors are linearly independent and so they form a basis for R^n. In some way this set of vectors is the simplest and so we call them the standard basis vectors for R^n.

We also have a set of standard basis vectors for a couple of the other vector spaces.

Example 2: The set $V_1 = \begin{bmatrix} 1 & 0 \\ 0 & 0 \end{bmatrix}$, $V_2 = \begin{bmatrix} 0 & 0 \\ 1 & 0 \end{bmatrix}$, $V_3 = \begin{bmatrix} 0 & 1 \\ 0 & 0 \end{bmatrix}$ and

$$V_4 = \begin{bmatrix} 0 & 0 \\ 0 & 1 \end{bmatrix}$$ is a basis for M_{22} and is usually called

the standard basis for M_{22}.

Set up the following equation

$$c_1 \begin{bmatrix} 1 & 0 \\ 0 & 0 \end{bmatrix} + c_2 \begin{bmatrix} 0 & 0 \\ 1 & 0 \end{bmatrix} + c_3 \begin{bmatrix} 0 & 1 \\ 0 & 0 \end{bmatrix} + c_4 \begin{bmatrix} 0 & 0 \\ 0 & 1 \end{bmatrix} = \begin{bmatrix} 0 & 0 \\ 0 & 0 \end{bmatrix}$$

$$\begin{bmatrix} c_1 & c_3 \\ c_2 & c_4 \end{bmatrix} = \begin{bmatrix} 0 & 0 \\ 0 & 0 \end{bmatrix}$$

4.6 CHANGE OF BASIS

In Example1 of the previous section, we saw that the vectors $u_1 = (1, -1, 1)$, $u_2 = (0, 1, 2)$ and $u_3 = (3, 0, -1)$ formed a basis for R^3. This means that every vector in R^3, for example, the vector $x = (10, 5, 0)$, can be written as a linear combination of these three vectors. Of course, this is not the only basis for R^3. There are many other bases for R^3, not the least of which is the standard basis for R^3

$$e_1 = (1, 0, 0), \quad e_2 = (0, 1, 0) \text{ and } e_3 = (0, 0, 1)$$

Definition 1: Suppose that $S = \{u_1, u_2,..., u_n\}$ is a basis for a vector space U. Since u is a vector in U, it can be expressed as a linear combination of the vectors from S as follows

$$u = c_1 u_1 + c_2 u_2 + ... + c_n u_n$$

The scalars $c_1, c_2,..., c_n$ are called the coordinates of u relative to the basis S. The coordinate vector of u relative to S is denoted by $(u)_s$ and defined to be the following vector in R^n

$$(u)_s = (c_1, c_2,..., c_n)$$

Example 1: Determine the coordinate vector of $x = (10, 5, 0)$ relative to the following bases.

(a) The standard basis vectors for R^3, $S = \{e_1, e_2, e_3\}$.
(b) The basis $A = \{u_1, u_2, u_3\}$, where $u_1 = (1, -1, 1)$, $u_2 = (0, 1, 2)$ and $u_3 = (3, 0, -1)$.

Solution:
Determine to write $x = (10, 5, 0)$ as a linear combination of the given basis vectors.

(a) The standard basis vectors for R^3, $S = \{e_1, e_2, e_3\}$.
In this case, the linear combination is

$$x = (10, 5, 0) = 10e_1 + 5e_2 + 0e_3$$

So the coordinate vector for x relative to the standard basis vectors for R^3 is

$$(x)_s = (10, 5, 0)$$

So, in the case of the standard basis vectors $(X)_s = (10, 5, 0) = x$
The coordinate vector relative to the standard basis vector is just the vector itself.

(b) The basis $A = \{u_1, u_2, u_3\}$, where $u_1 = (1, -1, 1)$, $u_2 = (0, 1, 2)$ and $u_3 = (3, 0, -1)$.

Vector equation $(10, 5, 0) = c_1(1, -1, 1) + c_2(0, 1, 2) + c_3(3, 0, 1)$ and need to determine the scalars c_1, c_2 and c_3. The following system of equations is

$$c_1 + 3c_3 = 10$$
$$-c_1 + c_2 = 5$$
$$c_1 + 2c_2 - c_3 = 0$$

The solution to this system is

$$c_1 = -2, \quad c_2 = 3, \quad c_3 = 4$$

The coordinate vector for x relative to A is

$$(x)_A = (-2, 3, 4)$$

Example 2: Determine the coordinate vector of $p = 4 - 2x + 3x^2$ relative to the following bases.

(a) The standard basis for P_2 $S = \{1, x, x^2\}$.

(b) The basis for P_2, $A = \{p_1, p_2, p_3\}$, where $p_1 = 2, p_2 = -4x$, and $p_3 = 5x^2 - 1$.

Solution:

(a) The standard basis for P_2 $S = \{1, x, x^2\}$.

So, we need to write p as a linear combination of the standard basis vectors in this case. So, the coordinate vector for p relative to the standard basis vector is

$$(p)_s = (4, -2, 3)$$

We can write down this vector as the set of vectors which is the standard basis vectors for P_2.

(b) The basis for P_2, $A = \{p_1, p_2, p_3\}$, where $p_1 = 2$, $p_2 = -4x$ and $p_3 = 5x^2 - 1$.

We will need to find scalars c_1, c_2 and c_3 for the following linear combination.

$$4 - 2x + 3x^2 = c_1 p_1 + c_2 p_2 + c_3 p_3 = c_1(2) + c_2(-4x) + c_3(5x^2 - 1)$$

This means solving the following system of equations

$$2c_1 - c_3 = 4$$
$$-4c_2 = -2$$
$$5c_3 = 3$$

This is not a difficult system to solve. Here is the solution

$$c_1 = \frac{23}{10} \qquad c_2 = \frac{1}{2} \qquad c_3 = \frac{3}{5}$$

The coordinate vector for p relative to this basis is then,

$$(p)_A = \left[\frac{23}{10}, \frac{1}{2}, \frac{3}{5} \right]$$

Example 3: Determine the coordinate vector of $\begin{bmatrix} -1 & 0 \\ 1 & -4 \end{bmatrix}$ relative to the following bases.

(a) The standard basis of M_{22}, $S = \left\{ \begin{bmatrix} 1 & 0 \\ 0 & 0 \end{bmatrix}, \begin{bmatrix} 0 & 0 \\ 1 & 0 \end{bmatrix}, \begin{bmatrix} 0 & 1 \\ 0 & 0 \end{bmatrix}, \begin{bmatrix} 0 & 0 \\ 0 & 1 \end{bmatrix} \right\}$

(b) The basis for M_{22}, $A = \{u_1, u_2, u_3, u_4\}$, where

$$v_1 = \begin{bmatrix} 1 & 0 \\ 0 & 0 \end{bmatrix}, \ v_2 = \begin{bmatrix} 2 & 0 \\ -1 & 0 \end{bmatrix}, \ v_3 = \begin{bmatrix} 0 & 1 \\ 0 & 1 \end{bmatrix} \text{ and } v_4 = \begin{bmatrix} -3 & 0 \\ 0 & 2 \end{bmatrix}.$$

Solution:

(a) The standard basis of M_{22}, $S = \left\{ \begin{bmatrix} 1 & 0 \\ 0 & 0 \end{bmatrix}, \begin{bmatrix} 0 & 0 \\ 1 & 0 \end{bmatrix}, \begin{bmatrix} 0 & 1 \\ 0 & 0 \end{bmatrix}, \begin{bmatrix} 0 & 0 \\ 0 & 1 \end{bmatrix} \right\}.$

$$\begin{bmatrix} -1 & 0 \\ 1 & -4 \end{bmatrix} = (-1) \begin{bmatrix} 1 & 0 \\ 0 & 0 \end{bmatrix} + (1) \begin{bmatrix} 0 & 0 \\ 1 & 0 \end{bmatrix} + (0) \begin{bmatrix} 0 & 1 \\ 0 & 0 \end{bmatrix} + (-4) \begin{bmatrix} 0 & 0 \\ 0 & 1 \end{bmatrix}$$

The coordinate vector for u relative to the standard basis is

$$(u)_s = (-1, 1, 0, -4)$$

(b) The basis for M_{22}, $A = \{u_1, u_2, u_3, u_4\}$, where

$$v_1 = \begin{bmatrix} 1 & 0 \\ 0 & 0 \end{bmatrix}, v_2 = \begin{bmatrix} 2 & 0 \\ -1 & 0 \end{bmatrix}, v_3 = \begin{bmatrix} 0 & 1 \\ 0 & 1 \end{bmatrix} \text{ and } v_4 = \begin{bmatrix} -3 & 0 \\ 0 & 2 \end{bmatrix}$$

To find scalars c_1, c_2, c_3, c_4 for the following linear combination

$$\begin{bmatrix} -1 & 0 \\ 1 & -4 \end{bmatrix} = c_1 \begin{bmatrix} 1 & 0 \\ 0 & 0 \end{bmatrix} + c_2 \begin{bmatrix} 2 & 0 \\ -1 & 0 \end{bmatrix} + c_3 \begin{bmatrix} 0 & 1 \\ 0 & 1 \end{bmatrix} + c_4 \begin{bmatrix} -3 & 0 \\ 0 & 2 \end{bmatrix}$$

Adding the matrices on the right into a single matrix and setting components equal yields the following system of equations

$$c_1 + 2c_2 - 3c_4 = -1$$
$$-c_2 = 1$$
$$-c_3 = 0$$
$$c_3 + 2c_4 = -4$$

Here is the solution.

$$c_1 = -5, \quad c_2 = -1, \quad c_3 = 0, \quad c_4 = -2$$

The coordinate vector for u relative to this basis is

$$(u)_A = (-5, -1, 0, -2)$$

Example 4: The vectors $u_1 = (1, -1, 1)$, $u_2 = (0, 1, 2)$ and $u_3 = (3, 0, -1)$ form a basis for R^3. Let $A = \{u_1, u_2, u_3\}$ and $B = \{u_2, u_3, u_1\}$ be different orderings of these vectors and determine the vector in R^3 that has the following coordinate vectors.

(a) $(x)_A = (3, -1, 8)$ (b) $(x)_B = (3, -1, 8)$

Solution

(a) Here $x = 3(1, -1, 1) + (-1)(0, 1, 2) + (8)(3, 0, -1) = (27, -4, -7)$
(b) $x = 3(0, 1, 2) + (-1)(3, 0, -1) + (8)(1, -1, 1) = (5, -5, 15)$

So, clearly rearranging the order of the vectors in our basis.

Definition 2: Suppose that U is a n-dimensional vector space and further suppose that $B = \{u_1, u_2,..., u_n\}$ and $C = \{w_1, w_2,...,w_n\}$ are two bases for U. The transition matrix from C to B is defined to be the ith column of p is the coordinate matrix of w_1 relative to B.

The coordinate matrix of a vector u in U, relative to B, is then related to the coordinate matrix of u relative to C by the following equation.

$$[u]_B = P[u]_c$$

We should probably take a look at an example at this point.

Example 5: Consider the standard basis for R^3, $B = \{e_1, e_2, e_3\}$ and the basis $C = \{u_1, u_2, u_3\}$, where $u_1 = (1, -1, 1)$, $u_2 = (0, 1, 2)$ and $u_3 = (3, 0, -1)$.

(a) Find the transition matrix from C to B.
(b) Find the transition matrix from B to C.
(c) Use the result of part (a) to compute $[u]_B$ given $(u)_C = (-2, 3, 4)$.
(d) Use the result of part (a) to computer $[u]_B$ given $(u)_C = (9, -1, -8)$.
(e) Use the result of part (b) to compute $[u]_C$ given $(u)_B = (10, 5, 0)$.
(f) Use the result of part (b) to compute $[u]_C$ given $(u)_B = (-6, 7, 2)$.

Solution:

(a) Find the transition matrix from C to B.
   When the standard basis vectors for the vector space computing the transition matrix. Recall that the columns of P are just the coordinate matrices of the vectors in C relative to B. However, when B is the standard basis vectors, the coordinate matrix in this case is

$$P = \begin{bmatrix} 1 & 0 & 3 \\ -1 & 1 & 0 \\ 1 & 2 & -1 \end{bmatrix}$$

(b) Find the transition matrix from B to C.

First, the transition matrix will be the same as the transition matrix from part (a). To find this transition matrix, we need the coordinate matrices of the standard basis vectors relative to C. This means that we need to write each of the standard basis vectors as linear combinations of the basis vectors from C. Verify the following linear combinations.

$$e_1 = \frac{1}{10}v_1 + \frac{1}{10}v_2 + \frac{3}{10}v_3$$

$$e_2 = -\frac{3}{5}v_1 + \frac{2}{5}v_2 + \frac{1}{5}v_3$$

$$e_3 = \frac{3}{10}v_1 + \frac{3}{10}v_2 - \frac{1}{10}v_3$$

This is coordinate matrices.

(c) Use the result of part that we converted to get $[u]_B$ given $(u)_C = (-2, 3, 4)$.

$$[u]_B = \begin{bmatrix} 1 & 0 & 3 \\ -1 & 1 & 0 \\ 1 & 2 & -1 \end{bmatrix} \begin{bmatrix} -2 \\ 3 \\ 4 \end{bmatrix} = \begin{bmatrix} 10 \\ 5 \\ 0 \end{bmatrix}$$

We got the coordinate matrix for the point that we converted to get $(u)_C = (-2, 3, 4)$ from Example 1.

(d) Use the result of part (a) to compute $[u]_B$ given $(u)_C = (9, -1, -8)$.

The matrix multiplication is

$$[u]_B = \begin{bmatrix} 1 & 0 & 3 \\ -1 & 1 & 0 \\ 1 & 2 & -1 \end{bmatrix} \begin{bmatrix} 9 \\ -1 \\ -8 \end{bmatrix} = \begin{bmatrix} -15 \\ -10 \\ 15 \end{bmatrix}$$

$$u = (-15, -10, 15)$$

(e) Use the result of part (b) to compute $[u]_C$ given $[u]_C = (10, 5, 0)$.

Here is the matrix multiplication

$$[u]_c = \begin{bmatrix} \dfrac{1}{10} & -\dfrac{3}{5} & \dfrac{3}{10} \\ \dfrac{1}{10} & \dfrac{2}{5} & \dfrac{3}{10} \\ \dfrac{3}{10} & \dfrac{1}{5} & -\dfrac{1}{10} \end{bmatrix} \begin{bmatrix} 10 \\ 5 \\ 0 \end{bmatrix} = \begin{bmatrix} -2 \\ 3 \\ 4 \end{bmatrix}$$

(f) Use the result of part (b) to compute $\left[u\right]_c$ given $(u)_B = (-6,7,2)$.

Here is the matrix multiplication.

$$\left[u\right]_c = \begin{bmatrix} \dfrac{1}{10} & -\dfrac{3}{5} & \dfrac{3}{10} \\ \dfrac{1}{10} & \dfrac{2}{5} & \dfrac{3}{10} \\ \dfrac{3}{10} & \dfrac{1}{5} & -\dfrac{1}{10} \end{bmatrix} \begin{bmatrix} -6 \\ 7 \\ 2 \end{bmatrix} = \begin{bmatrix} -\dfrac{21}{5} \\ \dfrac{14}{5} \\ -\dfrac{3}{5} \end{bmatrix}$$

$\left[u\right]_c = \left(-\dfrac{21}{5}, \dfrac{14}{5}, -\dfrac{3}{5}\right)$. Also B is the standard basis vectors. We know that the vector from that we are starting with (–6, 7, 2).

The coordinate matrix/vector that we just found is the vector as a linear combination of vectors from the basis C gives

$$(-6, 7, 2) = -\frac{21}{5}v_1 + \frac{14}{5}v_2 - \frac{3}{5}v_3$$

Example 6: Consider the standard basis for P_2, $B = \{1, x, x^2\}$ and the basis $C = \{p_1, p_2, p_3\}$,

where $p_1 = 2$, $p_2 = -4x$ and $p_3 = 5x^2 - 1$.

(a) Find the transition matrix from C to B

(b) Determine the polynomial that has the coordinate vector

$$(p)_c = (-4, 3, 11)$$

Solution:

(a) Find the transition matrix from C to B

Now, since B is the standard basis vectors, the transition matrix is given by

$$P = \begin{bmatrix} 2 & 0 & -1 \\ 0 & -4 & 0 \\ 0 & 0 & 5 \end{bmatrix}$$

Each column of P will be the coefficients of the vectors from C, since those will also be the coordinates of each of those vectors relative to the standard basis vectors. The first row will be constant terms from each basis vector, the second row will be the coefficient of x^2 from each basis vector.

(b) Determine the polynomial that coordinate vector

$$(p)_c = (-4, 3, 11)$$

$$[p]_B = P[p]_C$$

$$= \begin{bmatrix} 2 & 0 & -1 \\ 0 & -4 & 0 \\ 0 & 0 & 5 \end{bmatrix} \begin{bmatrix} -4 \\ 3 \\ 11 \end{bmatrix} = \begin{bmatrix} -19 \\ -12 \\ 55 \end{bmatrix}$$

So the coordinate vector for u relative to the standard basis vectors is

$$(P)_B = (-19, -12, 55)$$

Therefore, the polynomial is

$$P(x) = -19 - 12x + 55x^2$$

Note that, as mentioned above, we can also do this problem as follows

$$P(x) = -4p_1 + 3p_2 + 11p_3 = -4(2) + 3(-4x) + 11(5x^2 - 1) = -19 - 12x + 55x^2$$

Example 7: Consider the standard basis for M_{22}

$$B = \left\{ \begin{bmatrix} 1 & 0 \\ 0 & 0 \end{bmatrix}, \begin{bmatrix} 0 & 0 \\ 1 & 0 \end{bmatrix}, \begin{bmatrix} 0 & 1 \\ 0 & 0 \end{bmatrix}, \begin{bmatrix} 0 & 0 \\ 0 & 1 \end{bmatrix} \right\} \text{ and the basis } C = \{u_1, u_2, u_3, u_4,\}$$

where $u_1 = \begin{bmatrix} 1 & 0 \\ 0 & 0 \end{bmatrix}, u_2 = \begin{bmatrix} 2 & 0 \\ -1 & 0 \end{bmatrix}, u_3 = \begin{bmatrix} 0 & 1 \\ 0 & 1 \end{bmatrix}$ and $u_4 = \begin{bmatrix} -3 & 0 \\ 0 & 2 \end{bmatrix}$

(a) Find the transition matrix from C to B.

(b) Determine the matrix that has the coordinate vector $(u)_C = (-8, 3, 5, -2)$.

Solution:

(a) Find the transition matrix from C to B.

Now, B is the standard basis vectors to find a linear combination of the standard basis vectors.

$$\begin{bmatrix} -3 & 0 \\ 0 & 2 \end{bmatrix} = (-3) \begin{bmatrix} 1 & 0 \\ 0 & 0 \end{bmatrix} + (0) \begin{bmatrix} 0 & 0 \\ 1 & 0 \end{bmatrix} + (0) \begin{bmatrix} 0 & 1 \\ 0 & 0 \end{bmatrix} + (2) \begin{bmatrix} 0 & 0 \\ 0 & 1 \end{bmatrix}$$

So, the coordinate matrix for u_4 relative to B and hence the fourth column of P is

$$[u_4]_B = \begin{bmatrix} -3 \\ 0 \\ 0 \\ 2 \end{bmatrix}$$

Here is the transition matrix for this problem.

$$P = \begin{bmatrix} 1 & 2 & 0 & -3 \\ 0 & -1 & 0 & 0 \\ 0 & 0 & 1 & 0 \\ 0 & 0 & 1 & 2 \end{bmatrix}$$

(b) Determine the matrix that has the coordinate vector$(u)_C = (-8, 3, 5, -2)$. So, the coordinate vector is for the non-standard basis vectors. As with the previous problem we could just write down in linear combination of the vectors from C.

$$[v]_B = \begin{bmatrix} 1 & 2 & 0 & -3 \\ 0 & -1 & 0 & 0 \\ 0 & 0 & 1 & 0 \\ 0 & 0 & 1 & 2 \end{bmatrix}\begin{bmatrix} -8 \\ 3 \\ 5 \\ -2 \end{bmatrix} = \begin{bmatrix} 4 \\ -3 \\ 5 \\ 1 \end{bmatrix}$$

The coordinate for u relative to the standard basis we can write down u.

$$u = \begin{bmatrix} 4 & 5 \\ -3 & 1 \end{bmatrix}$$

Example 8: Consider the two bases for R^2, $B = \{(1, -1), (0, 6)\}$ and $C = \{(2,1), (-1, 4)\}$.

(a) Find the transition matrix from C to B.

(b) Find the transition matrix from B to C.

Solution:

(a) Find the transition matrix from C to B.

The vectors from C as linear combinations of the vectors from B. Here, are those linear combinations

$$(2,1) = 2(1,-1) + \frac{1}{2}(0,6)$$

$$(-1,4) = -(1,1) + \frac{1}{2}(0,6)$$

The two coordinate matrices are

$$[(2,1)]_B = \begin{bmatrix} 2 \\ \frac{1}{2} \end{bmatrix} \qquad [(-1,4)]_B = \begin{bmatrix} -1 \\ \frac{1}{2} \end{bmatrix}$$

and the transition matrix is

$$P = \begin{bmatrix} 2 & -1 \\ \dfrac{1}{2} & \dfrac{1}{2} \end{bmatrix}$$

(b) Find the transition matrix from B to C.

$$(1,-1) = \frac{1}{3}(2,1) - \frac{1}{3}(-1,4)$$

$$(0,6) = -\frac{2}{3}(2,1) + \frac{4}{3}(-1,4)$$

The coordinate matrices are

$$[(1,-1)]_C = \begin{bmatrix} \dfrac{1}{3} \\ \dfrac{-1}{3} \end{bmatrix} \quad [(0,6)]_C = \begin{bmatrix} \dfrac{2}{3} \\ \dfrac{4}{3} \end{bmatrix}$$

The transition matrix is

$$P' = \begin{bmatrix} \dfrac{1}{3} & \dfrac{2}{3} \\ \dfrac{-1}{3} & \dfrac{4}{3} \end{bmatrix}$$

4.7 FUNDAMENTAL SUBSPACES

Given an $n \times m$ matrix

$$A = \begin{bmatrix} a_{11} & a_{12} & \cdots & a_{1m} \\ a_{21} & a_{22} & \cdots & a_{2m} \\ \vdots & \vdots & & \vdots \\ a_{n1} & a_{n2} & \cdots & a_{nm} \end{bmatrix}$$

The **row vectors** are the vectors in R^m formed out of the rows of A. The column vectors (again we called them column matrices at the time) are the vectors in R^n that are formed out of the columns of A.

Example 1: Write down the row vectors and column vectors for

$$A = \begin{bmatrix} -1 & 5 \\ 0 & -4 \\ 9 & 2 \\ 3 & -7 \end{bmatrix}$$

Solution:

The row vectors are $r_1 = [-1\ 5]$ $r_2 = [0,\ 4]$

$$r_3 = [9\ 2] \quad r_4 = [3\ -7]$$

The column vectors are

$$c_1 = \begin{bmatrix} -1 \\ 0 \\ 9 \\ 3 \end{bmatrix} \quad c_2 = \begin{bmatrix} 5 \\ -4 \\ 2 \\ -7 \end{bmatrix}$$

Definition 1: Suppose that A is an $n \times m$ matrix.

(a) The subspace of R^m that is spanned by the row vectors of A is called the **row space** of A.

(b) The subspace of R^n that is spanned by the column vectors of A is called the **column space** of A.

(c) The set of all x in R^m such that $Ax = 0$ (which is a subspace of R^m by Theorem 2 from the subspaces section) is called the **null space** of A.

Definition 2: The dimension of the null space of A is called the nullity of A and is denoted by nullity(A).

Example 2: Determine a basis for the null space of the following matrix.

$$A = \begin{bmatrix} 2 & -4 & 1 & 2 & -2 & -3 \\ -1 & 2 & 0 & 0 & 1 & -1 \\ 10 & -4 & -2 & 4 & -2 & 4 \end{bmatrix}$$

Solution:

So, to find the null space we need to solve the following system of equations

$$2x_1 - 4x_2 + x_3 + 2x_4 - 2x_5 - 3x_6 = 0$$

$$-x_1 + 2x_2 + x_5 - x_6 = 0$$

$$10x_1 - 4x_2 - 2x_3 + 4x_4 - 2x_5 + 4x_6 = 0$$

Verify that the solution is given by

$$x_1 = -t + r \quad x_2 = -\frac{1}{2}t - \frac{1}{2}s + r \quad x_3 = -2t + 5r$$

$$x_4 = t$$

$$x_5 = s$$

$x_6 = r$, where t, s, r are any real numbers.

In matrix form the solution can be written as

$$x = \begin{bmatrix} -t+r \\ -\dfrac{1}{2}t - \dfrac{1}{2}s + r \\ -2t + 5r \\ t \\ s \\ r \end{bmatrix} = t \begin{bmatrix} -1 \\ -\dfrac{1}{2} \\ -2 \\ 1 \\ 0 \\ 0 \end{bmatrix} + s \begin{bmatrix} 0 \\ -\dfrac{1}{2} \\ 0 \\ 0 \\ 1 \\ 0 \end{bmatrix} + r \begin{bmatrix} 1 \\ 1 \\ 5 \\ 0 \\ 0 \\ 1 \end{bmatrix}$$

So, the solution can be written as a linear combination of the three linearly independent vectors.

$$x_1 = \begin{bmatrix} -1 \\ -\dfrac{1}{2} \\ -2 \\ 1 \\ 0 \\ 0 \end{bmatrix} \qquad x_2 = \begin{bmatrix} 0 \\ -\dfrac{1}{2} \\ 0 \\ 0 \\ 1 \\ 0 \end{bmatrix} \qquad x_3 = \begin{bmatrix} 1 \\ 1 \\ 5 \\ 0 \\ 0 \\ 1 \end{bmatrix}$$

nullity $(A) = 3$

Theorem 1: Suppose that the matrix U is in the row-echelon form. The row vectors containing leading 1's (so the non-zero row vectors) will form a basis for the row space of U. The column vectors that contain the leading 1's from the row vectors will form a basis for the column space of U.

Example 3: Find the basis for the row and column space of the following matrix.

$$U = \begin{bmatrix} 1 & 5 & -2 & 3 & 5 \\ 0 & 0 & 1 & -1 & 0 \\ 0 & 0 & 0 & 0 & 1 \\ 0 & 0 & 0 & 0 & 0 \end{bmatrix}$$

Solution:

The basis for the row space is simply all the row vectors that contain a leading 1. So, for this matrix the basis for the row space is

$$r_1 = [1\ 5\ -2\ 3\ 5] \qquad r_2 = [0\ 0\ 1\ -1\ 0]$$

$$r_3 = [0\ 0\ 0\ 0\ 1]$$

We can also see that the dimension of the row space will be 3.

The basis for the column space will be the columns that contain leading 1's and so for this matrix the basis for the column space will be

$$c_1 = \begin{bmatrix} 1 \\ 0 \\ 0 \\ 0 \end{bmatrix} \qquad c_2 = \begin{bmatrix} -2 \\ 1 \\ 0 \\ 0 \end{bmatrix} \qquad c_3 = \begin{bmatrix} 5 \\ 0 \\ 1 \\ 0 \end{bmatrix}$$

Theorem 2: Suppose that A is matrix and U is a matrix in row-echelon form that has been obtained by performing row operations on A. Then the row space of A and the row space of U are the same space.

Example 4: Find a basis for the null space, row space and column space of the following matrix. Determine the rank and nullity of the matrix.

$$A = \begin{bmatrix} -1 & 2 & -1 & 5 & 6 \\ 4 & -4 & -4 & -12 & -8 \\ 2 & 0 & -6 & -2 & 4 \\ -3 & 1 & 7 & -2 & 12 \end{bmatrix}$$

Solution:

Solve the following system of equations

$$-x_1 + 2x_2 - x_3 + 5x_4 + 6x_5 = 0$$
$$4x_1 - 4x_2 - 4x_3 - 12x_4 - 8x_5 = 0$$
$$2x_1 - 6x_3 - 2x_4 + 4x_5 = 0$$
$$-3x_1 + x_2 + 7x_3 - 2x_4 + 12x_5 = 0$$

You should verify that the solution is

$$x_1 = 3t, \quad x_2 = 2t - 8s, \quad x_3 = t, \quad x_4 = 2s, \quad x_5 = s$$

where s and t are any real numbers.

The null space is then given by

$$x = \begin{bmatrix} 3t \\ 2t - 8s \\ t \\ 2s \\ s \end{bmatrix} = t \begin{bmatrix} 3 \\ 2 \\ 1 \\ 0 \\ 0 \end{bmatrix} + s \begin{bmatrix} 0 \\ -8 \\ 0 \\ 2 \\ 1 \end{bmatrix}$$

and so we can see that a basis for the null space is

$$x_1 = \begin{bmatrix} 3 \\ 2 \\ 1 \\ 0 \\ 0 \end{bmatrix} \quad x_2 = \begin{bmatrix} 0 \\ -8 \\ 0 \\ 2 \\ 1 \end{bmatrix}$$

Therefore, we now know that nullity(A) = 2. At this point we know the rank of A. According to nullity theorem, rank (A) = columns–nullity (A) = 5–2 = 3. We find a basis for the row space and the column space. We now know that each should contain three vectors.

We will need to reduce A to row-echelon form first.

$$U = \begin{bmatrix} 1 & -2 & 1 & -5 & -6 \\ 0 & 1 & -2 & 2 & 4 \\ 0 & 0 & 0 & 1 & -2 \\ 0 & 0 & 0 & 0 & 0 \end{bmatrix}$$

The rows containing leading 1's will form a basis for the row space of A and so this basis is

$$r_1 = [1 \ -2 \ 1 \ -5 \ -6] \quad r_2 = [0 \ 1 \ -2 \ 2 \ 4] \quad r_3 = [0 \ 0 \ 0 \ 1 \ -2]$$

Next, the first, second and fourth columns of U contain leading 1's and so will form a basis for the column space of U and that the first, second and fourth columns of A will form a basis for the column space of A. Here is that basis.

$$c_1 = \begin{bmatrix} -1 \\ 4 \\ 2 \\ -3 \end{bmatrix} \quad c_2 = \begin{bmatrix} 2 \\ -4 \\ 0 \\ 1 \end{bmatrix} \quad c_4 = \begin{bmatrix} 5 \\ -12 \\ -2 \\ -2 \end{bmatrix}$$

Note that the dimension of each of these is 3 as we noted above.

4.8 FIELDS

Definition: Let $(F, +, .)$ be a field. The elements of F are called scalars. Let V be a non-empty set whose elements are called vectors, then V is a vector space over the field F if

1. A rule (or operation), called vector addition which associates with each pair of vectors α, β in V, a vector $(\alpha + \beta)$ in V called the sum of α and β in such a way that
   (i) Addition is commutative, i.e. $\alpha + \beta = \beta + \alpha \quad \forall \alpha, \beta \in V$.
   (ii) Addition is associative, i.e. $\alpha + (\beta + \gamma) = (\alpha + \beta) + \gamma \quad \forall \alpha, \beta, \gamma \in V$.

(iii) There is an element or a unique vector 0 in V called zero vector such that $\alpha + 0 = \alpha, \; \forall \; \alpha \in V$.

(iv) To every vector $\alpha \in V$, there is a unique vector $-\alpha$ in V such that $\alpha + (-\alpha) = 0$.

2. A rule (or operation), called scalar multiplication which associates with each scalar c in F and a vector α in V, a vector $c\alpha$ in V called the product of c and α in such a way that

(a) $1\alpha = \alpha$ for every α in V

(b) $(c_1 c_2) \alpha = c_1 (c_2 \alpha), \; \forall \; c_1, c_2 \in F$ and $\alpha \in V$

(c) $c_1(\alpha + \beta) = c\alpha + c\beta, \; \forall \; \alpha, \beta \in V$ and $c \in F$

(d) $(c_1 + c_2)\alpha = c_1\alpha + c_2\alpha, \; \forall \; c_1, c_2 \in F$ and $\alpha \in V$

Example 1: The n-tuple space, F^n or $V_n(F)$ is a vector space over the field F,

i.e. let V be the set of all n-tuples.

With $\alpha = (x_1, x_2,..., x_n)$ of scalars x_i in F and $\beta = (y_1, y_2,..., y_n)$ with y_i in F, the sum of α and β is defined by

$$\alpha + \beta = (x_1 + y_1, x_2 + y_2,..., x_n + y_n)$$

The product of a scalar c and vector α is defined by

$$c\alpha = (cx_1, cx_2,...,cx_n)$$

Example 2: The space of $m \times n$ matrices, $F^{m \times n}$. Let $F^{m \times n}$ be the set of all $m \times n$ matrices over the field F. Then

the sum of two matrices A and B in $F^{m \times n}$ is defined by

$$(A + B)_{ij} = A_{ij} + B_{ij}$$

The product of a scalar c and the matrix A is defined by $(cA)_{ij} = cA_{ij}$

Example 3: The space of functions from a set to a field.

Let F be any field and S be any non-empty set. Let V be the set of all functions from the set S into F. The sum of two vectors f and g in V is the vector $f + g$,

i.e. the function from S into F defined by

$$(f + g) \, S = f(S) + g(S)$$

The product of the scalar c and the function f is a function and it is defined by

$$(cf)S = cf(S)$$

Example 4: The space of polynomial functions over a field F. Let F be a field and V be the set of all functions f

$$\therefore \qquad f(x) = c_0 + c_1 x + ... + c_n x^n$$

where $c_0, c_1, c_2,...,c_n$ are fixed scalars in F.

A function of this type is called a polynomial function on F.

Example 5:

If F is a field, verify that $F^n - n$ tuple space is a vector space over the field F.

Solution: Let F be a field.

An ordered set $A = (a_1, a_2,...,a_n)$ of n-elements of F is called an n-tuple over F.

Let $V_n(F) = V = \{(a_1, a_2,...,a_n): a_1, a_2,...,a_n \in F\}$

[Now we shall give a vector space structure to V over the field F. For this we define equality of two n-tuples, addition of two n-tuples and multiplication of n-tuples by a scalar as follows]

Two elements $a = (a_1, a_2,...,a_n)$ and $b = (b_1, b_2,...,b_n)$ of V are said to be equal

iff $a_i = b_i$ for each $i = 1, 2,...,n$

i.e. $a_1 = b_1, a_2 = b_2, a_3 = b_3,...,a_n = b_n$

Define addition and Scalar multiplication as below:

1. $\alpha + \beta = (a_1 + b_1, a_2 + b_2,...,a_n + b_n)$
   $\forall \, \alpha = (a_1,...,a_m), \beta = (b_1,...,b_n) \in V$
   Since $a_1 + b_1, a_2 + b_2,...,a_n + b_n$ are all elements of F
   $\Rightarrow a + b \in V$
   $\Rightarrow V$ is closed w.r.t addition of n-tuples
2. We define $a\alpha = (aa_1 \, aa_2,...,aa_n) \, \forall \, a \in F, \alpha = (a_1, a_2,..., a_n) \in V$
   Since $aa_1, aa_2,..., aa_n$ are all elements of F
   $\therefore \, a\alpha \in V$ and thus V is closed w.r.t scalar multiplication.
   $\Rightarrow$ Now we shall see that V is a vector space for these two compositions or operations.

Associativity of addition in V:

We have $\alpha = (a_1, a_2,...,a_n), \beta = (b_1, b_2,...,b_n), \gamma = (c_1, c_2,...,c_n)$

$\therefore \, \alpha + (\beta + \gamma) = (\alpha + \beta) + \gamma$

$(a_1, a_2,...,a_n) + [(b_1, b_2,...,b_n) + (c_1, c_2,...,c_n)]$

$= (a_1, a_2,...,a_n) + [(b_1 + c_1), (b_2 + c_2),...,(b_n + c_n)]$

$= [a_1 + (b_1 + c_1), a_2 + (b_2 + c_2),...,a_n + (b_n + c_n)]$

$= ([a_1 + b_1] + c_1, [a_2 + b_2] + c_2,...,[a_n + b_n] + c_n)$

$= (a_1 + b_1, a_2 + b_2,...,a_n + b_n) + (c_1 + c_2,...,c_n)$

$= [(a_1, a_2,...,a_n) + (b_1 + b_2 +...+ b_n)] + (c_1, c_2 + ... + c_n)$

$= [\alpha + \beta] + \gamma$

Commutativity in addition in V:

$\alpha + \beta = \beta + \alpha$

$\alpha + \beta = (a_1, a_2,...,a_n) + (b_1, b_2,...,b_n) = (a_1 + b_1, a_2 + b_2,...,a_n + b_n)$

$$= b_1 + a_1, b_2 + a_2,..., b_n + a_n$$
$$= (b_1,...,b_n) + (a_1,...,a_n)$$
$$= \beta + \alpha$$

Existence of additive identity in V:

Let $(0, 0,...,0) \in V$. Also if $(a_1, a_2,...,a_n) \in V$, then
$$(a_1, a_2,..., a_n) + (0, 0, 0,...,0) = (a_1 + 0, a_2 + 0,...,a_n + 0)$$
$$= (a_1, a_2,...,a_n)$$
$$\Rightarrow (0, 0,...,0) \text{ is additive identity.}$$

Existence of additive inverse of each element of V:

If $(a_1, a_2,...,a_n) \in V$, then $(-a_1, -a_2,..., -a_n) \in V$
$$\text{Thus } (-a_1, -a_2,..., -a_n) + (a_1 + a_2,...,a_n)$$
$$= (-a_1 + a_1, -a_2 + a_2,..., -a_n + a_n)$$
$$= (0, 0, 0,...,0)$$
$$\therefore (-a_1, -a_2,..., -a_n) \text{ is additive inverse of } (a_1,a_2,...,a_n).$$

Thus V is an abelian group w.r.t addition.

Further we observe that

1. If $a \in F$ and $\alpha = (a_1,a_2,...,a_n)$, $\beta = (b_1,b_2,...,b_n) \in V$, then
$$a[\alpha + \beta] = a[a_1 + b_1, a_2 + b_2,...,a_n + b_n]$$
$$= [aa_1 + ab_1, aa_2 + ab_2,...,aa_n + ab_n]$$
$$= (aa_1, aa_2,...,aa_n) + (ab_1, ab_2,...,ab_n)$$
$$= a(a_1, a_2,...,a_n) + a(b_1, b_2,...,b_n)$$
$$= a\alpha + a\beta$$
$$a(\alpha + \beta) = a\alpha + a\beta$$

2. Let $a, b \in F$ and $\alpha = (a_1, a_2,...,a_n) \in V$, then
$$(a + b)\alpha = [(a + b)a_1, (a + b)a_2,...,(a + b)a_n]$$
$$= [aa_1 + ba_1, aa_2 + ba_2,...,aa_n + ba_n]$$
$$= (aa_1, aa_2,...,aa_n) + (ba_1, ba_2,...,ba_n)$$
$$= a(a_1, a_2,...,a_n) + b(a_1, a_2,...,a_n)$$
$$= a\alpha + b\alpha$$
$$(a + b)\alpha = a\alpha + b\alpha$$

3. Let $a, b \in F$ and $\alpha = (a_1, a_2,...,a_n) \in V$, then
$$(ab)\alpha = [(ab)a_1, (ab)a_2,...,(ab)a_n]$$
$$= [a(ba_1), a(ba_2),...,a(ba_n)]$$
$$= a[ba_1, ba_2,...,ba_n]$$
$$= a[b(a_1,...,a_n)]$$
$$= a(b\alpha)$$
$$(ab)\alpha = a(b\alpha)$$

4. If 1 is unity in F and $\alpha = (a_1,...,a_n) \in V$, then

   1. $\alpha = 1(a_1,...,a_n)$

$$= (1.a_1, \ 1.a_2,...,1.a_n)$$

$$= a_1, \ a_2,...,a_n$$

$$= \alpha$$

   1. $\alpha = \alpha$

Hence V is a vector space over F.

This vector space of all ordered n-tuples over the field F is denoted by $V_n(F)$ or $F^{(n)}$ or F_n. Here zero vector 0 is the n-tuple $(0, 0,...,0)$

Note:

$V_2(F) = \{(a_1, a_2): a_1, a_2 \in F\} \rightarrow$ vector space of ordered pairs.

$V_3(F) = \{(a_1, a_2, a_3): a_1, a_2, a_3 \in F\} \rightarrow$ vector space of ordered triads over F.

Example 6: Let V be the set of all pairs (x, y) of real numbers and let F be the field of real numbers. Define

$$(x, y) + (x_1, y_1) = (x + x_1, 0)$$

$$C(x, y) = (Cx, 0)$$

Is V, with these operations, a vector space over the field of real numbers?

Solution: If any one of the postulates of vector space is not satisfied, then V will not be vector space. We shall show that for the operation of addition of vectors as defined in this problem, the identity element does not exist.

Suppose the ordered pair (x_1, y_1) is to be the identity element for the operation of addition of vectors.

Then, we must have

$$(x, y) + (x_1, y_1) = (x, y) \ \ \forall x, \ y \in R$$

$\Rightarrow$ $(x + x_1, 0) = (x, y) \ \ \forall x, y \in R$

But if $y \neq 0$, then we cannot have $(x + x_1, 0) = (x, y)$

Thus, there is no element (x_1, y_1) of V.

such that $(x, y) + (x_1, y_1) = (x, y) \ \ \forall x, y \in V$

$\therefore$ The identity element does not exist and V is not a vector space over the field R.

Example 7: Let V be the set of all pairs (x, y) of real numbers and let F be the field of real numbers. Examine in each of the following cases whether V is a vector space over the field of real numbers or not.

   1. $(x, y) + (x_1, y_1) = (x + x_1, y + y_1)$

        $C(x, y) = (|C|x, |C|y)$

2. $(x, y) + (x_1, y_1) = (x + x_1, y + y_1)$

   $C(x, y) = (0, Cy)$

3. $(x, y) + (x_1, y_1) = (x + x_1, y + y_1)$

   $C(x, y) = (C^2x, C^2y)$

4. $(x, y) + (x_1, y_1) = (x + x_1, y + y_1)$

   $C(x, y) = (Cx, y)$

Solution:

1. We shall show that in this case the postulate

   $(a + b)\alpha = a\alpha + b\alpha \ \ \forall \ a, b \in F$ and $a \in V$ fails.

   Let $\alpha = (x, y)$ and $a, b \in R$

   We have $(a + b)\alpha = (a + b) (x, y) = (\ |a + b| \ x, |a + b| \ y)$ \qquad ... (1)

   Also $a\alpha + b\alpha = a(x, y) + b(x, y)$

   $= (|a| \ x, |a| \ y) + (|b| \ x, |b| \ y)$ \qquad (by def. of scalar multiple)

   $= (|a| \ x + |b| \ x, |a| \ y + |b| \ y)$ \qquad (by def. of vectors)

   $= \{(|a| + |b|)x, (|a| + |b|)y\}$ \qquad ... (2)

   Since $|a + b| \leq |a| + |b|$

   $\therefore$ From equations (1) and (2) we conclude that $(a + b) \alpha \neq a\alpha + b\alpha$

   Hence $V(R)$ is not vector space.

2. We shall show that in this case the postulate 1. $\alpha = \alpha \ \ \forall \ \alpha \in V$ fails.

   Let $\alpha = (x, y)$, where $x, y \in R$

   By definition of scalar multiplication we have $1.\alpha = 1, (x, y) = (0, 1y)$

   $= (0, y)$

   But $(0, y) \neq (x, y)$ if $x \neq 0$. Thus there exist $\alpha \in V$ such that $1\alpha \neq \alpha$.

   Hence $V(R)$ is not vector space.

3. Show that in this case the postulate $(a + b)\alpha = a\alpha + b\alpha \ \ \forall \ a, b \in F$ and $\alpha \in V$ fails.

   Note that in general $(a + b)^2 \neq a^2 + b^2$

4. This is similar to the above.

General properties of vector spaces:

Let $V(F)$ be a vector space and 0 be the zero vector of V, then

(i) $a \ 0 = 0 \ \forall \ a \in V$

(ii) $0 \ \alpha = 0 \ \forall \ \alpha \in F$

(iii) $a(-\alpha) = -(a\alpha) \ \forall \ a \in F, \ \forall \ \alpha \in V$

(iv) $(-a)\alpha = -(a\alpha) \ \forall \ a \in F, V\alpha \in V$

(v) $a(\alpha - \beta) = a\alpha - a\beta, \ \forall \ a \in F, V\alpha, \ \beta \in V$

(vi) $a\alpha = 0 \Rightarrow a = 0$ or $\alpha = 0$

4.9 VECTOR SUBSPACES

Let V be a vector space over the field F and let $W \subseteq V$. Then W is called a subspace of V, if W itself is a vector space over F w.r.t to the operation of vector addition and scalar multiplication in V.

Theorem: The necessary and sufficient conditions for a non-empty subset W of a vector space $V(F)$ to be a subspace of V are

(i) $\alpha \in W, \beta \in W \qquad \Rightarrow \qquad \alpha - \beta \in W$

(ii) $a \in F, \alpha \in W \qquad \Rightarrow \qquad a\alpha \in W$

Proof:

The conditions are necessary: If W is a subspace of V, then W is an abelian group w.r.t vector addition.

$\therefore \ \alpha \in W, \beta \in W \qquad \Rightarrow \qquad \alpha - \beta \in W$

Also W must be closed under scalar multiplication.

$\therefore$ Condition (ii) is also necessary.

The conditions are sufficient: Now suppose W is a non-empty subset of V satisfying the two given conditions.

From condition (1), we have $\alpha \in W, \alpha \in W \Rightarrow \alpha - \alpha \in W \Rightarrow 0 \in W$

Thus, the zero vector of V belongs to W and it will also be the zero vector of W.

Now, $0 \in W, \alpha \in W \Rightarrow 0 - \alpha \in W \Rightarrow -\alpha \in W$

Thus the additive inverse of each element of W is also in W.

Again $\alpha \in W, \beta \in W \Rightarrow \alpha \in W, -\beta \in W \Rightarrow \alpha - (-\beta) \in w \Rightarrow \alpha + \beta \in W$

Thus W is closed w.r.t vector addition.

Since the elements of W are also the elements of V,

$\therefore$ Vector addition will be commutative as well as associative in W.

Hence W is the abelian group under vector addition.

From condition (ii), W is closed under scalar multiplication. The remaining postulates of a vector space will hold in W since they hold in V of which W is a subset.

Hence W is subspace of V.

Example 1: The set W of ordered triads $(a_1, a_2, 0)$, where $a_1, a_2 \in F$ is a subspace of $V_3(F)$.

Solution: Let $\alpha = (a_1, a_2, 0)$ and $\beta = (b_1, b_2, 0)$ be any two elements of W and $\forall \ a_1, a_2, b_1, b_2 \in F$.

If $a, b \in F$, then we have

$$a\alpha + b\beta = a(a_1, a_2, 0) + b(b_1, b_2, 0)$$

$$= (aa_1, aa_2, 0) + (bb_1, bb_2, 0)$$

$$= (aa_1 + bb_1, aa_2 + bb_2, 0)$$

Since $aa_1 + bb_1$, $aa_2 + bb_2 \in F$ and the last coordinate of this triad is zero,

$\Rightarrow W$ is subspace of $V_3(F)$.

Example 2: Prove that the set of all solutions (a, b, c) of the equation $a + b + 2c = 0$ is a subspace of the vector space $V_3(R)$.

Solution: Let $W = \{(a, b, c): a, b, c \in R$ and $a + b + 2c = 0\}$

To prove that W is subspace of $V_3(R)$ or R^3.

Let $\alpha = (a_1, b_1, c_1)$ and $\beta = (a_2, b_2, c_2)$ be any two elements of W.

Then $a_1 + b_1 + 2c_1 = 0$ ...(1)

$\qquad a_2 + b_2 + 2c_2 = 0$ ...(2)

If a and b be any elements of R, we have

$a\alpha + b\beta = a(a_1, b_1, c_1) + b(a_2, b_2, c_2)$

$\qquad = (aa_1, ab_1, ac_1) + (ba_2, bb_2, bc_2)$

$\qquad = (aa_1 + ba_2, ab_1 + bb_2, ac_1 + bc_2)$

Now consider

$\qquad = (aa_1 + ba_2) + (ab_1 + bb_2) + 2(ac_1 + bc_2)$

$\qquad = a(a_1 + b_1 + 2c_1) + b(a_2 + b_2 + 2c_2) = a \cdot 0 + b \cdot 0 = 0$

$\therefore \qquad a\alpha + b\beta = (aa_1 + ba_2, ab_1 + bb_2, ac_1 + bc_2) \in W$

Thus $\alpha, \beta \in W$ and $a, b \in R$

$\Rightarrow \quad a\alpha + b\alpha \in W$

$\Rightarrow \quad W$ is subspace of $V_3(R)$.

Example 3: Let R be the field of real numbers.

Which of the following are subspaces of $V_3(R)$.

(i) $\{(x, 2y, 3z): x, y, z \in R\}$ (ii) $\{(x, y, z): x, y, z$ are rational numbers$\}$

Solution:

(i) Let $W = \{(x, 2y, 3z): x, y, z \in R\}$

Let $\alpha = (x_1, 2y_1, 3z_1)$, $\beta = (x_2, 2y_2, 3z_2)$ be two elements of W.

$x_1, y_1, z_1, x_2, y_2, z_2 \in R$

If a, b are any two real numbers, then

$\qquad a\alpha + b\beta = a(x_1, 2y_1, 3z_1) + b(x_2, 2y_2, 3z_2)$

$\qquad\qquad = (ax_1, 2ay_1, 3az_1) + (bx_2, 2by_2, 3bz_2)$

$\qquad\qquad = (ax_1 + bx_2, 2ay_1 + 2by_2, 3az_1 + 3bz_2)$

$\qquad\qquad = [ax_1 + bx_2, 2(ay_1 + by_2), 3(az_1 + bz_2)] \in W$

Since $ax_1 + bx_2$, $ay_1 + by_2$, $az_1 + bz_2$, are all real numbers, thus we have proved $a, b \in R$ and $\alpha, \beta \in W$

$\Rightarrow \quad a\alpha + b\alpha \in W$

$\Rightarrow \quad W$ is subspace of $V_3(R)$

(ii) Let $W = \{(x, y, z) : x, y, z$ are rational numbers$\}$

Now $\alpha = (3, 4, 5)$ is an element of W.

Let also $a = \sqrt{7} \in R$

Consider $a\alpha = \sqrt{7}\,(3, 4, 5)$

$$= (3\sqrt{7}, 4\sqrt{7}, 5\sqrt{7}) \notin W$$

$\because 3\sqrt{7}, 4\sqrt{7}, 5\sqrt{7}$ are not rational numbers.

Since it is not closed under scalar multiplication and also it is not subspace of $V_3(R)$

$\therefore V_3(R) \Rightarrow W$

Example 4: The set of vectors $\alpha = (a_1, a_2, ..., a_n)$ in R^n

such that $a_1 + 3a_2 = a_3$ is subspace of R^n $(n \geq 3)$.

Solution: Let $W = \{\alpha : \alpha \in R^n$ and $a_1 + 3a_2 = a_3\}$

Let $\alpha = (a_1, a_2, ..., a_n)$, $\beta = (b_1, b_2, ..., b_n)$ be any two members of W.

Then $a_1 + 3a_2 = a_3$ and $b_1 + 3b_2 = b_3$.

If $a, b \in R$, then $a\alpha + b\beta = (aa_1 + bb_1, aa_2 + bb_2 + ... + aa_n + bb_n)$

Now $aa_1 + bb_1 + 3(aa_2 + bb_2) = a(a_1 + 3a_2) + b(b_1 + 3b_2) = aa_3 + bb_3$

$\Rightarrow a\alpha + b\beta \in W$ according to the definition of W.

Thus $\alpha, \beta \in W$, $a, b \in R \Rightarrow a\alpha + b\beta \in W$

$\Rightarrow W$ is a subspace of R^n.

4.10 ALGEBRA OF SUBSPACES

Theorem: The intersection of any two subspaces W_1 and W_2 is a vector space $V(F)$ is also a subspace of $V(F)$.

Proof: Since $0 \in W_1$ and W_2 both, $W_1 \cap W_2$ is not empty.

Let $\alpha, \beta \in W_1 \cap W_2$ and $a, b \in F$

Now $\alpha \in W_1 \cap W_2 \Rightarrow \alpha \in W_1$ and $\alpha \in W_2$

$\beta \in W_1 \cap W_2 \Rightarrow \beta \in W_1$ and $\beta \in W_2$

Since W_1 is a subspace, therefore $a, b \in F$, $\alpha, \beta \in W_1$

$\Rightarrow a\alpha + b\beta \in W_1$

Similarly $a, b \in F$ and $\alpha, \beta \in W_2 \Rightarrow a\alpha + b\beta \in W_2$

Now $a\alpha + b\beta \in W_2$

$a\alpha + b\beta \in W_2 \Rightarrow a\alpha + b\beta \in W_1 \cap W_2$

Thus, $a, b \in F$ and $\alpha, \beta \in W_1 \cap W_2 \Rightarrow a\alpha + b\beta \in W_1 \cap W_2$

Hence $W_1 \cap W_2$ is a subspace of $V(F)$.

Note: The union of two subspaces of $V(F)$ may not be a subspace of $V(F)$.

Example: If R be the field of real numbers, then $W_1 = \{(0, 0, z) : z \in R\}$ and $W_2 = \{(0, y, 0) : y \in R\}$ are two subspace of $V_3(R)$

We have $(0, 0, 3) \in W_1$ and $(0, 5, 0) \in W_2$

But $(0, 0, 3) + (0, 5, 0) = (0, 5, 3) \notin W_1 \cap W_2$

Since neither $(0, 5, 3) \in W_1$ nor $(0, 5, 3) \in W_2$, therefore $W_1 \cap W_2$ is not closed under vector addition.

Hence $W_1 \cap W_2$ is not subspace of $V_3(R)$.

4.11 LINEAR COMBINATION OF VECTORS

Linear Span of a Set

Definition: Let $V(F)$ be a vector space. If $\alpha_1, \alpha_2,...,\alpha_n \in V$, then any vector $\alpha = a_1\alpha_1 + a_2\alpha_2 + ... + a_n\alpha_n$, where $a_1, a_2,...,a_n \in F$ is called a linear combination of the vectors $\alpha_1, \alpha_2,...,\alpha_n$.

Linear span: Let $V(F)$ be a vector space and S be any non-empty subset of V.

Then the linear span of S is the set of all linear combinations of finite sets of elements of S and is denoted by $L(S)$.

Thus we have $L(S) = \{a_1\alpha_1 + a_2\alpha_2 + ... + a_n\alpha_n : \alpha_1, \alpha_2,...,\alpha_n\}$ is any arbitrary finite subset of S and $a_1, a_2,...,a_n$ is any arbitrary finite subset of S and $a_1, a_2,...,a_n$ is any arbitrary finite subset of F.

Linearly Dependent and Linearly Independent Sets

Linearly dependent: Let $V(F)$ be a vector space.

A finite set $\{\alpha_1, \alpha_2,...,\alpha_n\}$ of vectors in V is said to be linearly dependent if scalars $a_1, a_2,...,a_n \in F$ not all of them are zero (some of them may be zero) such that $a_1\alpha_1 + a_2\alpha_2 + a_3\alpha_3 + ... + a_n\alpha_n = 0$.

Linearly independent: Let $V(F)$ be a vector space.

A finite set $\{\alpha_1, \alpha_2,...,\alpha_n\}$ of vectors V is said to be linearly independent, if every relation of the form $a_1\alpha_1 + a_2\alpha_2 + a_3\alpha_3 + ... + a_n\alpha_n = 0$, $a_i \in F$, $1 \le i \le n \Rightarrow a_i = 0$ for each $1 \le i \le n$, $(a_1 = a_2 = ... a_n = 0)$.

Any infinite set of vectors in V is said to be linearly independent, if its every finite subset is linearly independent, otherwise it is linearly dependent.

Example 1: In the vector space $V_n(F)$ the systems of 'n' vectors $e_1 = (1, 0, 0,...,0)$, $e_2 = (0, 1, 0,...,0)$, ..., $e_n = (0, 0, 0,...,1)$ is linearly independent, where 1 denotes the unity of the field F.

Solution: If $a_1, a_2,...,a_n$ be any scalars, then

$$a_1e_1 + a_2e_2 + ... + a_ne_n = 0$$

$\Rightarrow a_1(1, 0, 0,...,0) + a_2(0, 1, 0,...,0) + a_n(0, 0, 0,...,0, 1) = 0$

$\Rightarrow (a_1, a_2,...,a_n) = 0 = (0, 0,...,0)$

$\Rightarrow a_1 = 0, a_2 = 0,...,a_n = 0$

$\therefore$ The given set of n vectors is linearly independent.

Note:

1. $\{(1, 0, 0), (0, 1, 0), (0, 0, 1)\}$ is linearly independent subset of $V_3(F)$.
2. A set of vectors which contains the zero vector is necessarily linearly dependent for $1.0 = 0$.

Example 2: Show that $S = \{(1, 2, 4), (1, 0, 0), (0, 1, 0), (0, 0, 1)\}$ is linearly dependent subset of the vector space $V_3(R)$, where R is the field of real numbers.

Solution:

We have $1(1, 2, 4) + (-1)(1, 0, 0) + (-2)(0, 1, 0) + (-4)(0, 0, 1)$

$= (1, 2, 4) + (-1, 0, 0) + (0, -2, 0) + (0, 0, -4)$

$= (0, 0, 0) \rightarrow$ zero vectors

Since the scalar coefficients $1, -1, -2, -4$ are not all zero,

$\therefore$ The given system S is linear dependent.

Example 3: Whether $S = \{(2, 1, 2), (8, 4, 8)\}$ is dependent or independent?

$$= 4(2, 1, 2) + (-1)(8, 4, 8)$$
$$= (8, 4, 8), (-8, -4, -8)$$
$$= (0, 0, 0)$$

$\therefore$ S is linearly independent.

Example 4: In $V_3(R)$, where R is the field of real numbers, examine each of the following sets of vectors for linear dependence.

(i) $(1, 2, 0), (0, 3, 1), (-1, 0, 1)$

Let a, b, c be scalars real numbers such that

$a(1, 2, 0) + b(0, 3, 1) + c(-1, 0, 1) = (0, 0, 0)$

$\Rightarrow (a, 2a, 0) + (0, 3b, b) + (-c, 0, c) = (0, 0, 0)$

$\Rightarrow (a + 0 - c, 2a + 3b + 0, 0 + b + c) = (0, 0, 0)$

$\Rightarrow \qquad (a - c, 2a + 3b, b + c) = (0, 0, 0)$

$\Rightarrow \qquad\qquad\qquad a - c = 0$

$$2a + 3b = 0$$
$$b + c = 0$$

These will have non-zero solutions, i.e. a solution in which a, b, c are not all zero, if the rank of the coefficient matrix is less than three, i.e. number of unknowns a, b, c.

If rank is 3, then zero solution, $a = b = c = 0$ will be the only solution.

Thus coefficient matrix $A = \begin{bmatrix} 1 & 0 & -1 \\ 2 & 3 & 0 \\ 0 & 1 & 1 \end{bmatrix}$

$|A| = 1(3 - 0) - 2(0 + 1) = 1 \neq 0$

$\Rightarrow \text{rank} = 3$

$$\sim \begin{bmatrix} 1 & 0 & -1 \\ 0 & 3 & +2 \\ 0 & 1 & 1 \end{bmatrix}$$

$R_2 \rightarrow R_2 - 2R_1$

$R_3 \rightarrow R_3 - 3R_2$

$$\begin{bmatrix} 1 & 0 & -1 \\ 0 & 3 & 2 \\ 0 & 0 & -5 \end{bmatrix} \rightarrow \text{number of non-zero row, Rank} = 3$$

$\therefore$ Rank $= 3 \Rightarrow a = 0, b = 0, c = 0$ is the only solution.

$\Rightarrow$ System is linearly independent.

(ii) $\{(-1, 2, 1), (3, 0, -1), (-5, 4, 3)\}$

Let (a, b, c) be scalars such that

$$a(-1, 2, 1) + b(3, 0, -1) + c(-5, 4, 3) = (0, 0, 0)$$

$\Rightarrow (-a + 3b - 5c, 2a + 0b + 4c, a - b + 3c) = (0, 0, 0)$

$\Rightarrow$
$$-a + 3b - 5c = 0$$
$$2a + 0b + 4c = 0$$
$$a - b + 3c = 0$$

Coefficient matrix

$$A = \begin{bmatrix} -1 & 3 & -5 \\ 2 & 0 & 4 \\ 1 & -1 & 3 \end{bmatrix} \quad |A| = -1(0 + 4) - 3(6 - 4) - 5(2 - 0) = 0$$

$|A| = 0$

$\Rightarrow$ Rank is less than 3

and number of unknowns are $3 \Rightarrow a, b, c$

$\Rightarrow$ The system will possess a non-zero solution.

$a = -2, b = 1, c = 1$ is a non-zero solution

$\Rightarrow$ System of vectors is linearly dependent.

(iii) $\{(2, 3, 5), (4, 9, 25)\}$

$\Rightarrow \qquad a(2, 3, 5) + b(4, 9, 25) = (0, 0, 0)$

$\Rightarrow (2a + 4b, 3a + 9b, 5a + 25b) = (0, 0, 0)$

$$2a + 4b = 0$$
$$3a + 9b = 0$$
$$5a + 25b = 0$$

$$A = \begin{bmatrix} 2 & 4 \\ 3 & 9 \\ 5 & 25 \end{bmatrix}$$

Obviously, rank = 2 and number of unknowns are 2, i.e. a and b.
These equations have only solution $a = 0$, $b = 0$.

$\Rightarrow$ Given set is linearly independent.

(iv) $\{(1, 3, 2), (1, -7, -8), (2, 1, -1)\}$

$\Rightarrow a(1, 3, 2) + b(1, -7, -8) + c(2, 1, -1) = (0, 0, 0)$

$\Rightarrow \quad (a + b + 2c, 3a - 7b + c, 2a - 8b - c) = (0, 0, 0)$

$$a + b + 2c = 0$$

$$3a - 7b + c = 0$$

$$2a - 8b - c = 0$$

$$A = \begin{bmatrix} 1 & 1 & 2 \\ 3 & -7 & 1 \\ 2 & -8 & -1 \end{bmatrix}$$

$|A| = 1(7 + 8) - 1(-3 - 2) + 2(-24 + 14) = 0$

$\Rightarrow$ Rank $(A) < 3$. No. of unknowns are a, b, c

$\Rightarrow$ System will possess non-zero solution.

$\Rightarrow a = 3, b = 1, c = -2$ are the solutions.

$\Rightarrow$ System is linearly dependent.

(v) $\{(1, 2, 1), (3, 1, 5), (3, -4, 7)\}$

$\Rightarrow a(1, 2, 1) + b(3, 1, 5) + c(3, -4, 7) = (0, 0, 0)$

$\Rightarrow (a + 3b + 3c, 2a + b - 4c, a + 5b + 7c) = (0, 0, 0)$

$$a + 3b + 3c = 0 \qquad \qquad \text{...(1)}$$

$$2a + b - 4c = 0 \qquad \qquad \text{...(2)}$$

$$a + 5b + 7c = 0 \qquad \qquad \text{...(3)}$$

$$(1) \times (2), 2a + 6b + 6c = 0 \qquad \qquad \text{...(4)}$$

Subtracting Eq. (4) from Eq. (2),

$$-5b - 10c = 0$$

$$b + 2c = 0 \qquad \qquad \text{...(5)}$$

Again subtracting Eq. (3) from Eq. (1), we get

$$-2b - 4c = 0 \Rightarrow b + 2c = 0 \qquad \qquad \text{...(6)}$$

$$\Rightarrow b = -2c$$

Put $b = -2c$ in Eq. (1) $\Rightarrow a = 3c$ put $c = 1 \Rightarrow a = 3$

$a = 3, b = -2, c = 1$, so non-zero solution of system

$\Rightarrow$ Set is linearly dependent

$$a(1, 2, 1) + b(3, 1, 5) + c(3, -4, 7) = (0, 0, 0)$$

$\Rightarrow \qquad\qquad a = 3, b = -2, c = 1$

Example 5: Is the vector $(2, -5, 3)$ in the subspace of R^3 spanned by the vectors $(1, -3, 2), (2, -4, -1), (1, -5, 7)$?

Solution: Let $\alpha = (2, -5, 3)$, $\alpha_1 = (1, -3, 2)$, $\alpha_2 = (2, -4, -1)$, $\alpha_3 = (1, -5, 7)$

If α can be expressed as a linear combination of vectors $\alpha_1, \alpha_2, \alpha_3$, then it will be in the subspace of R^3 spanned by three vectors, otherwise it will not be.

Let $\quad \alpha = a_1\alpha_1 + a_2\alpha_2 + a_3\alpha_3, \qquad a_1, a_2, a_3 \in R$

$\Rightarrow \qquad (2, -5, 3) = a_1(1, -3, 2) + a_2(2, -4, -1) + a_3(1, -5, 7)$

$$= (a_1 + 2a_2 + a_3, -3a_1 - 4a_2 - 5a_3, 2a_1 - a_2 + 7a_3)$$

$\therefore \qquad a_1 + 2a_2 + a_3 = 2 \qquad\qquad\qquad\qquad\qquad ...(1)$

$\qquad -3a_1 - 4a_2 - 5a_3 = -5 \qquad\qquad\qquad\qquad ...(2)$

$\qquad 2a_1 - a_2 + 7a_3 = 3 \qquad\qquad\qquad\qquad\qquad ...(3)$

$$3(1) + (2) \Rightarrow 2a_2 - 2a_3 = 1 \Rightarrow a_2 - a_3 = \frac{1}{2} \qquad\qquad ...(4)$$

$$2(1) - (3) \Rightarrow 5a_2 - 5a_3 = 1 \Rightarrow a_2 - a_3 = \frac{1}{5} \qquad\qquad ...(5)$$

We note that equations (4) and (5) are inconsistent.

$\Rightarrow$ Vector α cannot be expressed as a linear combination of $\alpha_1, \alpha_2, \alpha_3$.

$\Rightarrow \alpha$ is not in the subspace of R^3 generated by the vectors $\alpha_1, \alpha_2, \alpha_3$.

Example 6: Are the vectors $(1, 1, 2, 4), (2, -1, -5, 2) (1, -1, -4, 0)$ and $(2, 1, 1, 6)$ linearly independent on R^4?

Solution:

$$(1, 1, 2, 4) = a(2, -1, -5, 2) + b(1, -1, -4, 0) + c(2, 1, 1, 6)$$

$\Rightarrow \qquad 2a + b + 2c = 1$

$\qquad\qquad -a - b + c = 1$

$\qquad\qquad -5a - 4b + c = 2$

$\qquad\qquad 2a + 0b + 6c = 4$

Solving $a = 2, b = -3, c = 0$

$\therefore \quad (1, 1, 2, 4) = 2(2, -1, -5, 2) - 3(1, -1, -4, 0) + 0(2, 1, 1, 6)$

$\quad 1(1, 1, 2, 4) - 2(2, -1, -5, 2) + 3(1, -1, -4, 0) - 0(2, 1, 1, 6)$

$$= (0, 0, 0, 0)$$

$\Rightarrow$ Not all scalars $1, -2, 3, 0$ not all zero.

$\Rightarrow$ Given vectors are linearly dependent in R^4.

EXERCISE

1. Show that $(1, 1, 0, 0)$, $(0, 1, -1, 0)$, $(0, 0, 0, 3)$ are linearly independent.
2. Show that $(1, 3, 2)$, $(-1, -7, -8)$, $(2, 1, -1)$ are linearly dependent in $V_3(R)$.
3. Show that $(1, 1, -1)$, $(2, -3, 5)$, $(-2, 1, 4)$ of R^3 are linearly independent.

4.12 COORDINATES

Ordered Basis

Let $V(F)$ be a finite dimensional vector space of dimension n and let $B = \{b_1, b_2, ..., b_n\}$ be a basis for V. Then a list of length n (ordered n-tuples) of vectors in B is called an ordered basis for V.

Note that in an ordered basis the order of arrangements of vectors is very important. If there are n vectors in a basis of a vector space V, then corresponding to various arrangements of vectors we can obtain $n!$ ordered basis for V.

For example, $\left(e_1^{(3)}, e_2^{(3)}, e_3^{(3)}\right), \left(e_1^{(3)}, e_3^{(3)}, e_2^{(3)}\right), \left(e_3^{(3)}, e_1^{(3)}, e_2^{(3)}\right)$, etc. are ordered basis for the real vector spaces R^3 corresponding to a basis are

$$B = \left(e_1^{(3)}, e_2^{(3)}, e_3^{(3)}\right)$$

Let $a_1, a_2, ..., a_n$ be an ordered basis for a finite dimensional vector space $V(F)$, and let $\alpha \in V$, then there exists a unique n-tuples $(\alpha_1, \alpha_2, ..., \alpha_n)$ of scalars in F such that

$$\alpha = \alpha_1 a_1 + \alpha_2 a_2 + ... + \alpha_n a_n$$

The n-tuples $(\alpha_1, \alpha_2, ..., \alpha_n)$ is called the n-tuples of ordinates of V relative to the ordered basis B and the scalars α_i is called ith coordinate relative to the ordered basis $(a_1, a_2, ..., a_n)$.

The column matrix $\begin{bmatrix} \alpha_1 \\ \alpha_2 \\ \vdots \\ \alpha_n \end{bmatrix}_{n \times 1}$ is called the coordinates matrix. Coordinate vector relative to the ordered basis is

$A = \{a_1, a_2, ..., a_n\}$ and is denoted by $[\alpha]_A$.

Example 1: Relative to the basis $B = \{V_1, V_2\} = \{(1, 1), (2, 3)\}$ of R^2, find the coordinate matrix of
(i) $V = (4, -3)$ (ii) (a, b)

Solution: Let $x, y \in R$
such that $V = xV_1 + yV_2 = x(1, 1) + y(2, 3) = (x + 2y, x + 3y)$

(i) If $u = (4, -3)$, then

$$u = xu_1 + yu_2$$

$\Rightarrow (4, -3) = (x + 2y, x + 3y)$

$\Rightarrow x + 2y = 4, x + 3y = -3 \quad \Rightarrow \quad x = 18, y = -7$

Hence coordinate matrix $[V]_A$ of u relative to the basis A is given by

$$[V_A] = \begin{bmatrix} 18 \\ -7 \end{bmatrix}$$

(ii) If $v = (a, b)$

$v = xv_1 + yv_2$

$\Rightarrow (a, b) = (x + 2y, x + 3y)$

$\Rightarrow x + 2y = a, x + 3y = b$

$\Rightarrow x = 3a - 2b, y = -a + b$

Hence the coordinate matrix $[V]_A$ of v relative to the basis A is given by

$$[V_A] = \begin{bmatrix} 3a - 2b \\ -a + b \end{bmatrix}$$

Example 2: Find the coordinate vector of $v = (1, 1, 1)$ relative to the basis $B = \{v_1 = (1, 2, 3), v_2 = (-4, 5, 6), v_3 = (7, -8, 9)\}$ of vector space R^3.

Solution: Let $x, y, z \in R$ be such that $v = xv_1 + yv_2 + zv_3$

$\Rightarrow (1, 1, 1) = x(1, 2, 3) + y(-4, 5, 6) + z(7, -8, 9)$

$\Rightarrow x - 4y + 7z = 1, 2x + 5y - 8z = 1, 3x + 6y + 9z = 1$

$$x = \frac{7}{10}, \quad y = \frac{-2}{15}, \quad z = \frac{-1}{30}$$

Hence $[V]_B = \begin{bmatrix} \dfrac{-7}{10} \\ \dfrac{-2}{15} \\ \dfrac{-1}{30} \end{bmatrix}$ is the coordinate vector of V relative to basis B.

Example 3: Find the coordinates of the vector (a, b, c) in the real vector space R^3 relative to the ordered basis (b_1, b_2, b_3), where $b_1 = (1, 0, -1)$, $b_2 = (1, 1, 1)$, $b_3 = (1, 0, 0)$.

Solution: Let $\lambda, \mu, \gamma \in R$ be such that

$(a, b, c) = \lambda b_1 + \mu b_2 + \gamma b_3$

$(a, b, c) = \lambda(1, 0, -1) + \mu(1, 1, 1) + \gamma(1, 0, 0)$

$\Rightarrow (a, b, c) = (\lambda + \mu + \gamma, \mu, -\lambda + \mu)$

$$\Rightarrow \lambda + \mu + \gamma = a, \ \mu = b, \ -\lambda + \mu = c$$
$$\lambda = b - c, \quad \mu = b, \quad \gamma = a - 2b + c$$

Hence the coordinates of vector $(a, b, c) \in R^3$ relative to the given ordered basis are $(b - c, b, a - 2b + c)$.

Example 4: Let V be the vector space of all real polynomials of degree less than or equal to 2. For a fixed $c \in R$, let $f_1(x) = 1$, $f_2(x) = x + c$, $f_3(x) = (x + c)^2$, obtain the coordinates of $c_0 + c_1 x + c_2 x^2$ relative to the ordered basis (f_1, f_2, f_3) of V.

Solution: Let $\lambda, \mu, \gamma \in R$ be such that

$$c_0 + c_1 x + c_2 x^2 = \lambda f_1(x) + \mu f_2(x) + \gamma f_3(x)$$

Then,

$$c_0 + c_1 x + c_2 x^2 = (\lambda + \mu c + \gamma c^2) + (\mu + 2\gamma c) x + \gamma x^2$$
$$\Rightarrow \qquad \lambda + \mu c + \gamma c^2 = c_0, \ \mu + 2\gamma c = c_1, \ \gamma = c_2$$
$$\mu = c_1 - 2cc_2 \qquad \lambda = c_0 - c_1 c + c_2 c^2$$

Hence the coordinates of $c_0 + c_1 x + c_2 x^2$ relative to the ordered basis (f_1, f_2, f_3) are $(c_0 - c_1 c + c_2 c^2, c_1 - 2c_2 c, c_2)$.

Example 5: Consider the vector space $P_3(t)$ of polynomials of degree less than or equal to 3.
  (i) Show that $B = \{(t - 1)^3, (t - 1)^2, (t - 1), 1\}$ is a basis of $P_3(t)$.
  (ii) Find the coordinate matrix of $f(t) = 3t^3 - 4t^2 + 2t - 5$ relative to basis B.

Solution:
  (i) Consider the polynomials in B in the following order.

$$(t - 1)^3, (t - 1)^2, (t - 1), 1$$

We see that no polynomial is a linear combination of preceeding polynomials. So the polynomials are linearly independent and since $[R_3(t)] = 4$, therefore, B is a basis of $P_3[t]$.

  (ii) Let x, y, z, s be scalars such that

$$f(t) = x(t - 1)^3 + y(t - 1)^2 + z(t - 1) + s(1)$$
$$\Rightarrow f(t) = xt^3 + (-3x + y)t^2 + (3x - 2y + z)t + (-x + y - z + s)$$
$$\Rightarrow 3t^3 - 4t^2 + 2t - 5 = xt^3 + (-3x + y)t^2 + (3x - 2y + z) + (t - x + y - z + s)$$
$$\Rightarrow x = 3, y = 13, z = 19, s = 4$$

Hence the coordinates matrix of $f(t)$ relative to the given basis is $[f(t)]$

$$B = \begin{bmatrix} 3 \\ 13 \\ 19 \\ 4 \end{bmatrix}$$

Example 6: Let F be a field and n be a positive integer. Find the coordinates of the vector $(a_1, a_2, ..., a_n) \in F^n$ relative to the standard basis.

Solution: We know that the ordered set $\left(e_1^{(n)}, e_2^{(n)}, ..., e_n^{(m)}\right)$ is the standard basis for $F^n(F)$, where $e_1^{(n)} = (1, 0, 0, ..., 0)$, $e_2^{(n)} = (0, 1, 0, ..., 0)$, $e_3^{(n)} = (0, 0, 1, 0, ..., 0)$, ..., $e_n^{(n)} = (0, 0, ..., 1)$ and 1 is unity in F.

Let $\lambda, \lambda_2, ..., \lambda_n$ be scalars in F such that

$$(a_1, a_2, ..., a_n) = \lambda e_1^{(n)} + \lambda_2 e_2^{(n)} + \lambda_3 e_3^{(n)} + ... + \lambda_n e_n^{(n)}.$$

Then $(a_1, a_2, ..., a_n) = \lambda_1(1, 0, 0, ..., 0) + \lambda_2(0, 1, 0) +$
$$\lambda_3(0, 0, 1, 0), ..., \lambda_n(0, 0, ..., 1)$$

$\Rightarrow \qquad a_1, a_2, ..., a_n = (\lambda_1, \lambda_2, ..., \lambda_n)$
$\qquad (a_1, a_2, ..., a_n) = (\lambda_1, \lambda_2, ..., \lambda_n)$
$\Rightarrow \qquad a_1 = \lambda_1, a_2 = \lambda_2, ..., a_n = \lambda_n$

$\therefore$ The vector $(a_1, a_2, ..., a_n) \in F^n$ relative to the standard basis.

Example 7: Find the coordinate matrix $A = \begin{bmatrix} 2 & 3 \\ 4 & -7 \end{bmatrix}$ in the real vector space

$R^{2 \times 2}(R)$ relative to the basis.

(i) $B_1 = \left\{ E_{11} = \begin{bmatrix} 1 & 0 \\ 0 & 1 \end{bmatrix}, E_{12} = \begin{bmatrix} 0 & 1 \\ 0 & 0 \end{bmatrix}, E_{21} = \begin{bmatrix} 0 & 0 \\ 1 & 0 \end{bmatrix}, E_{22} = \begin{bmatrix} 0 & 0 \\ 0 & 1 \end{bmatrix} \right\}$

(ii) $B_2 = \left\{ P = \begin{bmatrix} 1 & 1 \\ 1 & 1 \end{bmatrix}, Q = \begin{bmatrix} 1 & -1 \\ 1 & 0 \end{bmatrix}, R = \begin{bmatrix} 1 & -1 \\ 0 & 0 \end{bmatrix}, S = \begin{bmatrix} 1 & 0 \\ 0 & 0 \end{bmatrix} \right\}$

Solution:

(i) Let x, y, z, t be scalars
such that $A = xE_{11} + yE_{12} + zE_{21} + tE_{22}$

$$\Rightarrow \begin{bmatrix} 2 & 3 \\ 4 & -7 \end{bmatrix} = \begin{bmatrix} x & y \\ z & t \end{bmatrix} \Rightarrow x = 2, y = 3, z = 4, t = -7$$

Hence the coordinate matrix of A relative to the usual basis B_1 is

$$[A]_{B_1} = \begin{bmatrix} 2 \\ 3 \\ 4 \\ -7 \end{bmatrix}$$

(ii) Let x, y, z, t be scalars such that $A = xP + yQ + zR + tS$.

$$\Rightarrow \begin{bmatrix} 2 & 3 \\ 4 & -7 \end{bmatrix} = x\begin{bmatrix} 1 & 1 \\ 1 & 1 \end{bmatrix} + y\begin{bmatrix} 1 & -1 \\ 1 & 0 \end{bmatrix} + z\begin{bmatrix} +1 & -1 \\ 0 & 0 \end{bmatrix} + t\begin{bmatrix} 1 & 0 \\ 0 & 0 \end{bmatrix}$$

$$\Rightarrow \begin{bmatrix} 2 & 3 \\ 4 & -7 \end{bmatrix} = \begin{bmatrix} x+y+z+t & x-y-z \\ x+y & x \end{bmatrix}$$

$$\Rightarrow x+y+z+t=2, \qquad x-y-z=3, \qquad x+y=4, \qquad x=-7$$

$$t=30 \qquad\qquad z=-21 \qquad\qquad y=11$$

$$\Rightarrow x=-7, y=11, z=-21, t=30$$

Hence the coordinate matrix of A relative to the basis B_2 is

$$[A]_{B_2} = \begin{bmatrix} -7 \\ 11 \\ -21 \\ 30 \end{bmatrix}$$

EXERCISE

1. The vectors $V_1 = (1, 2, 0)$, $V_2 = (1, 3, 2)$, $V_3 = (0, 1, 3)$ form a basis of $R^3(R)$. Find the coordinate matrix of vector V relative to basis $B = \{V_1, V_2, V_3\}$, where (i) $V = (2, 7, -4)$ (ii) $(a, b, c) = V$

2. $B = \{t^3 + t^2, t^2 + t, t + 1, 1\}$ is an ordered basis of vector space $P_3[t]$. Find the coordinate matrix $f(t)$ relative to B, where:

   (i) $f(t) = 2t^3 + t^2 - 4t + 2$ (ii) $f(t) = at^3 + bt^2 + ct + d$

3. Consider the vector space $R_2(t)$ of all polynomials of degree less than or equal to 2. Show that the polynomials $f_1(t) = t - 1$, $f_2(t) = t - 1$, $f_3(t) = (t - 1)^2$ form a basis of $P_2[t]$. Find the coordinate matrix of polynomial $f(t) = 2t^2 - 5t + 9$ relative to the ordered basis $B = \{f_1(t), f_2(t), f_3(t)\}$.

4. Find the coordinate vector $V = (a, b, c)$ in $R^3(R)$ relative to the ordered basis $B = \{V_1, V_2, V_3\}$, where $V_1 = (1, 1, 1)$, $V_2 = (1, 1, 0)$, $V_3 = (1, 0, 0)$.

4.13 SUMMARY OF ROW EQUIVALENCE

Definition 1: Two matrices are row equivalent if one can be changed to the other by a sequence of elementary row operations. Alternatively, two $m \times n$ matrices are row equivalent if and only if they have the same row space. The concept is most commonly applied to matrices that represent systems of linear equations, in which case two matrices of the same size are row equivalent if and only if the corresponding homogeneous systems have the same set of solutions, or equivalently the matrices have the same null space.

Because elementary row operations are reversible, row equivalence is an equivalence relation. It is commonly denoted by a tilde (~).

Row Space

The row space of a matrix is the set of all possible linear combinations of its row vectors. If the rows of the matrix represent a system of linear equations, then the row space consists of all linear equations that can be deduced algebraically from those in the system. Two $m \times n$ matrices are row equivalent if and only if they have the same row space.

Properties

1. **Reflexive:** Every $m \times n$ matrix A is row equivalent to itself.
2. **Symmetric:** Let A and B be $m \times n$ matrices. Then matrices are symmetric if the matrix A is row equivalent to B and the matrix B is row equivalent to A.
3. **Transitive:** Let A, B and C be $m \times n$ matrices. Then matrices are transitive if matrix $A \sim B$, the matrix $B \sim C$ and the matrix $A \sim C$.

Application

Finite state machine minimization using row equivalence method.

Finite state machine minimization (minimum automata) is a well-known problem in formal languages and computer design.

But this row equivalence method of minimizing a machine does not always yield a minimum machine.

The row equivalence method of minimization on identification of equivalent rows in a state table is given below. It is based on the following definition.

Definition 2: In a state table two states are said to be equivalent if:

(a) The next states rows are identical.

(b) If the output is the same from each state on each input combination.

For two states A and B with identical output on all input combinations starting in either state, the two states are equivalent if either state, the two states are equivalent if either or both properties 1 and 2 are satisfied.

Property 1: The successor of state A on all input X is A and the successor of state B on all input X is B (each state has an edge that loops back to itselfy on all input X).

Property 2: If on some all input X the successor of state A is state B and the successor of state B is state A.

By inspection of the table, there are no identical rows. We then look at two rows that satisfy properties 1 or 2 as stated above on all input $X = 0$, rows D, E and F have loops (next state = present state). However, the next states are different on all input X. Hence property 1 fails. Note that state N is not considered since the all output from state N is 1.

We then check to see if property 2 holds true. For this property to hold true, we need to have two rows i and j (present states i and j) such that on some all input X from j is state i. In addition, the remaining elements of the rows should be identical. By inspection, we find this property does not hold true as well.

PS	NS		Z
	$X=0$	$X=1$	$X=0, 1$
A	F	B	0
B	E	C	0
C	D	A	0
D	D	M	0
E	E	L	0
F	F	K	0
K	N	C	0
L	N	B	0
M	N	A	0
N	N	N	1

Conclusion

We showed the row equivalence method does generally result in a minimum automation. The row equivalence method can be chosen as a preprocessing step in minimization. However, to guarantee minimum automation it needs to be appended by the implication method of minimization or the partition method based on the state successor method.

4.14 COMPUTATION CONCERNING SUBSPACES

Subspaces

A subspace is a vector space inside a vector space.

The subspace 'S' of a vector space 'V' is that 'S' which is a subset of V and that it has the following characteristics.

S is closed under scalar multiplication.

S is closed under addition.

S contains 'O', the zero vector.

Any subset with these characteristics is a vector space.

Application of subspaces : *Polynomical filtered Lanczos iterations with applications in Density Functional Theory.*

The most expensive part of all electronic structure calculations based on density functionality theory lies in computation of an invariant subspace associated with some of smallest eigenvalues of a discretized Hamilton operator.

The dimension of a subspace typically depends on the total number of valence electrons in the system and can easily reach hundreds or even thousands when large systems with many atoms are considered.

At the same time, discretization of Hamiltonians associated with large systems yields very large matrices, whether with plane-wave or real space discretization.

The combinations of these two factors results in one of the most significant bottlenecks in computational materials science.

In this experiment we show how to efficiently compute a large invariant subspace associated with smallest eigenvalues of a Hermition matrix using polynomially filtered lanczos iterations.

The proposed method constructs an orthogonal basis of invariant subspace by combining two main ingredients.

1. The first is filtering technique to dampen the undesirable contribution of larger eigenvalues at each matrix vector product in Lanczos algorithm.

This technique employs a well-selected low pass filter polynomial obtained in conjugate residual type algorithm in polynomial space.

2. The second ingredient is the **Lanczos algorithm with partial reorthogonalization.** The main rationale for this approach is that filtering will help reduce the size of the Krylev subspace required for convergence and this will result in substantial savings both in memory and in computational costs.

There are variety of ways to compute bases of large eigenspaces. Subspace iteration algorithm is probably the simplest. This computer dominant eigenspace which can be modified to compute the eigenspace associated with algebraically smallest eigenvalue by shifting the matrix.

In fact, subspace iteration algorithm is often used with Chebyshev acceleration. Specifically, one can use Lanczos procedure which are inexpensive form of reorthogonalisation. This method proposed here explain two distinct and complementary tools to solve problem. The first is filtering technique which need to dampen undesirable contribution of largest eigenvalue at each matrix product in Lanczos algorithm and the other is the Lanczos algorithm with partial reorthogonalization.

4.15 APPLICATIONS OF VECTOR SPACES
Advanced Coding Technique : Hamming Code

Transmitted messages, like data from a satellite, are always subject to noise. It is important, therfore, to be able to encode a message in such a way that after noise scrembles it, it can be decoded to its original form. This is sometimes done by repeating the message two or three times.

In 1950's, R.H. Hamming introduced an interesting single error-correcting code that became known as the Hamming code. This coding technique had the application of vector space.

The word "scalar" means a real or a complex number. This can be generalized to an arbitrary element of a certain "field".

Fields are Q (rational numbers), R (real numbers), C (complex numbers) and Z/PZ, if P is prime number.

$$Z/PZ = \{0, 1, \ldots, (P-1)\}$$

when $P = 2$, $Z/2Z = \{0, 1\}$

denoted by $Z_2 = \{0, 1\}$.

In Z_2 addition and multiplication rules are defined as follows:

$0 + 0 = 0$	$1 + 0 = 1$	$0 + 1 = 1$	$1 + 1 = 0$
$0 - 0 = 0$	$1.0 = 0$	$0.1 = 0$	$1.1 = 1$

Thus addition and subtraction are same in Z_2.

Using vector space structure of Rn over R.

[R is the set of all real numbers]

1. $(x_1, x_2, \ldots, x_n) + (y_1, y_2, \ldots, y_n) = (x_1 + y_1, \ldots x_n + y_n)$

2. $a(x_1, x_2, \ldots, x_n) = (ax_1, ax_2, \ldots, ax_n)$

The same structure can be defined on Z_2^n. We equip Z_2^n with an addition and a scalar multiplication.

Example 1: For Z_2^5, we have (10110)

$$(1, 0, 1, 1, 0) + (0, 1, 1, 1, 1) = (1, 1, 0, 0, 1)$$

$$0(1, 1, 0, 1, 0) = (0, 0, 0, 0, 0)$$

Equipped with these two operations, Z_2^n becomes a vector space over the field Z_2 (the scalars here are 0 and 1).

All the basic concepts of vector spaces like linear independence, spanning set, subspaces, dimension, row space, null space apply in this case. A big difference from the vector space R^n is that Z_2^n contains a finite number of vectors, namely 2^n vectors.

Hamming (7, 4) code

Given two integers $K \leq n$, a subspace Z_2^n of dimension K is called an (n, K) linear code. The elements of a linear code are called encoded words.

Consider matrix H over Z_2 whose columns $C_1, C_2,...,C_7$ are all the non-zero vectors of Z_2^3.

$$H = \begin{bmatrix} 0 & 0 & 0 & 1 & 1 & 1 & 1 \\ 0 & 1 & 1 & 0 & 0 & 1 & 1 \\ 1 & 0 & 1 & 0 & 1 & 0 & 1 \end{bmatrix}$$

The null space of H, Null (H) is called a Hamming (7, 4) code.

Null (H) is nothing but the set of all solutions to the homogeneous linear system $HX = 0$ that corresponds to H. We say that H is a parity check matrix for the code Null (H). By solving the system $HX = 0$ to find Null (H).

$$H = \begin{bmatrix} 0 & 0 & 0 & 1 & 1 & 1 & 1 \\ 0 & 1 & 1 & 0 & 0 & 1 & 1 \\ 1 & 0 & 1 & 0 & 1 & 0 & 1 \end{bmatrix}$$

since rank of $H = 3$, dimension Null $(H) = 7 - 3$

Null $(H) = 4$

The matrix G, generator matrix of Hamming (7, 4) code is

$$G = \begin{bmatrix} 1 & 0 & 0 & 0 & 0 & 1 & 1 \\ 0 & 1 & 0 & 0 & 1 & 0 & 1 \\ 0 & 0 & 1 & 0 & 1 & 1 & 0 \\ 0 & 0 & 0 & 1 & 1 & 1 & 1 \end{bmatrix}$$

Example 2: Suppose that the received message $W = 1100011$ encoded by Hamming (4, 7) code. Suppose that there is atmost one error in the transmission. Find the original message.

Solution :

$$
\begin{bmatrix} 0 & 0 & 0 & 1 & 1 & 1 & 1 \\ 0 & 1 & 1 & 0 & 0 & 1 & 1 \\ 1 & 0 & 1 & 0 & 1 & 0 & 1 \end{bmatrix}_{3 \times 7}
\begin{bmatrix} 1 \\ 1 \\ 0 \\ 0 \\ 0 \\ 1 \\ 1 \end{bmatrix}_{7 \times 1}
$$

$$
= \begin{bmatrix} 0 \\ 1 \\ 0 \end{bmatrix}_{3 \times 1}
$$

Since HW is equal to second column of H, changing the second component of W gives the encoded word 1000011. We conclude that the original message is 1000.

Conclusion

Vector spaces are mainly focussed on the properties and hence the applications of the vector space are applicable to the Hamming code and coding technique.

5

Basis and Dimension

5.1 INTRODUCTION

Basis

In our previous discussion, we introduced the concepts of span and linear independence. In a way, a set of vectors $S = \{V_1, V_2, ..., V_n\}$ span a vector space V, if there are enough of the right vectors in S, while they are linearly indpendent, if there are no renundancies. We now combine the two concepts.

Definition: If V is any vector space and $S = \{V_1, V_2, ..., V_n\}$ is a finite set of vectors in V, then S is called a basis if

(i) S is linearly independent.

(ii) S spans V.

Dimension

A non-zero vector space V is called finite dimensional if it contains a finite set of vectors $\{V_1, V_2, ..., V_n\}$ which forms a basis. If no such set exists, V is called infinite dimensional. In addition, we shall regard the zero vector space a finite dimensional even though it has no linearly independent sets and consequently no basis. The theorem is as follows, given the concept of dimension of vector space.

Theorem 1: If $S = \{V_1, V_2, ..., V_n\}$ is a basis for a vector space V and $T = \{W_1, W_2, ..., W_K\}$ is a linearly independent set of vectors in V, then $K \le n$.

Remark: If S and T are both bases for V, then $K = n$. This means that every basis has the same number of vectors. Hence the dimension is well defined.

The dimension of a vector space V is the number of vectors in a basis. If there is no finite basis, we call V an infinite dimensional vector space, otherwise, we call V a finite dimensional vector space.

Proof: If $K > n$, then we consider the set

$$R_1 = \{W_1, V_1, V_2, ..., V_n\}$$

Since S spans V, W can be written as a linear combination of V_i's.

$$W_1 = c_1 V_1 + c_2 V_2 + ... + c_n V_n$$

186

Since T is linearly independent, W_1 is non-zero and at least one of the coefficients c_i is non-zero. Without loss of generality, assume it is c_i. We can solve for V_1 and write V_1 as a linear combination of $W_1, V_2,...,V_n$.

Hence $T_1 = \{W_1, V_2,...,V_n\}$ is a basis for V. Now let
$$R_2 = \{W_1, W_2, V_2,...,V_n\}$$
Similarly, W_2 can be written as a linear combination of the rest and one of the coefficients is non-zero.

Hence $T_2 = \{W_1, W_2, V_3,...,V_n\}$ is a basis for V. Continuing this process, we see that

$T_n = \{W_1, W_2,...,W_n\}$ is a basis for V. But then T_n spans V and hence W_{n+1} is a linear combination of vectors in T_n. This is a contradiction, since the W's are linearly independent hence $n \geq K$.

Example1: $V_1 = (1, 2, 1)$, $V_2 = (2, 9, 0)$, $V_3 = (3, 3, 4)$ are vector spaces, show that the set $S = \{V_1, V_2, V_3\}$ is a basis for R^3.

Solution: To show that S is a basis for R^3, we must show that S is a linearly independent set and every vector of R^3 can be expressed as a linear combination of V_1, V_2, V_3.

To prove that S is linearly independent we must show that the only solution of
$$aV_1 + bV_2 + cV_3 = 0 \qquad ...(1)$$
is $\qquad\qquad a = b = c = 0$

Equation (1) implies that
$$a + 2b + 3c = 0$$
$$2a + 9b + 3c = 0$$
$$a + 4c = 0$$
which is the system of homogeneous equations. It has trivial solution.

$$|A| = \begin{vmatrix} 1 & 2 & 3 \\ 2 & 9 & 3 \\ 1 & 0 & 4 \end{vmatrix} = -1 \neq 0$$

Hence S is linearly independent.

Again, for an arbitrary element
$$B = (b_1, b_2, b_3)$$
$$B = aV_1 + bV_2 + cV_3 \qquad ...(2)$$
$$(b_1, b_2, b_3) = a\,(1, 2, 1) + b\,(2, 9, 0) + c(3, 3, 4)$$
$$a + 2b + 3c = b_1$$
$$2a + 9b + 3c = b_2$$
$$a + 4c = b_3$$

To show that S spans V, we must show that the system (2) has a solution for all choices of $B = (b_1, b_2, b_3)$. Since the determinant of the coefficient matrix A

$$|A| = \begin{vmatrix} 1 & 2 & 3 \\ 2 & 9 & 3 \\ 1 & 0 & 4 \end{vmatrix} = -1 \neq 0$$

A^T exists and the system (2) has unique solution for all $B = (b_1, b_2, b_3)$. Hence S spans V. Thus, S is a basis for R^3.

Theorem 2: If $S = \{V_1, V_2, ..., V_n\}$ is a basis for a vector space V, then every set with more than n-vectors is linearly dependent.

Proof: Let $S = \{W_1, W_2, ..., W_m\}$ be any set of m vectors in V, where $m > n$. We have to show that S is linearly dependent. Since $S = \{V_1, V_2, ..., V_n\}$ is a basis, each W_i can be expressed as a linear combination of the vectors of S, say

$$S = \begin{cases} W_1 = a_{11}v_1 + a_{21}v_2 + ... + ... + a_{n1}v_n \\ W_2 = a_{12}v_1 + a_{22}v_2 + ... + ... + a_{n2}v_n \\ .... \\ .... \\ W_m = a_{1m}v_1 + a_{2m}v_2 + ... + ... + a_{nm}v_n \end{cases} \quad ...(1)$$

To show that S is linearly dependent, we must find scalars, $a_1, a_2, ..., a_m$ not all zero such that

$$a_1 W_1 + a_2 W_2 + ... + a_m W_m = 0$$
$$\Rightarrow a_1(a_{11}V_1 + a_{21}V_2 + ... + a_{n1}V_n) + a_2(a_{12}V_1 + a_{22}V_2 + ... + a_{n2}V_n)$$
$$+ ... + a_m(a_{1m}V_1 + a_{2m}V_2 + ... + a_{nm}V_n) = 0$$
$$\Rightarrow (a_1 a_{11} + a_2 a_{12} + ... + a_{1m}a_m)V_1 +$$
$$(a_{21}a_1 + a_{22}a_2 + ... + a_{2m}a_m)V_2 +$$
$$... + (a_{n1}a_1 + a_{n2}a_2 + ... + a_{nm})V_n = 0$$

$$\Rightarrow \begin{cases} a_{11}a_1 + a_{12}a_2 + ... + a_{1m}a_m = 0 \\ a_{21}a_1 + a_{22}a_2 + ... + a_{2m}a_m = 0 \\ .... \\ .... \\ a_{n1}a_1 + a_{n2}a_2 + ... + a_{nm}a_m = 0 \end{cases} \quad ...(2)$$

The set S will be linearly dependent if the solution of n linear equations in m unknowns and $a_1, a_2, ..., a_n$ will have non-zero values. Thus S is linearly dependent.

Theorem 3: Any two bases for a finite dimension vector space have the same number of vectors.

Proof: Let $S = \{V_1, V_2, ..., V_n\}$ and $S_1 = \{U_1, U_2, ..., U_m\}$ be two bases of a finite dimension vector space V. Since S is a basis and S_1 is a linearly independent set, Theorem 1 gives that $m \le n$. Similarly, since S_1 is a basis and S is a linearly independent set, we have $n \le m$. So $m = n$.

Example 2: Is the vector $(3, -1, 0, -1)$ in the subspace of R^4 spanned by the vectors $(2, -1, 3, 2)$, $(-1, 1, 1, -3)$ and $(1, 1, 9, -5)$?

Solution: $\alpha = (3, -1, 0, -1)$, it can be expressed as a linear combination of $\alpha_1, \alpha_2, \alpha_3$

$$\alpha_1 = (2, -1, 3, 2)$$
$$\alpha_2 = (-1, 1, 1, -3)$$
$$\alpha_3 = (1, 1, 9, -5)$$

Then it will be the subspace of R^4 spanned by these vectors, otherwise, it will not be.

Let $\alpha = a\alpha_1 + b\alpha_2 + c\alpha_3$, where $a, b, c \in R$ do not have common solution, α cannot be expressed as a linear combination of $\alpha_1, \alpha_2, \alpha_3$.

$\Rightarrow \alpha$ is not in the span of R^4 generated by the vectors $\alpha_1, \alpha_2, \alpha_3$.

Example 3: Find a linearly independent subset of the set

$$S_1 = \{\alpha_1, \alpha_2, \alpha_3, \alpha_4\},$$

where $\alpha_1 = (1, 2, -1)$, $\alpha_2 = (-3, -6, 3)$, $\alpha_3 = (2, 1, 3)$, $\alpha_4 = (8, 7, 7) \in R^3$ which spans the same space as S.

Solution: First we observe that $\alpha_2 = -3\alpha_1$. So that the vectors α_1 and α_2 are linearly dependent.

$\therefore S_1 = \{\alpha_1, \alpha_2, \alpha_3, \alpha_4\}$ that the subspace spanned by S_1 is the same as that spanned by S such that $\alpha_3 = c\alpha_1$

$\therefore$ The vectors α_1 and α_3 are linearly independent.

$\therefore$ Let us see whether the vector α_4 lies in the subspace of R^3 spanned by the vectors α_1 and α_3 or not.

Let $\alpha_4 = a\alpha_1 + b\alpha_3$, where $a, b \in R$.

Then $(8, 7, 7) = a(1, 2, -1) + b(2, 1, 3)$

$$a + 2b = 8 \qquad \qquad ...(1)$$
$$2a + b = 7 \qquad \qquad ...(2)$$
$$-a + 3b = 7 \qquad \qquad ...(3)$$

Solving equations (1) and (2) $\Rightarrow a = 2$, $b = 3$

These values of a and b also satisfy equation (3)

$\therefore$
$$\alpha_4 = 2\alpha_1 + 3\alpha_3$$

Thus, the vector α_4 can be expressed as a linear combination of α_1 and α_3. So the subspace of R^3 spanned by the vectors α_1, α_3 and α_4 is the same as that of spanned by the vectors α_1 and α_3.

Hence $T = \{\alpha_1, \alpha_3\}$ is linearly independent subset of S which spans the same subspace of R^3 as spanned by S.

Example 4: A system S consisting of n vectors $e_1 = (1,0,0,...,0)$, $e_2 = (0,1,0,...,0),...,e_n = (0, 0,...,1)$ is a basis of $V_n(F)$.

Solution: First we should show that S is linearly independent set of vectors.

Now we should prove that $L(S) = V_n(F)$, i.e. $L(S) \subseteq V_n(F)$. So we should prove that $V_n(F) \subseteq L(S)$, i.e. each vector in $V_n(F)$ is a linear combination of elements of S.

Let $a = (a_1,...,a_n)$ be a vector in $V_n(F)$.

We can write

$$(a_1,...,a_n) = a_1(1,0,0,...,0) + a_2(0,1,0,...,) +...+a_n(0,0,...,1)$$

$$\alpha = a_1e_1 + a_2e_2 + ... + a_ne_n$$

Hence S is a basis of $V_n(F)$.

Note:

(i) The set $\{(1,0),(0,1)\}$ is basis of $V_2(F)$.

(ii) The set $\{(1,0,0),(0,1,0),(0,0,1)\} \rightarrow$ basis of $V_3(F)$.

(iii) As a particular case, a basis of $V(F)$ is the set consisting of only the unit elements of F.

5.2 FINITE DIMENSIONAL VECTOR SPACES

The vector space $V(F)$ is said to be finite dimensional or finitely generated if there exist a finite subset S of V such that $V = L(S)$.

Theorem 1: The vector space $V_n(F)$ of n-tuples is a finite dimensional vector space.

Or

If $V(F)$ is a finite dimension vector space, then any two bases of V have the same number of elements.

Proof: Suppose $V(F)$ is a finite dimensional vector space.

Let $S_1 = \{\alpha_1, \alpha_2,...,\alpha_m\}$

$S_2 = \{\beta_1, \beta_2, ..., \beta_n\}$ be two bases of V.

To prove that $m = n$.

Since $V = L(S_1)$ and $\beta_1 \in V$, therefore β_1 can be expressed as a linear combination of $\alpha_1, \alpha_2, ..., \alpha_m$. Consequently, the set

$S_3 = \{\beta_1, \alpha_1, \alpha_2, ..., \alpha_m\}$ which also generated $V(F)$ is linearly dependent.

$\therefore$ There exist a number $\alpha_i \neq \beta_1$ of this set S_3, such that α_i is a linear combination of the preceding vectors $\beta_1, \alpha_1, \alpha_2, ..., \alpha_i$.

If we omit the vector α_i from S_3, then V is also generated by the remaining set, i.e.

$$S_4 = \{\beta_1, \alpha_1, \alpha_2, ..., \alpha_{i-1}, \alpha_{i+1}, ..., \alpha_m\}$$

Since $V = L(S_4)$ and $\beta_2 \in V$, therefore β_2 can be expressed as a linear combination of the vectors that belongs to S_4.

Consequently, the set

$S_5 = \{\beta_2, \beta_1, \alpha_1, \alpha_2, ..., \alpha_{i-1}, \alpha_{i+1}, ..., \alpha_m\}$ is linearly dependent.

$\therefore$ There exist a number μ_i of the set S_5 such that α_i is a linear combination of the preceeding vectors.

Obviously, α_i will be different from β_1 and β_2 since $\{\beta_1, \beta_2\}$ is linearly dependent set.

If we exclude the vector α_i from S_5, then the remaning set will generate $V(F)$.

We can continue to proceed in this way. Here each step consists of the exclusion of an α and inclusion of a β in S_1.

Obviously, the set S_1 of α's cannot be exhausted before the set S_2 of β's otherwise, S_2 will become linearly dependent.

$\therefore$ We must have $m \leq n$.

Interchanging the rules of S_1 and S_2, we get $n \leq m \Rightarrow m = n$.

Theorem 2: If W_1, W_2 are two subspaces of a finite dimensional vector space $V(F)$, then

$$\dim(W_1 + W_2) = \dim W_1 + \dim W_2 - \dim(W_1 \cap W_2)$$

Proof: Let $\dim(W_1 \cap W_2) = k$

Let $S = \{r_1, r_2, ...r_k\}$ be a basis of $W_1 \cap W_2$.

$\therefore S \subseteq W_1$ and $S \subseteq W_2$

Since S is linearly independent and $S \subseteq W_1$, therefore S can be extended to form a basis of W_1.

Let $\{r_1, r_2, ..., r_k, \alpha_1, \alpha_2, ..., \alpha_m\}$ be a basis of W_1

$\Rightarrow \dim W_1 = k + m$

Similarly, let $\{r_1, r_2, ..., r_k, \beta_1, \beta_2, ..., \beta_t\}$ be a basis of W_2.

$\Rightarrow \dim W_2 = k + t$

$$\therefore \dim W_1 + \dim W_2 - \dim(W_1 \cap W_2) = (m+k) + (k+t) - k$$
$$= m + k + t \qquad \ldots(1)$$

Hence to prove the theorem, we must show that $\dim(W_1 + W_2) = m + k + t$

From Eq. (1), we claim that the set S_1

$$S_1 = \{r_1, r_2, \ldots, r_k, \alpha_1, \alpha_2, \ldots, \alpha_m, \beta_1, \beta_2, \ldots, \beta_t\}$$

be a basis of $W_1 + W_2$.

Now to show that (i) S_1 is linearly independent

(ii) $L(S_1) = W_1 + W_2$

Let $c_1 r_1 + c_2 r_2 + \ldots + c_k r_k + a_1 \alpha_1 + a_2 \alpha_2 + \ldots + a_m \alpha_m +$

$$b_1 \beta_1 + b_2 \beta_2 + \ldots + b_t \beta_t = 0 \qquad \ldots(2)$$

$$\Rightarrow \ b_1 \beta_1 + b_2 \beta_2 + \ldots + b_t \beta_t = -(c_1 r_1 + \ldots + c_k r_k + a_1 \alpha_1 + \ldots + a_m \alpha_m) \qquad \ldots(3)$$

Now $\qquad -(c_1 r_1 + \ldots + c_k r_k + a_1 \alpha_1 + \ldots + a_m \alpha_m) \in W_1$

since it is linear combination of basis of W_1.

Again $b_1 \beta_1 + b_2 \beta_2 + \ldots + b_t \beta_t \in W_2$ since it is linear combination of the elements belonging to a basis of W_2.

By Eq. (3)

$$b_1 \beta_1 + b_2 \beta_2 + \ldots + b_t \beta_t \in W_1 \cap W_2$$

$\therefore$ It can be expressed as a linear combination of the basis of $W_1 \cap W_2$. Thus,

$$b_1 \beta_1 + b_2 \beta_2 + \ldots + b_t \beta_t = d_1 r_1 + \ldots + d_k r_k$$

$\Rightarrow b_1 = 0, b_2 = 0, \ldots, b_t = 0$. Put these in equation (2) gives

$$c_1 r_1 + c_2 r_2 + \ldots + c_k r_k + a_1 \alpha_1 + a_2 \alpha_2 + \ldots + a_m \alpha_m = 0$$

$\Rightarrow c_1 = 0, c_2 = 0, \ldots, c_k = 0, a_1 = 0, a_2 = 0, \ldots, a_m = 0$

Since $r_1, r_2, \ldots, r_k, \alpha_1, \alpha_2, \ldots, \alpha_m$ vectors are linearly independent,

Equation (2) $\Rightarrow c_1 = 0, \ldots, c_k = 0, a_1 = 0, \ldots, a_m = 0, b_1 = 0, \ldots, b_t = 0$.

$\therefore$ The set S_1 of vectors $r_1, r_2, \ldots, r_k, \alpha_1, \ldots, \alpha_m, \beta_1, \ldots, \beta_t$ is linearly independent.

To show that $L(S_1) = W_1 + W_2$

Since $W_1 + W_2$ is a subspace of V and each element of S_1 belongs to $W_1 + W_2 \Rightarrow L(S_1) \subseteq W_1 + W_2$

Let α be any element of $W_1 + W_2$. Then

α = some element of W_1 + some element of W_2

= a linear combination of elements of basis of W_1 +
    a linear combination of elements of basis of W_2.

= a linear combination of elements of basis of S_1

$\therefore$ $\alpha \in L(S_1)$. Hence $W_1 + W_2 \subseteq L(S_1)$

$\therefore L(S_1) \subseteq W_1 + W_2$

$\therefore S_1$ is the basis of $W_1 + W_2$ and consequently

$$\dim(W_1 + W_2) = m + k + t \qquad \text{...(4)}$$

From equations (1) and (2), result follows.

Example 5: Let V be the vector space of all 2×2 matrices over the field F. Prove that V has dimension 4, by exhibiting a basis for V, which has 4 elements.

Solution: Let $\alpha = \begin{bmatrix} 1 & 0 \\ 0 & 0 \end{bmatrix}, \beta = \begin{bmatrix} 0 & 1 \\ 0 & 0 \end{bmatrix}, \eta = \begin{bmatrix} 0 & 0 \\ 1 & 0 \end{bmatrix}$

and $\delta = \begin{bmatrix} 0 & 0 \\ 0 & 1 \end{bmatrix}$ be four elements of V.

The subset $S = \{\alpha, \beta, \eta, \delta\}$ of V is linearly independent because $a\alpha + b\beta + c\eta + d\delta = 0$

$$\Rightarrow a\begin{bmatrix} 1 & 0 \\ 0 & 0 \end{bmatrix} + b\begin{bmatrix} 0 & 1 \\ 0 & 0 \end{bmatrix} + c\begin{bmatrix} 0 & 0 \\ 1 & 0 \end{bmatrix} + d\begin{bmatrix} 0 & 0 \\ 0 & 1 \end{bmatrix} = \begin{bmatrix} 0 & 0 \\ 0 & 0 \end{bmatrix}$$

$$\Rightarrow a\begin{bmatrix} a & b \\ c & d \end{bmatrix} + \begin{bmatrix} 0 & 0 \\ 0 & 0 \end{bmatrix} \Rightarrow a = b = c = d = 0$$

Also $L(S) = V$

$\therefore$ If $\begin{bmatrix} a & b \\ c & d \end{bmatrix} = a\alpha + b\beta + c\eta + d\delta$

$\Rightarrow S$ is a basis of V.

$\Rightarrow \dim V = 4$ since the number of elements in S is 4.

Example 6: Show that the vectors $(1, 2, 1), (2, 1, 0), (1, -1, 2)$ form a basis of R^3.

Solution: Let $S = \{(1, 2, 1), (2, 1, 0), (1, -1, 2)\}$

If we show that this set S is linearly independent, then this will form a basis for R^3 [we know that the set $\{(1, 0, 0), (0, 1, 0), (0, 0, 1)\}$ form the basis for R^3].
We have

$$a_1(1, 2, 1) + a_2(2, 1, 0) + a_3(1, -1, 2) = (0, 0, 0)$$

$$\Rightarrow a_1 + 2a_2 + a_3 = 0 \qquad \text{...(1)}$$

$$2a_1 + a_2 - a_3 = 0 \qquad \text{...(2)}$$

$$a_1 + 2a_3 = 0 \qquad \text{...(3)}$$

By solving equations (1), (2), (3), we get $a_1 = a_2 = a_3 = 0$

$\therefore$ The set S is linearly independent.

$\therefore$ S is basis for the given vectors.

Example 7: Determine whether or not the following vectors form a basis of R^3.

$\quad$ $(1, 1, 2), (1, 2, 5), (5, 3, 4)$.

Solution: We know that dim $R^3 = 3$

If the given set of vectors is linearly independent, then it will form a basis of R^3, otherwise not.

$$a_1(1,1,2) + a_2(1,2,5) + a_3(5,3,4) = (0,0,0)$$

$$\Rightarrow a_1 + a_2 + 5a_3 = 0 \quad \left. \begin{cases} a_1 = -7 \\ a_2 = 2 \\ a_3 = 1 \end{cases} \right\}$$

$$a_1 + 2a_2 + 3a_3 = 0$$

$$2a_1 + 5a_2 + 4a_3 = 0 \qquad \text{Non-zero solution of the given system.}$$

Therefore, given set is linearly dependent.

Hence, it does not form a basis of R^3.

Example 8: For the 3-dimensional space R^3 over the field of real numbers R, determine if the set $\{(2,-1,0),(3,5,1),(1,1,2)\}$ is a basis.

Solution: dim $R^3 = 3$. If the given set, containing three vectors, is linearly independent, it will form a basis of R^3, otherwise not.

$\Rightarrow a = 0$, $b = 0$, $c = 0$

$\Rightarrow$ Linearly independent

$\therefore$ It forms a basis of R^3.

Example 9: Show that the vectors $\alpha_1 = (1,0,-1), \alpha_2 = (1,2,1), \alpha_3 = (0,-3,2)$ form a basis for R^3. Express each of the standard basis vector as linear combination of $\alpha_1, \alpha_2, \alpha_3$.

Solution: Let $S = \{\alpha_1, \alpha_2, \alpha_3\}$

Let a, b, c be scalars (real nos) such that $a\alpha_1 + b\alpha_2 + c\alpha_3 = 0$

$$a(1,0,-1) + b(1,2,1) + c(0,-3,2) = (0,0,0)$$

$$a + b = 0 \qquad \qquad \text{...(1)}$$

$$2b - 3c = 0 \qquad \qquad \text{...(2)}$$

$$-a + b + 2c = 0 \qquad \qquad \text{...(3)}$$

By solving Eqs. (1), (2), (3), we get $a = b = c = 0$ as the only solution of the equations.

$\therefore$ $\qquad\qquad a\alpha_1 + b\alpha_2 + c\alpha_3 = 0 \Rightarrow a = 0, b = 0, c = 0$

$\therefore$ $\alpha_1, \alpha_2, \alpha_3$ are linearly independent.

Now to show $\alpha_1, \alpha_2, \alpha_3$ also generates R^3.

Let $\eta = (p, q, r)$ be any vector in R^3

i.e. $\eta = (p, q, r) = x\alpha_1 + y\alpha_2 + z\alpha_3 \ \forall \ x, y, z \in R$

$$= x(1, 0, -1) + y(1, 2, 1) + z(0, -3, 2)$$
$$(p, q, r) = (x + y, 2y - 3z, -x + y + 2z)$$
$$x + y = p \qquad \qquad \qquad \qquad \text{...(1)}$$
$$2y - 3z = q \qquad \qquad \qquad \qquad \text{...(2)}$$
$$-x + y + 2z = r \qquad \qquad \qquad \text{...(3)}$$

Adding equations (1) and (3), we get

$$2y + 2z = p + r \qquad \qquad \qquad \text{...(4)}$$

Solving Eqs. (2) and (4)

we get $z = \dfrac{1}{5}(p + r - q)$

Equation (4) becomes

$$2y = p + r - 2z$$
$$= p + r - \frac{2}{5}(p + r - q)$$
$$y = \frac{3}{10}p + \frac{1}{5}q + \frac{3}{10}r$$
$$x + y = p$$
$$x = p - y$$
$$x = \frac{7}{10}p - \frac{1}{5}q - \frac{3}{10}r$$

Thus $\eta = (p, q, r)$ is R^3 can be expressed as

$$\eta = x\alpha_1 + y\alpha_2 + z\alpha_3 \ \forall \ x, y, z \in R^3$$

Therefore, S generates R^3.

$\therefore$ S is linearly independent and S generates R^3.

$\therefore$ S is the basis of R^3.

[$\eta = (p, q, z)$ as a linear combination of $\alpha_1, \alpha_2, \alpha_3$]

The standard basis vectors are

$$e_1 = (1, 0, 0), e_2 = (0, 1, 0), e_3 = (0, 0, 1)$$

If $\eta = e_1$, then $p = 1, q = 0, r = 0$

$$\therefore \ x = \frac{7}{10}, \ y = \frac{3}{10}, \ z = \frac{1}{5}$$

$$\therefore \ e_1 = \frac{7}{10}\alpha_1 + \frac{3}{10}\alpha_2 + \frac{1}{5}\alpha_3$$

If $\eta = e_2$, then $p = 0, \ q = 1, \ r = 0 \ \Rightarrow \ x = -\frac{1}{5}, \ y = \frac{1}{5}, \ z = \frac{-1}{5}$

$$\therefore \ e_2 = -\frac{1}{5}\alpha_1 + \frac{1}{5}\alpha_2 - \frac{1}{5}\alpha_3$$

If $\eta = e_3$, then $p = 0, \ q = 0, \ r = 1 \ \Rightarrow \ x = -\frac{3}{10}, \ y = \frac{3}{10}, \ z = \frac{1}{5}$

$$\therefore \ e_2 = -\frac{3}{10}\alpha_1 + \frac{3}{10}\alpha_2 + \frac{1}{5}\alpha_3$$

Example 10: Show that a system X consisting of vectors $\alpha_1 = (1,0,0,0), \alpha_2 = (0,1,0,0), \alpha_3 = (0,0,1,0), \alpha_4 = (0,0,0,1)$ is a basis of $R^4(R)$.

Solution: First we show that X is linearly independent.

If a_1, a_2, a_3, a_4 be any scalars, then

$a_1\alpha_1 + a_2\alpha_2 + a_3\alpha_3 + a_4\alpha_4$ = zero vector

$$a_1(1,0,0,0) + a_2(0,1,0,0) + a_3(0,0,1,0) + a_4(0,0,0,1) = (0,0,0,0)$$

$$(a_1, a_2, a_3, a_4) = (0,0,0,0)$$

Therefore, $a_1 = a_2 = a_3 = a_4 = 0$

Therefore, the set X of 4 vectors are linearly independent.

Now we will show X generates R^4.

Each vector of R^4 can be expressed as a linear combination of the vectors of X.

Let (a, b, c, d) be any vectors in R^4.

$$(a, b, c, d) = a(1,0,0,0) + b(0,1,0,0) + c(0,0,1,0) + d(0,0,0,1)$$

$$= a_1\alpha_1 + a_2\alpha_2 + a_3\alpha_3 + a_4\alpha_4$$

$\Rightarrow X$ generates R^4 and hence it is a basis for R^4.

Example 11: Select any basis of $R^3(R)$ from the set $\{\alpha_1, \alpha_2, \alpha_3, \alpha_4\}$, where $\alpha_1 = (1,-3,2), \alpha_2 = (2,4,1), \alpha_3 = (3,1,3), \alpha_4 = (1,1,1)$

Solution: Let $S = \{\alpha_1, \alpha_2, \alpha_3, \alpha_4\}$

If any three vectors in S are linearly independent, then they form basis of R^3.

Let $S_1 = \{\alpha_1, \alpha_2, \alpha_3\}$ and a, b, c be any scalars such that

$$a\alpha_1 + b\alpha_2 + c\alpha_3 = (0,0,0)$$

$$a(1,-3,2) + b(2,4,1) + c(3,1,3) = (0,0,0)$$

$$a + 2b + 3c = 0$$

$$-3a + 4b + c = 0$$

$$2a + b + 3c = 0$$

Coefficient matrix $A = \begin{bmatrix} 1 & 2 & 3 \\ -3 & 4 & 1 \\ 2 & 1 & 3 \end{bmatrix}$

$\therefore$ det $(A) = 0$, rank A is less than 3.

$\therefore$ The vectors $\alpha_1, \alpha_2, \alpha_3$ are linearly dependent.

So they do not form basis.

Let $S_2 = \{\alpha_1, \alpha_2, \alpha_3\}$

The coordinates of vectors $\alpha_1, \alpha_2, \alpha_4$ is

$$\begin{vmatrix} 1 & 2 & 1 \\ -3 & 4 & 1 \\ 2 & 1 & 1 \end{vmatrix} = 2 \neq 0$$

Since $\{\alpha_1, \alpha_2, \alpha_4\}$ are linearly independent subset of R^3 containing three vectors, therefore it form a basis for R^3.

EXERCISE

1. Find a basis for the vector space V spanned by vectors $W_1 = (1,1,0)$,
$W_2 = (0,1,1)$, $W_3 = (2,3,1)$ and $W_4 = (1,1,1)$.

[**Ans.** General solution: $(C_1, C_2, C_3, C_4) = (-2t, -t, t, 0) \in R$

Particular solution: $(C_1, C_2, C_3, C_4) = (2, 1, -1, 0)$.]

2. Find a basis for the vector space V spanned by the vectors
$W_1 = (1,1,0)$, $W_2 = (0,1,1)$, $W_3 = (2,3,1)$ and $W_4 = (1,1,1)$.

[**Ans.** $\{W_1, W_2, W_4\}$ is a basis V.

$V_1 = (0,1,0), V_2 = (-2,0,1)$ are linearly independent.]

3. Determine a basis and the dimension of the solution space of

$$2x_1 + 2x_2 - x_3 + x_5 = 0$$

$$-x_1 + x_2 - 2x_3 - 3x_4 + x_5 = 0$$
$$x_1 + x_2 - 2x_3 - x_5 = 0$$
$$x_3 + x_4 + x_5 = 0$$

[**Ans.** Vectors $V_1 = \begin{bmatrix} -1 \\ 1 \\ 0 \\ 0 \\ 0 \end{bmatrix}$ and $V_2 = \begin{bmatrix} -1 \\ 0 \\ -1 \\ 0 \\ 1 \end{bmatrix}$ are linearly independent,

if they form a basis, the dimension of the solution space is 2.]

4. Let $V = \mathbb{R}^n$ and let $(a_1,...,a_n)$ be a fixed vector in V. Prove that the collection of elements $(x_1, x_2,...,x_n)$ of V with $a_1x_1 + a_2x_2 + ... + a_nx_n = 0$ is a subspace of V. Determine the dimension of this subspace and find a basis.

[**Ans.** Dimension is $n - 1$ and $\mathbb{R}^n$ is basis.]

5. Let V be the collection of polynomials in the variable x of degree at most 5 with coefficients in Q. Prove that V is a vector space over Q of dimension 6 with $1, x, x^2,..., x^5$ as basis. Prove that $1, 1 + x, 1 + x + x^2, ...,1 + x + x^2 + x^3 + x^4 + x^5$ is also a basis for V.

6. Determine whether the set $S = \{(3, -2), (4, 5)\}$ is basis for R^2.

[**Ans.** S is a basis for R^2.]

7. Determine whether the set $S = \{(1, 5, 3), (0, 1, 2), (0, 0, 6)\}$ is basis for R^3.

[**Ans.** S is basis for R^3.]

8. Determine whether the set $S = \{(0, 0, 0), (1, 5, 6), (6, 2, 1)\}$ is a basis for R^3.

[**Ans.** S cannot be a basis.]

9. Determine the dimension of the vector space P_7.

[**Ans.** Dimension of P_7 is 8, $\dim(P_n) = n + 1$.]

10. Determine the dimension of the space $M_{2,3}$.

[**Ans.** $\dim(D_{n,m})$.]

11. Let $W = \{(2t, t): t \in R\}$ be a subspace of R^2. Give a geometric description for W, find a basis for W, and find the dimension for W.

[**Ans.** Basis: $\{(2, 1)\}$ and $\dim(W) = 1$.]

12. Let $W = \{(2S - t, S, t, S): S, t \in R\}$ be a subspace of R^4. Give a geometric description for W, find a basis for W, and find the dimension of W.

[**Ans.** $\dim(W) = 2$, Basis: $\{(2, 1, 0, 1), (-1, 0, 1, 0)\}$.]

13. Prove that if $S = \{V_1, V_2,...,V_n\}$ is a basis for a vector space V and C is a non-zero scalar, thus the set $S_0 = \{CV_1, CV_2,...,CV_n\}$ is also a basis for V.

14. Let $\mathbb{R}^N$ be the vector space of sequences in $\mathbb{R}$. Consider the subsets.

$V = \{(a_n)_{n \in N} \in \mathbb{R}^n / \text{the equation}\}$

$a_{n+2} = a_{n+1} + a_n$ holds for all $n \in N\}$

$V = \{(a_n)_{n \in N} \in \mathbb{R}^n / \text{the equation}\}$

$a_{n+3} = a_n$ holds for all $n \in N\}$

(a) Show that V and W are subspaces of $\mathbb{R}^n$.

(b) Compute the dimensions of V and W.

(c) Compute $V \cap W$ and its dimension.

(d) Compute V + W and its dimension.

(e) Check your result using the formula

$$\dim(U + W) = \dim(U) + \dim(W) - \dim(U \cap W)$$

[**Ans.** $5 = 2 + 3 - 0$ and is valid.]

15. Determine a basis of the subspaces spanned by the vectors

$\alpha_1 = (1,2,3), \alpha_2 = (2,1,-1), \alpha_3 = (1,-1,-4), \alpha_4 = (4,2,-2)$

[**Ans.** α_1, α_2.]

6

Linear Transformations

6.1 INTRODUCTION

In this chapter, we are concerned with linear mappings from one vector space to another. Recall the special case, when the second vector space is the underlying field of the first vector space which was the subject of discussion in the last chapter. Our purpose here is to elaborate on those ideas and generalize the results.

Definition: Let V and V' be two vector spaces over the same field F. Then a mapping $T : V \to V'$ is called a linear transformation (or) a vector space homomorphism or simply a linear map if

(i) $T(u + v) = T(u) + t(v)$

(ii) $T(au) = a\, T(u)$ $\forall\, u, v \in V$ and $\forall\, a \in F$

Thus, $T : V \to V'$ is a linear transformation if it "preserves" the two basic operations of a vector space, that is, vector addition and scalar multiplication.

Monomorphism

Let V and V' be two vector spaces over the same field F. Then a linear transformation $T : V \to V'$ is called a monomorphism if it is one-to-one (or) one-one.

Epimorphism

Let V and V' be two vector spaces over the same field F. Then a linear transformation $T : V \to V'$ is called an epimorphism if T is onto.

Isomorphism

A linear transformation T from a vector space $V(F)$ to a vector space $V'(F)$ is an isomorphism if T is both one-one and onto, i.e. a bijection.

In such a case, we say that V is isomorphic to V' and we write $V \cong V'$.

Thus, two vector spaces V and V' over the same field F are isomorphic if there exists a bijection linear transformation $T : V \to V'$.

A linear transformation from a vector space to itself is called a **"linear operator"**.

Example 1: Let V be a vector space over a field F. Then the identity mapping I_V on V is a linear transformation. Moreover, it is an automorphism.

Solution: For any $u, v \in V$ and $a \in F$, we have

$$I_V(u + v) = u + v = I_V(u) + I_V(v) \quad \text{and}$$

$$I_V(au) = av = a\,I_V(u)$$

So I_V is a linear transformation.

We know that $I_V : V \to V$ is bijective. Hence I_V is an automorphism on V.

Example 2: Let V and V' be vector spaces over the same field F and let 'T' be the mapping that assigns every vector $v \in V$ to the zero vector $0v' \in V$. Show that T is a linear transformation.

Solution: For any $u, v \in V$ and $a \in F$, we have

$$T(u + v) = 0u' + 0v' = T(u) + T(v) \text{ and}$$

$$T(au) = a0u' = aT(u)$$

Thus $T : V \to V'$ is a linear transformation.

Remark: The above transformation is called the zero linear transformation or zero linear mapping and is denoted by 0.

Example 3: Let F be a field. Then the mapping $T : F^2 \to F^3$ given by $T(a, b) = (a, b, 0) \; \forall\, (a, b) \in F^2$ is a linear transformation.

Solution: Let $u = (a_1, b_1)$, $v = (a_2, b_2) \in F^2$

Then $\quad T(u + v) = T(a_1 + a_2, b_1 + b_2) = (a_1 + a_2, b_1 + b_2, 0)$

$\Rightarrow \qquad T(u + v) = (a_1, b_1, 0) + (a_2, b_2, 0) = T(u) + T(v)$ and

$$T(1u) = T(1a_1, 1b_1) = (1a_1, 1b_1, 0) = 1(a_1, b_1, 0) = 1T(u).$$

Hence $T : F^2 \to F^3$ is a linear transformation.

Example 4: Let $T : R^3 \to R^3$ be the mapping defined by

$$T(x, y, z) = (x, y, 0) \; \forall\, (x, y, z) \in R^3.$$

Show that T is a linear transformation.

Solution: For any $u = (a, b, c)$, $v = (a', b', c') \in R^3$, $1 \in R$

We have

$$T(u + v) = T(a + a', b + b', c + c') = (a + a', b + b', 0)$$

$\Rightarrow \quad T(u + v) = (a, b, 0) + (a', b', 0) = T(u) + T(v)$

and $\qquad T(1u) = T(1a, 1b, 1c) = (1a, 1b, 0) = 1(a, b, 0) = 1T(u).$

Thus 'T' is a linear transformation.

Example 5: Let $V = R[x]$ be the vector space of all polynomials over the field R and let $D : V \to V$ be the mapping associating each polynomial $f(x)$ to its derivative $\dfrac{d}{dx}\big(f(x)\big)$. Show that D is a linear transformation.

Solution: Let $f(x)$ and $g(x)$ be any two polynomials in $R[x]$ and $\lambda \in R$.

Then
$$D\big(f(x) + g(x)\big) = \frac{d}{dx}\big[f(x) + g(x)\big]$$

$$= \frac{d}{dx}\big(f(x)\big) + \frac{d}{dx}\big(g(x)\big)$$

$$= D\big(f(x)\big) + D\big(g(x)\big)$$

and
$$D\big(\lambda f(x)\big) = \frac{d}{dx}\big(\lambda f(x)\big) = \lambda \frac{d}{dx}\big(f(x)\big) = \lambda D\big(f(x)\big)$$

Thus $D : V \to V$ is a linear transformation and is known as the derivative mapping.

Note that it is not a monomorphism because $D(4x^2 + 3) = D(4x^2)$ but $4x^2 + 3 \neq 4x^2$.

Example 6: Let V be the real vector space of all continuous functions from R into itself. Show that a mapping $T : V \to V$ given by

$$T\big[f(x)\big] = \int_0^x f(t)\,dt \quad \text{for all } f(x) \in V \text{ and } \lambda \in R \text{ is a linear transformation}$$

from V into itself.

Solution: For any $f(x), g(x) \in V$ and $\lambda \in R$, we have

$$T\big(f(x) + g(x)\big) = \int_0^x \{f(t) + g(t)\}\,dt = \int_0^x f(t)\,dt + \int_0^x g(t)\,dt$$

$$\Rightarrow \quad T[f(x) + g(x)] = T\,f(x) + T\,g(x)$$

and
$$T\{\lambda f(x)\} = \int_0^x \lambda\, f(t)\,dt = \lambda \int_0^x f(t)\,dt = \lambda T f(x)$$

Thus, T is a linear mapping and is known as the integral mapping.

Example 7: Let A be an $m \times n$ real matrix and let $T_A : R^{n \times 1} \to R^{m \times 1}$ be a mapping defined by $T_A(U) = AU$ for all $U \in R^{n \times 1}$.

Show that T_A is a linear transformation.

Solution: For any $U, V \in R^{n \times 1}$ and $a \in R$, we have

$$T_A(U + V) = A(U + V) = AU + AV$$

$$\Rightarrow \quad T_A(U + V) = T_A(U) + T_A(V)$$

and
$$T_A(aU) = A(aU) = a(AU) = aT_A(U)$$

Hence, T_A is a linear transformation.

Example 8: Let C be the vector space of all complex numbers over the field of complex numbers and let $T : C \rightarrow C$ be a mapping given by $T(x + iy) = x$ for all $x + iy \in C$.

Show that T is not a linear transformation.

Solution: Let $z_1 = x_1 + iy_1, z_2 = x_2 + iy_2 \in C$.

Then
$$T(z_1 + z_2) = T[(x_1 + x_2 + i(y_1 + y_2)] = x_1 + x_2$$
$$= T(x_1 + iy_1) + T(x_2 + iy_2)$$
$$= T(z_1) + T(z_2)$$
$$\Rightarrow \quad T(z_1 + z_2) = T(z_1) + T(z_2)$$

So, T satisfies condition (i) in the definition of a linear transformation.

Now, $T\{(3 + i)(3 - i)\} = T(10) = 10$, but
$$(3 + i) T(3 - i) = (3 + i) 3 = 9 + 3i \neq 10$$
$$\therefore \quad T[(3 + i)(3 - i)] \neq (3 + i) T(3 - i)$$

So T does not satisfy condition (ii) in the definition of linear transformation. Hence, T is not a linear transformation.

Example 9: Let C be the field of complex numbers regarded as a vector space over the field R of real numbers. Then show that the mapping $T: C \rightarrow R$ given by $T(z) = (x^3 + y^3)^{1/3}$ for all $z = x + iy \in C$ is not a linear transformation.

Solution: For any $z = x + iy \in C$ and $1 \in R$
$$T(1z) = T(1x + i1y) = (1^3 x^3 + 1^3 y^3)^{1/3}$$
$$= 1(x^3 + y^3)^{1/3}$$
$$= 1 \, T(z)$$

So, T satisfies condition (ii) in the definition of linear transformation.

Now
$$T(2) = 2, \; T(3i) = 3 \text{ and } T(2 + 3i) = (8 + 27)^{1/3}$$
$$= (35)^{1/3}$$
$$\neq T(2) + T(3i)$$

So, T does not satisfy condition (ii) in the definition of a linear transformation.

Hence, T is not a linear transformation.

Example 10: $T : V_2(R) \rightarrow V_2(R)$ is defined by $T(x, y) = (3x + 2y, 3x - 4y)$. Verify whether T is a linear transformation.

Solution: Let $\alpha = (x_1, y_1)$ and $\beta = (x_2, y_2)$
$$\therefore \quad \alpha + \beta = (x_1 + x_2, y_1 + y_2)$$
$$\therefore \quad T(\alpha + \beta) = T(x_1 + x_2, y_1 + y_2)$$
$$= [3(x_1 + x_2) + 2(y_1 + y_2), 3(x_1 + x_2) - 4(y_1 + y_2)]$$

$$= \left(3x_1 + 2y_1 + 3x_2 + 2y_2, 3x_1 - 4y_1 + 3x_2 - 4y_2\right)$$
$$= \left(3x_1 + 2y_1, 3x_1 - 4y_1\right) + \left(3x_2 + 2y_2, 3x_2 - 4y_2\right)$$
$$= T\left(x_1, y_1\right) + T\left(x_2, y_2\right)$$
$$= T\left(\alpha\right) + T\left(\beta\right)$$

and $\qquad c\alpha = c\left(x_1, y_1\right) = \left(cx_1, cy_1\right)$

$\therefore \qquad T(c\alpha) = T(cx_1, cy_1)$

$$= [3\left(cx_1\right) + 2\left(cy_1\right), 3\left(cx_1\right) - 4\left(cy_1\right)]$$
$$= [c\left(3x_1 + 2y_1\right), c\left(3x_1 - 4y_1\right)]$$
$$= cT\left(x_1, y_1\right) = cT\left(\alpha\right)$$

$\therefore \qquad T : V_2(R) \to V_2(R)$ is a linear transformation and hence a linear map on $V_2(R)$.

Example 11: Define $T : R^3 \to R^3$ by $T\left(x, y, z\right) = \left(2x + y, y - z, 2y + 4z\right)$. Verify whether T is a linear transformation.

Solution:

(i) $\quad T(\alpha + \beta) = T\left(\alpha\right) + T\left(\beta\right)$

Let $\qquad \alpha = \left(x_1, y_1, z_1\right)$ and $\beta = \left(x_2, y_2, z_2\right)$

$$\alpha + \beta = \left(x_1 + x_2, y_1 + y_2, z_1 + z_2\right)$$

$\therefore \quad T(\alpha + \beta) = [2(x_1 + x_2) + \left(y_1 + y_2\right), \left(y_1 + y_2\right)$
$$- \left(z_1 + z_2\right), 2\left(y_1 + y_2\right) + 4\left(z_1 + z_2\right)]$$
$$= (2x_1 + y_1 + 2x_2 + y_2, y_1 - z_1 + y_2 - z_2 ,$$
$$2y_1 + 4z_1 + 2y_2 + 4z_2)$$
$$= \left(2x_1 + y_1, y_1 - z_1, 2y_1 + 4z_1\right) +$$
$$\left(2x_2 + y_2, y_2 - z_2, 2y_2 + 4z_2\right)$$
$$= T\left(x_1, y_1, z_1\right) + T\left(x_2, y_2, z_2\right)$$
$$= T\left(\alpha\right) + T\left(\beta\right)$$

(ii) $\quad c.\alpha \quad = c\left(x_1, y_1, z_1\right) = \left(cx_1, cy_1, cz_1\right)$

$\therefore \quad T\left(c\alpha\right) = T\left(cx_1, cy_1, cz_1\right)$

$$= \left(2cx_1 + cy_1, cy_1 - cz_1, 2cy_1 + 4cz_1\right)$$
$$= [c\left(2x_1 + y_1\right), c\left(y_1 - z_1\right), c\left(2y_1 + 4z_1\right)]$$
$$= c\left(2x_1 + y_1, y_1 - z_1, 2y_1 + 4z_1\right)$$
$$= cT\left(x_1, y_1, z_1\right) = cT(\alpha)$$

$\therefore$ T is a linear transformation and hence a linear map on R^3.

Example 12: Define $T : V_1(R) \to V_3(R)$ is defined by $T(x) = (x, 2x^2, x^3)$. Verify whether T is a linear transformation.

Solution: Let $\alpha = x$, $\beta = y$

$\therefore$ $\quad T(\alpha + \beta) = T(x + y)$

i.e. $\quad T(\alpha + \beta) = T[x + y, 2(x + y)^2, (x + y)^3]$ $\qquad$ ...(1)

$\quad T(\alpha) + T(\beta) = T(x) + T(y) = (x, 2x^2, x^3) + (y, 2y^2, y^3)$

i.e. $T(\alpha) + T(\beta) = (x + y, 2(x^2 + y^2), x^3 + y^3)$ $\qquad$ ...(2)

From Eq. (1) and (2) it is clear that

$$T(\alpha + \beta) \neq T(\alpha) + T(\beta)$$

Hence, T is not a linear transformation.

Example 13: Define a mapping $T : V_3(F) \to V_2(F)$ by $T(a_1, a_2, a_3) = (a_2, a_3)$. Verify whether T is a linear transformation.

Solution: Let $\alpha = (a_1, a_2, a_3)$, $\beta = (b_1, b_2, b_3)$

$\alpha + \beta = (a_1 + b_1, a_2 + b_2, a_3 + b_3)$

$T(\alpha + \beta) = T(a_1 + b_1, a_2 + b_2, a_3 + b_3)$

$\qquad = (a_2 + b_2, a_3 + b_3)$

$\qquad = (a_2, a_3) + (b_2, b_3) = T(a_1, a_2, a_3) + T(b_1, b_2, b_3)$

$\qquad = T(\alpha) + T(\beta)$

$c\alpha = c(a_1, a_2, a_3) = (ca_1, ca_2, ca_3)$

$T(c\alpha) = T(ca_1, ca_2, ca_3)$

$\qquad = (ca_2, ca_3)$

$\qquad = c(a_2, a_3)$

$\qquad = cT(a_1, a_2, a_3)$

$\qquad = cT(\alpha)$

$\therefore$ T is a linear transformation.

Example 14: Define a mapping $T : V_2(R) \to V_2(R)$ by

$T(x, y) = (x\cos\theta - y\sin\theta, x\sin\theta + y\cos\theta)$. Verify whether T is a linear transformation.

Solution: Let $\alpha = (x_1, y_1)$, $\beta = (x_2, y_2)$

$T(\alpha + \beta) = T(x_1 + x_2, y_1 + y_2)$

$$= (x_1 + x_2)\cos\theta - (y_1 + y_2)\sin\theta,$$
$$(x_1 + x_2)\sin\theta + (y_1 + y_2)\cos\theta$$
$$= (x_1\cos\theta - y_1\sin\theta, x_1\sin\theta + y_1\cos\theta)$$
$$+ (x_2\cos\theta - y_2\sin\theta, x_2\sin\theta + y_2\cos\theta)$$
$$= T(x_1, y_1) + T(x_2, y_2)$$
$$= T(\alpha) + T(\beta)$$
$$T(C\alpha) = T(cx_1, cy_1)$$
$$= (cx_1\cos\theta - cy_1\sin\theta, cx_1\sin\theta + cy_1\cos\theta)$$
$$= c(x_1\cos\theta - y_1\sin\theta, x_1\sin\theta + y_1\cos\theta)$$
$$= cT(\alpha)$$

$\therefore$ T is a linear transformation and hence a linear map on $V_2(R)$.

Example 15: Let $M(R)$ be the vector space of all 2×2 matrices over R and B be a fixed non-zero element of $M(R)$. Show that the mapping $T : M(R) \to M(R)$ defined by $T(A) = AB + BA$, $\forall A \in M(R)$ is a linear transformation.

Solution: Let $A, C \in M(R)$ be any arbitrary elements
$$T(A + C) = (A + C)B + B(A + C)$$
$$= AB + CB + BA + BC$$
$$= (AB + BA) + (CB + BC)$$
$$= T(A) + T(C)$$

Let $k \in R$
$$T(k \cdot A) = (k \cdot A)B + B(k \cdot A)$$
$$= k(AB + BA)$$
$$= kT(A)$$

$\therefore$ T is a linear transformation.

6.2 PROPERTIES OF A LINEAR TRANSFORMATION

Theorem 1: If $T : U \to V$ is a linear transformation, then

(i) $T(0) = 0'$, where 0 and 0' are zero vectors of U and V respectively.

(ii) $T(-\alpha) = -T(\alpha), \forall \alpha \in U$

(iii) $T(c_1\alpha_1 + c_2\alpha_2 + ... + c_n\alpha_n) = c_1T(\alpha_1) + c_2T(\alpha_2) + ... + c_nT(\alpha_n)$

Proof:

(i) $\forall \alpha \in U$
$$T(\alpha + 0) = T(\alpha) + T(0) \text{ since } T \text{ is a linear transformation.}$$
$$\Rightarrow \quad T(\alpha) = T(\alpha) + T(0)$$

$\Rightarrow T(\alpha) + 0' = T(\alpha) + T(0')$

$\Rightarrow \qquad\qquad 0' = T(0)$ (by left cancellation law in V)

$\Rightarrow \qquad\quad T(0) = 0'$

(ii) $T\big(\alpha + (-\alpha)\big) = T(\alpha) + T(-\alpha)$ since T is a linear transformation.

i.e. $\qquad T(0) = T(\alpha) + T(-\alpha)$

i.e. $\qquad 0' = T(\alpha) + T(-\alpha)$

Similarly $\quad 0' = T(-\alpha) + T(\alpha) \qquad\qquad\qquad [\because T(0) = 0']$

$\therefore\ T(-\alpha)$ is the additive inverse of $T(\alpha)$.

i.e. $\qquad T(-\alpha) = -T(\alpha)$

(iii) Let us prove this result by mathematical induction.

Let $P(n): T\big(c_1\alpha_1 + c_2\alpha_2 + ... + c_n\alpha_n\big) =$

$$c_1 T(\alpha_1) + c_2 T(\alpha_2) + ... + c_n T(\alpha_n)$$

If $n = 1$, $P(1) = T\big(c_1\alpha_1\big) = c_1 T(\alpha_1)$

Since T is linear, $P(1)$ is true

Let $n = m$, $P(m): T\big(c_1\alpha_1 + c_2\alpha_2 + ... + c_m\alpha_m\big)$

$$= c_1 T(\alpha_1) + c_2 T(\alpha_2) + ... + c_m T(\alpha_m)$$

Since T is linear, $P(m)$ is true. We have to show that $P(m+1)$ is true.

$T\big(c_1\alpha_1 + c_2\alpha_2 + ... + c_m\alpha_m + c_{m+1}\alpha_{m+1}\big)$

$$= T\big(c_1\alpha_1 + c_2\alpha_2 + ... + c_m\alpha_m + c_{m+1}\alpha_{m+1}\big)$$

$$= c_1 T(\alpha_1) + c_2 T(\alpha_2) + ... + c_m T(\alpha_m) + c_{m+1} T(\alpha_{m+1})$$

$\therefore\ P(m+1)$ is true.

Since $P(1)$, $P(m)$, $P(m+1)$ is true, therefore by mathematical induction $P(n)$ is true for all integers 'n'.

Theorem 2: If $\beta_1, \beta_2, ..., \beta_m$ is any basis of the vector space U and $\alpha_1, \alpha_2, ..., \alpha_m$ are any m vectors of the vector space V, then there exists one and only one linear tranformation $T: U \to V$ such that $T(\beta_i) = \alpha_i$ for $i = 1, 2, ..., m$.

Proof: Let α be any arbitrary vector of U.

$\therefore \qquad \alpha = c_1\beta_1 + c_2\beta_2 + ... + c_m\beta_m$ for $c_1, c_2, ..., c_m \in F$

Define: $T: U \to V$ by

$$T(\alpha) = c_1\alpha_1 + c_2\alpha_2 + ... + c_m\alpha_m$$

We shall prove that this is the required linear transformation. For this we shall show that

(i) T is a linear transformation

(ii) $T(\beta_i) = \alpha_i$ for $i = 1, 2, ..., m$

(iii) T is unique

(i) Consider $\alpha, \beta \in U$

$\therefore \qquad \alpha = c_1\beta_1 + c_2\beta_2 + ... + c_m\beta_m$

$$\beta = d_1\beta_1 + d_2\beta_2 + ... + d_m\beta_m$$

$$\alpha + \beta = (c_1 + d_1)\beta_1 + (c_2 + d_2)\beta_2 + ... + (c_m + d_m)\beta_m$$

$$T(\alpha + \beta) = T\Big[(c_1 + d_1)\beta_1 + (c_2 + d_2)\beta_2 + ... + (c_m + d_m)\beta_m\Big]$$

$$= (c_1 + d_1)\alpha_1 + (c_2 + d_2)\alpha_2 + ... + (c_m + d_m)\alpha_m$$

$$= c_1\alpha_1 + d_1\alpha_1 + c_2\alpha_2 + d_2\alpha_2 + ... + c_m d_m + d_m\alpha_m$$

$$= T(c_1\alpha_1 + c_2\beta_2 + ... + c_m\beta_m) +$$

$$T(d_1\beta_1 + d_2\beta_2 + ... + d_m\beta_m)$$

$$= T(\alpha) + T(\beta)$$

$$c\alpha = c(c_1\beta_1 + c_2\beta_2 + ... + c_m\beta_m)$$

$$= cc_1\beta_1 + cc_2\beta_2 + ... + cc_m\beta_m$$

$$T(c\alpha) = T(cc_1\beta_1 + cc_2\beta_2 + ... + cc_m\alpha_m)$$

$$= cc_1\alpha_1 + cc_2\alpha_2 + ... + cc_m\beta_m$$

$$= c(c_1\alpha_1 + c_2\alpha_2 + ... + c_m\alpha_m)$$

$$= cT(c_1\beta_1 + c_2\beta_2 + ... + c_m\beta_m)$$

$$= cT(\alpha)$$

$\therefore$ T is a linear transformation.

(ii) $\qquad \beta_i = 0 \cdot \beta_1 + 0 \cdot \beta_2 + ... + 0 \cdot \beta_i + 1 \cdot \beta_i + 0 \cdot \beta_{i+1} + ... + 0 \cdot \beta_m$

$$T(\beta_i) = T(0 \cdot \beta_1 + 0 \cdot \beta_2 + ... + 0 \cdot \beta_i + 1 \cdot \beta_i + 0 \cdot \beta_{i+1} + ... + 0 \cdot \beta_m)$$

$$= 0 \cdot \alpha_1 + 0 \cdot \alpha_2 + ... + 0 \cdot \alpha_{i-1} + 1 \cdot \alpha_i + 0 \cdot \alpha_{i+1} + ... + 0 \cdot \alpha_m$$

$$= \alpha_i$$

$$T(\beta_i) = \alpha_i \text{ for } i = 1, 2, ..., m$$

(iii) If possible, let there be another linear transformation $S : U \rightarrow V$ such that $S(\beta_i) = \alpha_i$

$$S(\alpha) = S(c_1\beta_1 + c_2\beta_2 + ... + c_m\beta_m)$$

$$= c_1 S(\beta_1) + c_2 S(\beta_2) + ... + c_m S(\beta_m) \quad \because S \text{ is a linear}$$
$$\text{transformation}$$

$$= c_1\alpha_1 + c_2\alpha_2 + ... + c_m\alpha_m$$

$$= T\left(c_1\beta_1 + c_2\beta_2 + \ldots + c_m\beta_m\right)$$

$$= T(\alpha)$$

$\therefore$ $S(\alpha) = T(\alpha)$ for any arbitrary vector $\alpha \in U$

$\therefore$ $S = T$

Hence linear transformation is unique.

WORKED EXAMPLES

Example 1: Find a linear transformation $T : V_2(R) \rightarrow V_2(R)$ such that $T(1, 2) = (3, 0)$ and $T(2, 1) = (1, 2)$.

Solution: Let us express $(1, 2)$ and $(2, 1)$ as linear combinations of the basis vectors $e_1 = (1, 0)$ and $e_2 = (0, 1)$.

$$(1, 2) = 1(1, 0) + 2(0, 1) = 1e_1 + 2e_2$$

$$(2, 1) = 2(1, 0) + 1(0, 1) = 2e_1 + 1e_2$$

$\therefore$ $T(e_1 + 2e_2) = T(1, 2)$

$\quad\quad\quad T(2e_1 + 1e_2) = T(2, 1)$

i.e. $T\left(e_1\right) + 2T\left(e_2\right) = (3, 0)$ ... (1)

$\quad\quad 2T\left(e_1\right) + T\left(e_2\right) = (1, 2)$ ... (2)

Solving equations (1) and (2) for $T(e_1)$ and $T(e_2)$.

Multiply Eq. (2) by 2 and subtract from Eq. (1),

we get $-3T(e_1) = (3, 0) - (2, 4)$

i.e. $-3T(e_1) = (1, -4)$

$\therefore$ $T\left(e_1\right) = \left(\dfrac{-1}{3}, \dfrac{4}{3}\right)$

From Eq. (2), $T\left(e_2\right) = (1, 2) - 2T\left(e_1\right)$

$$= (1, 2) - 2\left(\dfrac{-1}{3}, \dfrac{4}{3}\right)$$

$$T\left(e_2\right) = \left(\dfrac{5}{3}, \dfrac{-2}{3}\right)$$

$$(x, y) = x(1, 0) + y(0, 1)$$

Now $T(x, y) = T\left[x(1, 0) + y(0, 1)\right]$

$$= T\left[xe_1 + ye_2\right]$$

$$= xT(e_1) + yT(e_2) \quad\quad (\because\ T \text{ is linear})$$

$$= x\left(\frac{-1}{3}, \frac{4}{3}\right) + y\left(\frac{5}{3}, \frac{-2}{3}\right)$$

$$= \left(\frac{-x}{3} + \frac{5y}{3}, \frac{4x}{3} - \frac{2y}{3}\right)$$

i.e. $T(x, y) = \left(\frac{-x+5y}{3}, \frac{4x-2y}{3}\right)$ is the required linear transformation.

Example 2: Find a linear transformation $T : V_3(R) \to V_2(R)$ such that $T(1, 0, 0) = (-1, 0)$, $T(0, 1, 0) = (1, 1)$, $T(0, 0, 1) = (0, -1)$.

Solution: $e_1 = (1, 0, 0)$, $e_2 = (0, 1, 0)$, $e_3 = (0, 0, 1)$

$\therefore \qquad T(e_1) = (-1, 0), \ T(e_2) = (1, 1), \ T(e_3) = (0, -1)$

Now $(x, y, z) = x(1,0,0) + y(0,1,0) + z(0,0,1)$

$$T(x, y, z) = T\left[x(1, 0, 0) + y(0, 1, 0) + z(0, 0, 1)\right]$$

$$= xT(e_1) + yT(e_2) + zT(e_3)$$

$$= x(-1, 0) + y(1, 1) + z(0, -1)$$

$$= (-x + y, y - z)$$

i.e. $\qquad T(x, y, z) = (y - x, y - z)$

Example 3: Find a linear transformation $T : R^2 \to R^3$ such that $T(-1, 1) = (-1, 0, 2)$ and $T(2, 1) = (1, 2, 1)$.

Solution: Let us express $(-1, 1)$ and $(2, 1)$ as linear combinations of $e_1 = (1, 0)$ and $e_2 = (0, 1)$.

$$(-1, 1) = -1(1,0) + 1(0,1) = -e_1 + e_2$$

$$(2, 1) = 2(1,0) + 1(0,1) = 2e_1 + e_2$$

$\therefore \ \ T(-e_1) + T(e_2) = (-1, 0, 2) \qquad\qquad\qquad \text{...(1)}$

$2T(e_1) + T(e_2) = (1, 2, 1) \qquad\qquad\qquad\qquad \text{...(2)}$

Solving equations (1) and (2) for $T(e_1)$ and $T(e_2)$:

Subtracting Eq. (1) from Eq. (2), we get

$$3T(e_1) = (2, 2, -1)$$

$$T(e_1) = \left(\frac{2}{3}, \frac{2}{3}, \frac{-1}{3}\right)$$

Substituting in Eq. (1), we get

$$T(e_2) = (-1, 0, 2) + \left(\frac{2}{3}, \frac{2}{3}, \frac{-1}{3}\right)$$

i.e. $\qquad T(e_2) = \left(\frac{-1}{3}, \frac{2}{3}, \frac{5}{3}\right)$

$$T(x, y) = T\left[x(e_1) + y(e_2)\right] = xT(e_1) + yT(e_2)$$

$$= x\left(\frac{2}{3}, \frac{2}{3}, \frac{-1}{3}\right) + y\left(\frac{-1}{3}, \frac{2}{3}, \frac{5}{3}\right)$$

$$= \left(\frac{2x - y}{3}, \frac{2x + 2y}{3}, \frac{-x + 5y}{3}\right)$$

$$T(x, y) = \left(\frac{2x - y}{3}, \frac{2(x + y)}{3}, \frac{5y - x}{3}\right)$$

Example 4: Find a linear transformation $T : R^3 \rightarrow R^3$ such that $T(1, 1, 1) = (1, 1, 1)$, $T(1, 2, 3) = (-1, -2, 3)$ and $T(1, 1, 2) = (2, 2, 4)$.

Solution: Let us express $(1, 1, 1), (1, 2, 3), (1, 1, 2)$ as linear combinations of $e_1 = (1, 0, 0)$, $e_2 = (0, 1, 0)$, $e_3 = (0, 0, 1)$.

$$(1, 1, 1) = 1e_1 + 1e_2 + 1e_3$$

$$(1, 2, 3) = 1e_1 + 2e_2 + 3e_3$$

$$(1, 1, 2) = 1e_1 + 1e_2 + 2e_3$$

$$T(1, 1, 1) = T(e_1 + e_2 + e_3)$$

$$T(1, 2, 3) = T(e_1 + 2e_2 + 3e_3)$$

$$T(1, 1, 2) = T(e_1 + e_2 + 2e_3)$$

$$T(e_1 + e_2 + e_3) = (1, 1, 1)$$

$$T(e_1) + T(e_2) + T(e_3) = (1, 1, 1) \qquad \ldots(1)$$

$$T(e_1 + 2e_2 + 3e_3) = (-1, -2, 3)$$

$$T(e_1) + 2T(e_2) + 3T(e_3) = (-1, -2, 3) \qquad \ldots(2)$$

$$T(e_1 + e_2 + 2e_3) = (2, 2, 4)$$

$$T(e_1) + T(e_2) + 2T(e_3) = (2, 2, 4) \qquad \ldots(3)$$

Solving equations (1), (2), (3) for $T(e_1)$, $T(e_2)$ and $T(e_3)$, we get

$$T(e_1) = (4, 5, 8), \quad T(e_2) = (-4, -5, -10), \quad T(e_3) = (1, 1, 3)$$

Now $\quad (x, y, z) = xe_1 + ye_2 + ze_3$

$$T(x, y, z) = xT(e_1) + yT(e_2) + zT(e_3)$$
$$= x(4, 5, 8) + y(-4, -5, -10) + z(1, 1, 3)$$

$T(-x, y, z) = (4x - 4y + z, 5x - 5y + z, 8x - 10y + 3z)$ is required linear transformation.

Example 5: If V is the vector space of all polynomials over R, then show that the mapping $f : V \rightarrow V$ defined by $f(p) = p(0)$ is a linear map.

Solution: Let $p, q \in V$

$\therefore \qquad\qquad\qquad\qquad p + q \in V$

$$f(p + q) = (p + q)(0) = p(0) + q(0) = f(p) + f(q)$$
$$f(cp) = (cp)(0) = c(p(0)) = cf(p)$$

$\therefore \ f : V \rightarrow V$ is a linear map.

Example 6: If $T : R^2 \rightarrow R^2$ is a linear transformation such that $T(1, 0) = (1, 1)$ and $T(0, 1) = (-1, 2)$. Show that T maps the square with vertices $(0, 0)$, $(1, 0)$, $(1, 1)$ and $(0, 1)$ into a parallelogram.

Solution: $T(1, 0) = (1, 1)$, $T(0, 1) = (-1, 2)$

Let $x, y \in R^2$

$\therefore \qquad (x, y) = x(1, 0) + y(0, 1)$

$\qquad T(x, y) = x\, T(1, 0) + y\, T(0, 1)$

$\qquad\qquad = x(1, 1) + y(-1, 2)$

$\qquad\qquad = (x - y, x + 2y)$

$\therefore \qquad T(x, y) = (x - y, x + 2y)$

$\qquad T(0, 0) = (0, 0) \equiv A$

$\qquad T(1, 0) = (1, 1) \equiv B$

$\qquad T(1, 1) = (0, 3) \equiv C$

$\qquad T(0, 1) = (-1, 2) \equiv D$

$\therefore$ A, B and C and D are the vertices of a quadrilateral, to show that $ABCD$ is a parallelogram. We will show that the diagonals AC and BD bisect each other.

Midpoint of $AC = \left(\dfrac{0 + 0}{2}, \dfrac{0 + 3}{2}\right) = \left(0, \dfrac{3}{2}\right)$

Midpoint of $BD = \left(\dfrac{1 - 1}{2}, \dfrac{1 + 2}{2}\right) = \left(0, \dfrac{3}{2}\right)$

$\therefore$ Diagonals bisect each other.

$\therefore$ $ABCD$ is a parallelogram.

6.3 MATRIX OF A LINEAR TRANSFORMATION

Let U and V be two vector spaces of dimensions m and n respectively.

Let $B_1 = \{\alpha_1, \alpha_2, ..., \alpha_m\}$ and $B_2 = \{\beta_1, \beta_2, ..., \beta_n\}$ be a basis of U and V respectively.

Let $T : U \to V$ be a linear transformation defined by

$$T(\alpha_1) = c_{11}\beta_1 + c_{12}\beta_2 + ... + c_{1n}\beta_n$$
$$T(\alpha_2) = c_{21}\beta_1 + c_{22}\beta_2 + ... + c_{2n}\beta_n$$
$$\vdots$$
$$T(\alpha_m) = c_{m1}\beta_1 + c_{m2}\beta_2 + ... + c_{mn}\beta_n$$

The coordinates of $T(\alpha_i)$, $i = 1, 2, ..., m$ w.r.t. the basis B_2 of V determines a $m \times n$ matrix.

$$A = \begin{bmatrix} c_{11} & c_{12} & \cdot\cdot & c_{1n} \\ c_{21} & c_{22} & \cdot\cdot & c_{2n} \\ \cdot\cdot & \cdot\cdot & \cdot\cdot & \cdot\cdot \\ \cdot\cdot & \cdot\cdot & \cdot\cdot & \cdot\cdot \\ c_{m1} & c_{m2} & \cdot\cdot & c_{mn} \end{bmatrix} = \begin{bmatrix} c_{11} & c_{21} & \cdot\cdot & c_{m1} \\ c_{12} & c_{22} & \cdot\cdot & c_{m2} \\ \cdot\cdot & \cdot\cdot & \cdot\cdot & \cdot\cdot \\ \cdot\cdot & \cdot\cdot & \cdot\cdot & \cdot\cdot \\ c_{1n} & c_{2n} & \cdot\cdot & c_{mn} \end{bmatrix}$$

This matrix A is called the matrix of linear transformation T relative to bases B_1 and B_2. We shall associate a linear transformation $T : U \to V$ where U and V are vector spaces of dimensions m and n respectively. Consider the bases $B_1 = \{\alpha_1, \alpha_2, ..., \alpha_m\}$ and $B_2 = \{\beta_1, \beta_2, ..., \beta_m\}$ of U and V respectively.

We shall define a linear transformation $T : U \to V$ by defining the values of T on the vectors of B_1 as:

$$T(\alpha_1) = c_{11}\beta_1 + c_{12}\beta_2 + ... + c_{1n}\beta_n$$
$$T(\alpha_2) = c_{21}\beta_1 + c_{22}\beta_2 + ... + c_{2n}\beta_n$$
$$\cdots\cdots\cdots\cdots\cdots\cdots$$
$$\cdots\cdots\cdots\cdots\cdots\cdots$$
$$T(\alpha_m) = c_{m1}\beta_1 + c_{m2}\beta_2 + ... + c_{mn}\beta_n$$

Now, we extend T linearly to the entire space V. Further, the linear transformation T is unique. Hence every matrix can be associated to a linear transformation.

WORKED EXAMPLES

Example 1: Find the matrix of the linear transformation $T : V_2'(R) \to V_2(R)$ defined by $T(x, y) = (x, -y)$ w.r.t. the standard basis of $V_2(R)$.

Solution:

$$T(x, y) = (x, -y)$$
$$T(e_1) = T(1, 0) = (1, 0)$$
$$T(e_2) = T(0, 1) = (0, -1)$$

∴ The matrix of linear transformation is $\begin{bmatrix} 1 & 0 \\ 0 & -1 \end{bmatrix}$

Example 2: Find the matrix of the linear transformation
$$T : V_2(R) \to V_3(R)$$
such that $T(-1, 1) = (-1, 0, 2)$ and $T(2, 1) = (1, 2, 1)$
Solution:

$$(-1, 1) = -1e_1 + 1e_2$$
$$(2, 1) = 2e_1 + 1e_2$$
$$T(1, 1) = T(-e_1 + e_2) \text{ and } T(2, 1) = T(2e_1 + e_2)$$

i.e. $T(e_1) + T(e_2) = (-1, 0, 2)$ ...(1)

$2T(e_1) + T(e_2) = (1, 2, 1)$ ...(2)

Solving these for $T(e_1)$ and $T(e_2)$
Subtracting Eq. (1) from Eq. (2)

$$3T(e_1) = (2, 2, -1)$$

$$T(e_1) = \left(\frac{2}{3}, \frac{2}{3}, \frac{-1}{3} \right)$$

$$T(e_2) = (-1, 0, 2) + \left(\frac{2}{3}, \frac{2}{3}, \frac{-1}{3} \right)$$

$$= \left(\frac{-1}{3}, \frac{2}{3}, \frac{5}{3} \right)$$

∴ The matrix of linear transformation is

$$\begin{bmatrix} \dfrac{2}{3} & \dfrac{2}{3} & \dfrac{-1}{3} \\ \dfrac{-1}{3} & \dfrac{2}{3} & \dfrac{5}{3} \end{bmatrix} = \begin{bmatrix} \dfrac{2}{3} & \dfrac{-1}{3} \\ \dfrac{2}{3} & \dfrac{2}{3} \\ \dfrac{-1}{3} & \dfrac{5}{3} \end{bmatrix}$$

Example 3: Find the matrix of the linear transformation $T : V_3(R) \to V_2(R)$ defined by $T(x, y, z) = (x + y, y + z)$ w.r.t. standard basis.

Solution: The standard basis are $(1, 0, 0), (0, 1, 0), (0, 0, 1)$

∴ $T(1, 0, 0) = (1 + 0, 0 + 0) = (1, 0)$

$$T(0, 1, 0) = (0 + 1, 1 + 0) = (1, 1)$$
$$T(0, 0, 1) = (0 + 0, 0 + 1) = (0, 1)$$

$\therefore$ The matrix of the linear transfromation is

$$\begin{bmatrix} 1 & 0 \\ 1 & 1 \\ 0 & 1 \end{bmatrix} = \begin{bmatrix} 1 & 1 & 0 \\ 0 & 1 & 1 \end{bmatrix}$$

Example 4: Find the matrix of the linear transformation $T : R_4 \to R_3$ defined by

$T(x_1, x_2, x_3, x_4) = (x_1 + x_2 + 2x_3 + 3x_4, x_1 + x_3 - x_4, x_1 + 2x_2)$ w.r.t. the basis $B_1 = \{(1, 1, 1, 2), (1, -1, 0, 0), (0, 0, 1, 1), (0, 1, 0, 0)\}$ and $B_2 = \{(1, 2, 3), (1, -1, 1), (2, 1, 1)\}$

Solution:

$$B_1 = \{(1,1,1,2),(1,-1,0,0),(0,0,1,1)(0,1,0,0)\}$$
$$B_2 = \{(1,2,3),(1,-1,1),(2,1,1)\}$$
$$T(1, 1, 1, 2) = (1+1+2+6, 1+1-2, 1+2) = (10, 0, 3)$$
$$T(1, -1, 0, 0) = (1-1+0+0, 1+0-0, 1-2) = (0, 1, -1)$$
$$T(0, 0, 1, 1) = (0+0+2+3, 1+0+-1, 0+0) = (5, 0, 0)$$
$$T(0, 1, 0, 0) = (0+1+0+0, 0+0-0, 0+2) = (1, 0, 2)$$

Now $(10, 0, 3) = a(1,2,3) + b(1,-1,1) + c(2,1,1)$

$$= (a+b+2c, 2a-b+c, 3a+b+c)$$

$\therefore \quad a+b+2c = 10$, $2a-b+c = 0$, $3a+b+c = 3$

Solving for a, b, c we get $a = \dfrac{-11}{9}$, $b = \dfrac{19}{9}$, $c = \dfrac{41}{9}$

$\therefore \quad (10, 0, 3) = \dfrac{-11}{9}(1,2,3) + \dfrac{19}{9}(1,-1,1) + \dfrac{41}{9}(2,1,1)$

$(0, 1, -1) = a(1,2,3) + b(1,-1,1) + c(2,1,1)$

$$= (a+b+2c, 2a-b+c, 3a+b+c)$$

$a+b+2c = 0$, $2a-b+c = 1$, $3a+b+c = -1$

Solving these equations, we get

$$a = \dfrac{-2}{9}, \quad b = \dfrac{-8}{9}, \quad c = \dfrac{5}{9}$$

$\therefore \quad (0, 1, -1) = \dfrac{-2}{9}(1,2,3) - \dfrac{8}{9}(1,-1,1) + \dfrac{5}{9}(2,1,1)$

Similarly, we have

$$(5, 0, 0) = (a + b + 2c, 2a - b + c, 3a + b + c)$$

$$a + b + 2c = 5, \quad 2a - b + c = 0, \quad 3a + b + c = 0$$

Solving these equations, we get $a = \dfrac{-10}{9}, \ b = \dfrac{5}{9}, \ c = \dfrac{25}{9}$

$$\therefore \quad (5, 0, 0) = -\frac{10}{9}(1,2,3) + \frac{5}{9}(1,-1,1) + \frac{25}{9}(2,1,1) \text{ and}$$

similarly, we have

$$(1, 0, 2) = (a + b + 2c, 2a - b + c, 3a + b + c)$$

$$a + b + 2c = 1, \ 2a - b + c = 0, \ 3a + b + c = 2$$

Solving these, we get $a = \dfrac{4}{9}, \ b = \dfrac{7}{9}, \ c = \dfrac{-1}{9}$

$$\therefore \quad (1, 0, 2) = \frac{4}{9}(1,2,3) + \frac{7}{9}(1,-1,1) - \frac{1}{9}(2,1,1)$$

∴ The matrix of the linear transformation is

$$\frac{1}{9}\begin{bmatrix} -11 & 19 & 41 \\ -2 & -8 & 5 \\ -10 & 5 & 25 \\ 4 & 7 & -1 \end{bmatrix} = \frac{1}{9}\begin{bmatrix} -11 & -2 & -10 & 4 \\ 19 & -8 & 5 & 7 \\ 41 & 5 & 25 & -1 \end{bmatrix}$$

Example 5: Find the linear transformation for the matrix $A = \begin{bmatrix} -1 & 0 \\ 2 & 0 \\ 1 & 3 \end{bmatrix}$ with

respect to

(i) $B_1 = \{(1,0,0),(0,1,0),(0,0,1)\}$ and

  $B_2 = \{(1,0),(0,1)\}$

(ii) $B_1 = \{(1,2,0),(0,-1,0),(1,-1,1)\}$ and

  $B_2 = \{(1,0),(2,-1)\}$

Solution:

(i) The given bases are:

  $B_1 = \{(1,0,0),(0,1,0),(0,0,1)\}$

  $B_2 = \{(1,0),(0,1)\}$

  Define the linear transformation

  $T : V_3 \to V_2(R)$ by

  $T(1, 0, 0) = (-1)(1, 0) + 0(0, 1) = (-1, 0)$

$$T(0, 1, 0) = 2(1, 0) + 0(0, 1) = (2, 0)$$
$$T(0, 0, 1) = 1(1, 0) + 3(0, 1) = (1, 3)$$
$$\therefore \quad T(e_1) = (-1, 0)$$
$$T(e_2) = (2, 0)$$
$$T(e_3) = (1, 3)$$

The matrix $A = \begin{bmatrix} -1 & 0 \\ 2 & 0 \\ 1 & 3 \end{bmatrix}$

Now
$$\begin{aligned} T(x, y, z) &= T(xe_1 + ye_2 + ze_3) \\ &= xT(e_1) + yT(e_2) + zT(e_3) \\ &= x(-1,0) + y(2,0) + z(1,3) \\ &= (-x + 2y + z, 3z) \\ T(x, y, z) &= (-x + 2y + z, 3z) \end{aligned}$$

(ii) The bases are $B_1 = \{(1,2,0),(0,-1,0),(1,-1,1)\}$
$$B_2 = \{(1,0),(2,-1)\}$$
Define the linear transformation $T : V_3(R) \to V_2(R)$ by
$$T(1, 2, 0) = (-1)(1, 0) + 0(2, -1) = (-1, 0)$$
$$T(0, -1, 0) = 2(1, 0) + 0(2, -1) = (2, 0)$$
$$T(1, -1, 1) = 1(1, 0) + 3(2, -1) = (7, -3)$$
Now
$$(1, 2, 0) = 1(1, 0, 0) + 2(0, 1, 0) + 0(0, 0, 1)$$
$$T(1, 2, 0) = T(1e_1 + 2e_2 + 0e_3)$$
i.e. $T(e_1) + 2T(e_2) = (-1, 0)$ ...(1)
$$(0, -1, 0) = 0(1, 0, 0) + (-1)(0, 1, 0) + 0(0, 0, 1)$$
$$= 0e_1 - 1e_2 + 0e_3$$
$$\therefore \quad T(0, -1, 0) = T(0e_1 - 1e_2 + 0e_3)$$
$$\Rightarrow \quad -T(e_2) = (2, 0) \qquad \text{...(2)}$$
$$(1, -1, 1) = 1(1, 0, 0) + (-1)(0, 1, 0) + 1(0, 0, 1)$$
$$= 1e_1 - 1e_2 + 1e_3$$
$$\therefore \quad T(1, -1, 1) = T(e_1 - e_2 + e_3)$$
$$\Rightarrow \quad T(e_1) - T(e_2) + T(e_3) = (7, -3) \qquad \text{...(3)}$$
Solving equations (1), (2) and (3), we get
From Eq. (2), $T(e_2) = (-2, 0)$
From Eq. (1), $T(e_1) + 2(-2, 0) = (-1, 0)$
$$\Rightarrow \quad T(e_1) = (3, 0)$$

From Eq. (3), we get $(3, 0) + (2, 0) + T(e_3) = (7, -3)$

$\therefore \qquad T(e_3) = (7, -3) - (3, 0) - (2, 0)$

$\Rightarrow \qquad T(e_3) = (2, -3)$

$\therefore \qquad T(x, y, z) = T(xe_1 + ye_2 + ze_3)$

$\qquad\qquad\qquad = xT(e_1) + yT(e_2) + zT(e_3)$

$\qquad\qquad\qquad = x(3, 0) + y(-2, 0) + z(2, -3)$

$\qquad\qquad\qquad = (3x - 2y + 2z, -3z)$

Example 6 : Find the linear transformation of the matrix $A = \begin{bmatrix} 0 & 1 & -1 \\ 1 & 0 & 0 \\ 1 & -1 & 0 \end{bmatrix}$

w.r.t. (i) standard bases $B_1 = B_2 = \{e_1, e_2, e_3\}$

(ii) $B_1 = B_2 = \{(0, 1, -1), (-1, 1, 0), (-1, -1, 0)\}$

Solution:

(i) Bases $B_1 = B_2 = \{(1, 0, 0), (0, 1, 0), (0, 0, 1)\} = \{e_1, e_2, e_3\}$

Define linear transformation $T : V_3(R) \to V_3(R)$ by

$T(e_1) = T(1, 0, 0) = 0e_1 + 1e_2 - 1e_3 = (0, 1, -1)$

$T(e_2) = T(0, 1, 0) = 1e_1 + -1e_2 - 0e_3 = (1, 0, 0)$

$T(e_3) = T(0, 0, 1) = 1e_1 + 0e_2 - 0e_3 = (1, -1, 0)$

$T(x, y, z) = T(xe_1 + ye_2 + ze_3)$

$\qquad\qquad = x(0, 1, -1) + y(1, 0, 0) + z(1, -1, 0)$

$\qquad\qquad = (y + z, x - z, -x)$ is the required linear transformation.

(ii) Bases $B_1 = B_2 = \{(0, 1, -1), (-1, 1, 0), (-1, -1, 0)\}$

Define the linear transformation $T : V_3(R) \to V_3(R)$ by

$T(0, 1, -1) = 0(0, 1, -1) + 1(-1, 1, 0) + (-1)(-1, -1, 0)$

$\qquad\qquad = (0, 2, 0)$

$T(-1, 1, 0) = 1(0, 1, -1) + 0(-1, 1, 0) + 0(-1, -1, 0)$

$\qquad\qquad = (0, 1, -1)$

$T(-1, -1, 0) = 1(0, 1, -1) - 1(-1, 1, 0) + 0(-1, -1, 0)$

$\qquad\qquad = (1, 0, -1)$

Now $\qquad (0, 1, -1) = 0e_1 + 1e_2 - 1e_3$

$\therefore \qquad T(0, 1, -1) = 0T(e_1) + 1T(e_2) - 1T(e_3)$

i.e. $T(e_2) - T(e_3) = (0, 2, 0)$ $\qquad\qquad\qquad\qquad$ ...(1)

$\qquad (-1, +1, 0) = -1e_1 + 1e_2 + 0e_3$

$\therefore \qquad T(-1, 1, 0) = -T(e_1) + T(e_2) + 0T(e_3)$

$\therefore \quad -T(e_1) + T(e_2) = (0, 1, -1)$ $\qquad\qquad\qquad$ ...(2)

$$(-1, -1, 0) = -1e_1 - 1e_2 + 0e_3$$

$$\therefore \quad T(-1, -1, 0) = -T(e_1) - T(e_2) + 0T(e_3)$$

i.e. $-T(e_1) - T(e_2) = (1, 0, -1)$ ...(3)

Solving equations (1), (2) and (3), we get

$$T(e_1) = \left(\frac{-1}{2}, \frac{-1}{2}, 1\right), \quad T(e_2) = \left(\frac{-1}{2}, \frac{-1}{2}, 0\right)$$

$$T(e_3) = \left(\frac{-1}{2}, \frac{-3}{2}, 0\right)$$

$$\therefore \quad T(x, y, z) = T(xe_1 + ye_2 + ze_3)$$

$$= x\left(\frac{-1}{2}, \frac{-1}{2}, +1\right) + y\left(\frac{-1}{2}, \frac{1}{2}, 0\right) + z\left(\frac{-1}{2}, \frac{-3}{2}, 0\right)$$

i.e. $\quad T(x, y, z) = \left(-\frac{x}{2} - \frac{y}{2} - \frac{z}{2}, -\frac{x}{2} + \frac{y}{2} - \frac{3z}{2}, x\right)$

is the linear transformation.

6.4 RANK NULLITY OF A LINEAR TRANSFORMATION

To a linear transformation $T : U \to V$, associated two sets are called the range space and the null space.

6.4.1 Range Space

Definition: Let $T : U \to V$ be a linear transformation. Then the range of T is the set of all images of the elements of U and is denoted by $R(T)$ $R(T) = \{T(\alpha) : \alpha \in U\}$, $R(T)$ is also called the **"range space"**. Clearly $R(T) \subseteq V$.

6.4.2 Null Space

Definition: Let $T : U \to V$ be a linear transformation. Then the kernel of T is the set of all elements of U whose images under T are the zero element of V and is denoted by $N(T)$. $N(T)$ is also called the "**null space**".

i.e. $\quad N(T) = \{\alpha \in U : T(\alpha) = 0'\}$

Clearly $N(T)$ is non-empty $\because 0 \in U : T(0) = 0'$ and $N(T) \subseteq U$

Theorem 1: If $T : U \to V$ is a linear transformation, then $R(T)$ is a subspace of V and $N(T)$ is a subspace of U.

Proof:

(i) To prove that $R(T)$ is a subspace of U.

Let $\quad\quad\quad\quad\quad v_1, v_2 \in R(T)$

$\therefore$ There exists $u_1, u_2 \in U$ such that

$$T(u_1) = v_1 \text{ and } T(u_2) = v_2$$

Now, $v_1 + v_2 = T(u_1) + T(u_2) = T(u_1 + u_2)$ $\because T$ is linear

$$= T(u)$$

$\therefore$ There exists some vector $u \in U$ such that

$$T(u) = v_1 + v_2$$

$$\therefore \qquad v_1 + v_2 \in R(T)$$

Let K be any scalar.

Then $Kv_1 \in V$ since V is a vector space.

$$\therefore \qquad Kv_1 = T(Ku_1)$$

$$\therefore \qquad Kv_1 \in R(T)$$

$R(T)$ is closed under addition and scalar multiplication. Hence, $R(T)$ is a subspace of V.

(ii) Let $u_1, u_2 \in N(T)$

$$\therefore T(u_1) = 0' \text{ and } T(u_2) = 0'$$

Now $T(u_1 + u_2) = T(u_1) + T(u_2)$ $\because T$ is linear

$$= 0' + 0'$$

$$= 0'$$

$\therefore u_1 + u_2 \in N(T)$

Let c be any scalar.

$$T(cu_1) = cT(u_1) \quad \because T \text{ is linear}$$

$$= C \cdot 0' = 0'$$

$\therefore cu_1 \in N(T)$

$\therefore N(T)$ is closed w.r.t. addition and scalar multiplication.

$\therefore N(T)$ is a subspace of U.

Theorem 2: Let $T : U \to V$ be a linear transformation. Then T is one-one if and only if $N(T) = \{0\}$, where 0 is the zero element of U.

Proof: Part I: Let T be one-one

$$T(\alpha_1) = T(\alpha_2) \Rightarrow \alpha_1 = \alpha_2 \quad \forall \alpha_1, \alpha_2 \in U$$

Let $\alpha \in N(T)$

$$\therefore \qquad T(\alpha) = 0' \text{ But } T(0) = 0'$$

$$\therefore \qquad T(\alpha) = T(0)$$

$\Rightarrow \alpha = 0$ as T is one-one

$\therefore$ We have proved that $\alpha \in N(T)$, then $\alpha = 0$

$$\therefore \qquad N(T) = \{0\}$$

Part II: Let $N(T) = \{0\}$

$$T(\alpha_1) = T(\alpha_2) \Rightarrow T(\alpha_1) - T(\alpha_2) = 0'$$

$$\Rightarrow T(\alpha_1) + (-T(\alpha_2)) = 0'$$

$$\Rightarrow T(\alpha_1) + T(-\alpha_2) = 0' \text{ since } -T(\alpha_2) = T(-\alpha_2)$$

$$\Rightarrow T(\alpha_1 - \alpha_2) = 0' \text{ since } T \text{ is linear}$$

$$\Rightarrow \alpha_1 - \alpha_2 \in N(T)$$

But $N(T) = \{0\}$ consisting of only one element 0

$$\therefore \quad \alpha_1 - \alpha_2 = 0$$

$$\therefore \quad \alpha_1 = \alpha_2$$

Hence $T(\alpha_1) = T(\alpha_2) \Rightarrow \alpha_1 = \alpha_2 \qquad \therefore \ T$ is one-one.

6.4.3 Nullity

Definition: If $T : U \to V$ is a linear transformation from a vector space U into another vector space V, then the dimension of the range space $R(T)$ is called the rank of T and is denoted by $r(T)$ and the dimension of the null space or the kernel of T is called the nullity of T and is denoted by $n(T)$.

Theorem 3: Let $T : U \to V$ be a linear transformation. If the vectors α_1, $\alpha_2,...,\alpha_m$ generates U, then the vectors $T(\alpha_1)$, $T(\alpha_2),...,T(\alpha_n)$ generates $R(T)$.

Proof: Let $S = \{\alpha_1, \alpha_2,...,\alpha_n\}$.

Since S spans U, every vector $\alpha \in U$ can be expressed as a linear combination of the vectors $\alpha_1, \alpha_2,...,\alpha_n$.

Now $T(\alpha_1), T(\alpha_2),...,T(\alpha_n) \in R(T)$

Since $R(T)$ is a subspace, any linear combination of these vectors is also $R(T)$.

Let $\beta \in R(T)$. This implies that there exists an $\alpha \in U$ such that $T(\alpha) = \beta$.

Since $\alpha \in U$, $\alpha = c_1\alpha_1 + c_2\alpha_2 + ... + c_n\alpha_n$

Since $\beta \in R(T)$

$$\beta = T(\alpha) = T(c_1\alpha_1 + c_2\alpha_2 + ... + c_n\alpha_n)$$

$$= c_1 T(\alpha_1) + c_2 T(\alpha_2) + ... + c_n T(\alpha_n) \text{ since } T \text{ is linear}$$

$\therefore \ \beta \in R(T) \Rightarrow \beta$ is a linear combination of $T(\alpha_1), T(\alpha_2),...,T(\alpha_n)$

i.e. $\beta \in R(T) \Rightarrow \beta$ is the linear span of $T(\alpha_1), T(\alpha_2),...,T(\alpha_n)$

$\therefore \ R(T)$ is in the span of $T(\alpha_1)$, $T(\alpha_2),...,T(\alpha_n)$

$\therefore \ T(\alpha_1)$, $T(\alpha_2),...,T(\alpha_n)$ generates $R(T)$

Theorem 4: Rank-Nullity Theorem

Let $T : U \to V$ be a linear transformation and U be a finite dimensional vector space.

Then $\dim R(T) + \dim N(T) = \dim U$

i.e. $r(T) + n(T) = \dim U$

or rank + nullity = dim (domain)

Proof: Let U be a vector space of dimension m, i.e. dim $U = m$.

Since $N(T)$ is a subspace of the finite dimensional vector space U, dimension of $N(T)$ is also finite.

Let dim$\left[n(T)\right] = n$, i.e. nullity $n(T) = n$

Since $N(T)$ is a subspace of U, $n \leq m$.

Let $B_1 = \{\alpha_1, \alpha_2, ..., \alpha_n\}$ be a basis of $N(T)$.

$\therefore B_1$ is linearly independent in $N(T)$ and hence is linearly independent in U.

We shall extend this set B_1 to a basis of the vector space U.

Let this basis of U be

$$B_2 = \{\alpha_1, \ \alpha_2, ..., \alpha_n, \ \beta_1, \ \beta_2, \beta_3, ..., \beta_s\}$$

Clearly $\quad n + s = m$ ...(1)

Now $\qquad T(\alpha_1), T(\alpha_2), ..., T(\alpha_n), T(\beta_1), T(\beta_2), ..., T(\beta_s)$

But $\qquad T(\alpha_1) = 0'$, $T(\alpha_1) = 0', ..., T(\alpha_n) = 0'$

Since $\qquad \alpha_1, \alpha_2, ..., \alpha_n \in N(T)$

Let $\qquad S = \{T(\beta_1), T(\beta_2), ..., T(\beta_s)\}$

We shall show that this set S of s vectors is a basis of $R(T)$

(i) S spans $R(T)$

Since B_2 is a basis of U, it spans U. Hence the set

$$\{T(\alpha_1), T(\alpha_2), ..., T(\alpha_n), T(\beta_1), T(\beta_2), ..., T(\beta_s)\}$$

spans $R(T)$

Since $T(\alpha_1) = T(\alpha_2) = ... = T(\alpha_n) = 0'$

$\therefore$ The set $S = \{T(\beta_1), T(\beta_2), ..., T(\beta_s)\}$

(ii) S is linearly independent

Consider $c_1 T(\beta_1) + c_2 T(\beta_2) + ... + c_s T(\beta_s) = 0$

$\Rightarrow (c_1\beta_1) + c_2(\beta_2) + ... + c_s T(\beta_s) = 0 \quad \because T$ is linear

$\Rightarrow c_1\beta_1 + c_2\beta_2 + ... + c_s\beta_s$ can be expressed as linear combination of the elements of the basis B_1 of $N(T)$

$\therefore \ c_1\beta_1 + c_2\beta_2 + ... + c_s\beta_s = d_1\alpha_1 + d_2\alpha_2 + ... + d_n\alpha_n$

$\Rightarrow d_1\alpha_1 + d_2\alpha_2 + ... + d_n\alpha_n - c_1\beta_1 - c_2\beta_2, -..., -c_s\beta_s = 0$

Since B_2 is a basis of U, it is linearly independent

$\therefore \ d_1 = 0$, $d_2 = 0, ..., d_n = 0$, $c_1 = 0$, $c_2 = 0, ..., c_s = 0$

$\therefore \ c_1 T(\beta_1) + c_2 T(\beta_2) + ... + c_s T(\beta_s) = 0$

$\Rightarrow c_1 = 0$, $c_2 = 0, ..., c_s = 0$

∴ S is linearly independent.

∴ S is a basis of $R(T)$.

∴ $\dim[R(T)] = s$

Hence from Eq. (1), we get

$$\dim[N(T)] + \dim[R(T)] = \dim U$$

i.e. $\qquad n(T) + r(T) = m$

(or) rank + nullity = dim (domain)

WORKED EXAMPLES

Example 1: Find the range space, kernel, rank and nullity of the following linear transformations. Also verify the rank-nullity theorem.

$$T : V_2(R) \to V_2(R) \text{ defined by } T(x_1, x_2) = (x_1 + x_2, x_1)$$

Solution: We shall find the matrices of T w.r.t. the standard basis $\{(1, 0),$ $(0, 1)\}$ of $V_2(R)$

$$T(1, 0) = (1 + 0, 1) = (1, 1)$$
$$T(0, 1) = (0 + 1, 0) = (1, 0)$$

∴ The matrix A of T is $\begin{bmatrix} 1 & 1 \\ 1 & 0 \end{bmatrix}$

$$A = \begin{bmatrix} 1 & 1 \\ 1 & 0 \end{bmatrix} \simeq \begin{bmatrix} 1 & 1 \\ 0 & -1 \end{bmatrix} \quad [R_1 \to R_2 - R_1]$$

This is in the echelon form.

There are two non-zero rows.

∴ Rank of $T = 2$

Hence $R(T)$ is the subspace generated by $(1, 1)$ and $(0, -1)$

$$R(T) = \{x_1(1, 1) + x_1(0, -1)\}$$
$$= \{(x_1, x_2) + (0, -x_2)\}$$
$$= \{x_1, x_1 - x_2\} \text{ for all } x_1, x_2 \in R$$

i.e. the range space = $\{x_1, x_1 - x_2\} = V_2(R)$

To find $N(T)$

Let $\qquad T(x_1, x_2) = 0$

$\Rightarrow \quad (x_1 + x_2, x_1) = (0, 0)$

$\Rightarrow x_1 + x_2 = 0, \ x_1 = 0$

$\Rightarrow \quad x_1 = 0, \ x_2 = 0$

∴ $N(T)$ contains only zero element of $V_2(R)$.

∴ $\qquad N(T) = \{(0, 0)\}$

i.e. the null space = $\{(0, 0)\}$

$\therefore \qquad \dim[N(T)] = 0$, i.e. nullity $= 0$

$\therefore$ Rank + nullity $= 2 + 0 = 2 = \dim V_2(R)$

Hence the rank-nullity theorem is verified.

Example 2: $T : R^3 \to R^3$ defined by $T(x, y, z) = (x + y, x - y, 2x + z)$. Find the range space, null-space, rank and nullity of T and verify rank of T + nullity of $T = \dim(R^3)$.

Solution: Let us find the matrix A of the linear transformation w.r.t. the standard basis $\{(1, 0, 0), (0, 1, 0), (0, 0, 1)\}$

$$T(1, 0, 0) = (1 + 0, 1 - 0, 2 + 0) = (1, 1, 2)$$
$$T(0, 1, 0) = (0 + 1, 0 - 1, 0 + 0) = (1, -1, 0)$$
$$T(0, 0, 1) = (0 + 0, 0 - 0, 0 + 1) = (0, 0, 1)$$

$\therefore$ The matrix A of T is $A = \begin{bmatrix} 1 & 1 & 2 \\ 1 & -1 & 0 \\ 0 & 0 & 1 \end{bmatrix} R_2 \to R_2 - R_1$

$$\simeq \begin{bmatrix} 1 & 1 & 2 \\ 0 & -2 & -2 \\ 0 & 0 & 1 \end{bmatrix}$$

This is in echelon form and there are three non-zero rows.

$\therefore \qquad \dim[R(T)] = 3$, i.e. rank of $T = 3$

$\therefore R(T) =$ the subspace generated by $(1, 1, 2), (0, -2, -2), (0, 0, 1)$

$\qquad = x_1(1,1,2) + x_2(0,-2,-2) + x_3(0,0,1)$

$\qquad = (x_1, x_1 - 2x_2, 2x_1 - 2x_2 + x_3) : x_1, x_2, x_3 \in R$

i.e. the range space $= \{(x_1, x_1 - 2x_2, 2x_1 - 2x_2 + x_3) : x_1, x_2, x_3 \in R\} = R^3$

To find $N(T)$

Consider $T(x_1, x_2, x_3) = (x_1 + x_2, x_1 - x_2, 2x_1 + x_3) = (0,0,0)$

$\qquad\qquad\qquad = x_1 + x_2 = 0, \; x_1 - x_2 = 0, \; 2x_1 + x_3 = 0$

$\Rightarrow x_1 = 0, \; x_2 = 0, \; x_3 = 0$

$\therefore T(x_1, x_2, x_3) = \{(0,0,0)\}$ consisting of only zero elements.

$\therefore \dim[N(T)] = 0$, i.e. nullity $= 0$

$\qquad$ and $N(T) = \{(0, 0, 0)\}$

i.e. null space $= \{(0, 0, 0)\}$

Rank + nullity $= 3 + 0 = 3 = \dim(R^3)$

Hence the rank-nullity theorem is verified.

Example 3: $T : V_3(R) \to V_4(R)$ is defined by

$$T(e_1) = (0, 1, 0, 2)$$
$$T(e_2) = (0, 1, 1, 0)$$
$$T(e_3) = (0, 1, -1, 4)$$

Find range space, null space, rank and nullity of T and verify the rank-nullity theorem.

Solution: The matrix A of linear transformation is

$$A = \begin{bmatrix} 0 & 1 & 0 & 2 \\ 0 & 1 & 1 & 0 \\ 0 & 1 & -1 & 4 \end{bmatrix} \begin{matrix} \\ R_2 \to R_2 - R_1 \\ R_3 \to R_3 - R_1 \end{matrix}$$

$$\simeq \begin{bmatrix} 0 & 1 & 0 & 2 \\ 0 & 0 & 1 & -2 \\ 0 & 0 & -1 & 2 \end{bmatrix} R_3 \to R_3 + R_2$$

$$\simeq \begin{bmatrix} 0 & 1 & 0 & 2 \\ 0 & 0 & 1 & -2 \\ 0 & 0 & 0 & 0 \end{bmatrix}$$

This is in the echelon form.

These are two non-zero rows.

Hence $\dim[R(T)] = 2$, i.e. rank $T = 2$

$R(T)$ = the subspace generated by $(0, 1, 0, 2)$ and $(0, 0, 1, -2)$

$$= \{x_1(0,1,0,2) + x_2(0,0,1,-2) : x_1, x_2 \in R\}$$

$$= \{(0, x_1, x_2, 2x_1 - 2x_2) : x_1, x_2 \in R\}$$

To find $N(T)$

$$T(x_1, x_2, x_3) = 0 \Rightarrow T[x_1(1,0,0) + x_2(0,1,0) + x_3(0,0,1)] = (0,0,0,0)$$
$$x_1 T(1,0,0) + x_2 T(0,1,0) + x_3 T(0,0,1) = (0,0,0,0)$$
$$x_1(0,1,0,2) + x_2(0,1,1,0) + x_3(0,1,-1,4) = (0,0,0,0)$$
$$(0, x_1 + x_2 + x_3, x_2 - x_3, 2x_1 + 4x_3) = (0,0,0,0)$$
$$x_1 + x_2 + x_3 = 0, \ x_2 - x_3 = 0, \ 2x_1 + 4x_3 = 0$$
$$x_1 = -2x_3, \ x_2 = x_3, \ 2x_1 + 4x_3 = 0$$
$$x_1 = -2x_3, \ x_2 = x_3, \ x_3 = x_3$$

$\therefore N(T) = \{(-2x_3, x_3, x_3) : x_3 \in R\}$

$\therefore$ dim$[N(T)] = 1$, i.e. nullity of $T = 1$

$\therefore$ rank of $T +$ nullity of $T = 2 + 1 = 3 = $ dim$[V_3(R)]$

Hence the rank-nullity theorem is verified.

Example 4: $T : V_3(R) \rightarrow V_2(R)$ is defined by

$T(e_1) = (2, 1)$

$T(e_2) = (0, 1)$

$T(e_3) = (1, 1)$

Find the range space, kernel, rank and nullity of T and verify rank + nullity = dim(domain).

Solution: The matrix of T w.r.t. $\{e_1, e_2, e_3\}$ is

$$A = \begin{bmatrix} 2 & 1 \\ 0 & 1 \\ 1 & 1 \end{bmatrix} \quad R_1 \leftrightarrow R_3$$

$$\sim \begin{bmatrix} 1 & 1 \\ 0 & 1 \\ 2 & 1 \end{bmatrix} \quad R_3 \rightarrow R_3 - 2R_1$$

$$\sim \begin{bmatrix} 1 & 1 \\ 0 & 1 \\ 0 & -1 \end{bmatrix} \quad R_3 \rightarrow R_2 + R_1$$

$$\sim \begin{bmatrix} 1 & 1 \\ 0 & 1 \\ 0 & 0 \end{bmatrix}$$

This is the echelon form and there are 2 non-zero rows in it.

$\therefore$ dim$[R(T)] = 2$, i.e. rank of $T = 2$

$\therefore$ Range space $= \{x_1(1,1) + x_2(0,1)\}$

$\qquad\qquad\quad = \{x_1, x_2 + x_2 : x_1, x_2 \in R\}$

To find kernel,

$T(x_1, x_2, x_3) = T(x_1 e_1 + x_2 e_2 + x_3 e_3)$

$\qquad\qquad\quad = x_1 T(e_1) + x_2 T(e_2) + x_3 T(e_3)$

$\qquad\qquad\quad = x_1(2,1) + x_2(0,1) + x_3(1,1)$

$\qquad\qquad\quad = (2x_1 + x_3, x_1 + x_2 + x_3)$

$$T(x_1, x_2, x_3) = 0 \Rightarrow (2x_1 + x_3, x_1 + x_2 + x_3) = (0, 0)$$

$$\Rightarrow \quad 2x_1 + x_3 = 0, \; x_1 + x_2 + x_3 = 0$$

$$\Rightarrow \quad x_1 = x_1, \; x_2 = x_1, \; x_3 = -2x_1$$

$$\therefore \quad T(x_1, x_2, x_3) = 0 \Rightarrow (x_1, x_2, x_3) = (x_1, x_1, -2x_1)$$

$$\therefore \qquad N(T) = \left\{ (x_1, x_1, -2x_1) : x_1 \in R \right\}$$

In particular, if $x_1 = 1$, $N(T) = \left\{ 1, 1, -2 \right\}$

$\therefore \; \dim[N(T)] = 1$, i.e. nullity of $T = 1$

$\therefore$ rank + nullity = 2 + 1 = 3 = dim (domain)

Hence the rank-nullity theorem is verified.

Example 5: Find the linear transformation $T : V_3(R) \to V_2(R)$ whose images are generated by the vectors $(0, 1)$, $(1, 1)$.

Solution: Consider the standard basis $\{(1, 0, 0), (0, 1, 0), (0, 0, 1)\}$ of $V_3(R)$.

Define $T(1, 0, 0) = (0, 1)$

$\qquad T(0, 1, 0) = (1, 1)$

$\qquad T(0, 0, 1) = (0, 0)$

$$T(x, y, z) = T[x(1, 0, 0) + y(0, 1, 0) + z(0, 0, 1)]$$

$$= xT(1, 0, 0) + yT(0, 1, 0) + zT(0, 0, 1)$$

$$= x(0, 1) + y(1, 1) + z(0, 0) = (0 + y + 0, x + y + 0)$$

i.e. $\qquad T(x, y, z) = (y, x + y)$

Example 6: Find the linear transformation $T : R^4 \to R^3$ whose null space is generated by $(1, 2, 0, -4)$, $(2, 0, -1, -3)$.

Solution: Define $T : R^4 \to R^3$ such that

$\qquad T(1, 2, 0, -4) = (0, 0, 0)$ and

$\qquad T(2, 0, -1, -3) = (0, 0, 0)$

Consider the basis of R^4 with $(1, 2, 0, -4)$ and $(2, 0, -1, -3)$ as two vectors and including $(1, 0, 0, 0)$, $(0, 1, 0, 0)$, $(0, 0, 1, 0)$ and $(0, 0, 0, 1)$ to them.

That is $S = \{(1, 2, 0, -4), (2, 0, -1, -3), (1, 0, 0, 0), (0, 1, 0, 0), (0, 0, 1, 0), (0, 0, 0, 1)\}$ spans R^4 but linearly dependent.

To make it linearly independent, delete those vectors in 'S' which can be expressed as linear combination of the preceding ones so that we get the required basis.

Consider

$\qquad (2, 0, -1, -3) = a(1, 2, 0, -4)$

$\Rightarrow (2, 0, -1, -3) = (a, 2a, 0, -4a)$

$\Rightarrow a = 2, 2a = 0, 0 = -1, -4a = -3$ which is impossible.

Consider

$(1, 0, 0, 0) = a(1, 2, 0, -4) + b(2, 0, -1, -3)$
$$= (a + 2b, 2a - b, -4a - 3b)$$

$\Rightarrow a + 2b = 1, 2a = 0, -b = 0, -4a - 3b = 0$

$\Rightarrow a = 1, a = 0, b = 0$, which is impossible.

Consider $(0, 1, 0, 0) = a(1, 2, 0, -4) + b(2, 0, -1, -3) + c(1, 0, 0, 0)$

$\Rightarrow (0, 1, 0, 0) = (a + 2b + c, 2a - b, -4a - 3b)$

$\Rightarrow a + 2b + c = 0, 2a = 1, -b = 0, -4a - 3b = 0$

$\Rightarrow a = 1/2, b = 0, a = 0$ which is impossible.

Consider

$(0, 0, 1, 0) = a(1, 2, 0, -4) + b(2, 0, -1, -3) + c(1, 0, 0, 0) + d(0, 1, 0, 0)$

$\Rightarrow (0, 0, 1, 0) = (a + 2b + c, 2a + d, -b, -4a - 3b)$

$\Rightarrow a + 2b + c = 0, 2a + d = 0, -b = 1, -4a - 3b = 0$

$\Rightarrow a = 3/4, b = -1, c = 5/4, d = 3/2$

$\therefore (0, 0, 1, 0)$ is expressed as a linear combination of its preceding ones.

Hence $\{(1, 2, 0, -4), (2, 0, -1, -3), (1, 0, 0, 0), (0, 1, 0, 0)\}$ is a basis of R^4.

For this basis $T : R^4 \rightarrow R^3$ is defined as

$T(1, 2, 0, -4) = (0, 0, 0), T(2, 0, -1, -3) = (0, 0, 0)$

$T(1, 0, 0, 0) = (1, 0, 0), T(0, 1, 0, 0) = (0, 1, 0)$

$\therefore T$ is linear.

$T(x_1, x_2, x_3, x_4) = (0, 0, 0)$

$\Rightarrow x_1 T(1, 2, 0, -4) + x_2 T(2, 0, -1, -3) + x_3 T(1, 0, 0, 0) +$
$$x_4 T(0, 1, 0, 0) = (0, 0, 0)$$

$\Rightarrow x_1(0, 0, 0) + x_2(0, 0, 0) + x_3(1, 0, 0) + x_4(0, 1, 0) = (0, 0, 0)$

$\Rightarrow (x_3, x_4, 0) = (0, 0, 0)$

$\Rightarrow x_3 = 0, x_4 = 0$

$\therefore (x_1, x_2, x_3, x_4) = (x_1, x_2 0, 0) = x_1(1, 0, 0, 0) + x_2(0, 1, 0, 0)$

$\therefore N(T)$ is spanned by $\{(1, 0, 0, 0), (0, 1, 0, 0)\}$ which is linear transformation.

$\therefore$ Nullity of $T = 2$

But $(1, 2, 0, -4), (2, 0, -1, -3)$ also belong to $N(T)$ and are linear transformation. Hence they also form a basis of $N(T)$.

$\therefore N(T)$ is generated by $(1, 2, 0, -4)$ and $(2, 0, -1, 3)$.

6.5 SINGULAR AND NON-SINGULAR LINEAR TRANSFORMATIONS

Definition: Let U and V be two vector spaces over the same field F. A linear transformation $T:U \to V$ is said to be singular, if there exists a non-zero vector α such that $T(\alpha) = 0'$ and $T:U \to V$ is said to be non-singular if $T(\alpha) = 0' \Rightarrow \alpha = 0$ where 0 is the zero vector of U and $0'$ is the zero vector of V.

Theorem 1: A linear transformation $T:U \to V$ of vector U and V over the same field F is non-singular if and only if T maps every linearly independent subset of U onto a linearly independent subset of V.

Proof:

(i) Let T be non-singular.

Let $S = \{\alpha_1, \alpha_2,..., \alpha_n\}$ be a linear independent subset of U. We shall show that

$S' = \{T(\alpha_1), T(\alpha_2),..., T(\alpha_n)\}$ is linearly independent.

Consider $a_1 T(\alpha_1) + a_2 T(\alpha_2) +...+ a_n T(\alpha_n) = 0'$

$\Rightarrow T(a_1\alpha_1 + a_2\alpha_2 +...+ a_n\alpha_n) = 0'$

$\because T$ is linear

$\Rightarrow a_1\alpha_1 + a_2\alpha_2 +....+ a_n\alpha_n = 0$

$\because T$ is non-singular.

$\Rightarrow a_1 = 0, \ a_2 = 0, \ .... \ a_n = 0$

$\because S$ is linearly independent

$\therefore S'$ is linearly independent.

(ii) Conversely, let T map every linearly independent subset of U onto a linearly independent subset of V.

If α is a non-zero vector of U, then $\{\alpha\}$ is linearly independent and hence by hypothesis $\{T(\alpha)\}$ is linearly independent.

Consequently $T(\alpha) \neq 0'$

Hence $T(\alpha) = 0' \Rightarrow \alpha = 0$

6.6 EIGENVALUES AND EIGENVECTORS OF A LINEAR TRANSFORMATION

Definition: Let A be a square matrix over a field F. The matrix $[A - \lambda I]$, where I is the unit matrix of the same order as that of A and λ is the indeterminate is called the characteristic matrix of A.

Definition: If A is a square matrix of order $n \times n$, then the determinant $|A - \lambda I|$ is a non-zero polynomial of degree n in λ. This polynomial is called the characteristic polynomial of A.

Definition: The equation $|A - \lambda I| = 0$ is called the characteristic equation of A or eigenequation of A.

If $A = \begin{bmatrix} a_{11} & a_{12} & ... & a_{1n} \\ a_{21} & a_{22} & ... & a_{2n} \\ ... & ... & ... & ... \\ ... & ... & .... & ... \\ a_{n1} & a_{n2} & ... & a_{nn} \end{bmatrix}$

then $|A - \lambda I| = 0$

$$\Rightarrow \begin{vmatrix} a_{11} - \lambda & a_{12} & ... & a_{1n} \\ a_{21} & a_{22} - \lambda & ... & a_{2n} \\ ... & ... & ... & ... \\ ... & ... & .... & ... \\ a_{n1} & a_{n2} & ... & a_{nm} - \lambda \end{vmatrix} = 0$$

Example: Let $A = \begin{bmatrix} 1 & 0 & -1 \\ 1 & 2 & 1 \\ 2 & 2 & 3 \end{bmatrix}$

$$\therefore |A - \lambda I| = 0 \Rightarrow \begin{vmatrix} 1 - \lambda & 0 & -1 \\ 1 & 2 - \lambda & 1 \\ 2 & 2 & 3 - \lambda \end{vmatrix} = 0$$

$$\Rightarrow (1 - \lambda)[(2 - \lambda)(3 - \lambda) - 2] - 1[2 - 2(2 - \lambda)] = 0$$

$$\Rightarrow (1 - \lambda)(\lambda^2 - 5\lambda + 6) + (-2 + 2\lambda) = 0$$

$$\Rightarrow \lambda^3 - 6\lambda^2 + 9\lambda - 4 = 0$$

$$\Rightarrow \lambda = 1, 2, 3$$

$\therefore$ The eigenvalues are 1, 2, 3.

Theorem 1: If A is any square matrix, then prove that A and A^T have the same eigenvalues.

Proof: Consider $(A - \lambda I)^T = A^T - (\lambda I)^T$

$$= A^T - \lambda I$$

But $\qquad |A - \lambda I| = |(A - \lambda I)^T| = |A^T - \lambda I|$

$\therefore$ A and A^T have the same characteristic (or eigen) equation and hence the same eigenvalues.

Definition: Let $T : V \to V$ be linear transformation of an n dimensional vector space V and A be the matrix of the linear transformation T. Then the characteristic equation (or eigenequation) of T is defined as the characteristic equation of A, i.e. $|A - \lambda I| = 0$. The roots of the characteristic equation (or the eigenequation) $|A - \lambda I| = 0$

Then to find the eigenvector corresponding to λ, put $\lambda = \lambda_1$, in $[A - \lambda I] x = 0$. We get n equations in n unknowns. The solution of this system of equations will give the eigenvectors $\{x_1, x_2, ..., x_n\}$ corresponding to λ_1.

Similarly, determine the eigenvectors corresponding to $\lambda = \lambda_2, \lambda = \lambda_3, ...,$ etc.

WORKED EXAMPLES

Example 1: Find the basis for the eigen space of the linear transformation $T : R^2 \to R^2$ defined by $T(x, y) = (x + y, y)$.

Solution: First, we shall find the matrix of T w.r.t. the standard basis $\{(1, 0), (0, 1)\}$

$$T(1, 0) = (1, 0)$$
$$T(0, 1) = (1, 1)$$

$\therefore$ The matrix of the linear transformation is $A = \begin{bmatrix} 1 & 0 \\ 1 & 1 \end{bmatrix}$

Eigenequation of A is $|A - \lambda I| = 0$

i.e.
$$\begin{bmatrix} 1 - \lambda & 0 \\ 1 & 1 - \lambda \end{bmatrix} = 0$$

$\Rightarrow \qquad (1 - \lambda)(1 - \lambda) - 0 = 0$

$$\lambda = 1, 1$$

Let $x = (x_1, x_2)$ be a vector in R^2, then $Ax = \lambda x$

$\Rightarrow \quad (A - \lambda I) X = 0$

$\Rightarrow \begin{bmatrix} 1 - \lambda & 0 \\ 1 & 1 - \lambda \end{bmatrix} \begin{bmatrix} x_1 \\ x_2 \end{bmatrix} = \begin{bmatrix} 0 \\ 0 \end{bmatrix}$

$\Rightarrow \begin{bmatrix} (1 - \lambda) & x_1 \\ x_1 + (1 - \lambda) & x_2 \end{bmatrix} = \begin{bmatrix} 0 \\ 0 \end{bmatrix}$

i.e.
$$\begin{bmatrix} 2 - \lambda & 0 & 0 \\ 1 & 1 - \lambda & 2 \\ 0 & -1 & 4 - \lambda \end{bmatrix} \begin{bmatrix} x_1 \\ x_2 \\ x_3 \end{bmatrix} = \begin{bmatrix} 0 \\ 0 \\ 0 \end{bmatrix}$$

i.e. $(2 - \lambda)x_1 + 0x_2 + 0x_3 = 0 \Rightarrow x_1 = 0$

$\quad x_1 + (1 - \lambda)x_2 + 2x_3 = 0 \Rightarrow (1 - \lambda)x_2 + 2x_3 = 0$

$\quad 0x_1 - x_2 + (4 - \lambda)x_3 = 0 \Rightarrow -x_2 + (4 - \lambda)x_3 = 0$

Put $\lambda = 2$ $\therefore$ $-x_2 + 2x_3 = 0 \Rightarrow x_2 = 2x_3$

If $x_3 = k$, then $x_2 = 2k$

∴ The vector is $(0, 2k, k)$ ∴ $(0, 2, 1)$ is a basis of the eigenspace corresponding to $\lambda = 2$.

Put $\lambda = 3$, then $-2x_2 + 2x_3 = 0 \Rightarrow -x_2 + x_3 = 0$ and

$-x_2 + x_3 = 0 \Rightarrow x_2 = x_3 = k$

∴ The vector is $(0, k, k)$.

∴ $(0, 1, 1)$ is a basis of the eigenspace corresponding to $\lambda = 3$.

Example 2: Find the eigenvalues and eigenvectors of the linear transformation $T : R^3 \rightarrow R^3$ defined by $T(e_1) = (1, 1, 0)$, $T(e_2) = (0, 1, 1)$, $T(e_3) = (1, 2, 1)$

Solution: The matrix of the linear transformation is

$$A = \begin{bmatrix} 1 & 1 & 0 \\ 0 & 1 & 1 \\ 1 & 2 & 1 \end{bmatrix}$$

∴ The eigen equation is $|A - \lambda I| = 0$

$$\Rightarrow \begin{bmatrix} 1-\lambda & 1 & 0 \\ 0 & 1-\lambda & 1 \\ 1 & 2 & 1-\lambda \end{bmatrix} = 0$$

Put $\lambda = \dfrac{3+\sqrt{5}}{2}$ ∴ $\left(1 - \dfrac{3+\sqrt{5}}{2}\right) x_1 + x_2 = 0$ ...(1)

$$\left(1 - \dfrac{3+\sqrt{5}}{2}\right) x_2 + x_3 = 0 \qquad \text{...(2)}$$

$$x_1 + 2x_2 + \left(1 - \dfrac{3+\sqrt{5}}{2}\right) x_3 = 0 \qquad \text{.. (3)}$$

From Eq. (1), $x_2 = -\left(1 - \dfrac{3+\sqrt{5}}{2}\right) x_1 = \left(\dfrac{1+\sqrt{5}}{2}\right) x_1$

From Eq. (2), $x_3 = -\left(1 - \dfrac{3+\sqrt{5}}{2}\right) x_2 = \left(\dfrac{1+\sqrt{5}}{2}\right) x_2$

$$= \left(\dfrac{1+\sqrt{5}}{2}\right)\left(\dfrac{1+\sqrt{5}}{2}\right) x_1$$

$$x_3 = \dfrac{6+2\sqrt{5}}{4} x_1$$

$\therefore$ The vector is $\left[x_1, \left(\dfrac{1+\sqrt{5}}{2} \right) x_1, \left(\dfrac{\sqrt{5}+3}{2} \right) x_1 \right]$

$= x_1 \left[1, \dfrac{1+\sqrt{5}}{2}, \dfrac{\sqrt{5}+3}{2} \right]$

$\therefore \qquad \left[1, \dfrac{1+\sqrt{5}}{2}, \dfrac{\sqrt{5}+3}{2} \right]$ is basis of the subspace.

Put $\qquad \lambda = \dfrac{3-\sqrt{5}}{2}$

$\therefore \qquad \left(1 - \dfrac{3-\sqrt{5}}{2} \right) x_1 + x_2 = 0 \qquad \qquad \text{...(4)}$

$\qquad \left(1 - \dfrac{3-\sqrt{5}}{2} \right) x_2 + x_3 = 0 \qquad \qquad \text{...(5)}$

$\qquad x_1 + 2x_2 + \left(1 - \dfrac{3-\sqrt{5}}{2} \right) x_3 = 0 \qquad \text{...(6)}$

$\qquad x_2 = -\left(\dfrac{-1+\sqrt{5}}{2} \right) x_1 = \left(\dfrac{1-\sqrt{5}}{2} \right) x_1$

$\qquad x_3 = -\left(\dfrac{-1+\sqrt{5}}{2} \right) x_2 = \left(\dfrac{1-\sqrt{5}}{2} \right) \left(\dfrac{1-\sqrt{5}}{2} \right) x_1$

$\qquad x_3 = \left(\dfrac{6-2\sqrt{5}}{4} \right) x_1 = \left(\dfrac{3-\sqrt{5}}{2} \right) x_1$

$\therefore$ The vectors $(x_1, x_2, x_3) = \left[x_1, \left(\dfrac{1-\sqrt{5}}{2} \right) x_1, \left(\dfrac{3-\sqrt{5}}{2} \right) x_1 \right]$

$\qquad \qquad = x_1 \left[1, \dfrac{1-\sqrt{5}}{2}, \dfrac{3-\sqrt{5}}{2} \right]$

$\therefore \left\{ \left[1, \dfrac{1-\sqrt{5}}{2}, \dfrac{3-\sqrt{5}}{2} \right] \right\}$ is a basis of the subspace.

6.7 ISOMORPHIC VECTOR SPACES

A vector space $V(F)$ is said to be isomorphic to a vector space V' (F) if there exists a bijective linear transformation of V onto V' $[T : V \to V']$

If V is isomorphic to V', then we write $V \cong V'$. It can be easily seen that the relation '$\cong$' is an equivalence relation on the set of all vector spaces over a field F.

Theorem 1: Every n-dimensional vector space will always mean a finite dimensional vector space.

Proof: Let V be an n-dimensional vector space over a field F and let $B = \{b_1, b_2, ..., b_n\}$ be an ordered basis for V. Then for each $v \in V$, there exists a unique list $(\lambda_1, \lambda_2, \lambda_3, ..., \lambda_n)$ of scalars in F such that

$$v = \lambda_1 b_1 + \lambda_2 b_2 + ... + \lambda_n b_n$$

Consider mapping $T : V \to F^n$ given by

$$T(v) = T\left(\lambda_1 b_1 + \lambda_2 b_2 + ... + \lambda_n b_n\right) = \left(\lambda_1 \lambda_2, ..., \lambda_n\right)$$

Since for each $v \in V$ there exists a unique list $\left(\lambda_1, \lambda_2, ..., \lambda_n\right) \in F_n$

$\therefore$ T is well defined.

T is Injective: Let u, v be any two vectors in V. Then there exists scalars λ_1, $\lambda_2, ..., \lambda_n, \mu_1, \mu_2, ..., \mu_n \in F$

such that

$$u = \lambda_1 b_1 + \lambda_2 b_2 + ... + \lambda_n b_n \text{ and}$$
$$v = \mu_1 b_1 + \mu_2 b_2 + ... + \mu_n b_n$$
$$T(u) = T(v)$$
$$T\left(\lambda_1 b_1 + \lambda_2 b_2 + ... + \lambda_n b_n\right) = T\left(\mu_1 b_1 + \mu_2 b_2 + ... + \mu_n b_n\right)$$
$$\Rightarrow \left(\lambda_1, \lambda_2, ..., \lambda_n\right) = \left(\mu_1, \mu_2, ..., \mu_n\right)$$
$$\Rightarrow \lambda_i = \mu_i \text{ for all } i \in N$$
$$\Rightarrow \sum_{i=1}^{n} \lambda_i b_i = \sum_{i=1}^{n} \mu_i b_i \Rightarrow u = v$$

Thus $T(u) = T(v) \Rightarrow u = v$ for all $u, v \in V$. So T is injective.

T is surjective: Let $(\lambda_1, \lambda_2, ..., \lambda_n)$ be an arbitrary element of F^n. Then there exists a vector $v = \lambda_1 b_1 + \lambda_2 b_2 + ... + \lambda_n b_n \in V$

such that

$$T(v) = T\left(\lambda_1 b_1 + \lambda_2 b_2 + ... + \lambda_n b_n\right)$$
$$= \left(\lambda_1, \lambda_2, ..., \lambda_n\right)$$

Thus, for each $\left(\lambda_1, \lambda_2, ..., \lambda_n\right) \in F^n$ there exists a vector $v \in V$ such that

$$T(v) = (\lambda_1, \lambda_2, ..., \lambda_n)$$

So T is surjective.

T is Linear Transformation: For any $u = \lambda_1 b_1 + \lambda_2 b_2 + ... + \lambda_n b_n$ and

$$v = \mu_1 b_1 + \mu_2 b_2 + ... + \mu_n b_n \in V \text{ and } \lambda, \mu \in F$$

$$T(\lambda u + \mu v) = T\{\lambda(\lambda_1 b_1 + \lambda_2 b_2 + ... + \lambda_n b_n) + \mu(\mu_1 b_1 + \mu_2 b_2 + ... + \mu_n b_n\}$$

$$= T\{(\lambda\lambda_1 + \mu\mu_1)b_1 + (\lambda\lambda_2 + \mu\mu_2)b_2 + ... + (\lambda\lambda_n + \mu\mu_n)b_n\}$$

$$T(\lambda u + \mu v) = \lambda\lambda_1 + \mu\mu_1, \lambda\lambda_2 + \mu\mu_2, ..., \lambda\lambda_n + \mu\mu_2$$

$$= (\lambda\lambda_1 + \lambda\lambda_2 + ... + \lambda\lambda_n) + (\mu\mu_1 + \mu\mu_2 + ... + \mu\mu_n)$$

$$= \lambda(\lambda_1, \lambda_2, ..., \lambda_n) + \mu(\mu_1, \mu_2, ..., \mu_n)$$

$$= \lambda T(u) + \mu T(v)$$

So, T is a linear transformation. Then $T: V \to F^n$ is an isomorphism of vector space. Hence, $V \cong F^n$

Theorem 2: Two finite dimensional vector spaces over the same field are isomorphic if they are of the same dimension.

Proof: Let V and V' be two finite dimensional vector spaces over the same field F such that $\dim V = \dim V' = n$, then we have to show that $V \cong V'$

Let $B = \{b_1, b_2, ..., b_n\}$ and $B' = \{b'_1, b'_2, ..., b'_n\}$ be bases for V and V' respectively.

Let $v \in V$, then there exist unique scalars $\lambda_1, \lambda_2, ..., \lambda_n$ such that

$$v = \lambda_1 b_1 + \lambda_2 b_2 + \lambda_3 b_3 + ... + \lambda_n b_n$$

Consider a mapping $T: V \to V'$ given by

$$T(v) = T(\lambda_1 b_1 + \lambda_2 b_2 + ... + \lambda_n b_n) = (\lambda_1 b'_1 + \lambda_2 b'_2 + ... + \lambda_n b'_n)$$

Clearly, $T: V \to V'$ is well defined.

T is injective: Let u, v be any two vectors in V. Then

$$u = \lambda_1 b_1 + \lambda_2 b_2 + ... + \lambda_n b_n$$

$$v = \mu_1 b_1 + \mu_2 b_2 + ... + \mu_n b_n \text{ for } \lambda_1, \lambda_2, ..., \lambda_n \text{ and }$$

$$\mu_1, \mu_2, ..., \mu_n \in F$$

$\therefore \qquad T(u) = T(v)$

$$\Rightarrow T(\lambda_1 b_1 + \lambda_2 b_2 + ... + \lambda_n b_n) = T(\mu_1 b_1 + \mu_2 b_2 + ... + \mu_n b_n)$$

$$\Rightarrow \lambda_1 b'_1 + \lambda_2 b'_2 + ... + \lambda_n b'_n = \mu_1 b'_1 + \mu_2 b'_2 + ... + \mu_n b'_n$$

$$\Rightarrow (\lambda_1 - \mu_1)b'_1 + (\lambda_2 - \mu_2)b'_2 + ... + (\lambda_n - \mu_n)b'_n = 0V'$$

$$\Rightarrow \lambda_1 - \mu_1 = 0, \ \lambda_2 - \mu_2 = 0, ..., \lambda_n - \mu_n = 0$$

$\Rightarrow \lambda_1 - \mu_1, \lambda_2 - \mu_2, ..., \lambda_n - \mu_n$

$\Rightarrow \lambda_1 b_1 + \lambda_2 b_2 + ... + \lambda_n b_n = \mu_1 b_1 + \mu_2 b_2 + ... + \mu_n b_n$

$\Rightarrow u = v$

Thus $T(u) = T(v) \Rightarrow u = v$ for all $u, v \in V$, so T is injective.

T is surjective : Let v' be any arbitrary vector in V', then there exists scalars $\lambda_1, \lambda_2, ..., \lambda_n \in F$ such that

$$v' = \lambda_1 b_1' + \lambda_2 b_2' + ... + \lambda_n b_n' \text{ (as } B' \text{ is basis for } V')$$

Consequently, there exists a vector

$$v = \lambda_1 b_1 + \lambda_2 b_2 + ... + \lambda_n b_n \in V$$

such that

$$T(v) = T\left(\lambda_1 b_1 + \lambda_2 b_2 + ... + \lambda_n b_n\right)$$
$$= T\left(\lambda_1 b_1' + \lambda_2 b_2' + ... + T\lambda_n b_n'\right) = V'$$

So T is surjective.

T is a linear transformation:

Let $\quad u = \lambda_1 b_1 + \lambda_2 b_2 + ... + \lambda_n b_n$

$\quad v = \mu_1 b_1 + \mu_2 b_2 + ... + \mu_n b_n$ be any two vectors in V and $\lambda, \mu \in F$

Then

$$T\left(\lambda u + \mu v\right) = T\{\lambda(\lambda_1 b_1 + \lambda_2 b_2 + ... + \lambda_n b_n) + ...$$
$$\mu(\mu_1 b_1 + \mu_2 b_2 + ... + \mu_n b_n)\}$$

$$T\left(\lambda u + \mu v\right) = T\{\left(\lambda\lambda_1 + \mu\mu_1\right)b_1 + \left(\lambda\lambda_2 + \mu\mu_2\right)b_2 + ...$$
$$+ \left(\lambda\lambda_n + \mu\mu_n\right)b_n\}$$

$$= \left(\lambda\lambda_1 + \mu\mu_1\right)b_1' + \left(\lambda\lambda_2 + \mu\mu_2\right)b_2' + ... + \left(\lambda\lambda_n + \mu\mu_n\right)b_n'$$

$$= \left(\lambda\lambda_1\right)b_1' + \left(\lambda\lambda_2\right)b_2' + ... + \left(\lambda\lambda_n\right)b_n' + \left(\mu\mu_1\right)b_1'$$

$$+ \left(\mu\mu_2\right)b_2' + ... + \left(\mu\mu_n\right)b_n'$$

$$T\left(\lambda u + \mu v\right) = \lambda\left(\lambda_1 b_1' + \lambda_2 b_2' + ... + \lambda_n b_n'\right) + \mu\left(\mu_1 b_1' + \mu_2 b_2' + ... + \mu_n b_n'\right)$$

$$= \lambda T(u) + \mu T(v)$$

Thus $T\left(\lambda u + \mu v\right) = \lambda T(u) + \mu T(v) \ \forall u, v \in V$ and $\lambda, \mu \in F$

So, T is a linear transformation.

Hence $T : V \to V'$ is an isomorphism.

Consequently $V \cong V'$

Conversely, let V and V' be two finite dimensional vector spaces over the same field F such that $V \cong V'$, then we have to show that $\dim V = \dim V'$.

Since V is isomorphic to V', therefore there exists an isomorphism T of V onto V'.

Let $B = \{b_1, b_2, ..., b_n\}$ be a basis for V.

Then $\dim V = n$

We shall now show that $B' = \{T(b_1), T(b_2), ..., T(b_n)\}$ is a basis for V'.

B' is linearly independent

Let $\lambda_1, \lambda_2, ..., \lambda_n$ be scalars is F such that

$$\lambda_1 T(b_1) + \lambda_2 T(b_2) + ... + \lambda_n T(b_n) = 0V'$$
$$\Rightarrow \quad T(\lambda_1 b_1 + \lambda_2 b_2 + ... + \lambda_n b_n) = T(0V)$$
$$\Rightarrow \quad \lambda_1 b_1 + \lambda_2 b_2 + ... + \lambda_n b_n = 0V$$
$$\Rightarrow \quad \lambda_1 = 0, \ \lambda_2 = 0, ..., \lambda_n = 0$$
$$\lambda_1 = \lambda_2 = ... = \lambda_n = 0$$

So, B' is linearly independent.

B' spans V': Since $T : V \to V'$ is subjective, therefore, for each $v' \in V'$ there exists $v \in V$ such that $T(v) = v'$

Now, $v \in V$

$\Rightarrow$ there exist scalars $\lambda_1, \lambda_2, ..., \lambda_n \in F$

such that $v = \lambda_1 b_1 + \lambda_2 b_2 + ... + \lambda_n b_n$

$$\Rightarrow \quad V' = T(V) = T(\lambda_1 b_1 + \lambda_2 b_2 + ... + \lambda_n b_n)$$
$$\Rightarrow \quad V' = \lambda_1 T(b_1) + \lambda_2 T(b_2) + ... + \lambda_n T(b_n)$$

$\Rightarrow V'$ is a linear combination of $T(b_1), T(b_2), ..., T(b_n)$. Thus, each vector in V' is a linear combination of vectors in B'. So B' spans V'.

Hence, B' is a basis for V'.

Consequently, $\dim V' = n$

Hence $\dim V = \dim V'$

Theorem 3: Let S be a subspace of a vector space $V(F)$. Then the quotient space V/S is homomorphic image of V with kernel S.

Proof: Consider a mapping $\phi : V \to V/S$ given by the rule $\phi(V) = v + s$ for all $v \in V$.

ϕ is a linear transformation: Let u, v be any two vectors in V and $\lambda, \mu \in F$

Then $\phi(\lambda u + \mu v) = (\lambda u + \mu v) + s$

$\Rightarrow \quad \phi(\lambda u + \mu v) = (\lambda u + s) + (\mu v + s)$ (by addition of V/S)

$\Rightarrow \quad \phi(\lambda u + \mu v) = \lambda(u + s) + u(v + s)$

[by scalar multiplication on V/S]

$\Rightarrow \quad \phi(\lambda u + \mu u) = \lambda \phi(u) + \mu \phi(v)$

So ϕ is a linear transformation.

ϕ is surjective: Let $v + s$ be an arbitrary element of V/S. Then there exists $v \in V$ such that $\phi(v) = v + s$

so, ϕ is surjective.

Hence $\phi : V \to V/S$ is an epimorphism

Consequently, V/S is homomorphic image of V.

Now, let $v \in V$ such that $v \in \ker(\phi)$.

Then $v \in \ker(\phi)$

$\Leftrightarrow \phi(v) = s$

$\Leftrightarrow v + s = s$

$\Leftrightarrow v \leftarrow s$. So, $\ker \phi = S$

Hence, V/S is homomorphic image of V with kernel.

Theorem 4: Let V be a finite dimensional vector space over a field F and let $T : V \to V$ be a monomorphism. Then T is an isomorphism.

Proof: Let $B = \{b_1, b_2, ..., b_n\}$ be a basis for V. First we establish that

$$B' = \{T(b_1), T(b_2), ..., T(b_n)\} \text{ is also a basis for } V.$$

B' is linearly independent: Let $\lambda_1, \lambda_2, ..., \lambda_n \in F$ be such that

$$\lambda_1 T(b_1) + \lambda_2 T(b_2) + ... + \lambda_n T(b_n) = 0v$$

Then $T(\lambda_1 b_1 + \lambda_2 b_2 + ... + \lambda_n b_n) = T(0v)$

$\qquad\qquad\qquad\qquad\qquad\qquad\qquad\qquad$ [$\because T : V \to V$ is linear]

$\Rightarrow \lambda_1 b_1 + \lambda_2 b_2 + ... + \lambda_n b_n = 0v \qquad\qquad$ [$\because T$ is injective]

$\Rightarrow \lambda_1 = \lambda_2 = ... = \lambda_n = 0 \qquad\qquad$ [$\because B$ is a basis for V]

So B' is linearly independent.

Since V is of dimension n and B' is a linearly independent set of n vectors in V, therefore B' is a basis of V.

Now let v be any arbitrary vector in V. Then there exist scalars $\lambda_1, \lambda_2, ..., \lambda_n \in F$

such that

$$v = \lambda_1 T(b_1) + \lambda_2 T(b_2) + ... + \lambda_n T(b_n) \qquad [\because B' \text{ is basis for } V]$$

$$\Rightarrow v = T(\lambda_1 b_1 + \lambda_2 b_2 + ... + \lambda_n b_n) \qquad\qquad [\because T \text{ is linear}]$$

$$\Rightarrow v = T(v) \text{ where } u = \sum_{i=1}^{n} \lambda_i b_i \in V$$

Thus for each $v \in V$, there exists $u \in V$

such that $T(u) = v$. Therefore, T is surjective.

Hence T is an isomorphism.

Theorem 5: Let $V(F)$ and V'' (F) be two finite dimension vector spaces such that $\dim V = \dim V'$ if $T : V \to V'$ is a monomorphism.

Proof: Same as above theorem.

6.8 LINEAR TRANSFORMATION AND ITS APPLICATIONS

Application I: Cryptology

Used in cryptology is the science of coding and decoding secret messages, mainly for secure communications.

Suppose that Mark and Susan are two under cover agents who want to communicate with each other by using a code because they suspect that their phone is being tapped and their mail is being intercepted. Mark wants to send Susan message a Meet Tomorrow.

For the security, we first code the alphabets as follows

$$A \quad B \quad C \quad D \text{---------} X \quad Y \quad Z$$
$$\updownarrow \quad \updownarrow \quad \updownarrow \quad \updownarrow \qquad \updownarrow \quad \updownarrow \quad \updownarrow$$
$$1 \quad 2 \quad 3 \quad 4 \text{---------} 24 \quad 25 \quad 26$$

Thus the code message is

$$M \quad E \quad E \quad T \quad T \quad O \quad M \quad O \quad R \quad R \quad O \quad W$$
$$13 \quad 5 \quad 5 \quad 20 \quad 20 \quad 15 \quad 13 \quad 15 \quad 18 \quad 18 \quad 15 \quad 23$$

The sequence

$$13 \ 5 \ 5 \ 20 \ 20 \ 15 \ 13 \ 15 \ 18 \ 18 \ 15 \ 23$$

is the original code message. To encrypt the original code message, we can apply a linear transformation to original code message.

When they under took the mission, they agreed on a 3×3 non-singular matrix such as

$$A = \begin{bmatrix} 1 & 2 & 3 \\ 1 & 1 & 2 \\ 0 & 1 & 2 \end{bmatrix}$$

Mark then breaks the message into 4 vectors in R^3. Thus we have the vectors

$$\begin{bmatrix} 13 \\ 5 \\ 5 \end{bmatrix}, \begin{bmatrix} 20 \\ 20 \\ 15 \end{bmatrix}, \begin{bmatrix} 13 \\ 15 \\ 18 \end{bmatrix}, \begin{bmatrix} 18 \\ 15 \\ 23 \end{bmatrix}$$

Mark now defines the linear transformation $L : R^3 \to R^3$ by $L(X) = AX$. So the message becomes

$$L \begin{bmatrix} 13 \\ 5 \\ 5 \end{bmatrix} = A \begin{bmatrix} 13 \\ 5 \\ 5 \end{bmatrix} = \begin{bmatrix} 38 \\ 28 \\ 15 \end{bmatrix}$$

$$L\begin{bmatrix} 20 \\ 20 \\ 15 \end{bmatrix} = A\begin{bmatrix} 20 \\ 20 \\ 15 \end{bmatrix} = \begin{bmatrix} 105 \\ 70 \\ 50 \end{bmatrix}$$

$$L\begin{bmatrix} 13 \\ 15 \\ 12 \end{bmatrix} = A\begin{bmatrix} 19 \\ 15 \\ 18 \end{bmatrix} = \begin{bmatrix} 97 \\ 64 \\ 51 \end{bmatrix}$$

$$L\begin{bmatrix} 18 \\ 15 \\ 23 \end{bmatrix} = A\begin{bmatrix} 18 \\ 15 \\ 23 \end{bmatrix} = \begin{bmatrix} 117 \\ 79 \\ 61 \end{bmatrix}$$

Now Mark transmitts the message

38, 28, 15, 105, 70, 50, 97, 64, 51, 117, 79, 61

Suppose Susan wants to encode the encrypted message code. Susan has to find the inverse matrix of A first.

$$A^{-1} = \begin{bmatrix} 1 & 2 & 3 \\ 1 & 1 & 2 \\ 0 & 1 & 2 \end{bmatrix}^{-1}$$

$$= \begin{bmatrix} 0 & 1 & -1 \\ 2 & -2 & -1 \\ -1 & 1 & 1 \end{bmatrix}$$

$$A^{-1}\begin{bmatrix} 38 \\ 28 \\ 15 \end{bmatrix} = \begin{bmatrix} 0 & 1 & -1 \\ 2 & -2 & -1 \\ -1 & 1 & 1 \end{bmatrix} = \begin{bmatrix} 13 \\ 5 \\ 5 \end{bmatrix}$$

$$A^{-1}\begin{bmatrix} 105 \\ 70 \\ 50 \end{bmatrix} = \begin{bmatrix} 20 \\ 20 \\ 15 \end{bmatrix}$$

$$A^{-1}\begin{bmatrix} 105 \\ 70 \\ 50 \end{bmatrix} = \begin{bmatrix} 20 \\ 20 \\ 15 \end{bmatrix}$$

$$A^{-1}\begin{bmatrix}97\\64\\51\end{bmatrix}=\begin{bmatrix}13\\15\\18\end{bmatrix}$$

$$A^{-1}\begin{bmatrix}117\\79\\61\end{bmatrix}=\begin{bmatrix}18\\15\\23\end{bmatrix}$$

Thus Susan can find the orginal message code.

Application II: Computer Graphics

Visual representation on some surfaces are graphics which are created using computers. Computer graphics play major role in (i) video games, (ii) special effects in the film industry, (iii) CAD (computer aided design) is automobile industry used to design a computer model of a product (e.g. car, engine).

(1) **Reflection** with respect to X-axis:

$Lb : R^2 \to R^2$ defined by $L(x, y) = (x_1 - y)$

$$A = \begin{bmatrix}1 & 0\\0 & -1\end{bmatrix}$$

$L(V) = AV$

$$\begin{bmatrix}1 & 0\\0 & -1\end{bmatrix}\begin{bmatrix}x\\y\end{bmatrix}=\begin{bmatrix}x\\-y\end{bmatrix}$$

To illustrate a reflection with respect to the X-axis, the computer graphics let the triangle T.

$$L\begin{bmatrix}-1\\4\end{bmatrix}=\begin{bmatrix}-1\\-4\end{bmatrix}$$

$$L\begin{bmatrix}3\\1\end{bmatrix}=\begin{bmatrix}3\\-1\end{bmatrix}$$

$$L\begin{bmatrix}2\\6\end{bmatrix}=\begin{bmatrix}2\\-6\end{bmatrix}$$

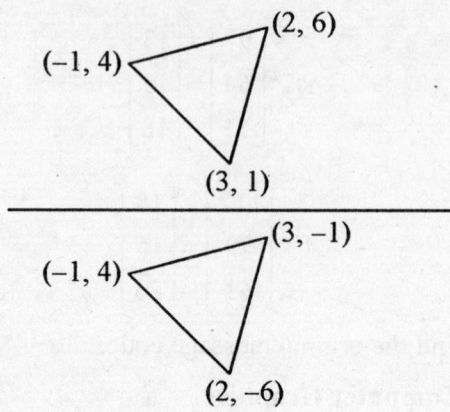

(ii) Reflection with respect to $y = -x$:

$Lb: R^2 \to R^2$ defined by $L(x, y) = (-y, -x)$

$$\Rightarrow \quad \begin{aligned} y &= -x \\ x &= -y \\ y &= -x \end{aligned}$$

$$L\begin{bmatrix} x \\ y \end{bmatrix} = A\begin{bmatrix} +y \\ +x \end{bmatrix}$$

$$= \begin{bmatrix} -1 & 0 \\ 0 & -1 \end{bmatrix}\begin{bmatrix} +y \\ +x \end{bmatrix} = \begin{bmatrix} -y \\ -x \end{bmatrix}$$

$$L\begin{bmatrix} -1 \\ 4 \end{bmatrix} = \begin{bmatrix} -4 \\ 1 \end{bmatrix}$$

$$L\begin{bmatrix} 3 \\ 1 \end{bmatrix} = \begin{bmatrix} -1 \\ -3 \end{bmatrix}$$

$$L\begin{bmatrix} 2 \\ 6 \end{bmatrix} = \begin{bmatrix} -6 \\ -2 \end{bmatrix}$$

The plot is given by

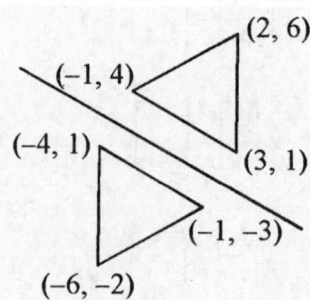

(2) Rotation:

A plane figure is rotated clockwise through an angle ϕ by using the matrix transformation.

$L : R^2 \rightarrow R^2$ defined by $L(v) = AV.$

$$A = \begin{bmatrix} \cos\phi & -\sin\phi \\ \sin\phi & \cos\phi \end{bmatrix}$$

Suppose we wish to rotate the triangle with vertices $(0, 0), (1, 0), (1, 1)$ through 90° in counter clockwise.

$$A = V_1 = (0, 0) \qquad V_2 = (1, 0) \qquad V_3 = (1, 1)$$

$$A = \begin{bmatrix} \cos(\pi/2) & -\sin\pi/2 \\ \sin\pi/2 & \cos\pi/2 \end{bmatrix} = \begin{bmatrix} 0 & -1 \\ 1 & 0 \end{bmatrix}$$

$$L[V_1] = AV_1 = \begin{bmatrix} 0 & -1 \\ 1 & 0 \end{bmatrix}\begin{bmatrix} 0 \\ 0 \end{bmatrix} = \begin{bmatrix} 0 \\ 0 \end{bmatrix}$$

$$L[V_2] = AV_2 = \begin{bmatrix} 0 & -1 \\ 1 & 0 \end{bmatrix}\begin{bmatrix} 1 \\ 0 \end{bmatrix} = \begin{bmatrix} 0 \\ 1 \end{bmatrix}$$

$$L[V_3] = AV_3 = \begin{bmatrix} 0 & -1 \\ 1 & 0 \end{bmatrix}\begin{bmatrix} 1 \\ 1 \end{bmatrix} = \begin{bmatrix} -1 \\ 1 \end{bmatrix}$$

The plot is given below

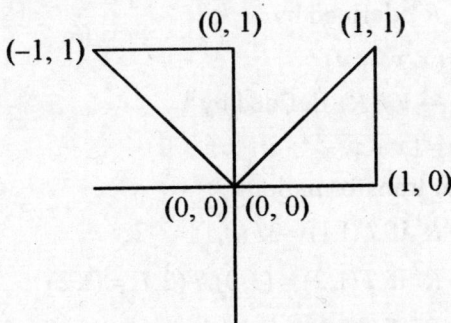

EXERCISE

1. Verify whether the following are linear transformation:

   (i) $T : V_2(R) \to V_3(R)$ defined by
   $$T(x, y) = (x, y, 0)$$

   (ii) $T : V_2(R) \to V_2(R)$ defined by
   $$T(x, y) = (2x, y)$$

   (iii) $T : V_2(R) \to V_2(R)$ defined by
   $$T(x, y) = (x^2, y)$$

   (iv) $T : V_2(R) \to V_2(R)$ defined by
   $$T(x, y) = (3x + 2y, 3x - 4y)$$

   (v) $T : V_2(R) \to V_2(R)$ defined by
   $$T(x, y) = (x + y, y)$$

   (vi) $T : R^2 \to R^2$ defined by
   $$T(x, y) = (2x + y, x - y)$$

   (vii) $T : R^3 \to R^1$ defined by
   $$T(x, y, z) = (2x + y, 3y - 4z)$$

   (viii) $T : R^3 \to R^1$ defined by
   $$T(x, y, z) = 2x - 3y + 4z$$

   (ix) $T : R^3 \to R^3$ defined by
   $$T(x, y, z) = (x, y, z)$$

   (x) $T : R^3 \to R^3$ defined by
   $$T(x, y, z) = (x + 2y - z, y + z, x + y - 2z)$$

   (xi) $T : R^2 \to R^3$ defined by
   $$T(x, y) = (x + y, 2y, x + 1)$$

   (xii) $T : R^2 \to R^4$ defined by
   $$T(x, y) = (x, y, y, y)$$

   (xiii) $T : V_3(R) \to V_2(R)$ defined by
   $$T(x, y, z) = (x + z, -x + y + z)$$

2. Find the linear transformation:

   (i) $T : R^2 \to R^1$ if $T(1, 1) = 3 T(0, 1) = -2$

   (ii) $T : R^2 \to R^2$ if $T(1, 2) = (3, 0), T(2, 1) = (1, 2)$

   (iii) $T : R^2 \to R^4$ if $T(1, 1) = (1, 1, 1, 1), T(1, -1) = (1, -1, -1, -1)$

(iv) $T: V_2(R) \to V_3(R)$ if $T(1,2) = (3,-1,5), T(0,1) = (2,1,-1)$

(v) $T: R^2 \to R^2$ if $T(2,1) = (3,4), T(-3,4) = (0,5)$

(vi) $T: R^2 \to R^4$ if $T(1,1) = (1,-1,1,-1), T(-1,2) = (-1,2,-1,-2)$

(vii) $T: R^3 \to R^3$ if $T(1,0,0) = (4,5,8)$
$$T(1,-1,0) = (8,10,18)$$
$$T(0,1,1) = (-3,-4,-7)$$

(viii) $T: R^3 \to R^3$ if $T(1,1,1) = (1,1,1)$
$$T(1,2,3) = (-1,-2,-3)$$
$$T(1,1,2) = (2,2,4)$$

(ix) $T: R^2 \to R^3$ if $T(1,0) = (1,0,1), T(0,1) = (-1,1,1)$

(x) $T: R^3 \to R^3$ if $T(1,1,1) = (2,1,1), T(1,2,1) = (3,2,1)$
$$T(1,0,0) = (1,0,0)$$

3. Let $M(R)$ be a vector space of all $n \times n$ matrices over R and B be any fixed non-zero matrix of $M(R)$. Show that the mapping $T: M(R) \to M(R)$ defined by

   (i) $T(A) = AB - BA$

   (ii) $T(A) = BA$

   (iii) $T(A) = AB^2 + BA$ are linear transformations and

   (iv) $T(A) = B + A$ is not linear unless B is a zero matrix.

4. (i) Show that $T: R^2 \to R^2$ defined by $T(x,y) = (x+2, y+3)$ is not linear.

   (ii) Show that $T: R \to R$ defined by $T(ab) = ab$ is not linear.

5. If V is the vector space of all real valued functions defined on $[0, 1]$ then show that $T: V \to R^2$ defined by $T(f) = (f(0), f(1))$ is linear.

6. Find the matrix of the following T.

   (i) $T: V_2(R) \to V_2(R)$ defined by
   $T(x,y) = (3x, x-y)$

   (ii) $T: V_3(R) \to V_3(R)$ defined by
   $T(x,y,z) = (z - 2y, x + 2y - z)$

   (iii) $T: V_3(R) \to V_3(R)$ defined by
   $T(x,y,z) = (x + y, 2y, 2y - x)$

   (iv) $T: R^3 \to R^3$ defined by
   $T(x,y) = (3x - y, 2x + 4y, 5x - 6y)$

   (v) $T: R^3 \to R^3$ defined by
   $T(x,y,z) = (x + 2y - z, y + z, x + y - 2z)$

(vi) $T: R^2 \to R^3$ defined by
$$T(-1,1) = (-1,0,2),\ T(2,1) = (1,2,1)$$

(vii) $T: R^2 \to R^2$ defined by
$$T(2,1) = (3,4),\ T(-3,4) = (0,5)$$

(viii) Defined by $T: R^3 \to R^2$
$$T(e_1) = 2f_1 - 2f_2,$$
$T(e_2) = f_1 + 2f_2,\ T(e_3) = 0$ where $\{e_1, e_2, e_3\}$ and $\{f_1, f_2\}$ are standard basis of R^3 and R^2.

(ix) $T: R^3 \to R^3$ such that $T(1,1,1) = (1,1,1)$
$T(1,2,3) = (-1,2,-3)$ and $T(1,1,2) = (2,2,4)$

(x) $T: R^2 \to R^3$ such that $T(-1,1) = (-1,0,2)$
$T(2,1) = (1,2,1)$ w.r.t. standard bases $\{e_1, e_2\}$ and $\{f_1, f_2\}$

(xi) $T: V_2(R) \to V_2(R)$ defined by $T(x,y,z) = (x+y, y+z)$ w.r.t. the bases

(a) $B_1 = \{e_1, e_2, e_3\}\ B_2 = \{f_1, f_2\}$

(b) $B_1 = \{(1,1,1), (1,0,0), (1,1,0)\}, B_2 = \{e_1, e_2\}$

(xii) $T: R^3 \to R^2$ defined by $T(x,y,z) = (2y+z, x-4y, 3x)$ w.r.t. the bases $\{(1,1,1), (1,1,0), (1,0,0)\}$

(xiii) $T: R^2 \to R^3$ defined by $T(x,y) = (-x+2y, y, 3y-3x)$ w.r.t. the bases $B_1 = \{(1,2), (-2,1)\}$
$$B_2 = \{(-1,0,2), (1,2,3), (1,-1,-1)\}$$

(xiv) $T: R^2 \to R^3$ defined by $T(x,y) = (x,y,0)$ w.r.t. the standard bases.

7. For the following matrices and bases, determine the linear transformations such that the matrix is the matrix of T. w.r.t. the bases.

(i) $\begin{bmatrix} 1 & -1 & 0 & 2 \\ 3 & 4 & 1 & -4 \end{bmatrix}$ w.r.t. the standard bases.

(ii) $\begin{bmatrix} 1 & 3 \\ -1 & 1 \\ 2 & 0 \end{bmatrix}$ w.r.t. the standard bases of R^3 and R^2.

(iii) $\begin{bmatrix} -1 & 2 & 1 \\ 1 & 0 & 3 \end{bmatrix}$ w.r.t. $B_1 = \{(1,2,0), (0,-1,0), (1,-1,1)\}$ and
$B_2 = \{(1,0), (2-1)\}$

(iv) $\begin{bmatrix} 2 & 1 \\ 0 & 1 \\ 3 & -3 \end{bmatrix}$ w.r.t. $B_1 = \{(-2,1),(1,2)\}$

$B_2 = \{(1,-1,-1),(1,2,3),(-1,0,2)\}$

(v) $\begin{bmatrix} 1 & 0 & 0 \\ 0 & 1 & 0 \\ 0 & 0 & 1 \end{bmatrix}$ w.r.t. (a) standard bases.

(b) $B_1 = \{(1,1,1,),(1,0,0),(0,1,0)\}$, $B_2 = \{(1,2,3),(1,-1,1),(2,1,1)\}$

(vi) $\begin{bmatrix} 1 & 2 \\ 0 & 1 \\ -1 & 3 \end{bmatrix}$ w.r.t. $B_1 = \{(1,1),(-1,1)\}$, $B_2 = \{(1,1,1),(1,-1,1),(0,0,1)\}$

8. For the following linear transformations, find the range space, null space, rank, nullity and verify the rank-nullity theorem.

(i) $T : V_3(R) \rightarrow V_3(R)$ defined by $T(x,y,z) = (x+y, x-y, 2x+z)$

(ii) $T : V_3(R) \rightarrow V_2(R)$ defined by $T(x,y,z) = (y-x, y-z)$

(iii) $T : V_3(R) \rightarrow V_3(R)$ defined by

$T(e_1) = e_1 + e_2 + e_3$, $T(e_2) = e_1 - e_2 + e_3$

$T(e_3) = e_1 - 3e_2 + 3e_3$

(iv) $T : R^3 \rightarrow R^4$ given by $T(1, 0, 0) = (0, 1, 0, 2)$

$T(0,1,0) = (0,1,1,0)$, $T(0,0,1) = (0,1,-1,4)$

(v) $T : R^3 \rightarrow R^3$ given by $T(x_1, x_2, x_3) = (x_1, x_3, x_2)$

(vi) $T : R^3 \rightarrow R^3$ given by $T(x,y,z) = (x+y, x+z, y+z)$

(vii) $T : R^3 \rightarrow R^3$ given by

$T(e_1) = e_1 - e_2$

$T(e_2) = 2e_1 - e_3$

$T(e_3) = e_1 - e_2 + e_3$

(viii) $T : R^3 \rightarrow R^2$

$T(e_1) = (2,1)$, $T(e_2) = (0,1)$, $T(e_3) = (1,1)$

(ix) $T : R^3 \rightarrow R^3$ given by

$T(1,0,0) = (1,-1,0)$, $T(0,1,0) = (2,0,1)$, $T(0,0,1) = (1,1,1)$

(x) $T : R^3 \rightarrow R^2$ given by

$T(x,y,z) = (x+y, y+z)$

9. Find a linear transformation $T:R^3 \to R^4$ whose range space is generated by $(1, 2, 0, -4)$ and $(2, 0, -1, -3)$.

10. Find the linear transformation $T:R^3 \to R^3$ whose range space is generated by $(1, 2, 3)$ and $(4, 5, 6)$.

11. Find the linear transformation $T:R^4 \to R^3$ whose kernel is generated by $(1, 2, 3, 4)$ and $(0, 1, 1,)$.

12. Find the linear transformation $T:R^3 \to R^3$ whose null space is generated by $(1, 1, -1), (1, 2, 2)$.

13. Find the linear transformation $T:R^3 \to R^3$ whose range space is spanned by $\{(1, 2, 2), (1, 0, -1)\}$.

14. Find the eigenvalues and eigenvectors of the following linear transformations:

   (i) $T:V_2(R) \to V_2(R)$ defined by $T(1, 0) = (1, 2), T(0, 1) = (3, 2)$

   (ii) $T:V_2(R) \to V_2(R)$ defined by $T(e_1) = (1, 4), T(e_2) = (2, 3)$

   (iii) $T:R^3 \to R^3$ defined by
   $T(e_1) = (4, 0, 1), T(e_2) = (-2, 1, 0), T(e_3) = (-2, 0, 1)$

   (iv) $T:R^3 \to R^3$ defined by $T(1, 0, 0) = (1, -3, 3)$
   $T(0, 0) = (3, -5, 3)$ defined by $T(1, 0, 0) = (1, -3, 3)$

   (v) $T:R^3 \to R^3$ defined by $T(1, 0, 0) = (-3, 1, 1)$
   $T(0, 1, 0) = (-7, 5, -1), T(0, 0, 1) = (-6, 6, 2)$

   (vi) $T:R^3 \to R^3$ given by
   $T(e_1) = (3, 2, 4), T(e_2) = (2, 0, 2), T(e_3) = (4, 2, 3)$

   (vii) $T:R^3 \to R^3$ given by
   $T(x, y, z) = (3x + 2y + z, x + 4y + z, x + 2y + 3z)$

   (viii) $T:V_3(R) \to V_3(R)$ given by
   $T(x, y, z) = (x, x + y, z)$

   (ix) $T:V_3(R) \to V_3(R)$ given by
   $T(x, y, z) = (3x, 2y + z, -5y - 2z)$

   (x) $T:R^3 \to R^3$ given by
   $T(x, y, z) = (x + 3z, 2x + y - z, x - y + z)$

Answers

1. iii, xi are not linear, the others are linear.

2. (i) $T(x, y) = 5x - 2y$ (ii) $T(x, y) = \left(\dfrac{5y - x}{3}, \dfrac{4x - 2y}{3} \right)$

   (iii) $T(x, y) = (x, y, y)$,   (iv) $T(x, y) = (-x + 2y, -3x + y, 7x - y)$

   (v) $T(x, y) = \left(\dfrac{12x + 9y}{11}, x + 2y \right)$

(vi) $T(x, y) = (x, -y, x, -y)$

(vii) $T(x, y, z) = (4x - 4y + z, 5x - 5y + z, 8x - 10y + 3z)$

(viii) $T(x, y, z) = (4x - 4y + z, 5x - 5y + z, 8x - 10y + 3z)$

(ix) $T(x, y) = (x - y, y, x + y)$

(x) $T(x, y) = (x + y, y, z)$

6.   (i) $\begin{bmatrix} 3 & 1 \\ 0 & -1 \end{bmatrix}$ (ii) $\begin{bmatrix} 0 & 1 \\ -2 & 2 \\ 1 & -1 \end{bmatrix}$

(iii) $\begin{bmatrix} 1 & 0 & -1 \\ 1 & 2 & 2 \\ 0 & 0 & 0 \end{bmatrix}$ (iv) $\begin{bmatrix} 3 & 2 & 5 \\ -1 & 4 & -6 \end{bmatrix}$

(v) $\begin{bmatrix} 1 & 0 & 1 \\ 2 & 1 & 1 \\ -1 & 1 & -2 \end{bmatrix}$ (vi) $\dfrac{1}{3}\begin{bmatrix} 2 & 2 & -1 \\ -1 & 2 & 5 \end{bmatrix}$

(vii) $\begin{bmatrix} \dfrac{12}{11} & 1 \\ \dfrac{9}{11} & 2 \end{bmatrix}$ (viii) $\begin{bmatrix} 2 & -1 \\ 1 & 2 \\ 0 & 0 \end{bmatrix}$

(ix) $\begin{bmatrix} 4 & 1 & 8 \\ -4 & -1 & -10 \\ 1 & 1 & 3 \end{bmatrix}$ (x) $\dfrac{1}{3}\begin{bmatrix} 2 & 2 & -1 \\ -1 & 2 & 5 \end{bmatrix}$

(xi) (a) $\begin{bmatrix} 1 & 0 \\ 1 & 1 \\ 0 & 1 \end{bmatrix}$ (b) $\begin{bmatrix} 2 & 2 \\ 1 & 0 \\ 2 & 1 \end{bmatrix}$ (xii) $\begin{bmatrix} 3 & -6 & 6 \\ 3 & -6 & 5 \\ 3 & -2 & -1 \end{bmatrix}$

(xiii) $\begin{bmatrix} -1 & 0 & 1 \\ 3 & 1 & 2 \end{bmatrix}$ (xiv) $\begin{bmatrix} 1 & 0 & 0 \\ 0 & 1 & 0 \end{bmatrix}$

7. (i) $T(x, y, z, t) = (x - y + 2t, 3x + 4y + 2z - 4t)$

(ii) $T(x, y, z) = (x - y + 2z, 3x + y)$

(iii) $T(x, y, z) = (5x - 2y, -x - 2z)$

(iv) $T(x,y) = \left(\dfrac{2x+4y}{5}, \dfrac{-x-2y}{5}, \dfrac{-17x+y}{5} \right)$

$\left(\dfrac{7x+9y}{5}, \dfrac{5x}{5}, \dfrac{-12x+4y}{5} \right)$

(v) (a) $T(x,y,z) = (x,y,z)$

    (b) $T(x,y,z) = (x, 2y, -2z, -x+y+2z, x+y+z)$

(vi) $T(x,y) = (2y-x, y, 3y-3x)$

8.(i) $R(T) = \{(x, x+y, 2x+y)\}, x, y \in R$

    $N(T) = \{(0,0,0)\}$, rank $= 3$, nullity $= 0$

(ii) $R(T) =$ subspace spanned by $\{(1,0),(0,1)\} = V_2(R)$

    $N(T) = \{(1,1,1)\}$, rank $= 2$, nullity $= 1$

(iii) $\{(1,1,1,),(1,-1,1)(1,-3,3)\}$, rank $= 3$, nullity $= 0$

(iv) $R(T) =$ subspace spanned by $\{(0,1,1,0),(0,1,1,0),(0,1,-1,4)\}$,

    $N(T) = \{(-1,2,1,1)\}$, rank $= 2$, nullity $= 1$

(v) $R(T) =$ subspace spanned by $\{(1,0,0),(0,1,0),(0,1,0),(0,0,1)\}$

    $N(T) = \{(0,0,0)\}$, rank $= 3$, nullity $= 0$

(vi) $R(T) = R_3 \quad N(T) = \{(0,0,0)\}$

    Rank $= 3$, nullity $= 0$

(vii) $R(T) =$ subspace spanned by $\{(1,-1,0),(2,0,1)\}$,

    $N(T) = \{(1,1,-1)\}$ rank $= 2$, nullity $= 1$

(viii) $R(T) =$ subspace spanned by $\{(0,1),(1,1)\}$,

    $N(T) = \{(1,1,-2)\}$ rank $= 2$, nullity $= 1$

(ix) $R(T) =$ subspace spanned by $\{(1,-1,0),(2,0,1)\}$,

    $N(T) = \{(1,1,-1)\}$ rank $= 2$, nullity $= 1$

(x) $R(T) =$ subspace spanned by $\{(1,0),(0,1)\}$,

    $N(T) = \{(1,-1,1)\}$ rank $= 2$, nullity $= 1$

9. $T(x,y,z) = (x+2y, 2x-y, -4x-3y)$

10. $T(x,y,z) = (x+4y, 2x+5y, 3x+6y)$

11. $T(x,y,z,t) = (x+y, -z, 2x+y-t, 0)$

12. $T(x, y, z) = \left(0, 0, \dfrac{4x - 3y + z}{4} \right)$

13. $T(x, y, z) = (x + y, 2y, 2y - x)$

14. (i) $\lambda = 4, -1$; $(2, 3), (1, -1)$

(ii) $\lambda = 5, -1; (1,1), (-2,1)$

(iii) $\lambda = 1, 2, 3; (0,1,0), (1,-2,-2)$

(iv) $\lambda = 4, -2; (1,1,2), (0,1,1)$

(v) $\lambda = 2, 4, -2; (1,1,-4), (1,1,0)$

(vi) $\lambda = 0, -1, 7; (1,2,-2)$

(vii) $\lambda = 2, 6; (1,2,-3), (1,2,1)$

(viii) $\lambda = 1; (1,0,2)$

(ix) $\lambda = 3; (1,0,0)$

(x) $\lambda = 2; (7,6,-15)$

Inner Product Spaces

7.1 INTRODUCTION

Untill now, we have been studying vector spaces over an arbitrary field F. In this chapter, we restrict F to be the real field R and in such a case V is called a real vector space. In the study of arbitrary vector space, the concepts of a vector, angle between two vectors, orthogonality of vectors did not appear. We shall do this by defining a certain type of scalar valued function from $V \times V$ to R which will be known as inner product on V. An inner product on a vector space V is a function with properties similar to those of the dot product in R^3 which helps us to know the relationship between linear algebra and geometry

7.2 INNER PRODUCT SPACES

Let us begin with the definition of inner product.

Inner Product

Let V be a real vector space. An inner product on V is a function [,], $\langle,\rangle : V \cdot V \to R$ which assigns each ordered pair (u,v) and $V \times V$ to a real number $\langle u, v \rangle$ in $(u, v) \in V \cdot V$ in such a way that following axioms hold:

(i) **Linearity:** $\langle au_1 + bu_2, v \rangle = a\langle u_1, v \rangle + b\langle u_2, v \rangle$

for all $u_1, u_2, v \in V$ and $a, b \in R$

(ii) **Symmetry:** $\langle u, v \rangle = \langle v, u \rangle \ \forall \ u, v \in V$

(iii) **Positive definiteness:** $\langle u, v \rangle = \langle v, u \rangle \ \forall u, v \in V \geq 0$ and $\langle u, u \rangle = u^2$ if $u = 0v$

A vector space equipped with an inner product is called an inner product space.

Example 1: Consider the vector space R^n. Prove that R^n is an inner product space with the inner product defined by

$$(u, v) = a_1b_1 + a_2b_2 + \dots + a_nb_n$$

where $u = (a_1, a_2, ..., a_n)$ and $v = (b_1, b_2, ..., b_n)$.

Solution: We observe the following properties of the product defined above.

(i) Linearity: Let $u = (a_1, a_2, ..., a_n)$,

$$v = (b_1, b_2, ..., b_n)$$
$$w = (c_1, c_2, ..., c_n) \in V \text{ and } \alpha, \beta \in R$$

Then, $\alpha u + \beta v = \alpha(a_1, a_2, ..., a_n) + \beta(b_1, b_2, ..., b_n)$

$$= (\alpha a_1 + \beta b_1, \ \alpha a_2 + \beta b_2 + ... + \alpha a_n + \beta b_n)$$

$\therefore \ \langle \alpha u + \beta v, w \rangle = (\alpha a_1 + \beta b_1)c_1 + (\alpha a_2 + \alpha b_2)c_2 + ... + (\alpha a_n + \beta b_n)c_n$

$$\langle \alpha u + \beta v, w \rangle = \{(\alpha a_1)c_1 + (\alpha a_2)c_2 + ... + (\alpha a_n)c_n\} +$$
$$\{(\beta b_1)c_1 + (\beta b_2)c_2 + ... + (\beta b_n)c_n\}$$
$$= \alpha(a_1 c_1 + a_2 c_2 + ... + a_n c_n) + \beta(b_1 c_1 + b_2 c_2 + ... + b_n c_n)$$

$\Rightarrow \langle \alpha u + \beta v, w \rangle = \alpha \langle u, w \rangle + \beta \langle v, w \rangle$

(ii) Symmetry: Let $u = (a_1, a_2, ..., a_n)$ and $v = (b_1, b_2, ..., b_n) \in R^n$

Then $\langle u, v \rangle = a_1 b_1 + a_2 b_2 + ... + a_n b_n$

$\Rightarrow \quad \langle v, u \rangle = b_1 a_1 + b_2 a_2 + ... + b_n a_n$

$\Rightarrow \quad \langle u, v \rangle = \langle v, u \rangle$

(iii) Positive definiteness: For any $u = (a_1, a_2, ..., a_n) \in R^n$, $u \neq 0$, we have
$\langle u, u \rangle = a_1^2 + a_2^2 + ... + a_n^2$

$\Rightarrow \langle u, u \rangle > 0$ $\qquad\qquad$ [$u \neq 0$, $a_i \neq 0$ for at least one a_i]

Thus, the given function is an inner product on R^n.

Hence, R^n is an inner product space for the defined product.

Example 2: Prove that R^2 is an inner product space with an inner product defined by $\langle u, v \rangle = a_1 b_1 - a_2 b_1 - a_1 b_2 + 2a_2 b_2$ where $u = (a_1, a_2)$, $v = (b_1, b_2) \in R^2$

Solution: Clearly, R^2 is a vector space over R. We observe the following properties of the function defined above.

(i) Linearity: For any $u = (a_1, a_2)$, $v = (b_1, b_2)$, $w = (c_1, c_2) \in R^2$ and $\alpha, \beta \in R$,

we have $\alpha u + \beta v = (\alpha a_1 + \beta b_1, \ \alpha a_2 + \beta b_2)$

$\langle \alpha u + \beta v, w \rangle = (\alpha a_1 + \beta b_1)c_1 - (\alpha a_2 + \beta b_2)c_1 - (\alpha a_1 + \beta b_1)c_2 +$
$$2(\alpha a_2 + \beta b_2)c_2$$
$$= \alpha(a_1 c_1 - a_2 c_1 - a_1 c_2 + 2a_2 c_2) + \beta(b_1 c_1 - b_2 c_1 -$$
$$b_1 c_2 + 2b_2 c_2)$$

$\langle \alpha u + \beta v, w \rangle = \alpha \langle u, w \rangle + \beta \langle v, w \rangle$

(ii) Symmetry: For any $u = (a_1, a_2)$, $v = (b_1, b_2) \in R^2$, we have

$\langle u, v \rangle = a_1 b_1 - a_2 b_1 - a_1 b_2 + 2a_2 b_2$

$\langle v, u \rangle = b_1 a_1 - b_1 a_2 - b_2 a_1 + 2b_2 a_2$

$\Rightarrow \langle u, v \rangle = \langle v, u \rangle$

(iii) Positive definiteness: For any non-zero $u = (a_1, a_2) \in R^2$ we have,

$\langle u, u \rangle = a_1 a_1 - a_2 a_1 - a_1 a_2 + 2a_2 a_2$

$$\langle u, u \rangle = a_1{}^2 - 2a_1a_2 + 2a_2{}^2 = (a_1 - a_2)^2 + a_2 > 0$$
$$[u \neq 0 \Rightarrow a_1 \neq 0 \text{ or } a_2 \neq 0]$$

Thus, the function defined above is an inner product on R^2.

Hence R^2 is an inner product space for the defined product.

Example 3: Consider the vector space $\in [a, b]$ of all continuous functions defined on the closed interval $[a, b]$. Prove that the following defines an inner product on $[a, b]$.

$$\langle \phi, \gamma \rangle = \int_b^a f(t)g(t)dt, \text{ where } f(t) \text{ and } g(t) \text{ are function in } [a, b].$$

Solution: We observe the following properties of the function defined above.

(i) Linearity: For any $f, g, h \in [a, b]$ and $\alpha, \beta \in R$, we have

$$\langle \alpha f + \beta g, h \rangle = \int_a^b (\alpha f + \beta g)t\, h(t)\, dt$$

$$= \int_a^b \{\alpha f(t)\, h(t) + \beta g(t)\, h(t)\}\, dt$$

$$\Rightarrow \quad \langle \alpha f + \beta g, h \rangle = \alpha \int_a^b f(t)\, h(t)\, dt + \beta \int_a^b g(t)\, h(t)\, dt$$

$$\Rightarrow \quad \langle \alpha f + \beta g, h \rangle = \alpha \langle f, h \rangle + \beta \langle g, h \rangle$$

(ii) Symmetry: For any $f, g \in [a, b]$, we have

$$\langle f, g \rangle = \int_a^b f(t)\, g(t)\, dt = \int_a^b g(t) f(t)\, dt = \langle g, f \rangle$$

(iii) Positive definiteness: For any non-zero function $f[a, b]$, we have

$$\langle f, f \rangle = \int_a^b f(t) f(t)\, dt = \int_a^b \{f(t)\}^2 dt > 0$$

$$\because f(t) \neq 0 \text{ for some } t \in [a, b]$$

Hence the given function is an inner product on $[a, b]$.

Example 4: Prove that the vector space $R^{m \times n}$ for all $m \times n$ matrices over R is an inner product space with an inner product defined on it by

$$\langle A, B \rangle = tr \langle B^T A \rangle \text{ for all } A, B \in R^{m \times n}$$

Solution: We observe the following properties of the function defined above.

(i) Linearity: For any $A, B, C \in R^{m \times n}$ and $a, b \in R$, we have

$$\langle aA + bB, C \rangle = tr\{C^T(aA + bB)\}$$
$$\Rightarrow \langle aA + bB, C \rangle = tr(aC^TA + bC^TB)$$
$$\Rightarrow \langle aA + bB, C \rangle = tr(aC^TA) + tr(bC^TB) \quad [\because tr(A + B) = tr(A) + tr(B)]$$
$$= a\,tr(C^TA) + b\,tr(C^TB) \quad [\because tr(\lambda A) = \lambda tr(A)]$$
$$= a\langle A, C \rangle + b\langle B, C \rangle$$

(ii) **Symmerty:** For any $A, B \in R^{m \times n}$, we have

$$\langle A, B \rangle = tr(B^T A)$$

$$\Rightarrow \quad \langle A, B \rangle = tr(B^T A)^T \qquad [\because tr(A) = tr(A^T)]$$

$$\Rightarrow \quad \langle A, B \rangle = tr(A^T B) \qquad [\because (B^T A)^T = A^T (B^T)^T = A^T B]$$

$$\Rightarrow \quad \langle A, B \rangle = \langle B, A \rangle$$

(iii) **Positive definiteness:** For any non-null matrix

$$A = [a_{ij}] \in R^{m \times n}, \text{we have}$$

$$\langle A, A \rangle = tr(A^T A)$$

$$\Rightarrow \quad \langle A, A \rangle = \sum_{i=1}^{n+m} (A^T A)_{ii}$$

$$= \sum_{i=1}^{n} \left(\sum_{r=1}^{m} (A^T A_{ir}(A)_{ri} \right)$$

$$\langle A, A \rangle = \sum_{i=1}^{n} \left(\sum_{r=1}^{m} a_{ri} a_{ri} \right)$$

$$= \sum_{i=1}^{n} \left(\sum_{r=1}^{m} (a_{ri})^2 \right) > 0 \ (\because A \neq 0)$$

$$(\therefore \text{atleast one } a_{ij} \neq 0)$$

Thus, the given function is an inner product and $R^{m \times n}$ is an inner product space.

Example 5: Find the value of K so that the following is an inner product on R^2.

$\langle u, v \rangle = x_1 y_1 - 3x_1 y_2 - 3x_2 y_1 + K x_2 y_2$, where $u = (x_1, x_2)$, $v = (y_1, y_2) \in R^2$.

Solution: The above function is an inner product on R^2. Therefore

$\langle u, u \rangle > 0$ for all $u = (x_1, x_2) \in R^2, u \neq 0$

$\Rightarrow x_1^2 - 3x_1 x_2 - 3x_2 x_1 + K x_2^2 > 0$ for all $x_1, x_2 \in R$

$$\Rightarrow x_2^2 \left\{ \left(\frac{x_1}{x_2} \right)^2 - 6 \left(\frac{x_1}{x_2} \right) + K \right\} > 0 \ \forall \ x_1, x_2 \in R$$

$$\Rightarrow \left(\frac{x_1}{x_2} \right)^2 - 6 \left(\frac{x_1}{x_2} \right) + K > 0 \ \forall \ x_1, x_2 \in R \qquad \left(\therefore a = \frac{x_1}{x_2} \right)$$

$\Rightarrow a^2 - 6a + K > 0$ for all $a \in R, a \neq 0$

$\Rightarrow 36 - 4K < 0 \qquad [\because ax^2 + bx + c > 0 \text{ for all } x \in R \Rightarrow a > 0]$

$\Rightarrow K > 9 \qquad [b^2 - 4ac > 0]$

Example 6: Let V be an inner product space and $u,\ v \in V$. Simplify $\langle 2u - 5v,\ 4u + 6v \rangle$.

Solution: Using linearity of the inner product, we have

$$\langle 2u - 5v,\ 4u + 6v \rangle = 2\langle u,\ 4u + 6v \rangle - 5\langle v,\ 4u + 6v \rangle$$

$$\Rightarrow \langle 2u - 5v,\ 4u + 6v \rangle = 2\{\langle u,\ 4u \rangle + \langle u,\ 6v \rangle\} - 5\{\langle v,\ 4u \rangle + \langle v,\ 6v \rangle\}$$

$$= 2\{4\langle u,\ u \rangle + 6\langle u,\ v \rangle\} - 5\{4\langle v,\ u \rangle + 6\langle v,\ v \rangle\}$$

$$= 8\langle u,\ u \rangle + 12\langle u,v \rangle - 20\langle v,\ u \rangle - 30\langle v,\ v \rangle$$

$$\Rightarrow \langle 2u - 5v,\ 4u + 6v \rangle = 8\langle u,\ u \rangle - 8\langle u,v \rangle - 30\langle v,\ v \rangle$$

Example 7: Let $\langle . \rangle$ be the standard inner product on R^2. If $u = (1,\ 2)$, $v = (-1,\ 1) \in R^2$, then find $w \in R^2$ satisfying $\langle u,\ w \rangle = -1$ and $\langle v,\ w \rangle = 3$.

Solution: Let $w = (a,\ b) \in R^2$, then

$$\langle u,w \rangle = -1 \text{ and } \langle v,w \rangle = 3$$

$$a + 2b = -1 \text{ and } -a + b = 3$$

$$\Rightarrow \qquad a = \frac{-7}{3},\ b = \frac{2}{3}$$

$$\Rightarrow \qquad w = \left(-\frac{7}{3}, \frac{2}{3} \right)$$

Example 8: Let $\langle , \rangle$ denote the standard inner product on R^2. Show that for any $u \in R^2$, we have $u = \left\langle u, e_1^{(2)} \right\rangle e_1^{(2)} + \left\langle u, e_1^{(2)} \right\rangle e_2^{(2)}$.

Solution: We have $e_1^{(2)} = (1,0)$ and $e_2^{(2)} = (0,\ 1)$

Let $\qquad u = (a,b) \in R^2$, then

$$\left\langle u, e_1^{(2)} \right\rangle = a \times 1 + b \times 0 = a \text{ and}$$

$$\left\langle u, e_2^{(2)} \right\rangle = a \times 0 + b \times 1 = b$$

$$\left\langle u, e_1^{(2)} \right\rangle e_1^{(2)} + \left\langle u, e_2^{(2)} \right\rangle e_2^{(2)} = ae_1^{(2)} + be_2^{(2)}$$

$$= a(1,0) + b(0,1) = (a,b) = u$$

Example 9: Let V be an inner product space with inner product $\langle , \rangle$. Then show that

(i) $\langle 0v,\ v \rangle = 0$ for all $v \in V$

(ii) If $\langle u,\ v \rangle = 0$ for all $v \in V$, then $u = 0v$

Solution:

(i) For any $v \in V$, we have

$$(0v,\ v) = \langle 00v_1,\ v \rangle$$

$$= 0\langle 0v_1, v\rangle = 0 \qquad\qquad [\because \langle au, v\rangle = a\langle u, v\rangle]$$

Hence $\langle 0v_1 v\rangle = 0$ for all $v \in V$

(ii) Let $\quad \langle u, v\rangle = 0$ for all $v \in V$

$$\Rightarrow \qquad \langle u, v\rangle = 0$$

$$\Rightarrow \qquad u = 0v \qquad\qquad\qquad [\text{Taking } v = u]$$

Example 10: Let V be an inner product space with $\langle,\rangle$ as an inner product and $u, w \in V$ for all $w \in V$.

Solution: First, let $u = v$. Then,

$$\langle u, v\rangle = \langle v, w\rangle \text{ for all } w \in V.$$

Conversely, let $u, v \in V$ such that

$$\langle u, v\rangle = \langle v, w\rangle \text{ for all } w \in V.$$

$$\Rightarrow \langle u, v\rangle - \langle v, w\rangle = 0 \text{ for all } w \in V.$$

$$\Rightarrow \qquad \langle u - v, w\rangle = 0 \qquad\qquad [\text{Taking } w = u - v]$$

$$\Rightarrow \qquad u - v = \text{ or } w = 0 \qquad\qquad [\because \langle u, u\rangle = 0 \Leftrightarrow u = 0]$$

$$\Rightarrow \qquad u = v$$

Example 11: Let $A = [a_{ij}]$ be a 2×2 matrix with real entries. For x, y in $R^{2\times 1}$ let $f_A(x, y) = y^T A x$.

Show that f_A is an inner product on $R^{2\times 1}$ iff

$$A^T = A,\ a_{11} > 0 \text{ and } |A| > 0.$$

Solution: First, let $A = [a_{ij}]$ be such that $A^T = A$, $a_{11} > 0$, $a_{22} > 0$ and $|A| = 0$. Then, we have to show that f_A is an inner product on $R^{2\times 1}$.

We observe the following properties of f_A:

(i) Linearity: Let $x, y, z \in R^{2\times 1}$ and $a, b \in R$. Then

$$f_A(ax + by, z) = z^T A(ax + by)$$

$$= af_A(x, z) + bf_A(y, z)$$

(ii) Symmetry: For any $x, y \in R^{2\times 1}$, we have

$$f_A(x, y) = y^T A x = y^T A^T (x^T)^T \qquad\qquad [\because A^T = A]$$

$$= (x^T A y)^T$$

$$= (x^T A y)$$

$$= f_A(y, x)$$

(iii) Positive definiteness: For any $x = \begin{bmatrix} x_1 \\ x_2 \end{bmatrix} \to k^{2\times 1}$ we have

$$f_A(x_1, x_2) = x^T A x$$

$$\Rightarrow \quad f_A(x_1, x_2) = a_{11} x_1^2 + a_{12} x_1 x_2 + a_{21} x_1 x_2 + a_{22} x_2^2$$

$$f_A(x_1, x_2) = a_{11} x_1^2 + 2a_{12} x_1 x_2 + a_{22} x_2^2 \quad [\because A^T = A \therefore a_{12} = a_{21}]$$

It is given that $a_{11} > 0$, $a_{22} > 0$ and $A < 0$

$\therefore a_{11} a_{22} a_{21} a_{12} > 0$

$\Rightarrow a_{11} a_{22} (a_{12})^2 > 0$

$\Rightarrow 4\{(a_{12})^2 a_{12} a_{12}\} < 0$

$\Rightarrow a_{11} x_1^2 (a_{12})^2 > 0$ $\qquad [\therefore a_{11} > 0]$

(Symmetry) $\qquad f_A(x_1, x) > 0$

Hence f_A is an inner product on $R^{2 \times 1}$.

Conversely, let f_A be an inner product on $R^{2 \times 1}$. Then

$f_A(x_1, y_1) = f_A(y_1, x_1)$ for all $x, y \to R^{2 \times 1}$ (symmetry)

$$\Rightarrow \qquad [y_1 y_2] \begin{bmatrix} a_{11} & a_{12} \\ a_{21} & a_{22} \end{bmatrix} \begin{bmatrix} x_1 \\ x_2 \end{bmatrix} = [x_1 x_2] \begin{bmatrix} a_{11} & a_{12} \\ a_{21} & a_{22} \end{bmatrix} \begin{bmatrix} y_1 \\ y_2 \end{bmatrix}$$

where $\qquad x = \begin{bmatrix} x_1 \\ x_2 \end{bmatrix}, y = \begin{bmatrix} y_1 \\ y_2 \end{bmatrix}$

$\Rightarrow a_{11} x_1 y_1 + a_{12} x_2 y_1 + a_{21} x_1 y_2 + a_{22} x_2 y_2$

$\qquad = a_{11} x_1 y_1 + a_{12} x_2 y_1 + a_{21} x_2 y_1 + a_{22} x_1 y_2 + a_{22} x_2 y_2$

$\Rightarrow (x_1 y_2 x_2 y_1 (a_{21} a_{12}) = 0 \; \forall \; x_1, x_2, y_1, y_2 \in R$

$\Rightarrow \qquad a_{21} a_{12} = 0 \Rightarrow a_{12} = a_{21} \Rightarrow A^T = A$

For any $x = \begin{bmatrix} x_1 \\ x_2 \end{bmatrix} \in R^{2 \times 1}$, we have

$f_A(x, x) > 0 \qquad$ (positive definiteness)

$\Rightarrow x^T A x > 0$

$\Rightarrow a_{11} x_1^2 + a_{12} x_1 x_2 + a_{21} x_2 x_2 + a_{22} x_2^2 > 0$

$\Rightarrow a_{11} x_1^2 + 2a_{12} x_1 x_2 + a_{22} x_2^2 > 0 \; \forall \; x_1, x_2 \in R \qquad [\because a_{12} = a_{21}]$

$\Rightarrow a_{11} > 0, a_{22} > 0$ and $4a_{12}^2 - 4a_{11} a_{22} < 0$

$\Rightarrow a_{11} > 0, a_{22} > 0$ and $a_{11} a_{22} - a_{12} a_{21} > 0 \qquad [\because a_{12} = a_{21}]$

$\Rightarrow a_{11} > 0, a_{22} > 0$ and $|A| > 0$

7.3 NORM OR LENGTH OF A VECTOR

In this section, we introduce the concept of length (norm) of a vector.

Norm of a vector

Let V be an inner product space and $u \in V$. Then non-negative square root of $\langle u, u \rangle$, i.e. $\sqrt{\langle u, u \rangle}$ is called the norm or length of u and is denoted by $\|u\|$.

Thus $\|u\| = \sqrt{\langle u, u \rangle}$

If $\|u\| = 1$ or equivalently $\langle u, u \rangle = 1$, then u is called a unit vector and is said to be normalized.

Note: Every non-zero vector u in an inner product space V can be normalized by multiplying it by the reciprocal of its length, i.e. $u = \dfrac{1}{\|u\|} \cdot u$

Clearly, u is a positive multiple of u. The process of getting unit vector u from a vector u is called normalized vector u.

Theorem 1: If V is an inner product space and $v \in V$, then

(i) $\|u\| \geq 0$ and $\|u\| = 0$ iff $u = 0v$

(ii) $\|au\| = |a| \|u\|$ for all $a \in \mathbb{R}$.

Proof:

(i) If $u \neq 0$, then $\langle u, u \rangle > 0$

$$\therefore \|u\| = \sqrt{\langle u, u \rangle} \Rightarrow \|u\|^2 = \langle u, u \rangle \Rightarrow \|u\|^2 > 0$$

If $u = 0v$, then

$$\langle u, u \rangle = \langle 0_v, 0_v \rangle = 0 \Rightarrow \|u\|^2 = 0 \text{ iff } u = 0v.$$

(ii) We have

$$\|au\|^2 = \langle au, au \rangle = a^2 \langle u, u \rangle = a^2 \|u\|^2$$

$$\Rightarrow \|au\| = |a| \|u\| \qquad \text{[taking square root of both sides]}$$

Theorem 2: (Cauchy-Schwarz inequality) For any two vectors u and v in an inner product space V, prove that $\langle u, v \rangle^2 \leq \langle u, u \rangle \langle v, v \rangle$ or $|\langle u, v \rangle| \leq \|u\| \|v\|$

Proof: If $u = 0v$, then both $\langle u, v \rangle = 0$ and $\|u\| \|v\| = 0$, so theorem holds good.

Then for any real number t, we have $\langle tu + v, tu + v \rangle \geq 0$

$$\text{[by positive definiteness]}$$

$\Rightarrow \quad \langle tu, tu \rangle + \langle tu, v \rangle + \langle v, tu \rangle + \langle v, v \rangle \geq 0$

$\Rightarrow \quad t^2 \langle u, u \rangle + t \langle u, v \rangle + t \langle v, u \rangle + \langle v, v \rangle \geq 0$

$\Rightarrow \quad t^2 \|u\|^2 + t \langle u, v \rangle + t \langle u, v \rangle + \|v\|^2 \geq 0$

$\Rightarrow \quad t^2 \|u\|^2 + 2t \langle u, v \rangle + \|v\|^2 \geq 0$

$\Rightarrow \quad 4\{\langle u, v \rangle\}^2 - 4\|u\|^2 \|v\|^2 \leq 0 \quad [\because ax^2 + bx + c > 0 \text{ for all } x \text{ and } a > 0$

$$\Rightarrow b^2 - 4ac \leq 0]$$

$\Rightarrow \quad \{\langle u, v \rangle\}^2 \leq \|u\|^2 \|v\|^2$

$\Rightarrow \quad |\langle u, v \rangle| \leq \|u\| \|v\| \qquad [\because x^2 \leq a^2 \Rightarrow |x| \leq a]$

Corollary 1: For any real numbers x_1, x_2, y_1 and y_2, prove that $|x_1 y_1 + x_2 y_2|$

$$\leq \left(x_1^2 + x_2^2\right)^{1/2} \left(y_1^2 + y_2^2\right)^{1/2}$$

Proof: Let $u = (x_1, x_2)$, $v = (y_1, y_2) \in R^2$.

Since R^2 is an inner product space with respect to the standard inner product, therefore by Cauchy-Schwarz inequality, we have $|\langle u, v \rangle| \leq \|u\| \, \|v\|$

$$\Rightarrow \quad |x_1 y_1 + x_2 y_2| \leq \left(x_1^2 + x_2^2\right)^{1/2} \left(y_1^2 + y_2^2\right)^{1/2}$$

Corollary 2: For any two vectors u and v in an inner product space V, prove that $|\langle u+v \rangle| \leq \|u\| + \|v\|$ (triangle inequality)

Proof: Using the definition of norm of a vector, we have

$$\|\langle u + v \rangle\|^2 = \langle u+v, \, u+v \rangle$$

$$\Rightarrow \quad \|\langle u+v \rangle\|^2 = \langle u, \, u + v \rangle \langle v, \, u + v \rangle$$

$$= \langle u, \, u \rangle + \langle u, \, v \rangle + \langle u, \, v \rangle + \langle v, \, v \rangle \qquad [\because \langle u, v \rangle = \langle v, u \rangle]$$

$$\Rightarrow \quad \|\langle u+v \rangle\|^2 = \|u\|^2 + 2\langle u, \, v \rangle + \|v\|^2$$

By Cauchy-Schwarz inequality, we have $\langle u, v \rangle \leq \|u\| \, \|v\|$

$$\Rightarrow 2 \langle u, v \rangle \leq 2 \| u \| \, \| v \|$$

$$\Rightarrow \|u\|^2 + 2\langle u, v \rangle + \|v\|^2 \leq \|u\|^2 + 2\|u\| \, \|v\| + \|v\|^2$$

$$\Rightarrow \|\langle u+v \rangle\|^2 \leq (\|u\| + \|v\|)^2 \qquad [\because x^2 \leq a^2 \Rightarrow |x| \leq a]$$

$$\Rightarrow \|\langle u+v \rangle\| \leq \|u\| + \|v\|$$

Theorem 3: Let V be an inner product space and $u, v \in V$, then

(i) $\|\langle u + v \rangle\|^2 - \|\langle u - v \rangle\|^2 = 4 \langle u, v \rangle$

(ii) $\|\langle u + v \rangle\|^2 + \|\langle u - v \rangle\|^2 = 2(\|u\|^2 + \|v\|^2)$ **(parallelogram law)**

Proof: By using the definition of norm of a vector, we have

$$\|u+v\|^2 = \langle u + v, u + v \rangle$$

$$= \langle u, \, u + v \rangle + \langle v, \, u+v \rangle$$

$$= \langle u, \, u \rangle + \langle u, \, v \rangle + \langle u, \, v \rangle + \langle v, \, v \rangle \qquad [\because \langle u, v \rangle = \langle v, u \rangle]$$

$$= \|u\|^2 + 2\langle u, \, v \rangle + \|v\|^2 \qquad \qquad \dots \text{(i)}$$

and

$$\|u - v\|^2 = \langle u - v, \, u-v \rangle$$

$$= \langle u, \, u - v \rangle + \langle -v, \, u - v \rangle$$

$$= \langle u, \, u \rangle - \langle u, \, v \rangle - \langle v, \, u \rangle + (-1)^2 \langle v, \, v \rangle$$

$$= \langle u, \, u \rangle - 2\langle u, \, v \rangle + \langle v, \, v \rangle$$

$$= \|u\|^2 - 2\langle u, \, v \rangle + \|v\|^2 \qquad \qquad \dots \text{(ii)}$$

On subtracting Eq. (ii) from Eq. (i) we get

$$\|u + v\|^2 - \|u - v\|^2 = 4\langle u, v \rangle$$

On adding Eq. (i) and (ii), we get

$$\|u + v\|^2 - \|u - v\|^2 = 2(\|u\|^2 + \|v\|^2)$$

Theorem 4: If u and v are vectors in an inner product space V, then

$$|\ \|u\| - \|v\|\ | \le \|u - v\|$$

Proof: We have

$$|\ \|u\| - \|v\|\ | = \|u\|^2 + \|v\|^2 - 2\|u\|\ \|v\|$$
$$= \langle u,\ u \rangle + \langle v,\ v \rangle - 2\|u\|\ \|v\|$$

By Cauchy-Schwarz inequality, we have $|\langle u,\ v \rangle| \le \|u\|\ \|v\|$

$\Rightarrow \quad -\|u\|\ \|v\| \le \langle u,\ v \rangle \le \|u\|\ \|v\| \qquad [\because |x| \le a \Leftrightarrow -a \le x \le a]$

$\Rightarrow \quad \langle u,\ v \rangle \le \|u\|\ \|v\|$

$\Rightarrow \quad -2\|u\|\ \|v\| \le -2 \langle u,\ v \rangle$

$\Rightarrow \quad \langle u,\ u \rangle + \langle v,\ v \rangle - 2\|u\|\ \|v\| \le \langle u,\ u \rangle + \langle v,\ v \rangle - 2\langle u, v \rangle$

$\Rightarrow \quad |\ \|u\| - \|v\|\ |^2 \le \langle u,\ u \rangle + \langle -v,\ -v \rangle + \langle u,\ -v \rangle + \langle -v,\ u \rangle$

$\Rightarrow \quad |\ \|u\| - \|v\|\ |^2 \le \langle u{-}v,\ u{-}v \rangle \qquad \left[\begin{array}{l} u\langle u, -v \rangle - v\langle -v, u \rangle \\ \langle u - v, -v + u \rangle \\ \|u - v\|^2 \end{array} \right.$

$\Rightarrow \quad |\ \|u\| - \|v\|\ |^2 \le \|u{-}v\|^2 \qquad \because$

$\Rightarrow \quad \|u\| - \|v\| \le \|u{-}v\|$

Example 1: Let u, v be vectors in an inner product space V, such that $|\langle u, v \rangle|$ = $\|u\| \cdot \|v\|$, i.e. Cauchy-Schwarz inequality is reduce to an equality. Show that u and v are linearly dependent vectors.

Solution: If one of the two vectors u and v is zero vector, then $|\langle u,\ v \rangle| = \|u\| \cdot \|v\|$ holds good and u and v form a linearly dependent set of vectors as any set containing zero vector is linearly dependent. So, let us assume that at least one of u and v is an non-zero vector. Let $u \ne 0v$.

Then $\|u\| > 0$.

Consider the vector

$$w = v - \frac{\langle u, v \rangle u}{\|u\|^2} = v - \lambda\, u \quad \text{where } \lambda = \frac{\langle u, v \rangle}{\|u\|^2}$$

$\Rightarrow \quad \langle w,\ w \rangle = \langle v - \lambda\, u,\ v - \lambda\, u \rangle$

$\qquad\qquad = \langle v,\ v \rangle + \langle v,\ -\lambda\, u \rangle + \langle -\lambda\, u, v \rangle + \langle -\lambda\, u,\ -\lambda\, u \rangle$

$\qquad\qquad = \langle v,\ v \rangle - \lambda \langle v,\ u \rangle - \lambda \langle u,\ v \rangle + \lambda^2 \langle u,\ u \rangle$

$\qquad\qquad = \|v\|^2 - 2\lambda \langle u,\ v \rangle + \lambda^2 \|u\|^2$

$\qquad\qquad = \|v\|^2 - \dfrac{2\{\langle u, v \rangle\}^2}{\|u\|^2} + \dfrac{\{\langle u, v \rangle\}^2}{\|u\|^2}$

$\qquad\qquad = \|v\|^2 - \|v\|^2$

$\qquad\qquad = 0 \qquad [\because |\langle u, v \rangle| = \|u\| \cdot \|v\| = \{\langle u,\ v \rangle\}^2 = \|u\|^2 \|v\|^2]$

$\qquad\qquad\qquad\qquad\qquad\qquad [\because |\langle u,\ v \rangle| = 0 \Rightarrow u = 0v]$

$$\Rightarrow \quad v - \frac{\langle u,v \rangle}{\|u\|^2} u = 0v$$

$$\Rightarrow \quad v = \frac{\langle u,v \rangle}{\|u\|^2} u$$

$\Rightarrow v$ is a scalar multiple of u.

$\Rightarrow u$ and v are linearly dependent vectors.

Example 2: Let u and v be two vectors in an inner product space V such that $\|u + v\| = \|u\| + \|v\|$. Prove that u and v are linearly dependent vectors. Give an example to show that the converse of this statement is not true.

Solution:

We have $\quad\quad\quad \|u + v\| = \|u\| + \|v\|$

$\Rightarrow \quad\quad\quad\quad \|u + v\|^2 = (\|u\| + \|v\|)^2$

$\Rightarrow \quad\quad \langle u + v, u + v \rangle = \|u\|^2 + \|v\|^2 + 2\|u\| \cdot \|v\|$

$\Rightarrow \langle u, u \rangle + 2\langle u, v \rangle + \langle v, v \rangle = |u\|^2 + \|v\|^2 + 2\|u\| \cdot \|v\|$

$\Rightarrow \quad\quad\quad\quad \langle u, v \rangle = \|u\| \cdot \|v\|$

$\Rightarrow u$ and v are linearly dependent vectors.

The converse is not true because vectors $u = (-1, 0, 1)$ and $v = (-2, 0, 2)$ in R^3 are linearly dependent as $v = 2u$.

But $\|u + v\| \neq (\|u\| + \|v\|)$.

7.4 ANGLE BETWEEN VECTORS

Let V be an inner product space. Let u and v be two non-zero vectors in V. The angle between u and v is defined as the angle θ such that $-\pi \leq \theta \leq \pi$

and $\cos\theta = \dfrac{\langle u,v \rangle}{\|u\| \, \|v\|}$

By the Cauchy-Schwarz inequality, we have

$$-\|u\| \, \|v\| \leq \langle u, v \rangle \leq \|u\| \, \|v\|$$

$$\Rightarrow \quad -1 \leq \frac{\langle u,v \rangle}{\|u\| \, \|v\|} \leq 1 \Rightarrow -1 \leq \cos\theta \leq 1$$

So $\cos\theta = \dfrac{\langle u,v \rangle}{\|u\| \, \|v\|}$ is meaningful and gives unique value of θ.

Example 1: R^3 is an inner product space with respect to standard inner product. Find the angle between the vector $u = (1, 1, 2)$ and $v = (2, -1, 1)$

Solution: Let θ be the angle between u and v. Then $\cos\theta = \dfrac{\langle u,v\rangle}{\|u\|\,\|v\|}$.

We have, $u=(1, 1, 2)$ and $v = (2, -1, 1)$

$\therefore \quad \langle u, v\rangle = 1{\cdot}2 + 1{\cdot}{-}1 + 2{\cdot}1 = 3$

$\|u\| = \sqrt{1+1+4} = \sqrt{6}$ and $\|v\|= \sqrt{4+1+1} = \sqrt{6}$

$\cos\theta = \dfrac{3}{\sqrt{6}\times\sqrt{6}} = \dfrac{1}{2} \Rightarrow \theta = \dfrac{\pi}{3}$

Example 2: In the inner product space R^4 with respect to standard inner product, find the angle between the vectors $u = (2, 1, 2, -3)$ and $v = (-2, 2, 1, 3)$.

Solution: We have

$u = (2, 1, 2, -3)$ and $v = (-2, 2, 1, 3)$

$\langle u, v\rangle = 2{\cdot}{-}2 + 1{\cdot}2 + 2{\cdot}1 + (-3){\cdot}3 = -9$

$\|u\| = \sqrt{4+1+4+9} = 3\sqrt{2}$,

$\|v\| = \sqrt{4+4+1+9} = 3\sqrt{2}$

If θ be the angle between u and v, then

$\cos\theta = \dfrac{\langle u,v\rangle}{\|u\|\,\|v\|} = \dfrac{-9}{(3\sqrt{2})\times(3\sqrt{2})} = \dfrac{-1}{3}$

$\Rightarrow \qquad \theta = \dfrac{2\pi}{3}$

Example 3: Find the angle between $f(t) = t-1$ and $g(t) = t$ in the polynomial space $p(t)$ with inner product $\langle f, g\rangle = \int_0^1 f(t)g(t)dt$.

Solution: $f(t) = t-1$ and $g(t) = t$

$\|f\|^2 = \langle f, f\rangle = \int_0^1 f^2(t)dt = \int_0^1 (t-1)^2\,dt = \left[\dfrac{(t-1)^3}{3}\right]_0^1 = \dfrac{1}{3}$

$\|g\|^2 = \langle g, g\rangle = \int_0^1 g^2(t)dt = \int_0^1 t^2\,dt = \dfrac{1}{3}$

and $\quad \langle f, g\rangle = \int_0^1 f(t)g(t)dt = \int_0^1 (t-1)t\,dt$

$= \left[\dfrac{t^3}{3} - \dfrac{t^2}{2}\right]_0^1 = \dfrac{-1}{6}$

Let 'θ' be the angle between f and g.

Then $\cos \theta = \dfrac{\langle f, g \rangle}{\|f\| \, \|g\|} = \dfrac{-\dfrac{1}{6}}{\sqrt{\dfrac{1}{3}} \times \sqrt{\dfrac{1}{3}}} = \dfrac{-1}{2} \Rightarrow \theta = \dfrac{2\pi}{3}$

Example 4: Consider the inner product space $R^{2\times 3}$ of all 2×3 matrices over R with the inner product defined by $\langle A, B \rangle = tr \langle B^T, A \rangle$ for all $A, B \in R^{2\times 3}$.

Find the angle between $A = \begin{bmatrix} 9 & 8 & 7 \\ 6 & 5 & 4 \end{bmatrix}$ and

$$B = \begin{bmatrix} 1 & 2 & 3 \\ 4 & 5 & 6 \end{bmatrix}$$

Solution: We have $\langle A, B \rangle = tr\langle B^T A \rangle = \sum_{i=1}^{3}(B^T A)_{ii} = \sum_{i=1}^{3}(\sum_{r=1}^{n} b_{ri} - a_{ri})$

 = sum of the product of corresponding elements of A and B.

$\Rightarrow \langle A, B \rangle = 9 \cdot 1 + 8 \cdot 2 + 7 \cdot 3 + 6 \cdot 4 + 5 \cdot 5 + 4 \cdot 6 = 119$

$$\|A\|^2 = \langle A, A \rangle = tr\langle A^T A \rangle = \sum_{i=1}^{3}(A^T A)_{ii} = \sum_{i=1}^{3}(\sum_{r=1}^{n} a_{ri}^2)$$

$\Rightarrow \quad \|A\|^2$ = sum of square of elements of A

 = $81 + 64 + 49 + 36 + 25 + 16 = 271$

$\Rightarrow \quad \|A\| = \sqrt{271}$

and

$\|B\|^2$ = sum of squares of elements of B

$\|B\| = 1 + 4 + 9 + 16 + 25 + 36 = 91$

$\|B\| = \sqrt{91}$

Let θ be the angle between A and B. Then

$$\cos \theta = \dfrac{\langle A, B \rangle}{\|A\| \, \|B\|} = \dfrac{199}{\sqrt{271} \times \sqrt{91}}$$

EXERCISE

1. Consider the inner product space R^3 with the standard inner product. If $u = (2, 3, 5)$ and $v = (1, -4, 3) \in R^3$ and θ is the angle between u and v, find $\cos \theta$.

Ans. $\dfrac{5}{\sqrt{26}\sqrt{38}}$

2. Find $\cos \theta$, where θ is the angle between $u = (1, 3, -5, 4)$ and $v = (2, -3, 4, 1)$ in inner product space R^4 with standard inner product.

Ans. $\dfrac{-23}{\sqrt{1530}}$

3. Let $p(t)$ be an inner product space of all polynomials with inner product defined by $\langle f, g \rangle = \int_0^1 f(t) g(t) dt$ for all $f, g \in p(t)$.

If $f(t) = 3t - 5$ and $g(t) = t^2$, then find the angle between f and g.

Ans. $\cos^{-1}\left(\dfrac{-55}{12\sqrt{65}} \right)$

7.5 ORTHOGONALITY

In this section, we shall discuss the concept of orthogonality and orthonormality of vectors in an inner product space. The same will be extended to orthogonal and orthonormal bases of an inner product space.

Orthogonal Vectors

Let V be an inner product space and vectors $u, v \in V$. Then vector u is said to be orthogonal to vector v if $\langle u, v \rangle = 0$.

If u is orthogonal to v, then we write $u \perp v$.

Let u, v be vectors in an inner product space V such that

$$u \perp v \Rightarrow \langle u, v \rangle = 0 \quad \Rightarrow \langle v, u \rangle = 0 \text{ (by symmetry)}$$
$$\Rightarrow v \perp u$$

Thus, the relation "is orthogonal to" an inner product space is a symmetric relation.

Let u be an arbitrary vector in an inner product space V.

Then $\langle u, 0v \rangle = 0$. So every vector in V is orthogonal to the null vector.

Let $u, v \in V$ such that $u \perp v$ and a be any scalar in R. Then

$$\langle au, v \rangle = a \langle u, v \rangle = a0 = 0 \qquad \because u \perp v \text{ and } \langle a, v \rangle = 0$$
$$\Rightarrow \quad au \perp v$$

Thus, if $u \perp v$, then every scalar multiple of u is also orthogonal to v.

Since $\langle u, v \rangle > 0$ for all $u \neq 0v$ and $\langle u, v \rangle = 0$ iff $u = 0v$. So the null vector is the only vector which is orthogonal to itself.

Now, let a vector $u \in V$ such that u is orthogonal to every vector in V. Then

$$\langle u, v \rangle > 0 \text{ for all } v \in V$$
$$\Rightarrow \quad u = 0v \text{ [taking } v = u]$$

Thus, two orthogonal vectors are always perpendicular to each other.

A vector u is said to be perpendicular or orthogonal to a subspace S of inner product space V if it is orthogonal to every vector in S, i.e. $\langle u, v \rangle = 0$ for all $v \in S$.

Consider the inner product space R^3 with standard inner product.

Let $u = (1, 2, -3)$, $v = (1, 1, 1)$ and $w = (-1, 4, -3) \in R$.

Then

$$\langle u, v \rangle = 1 \cdot 1 + 2 \cdot 1 + (-3) \cdot 1 = 0$$
$$\langle v, w \rangle = 1 \cdot -1 + 1 \cdot 4 + 1 \cdot -3) = 0$$

and $\quad \langle u, w \rangle = -1 + 8 + 9 = 16$

Thus, v is orthogonal to u and w but u and w are not orthogonal.

Example 1: Let $[-\pi, \pi]$ be the inner product space of all continuous functions defined on $[-\pi, \pi]$ with the inner product defined by

$$\langle f, g \rangle = \int_{-\pi}^{\pi} f(t)g(t)dt.$$

Prove that $\sin t$ and $\cos t$ are orthogonal function in $C\,[-\pi, \pi]$.

Solution: We have,

$$\langle f, g \rangle = \int_{-\pi}^{\pi} f(t)g(t)dt$$

$$\langle \sin t, \cos t \rangle = \int_{-\pi}^{\pi} \sin t \cos t\, dt = \frac{1}{2}\int_{-\pi}^{\pi} \sin 2t\, dt$$

$$= -\frac{1}{4}[\cos 2t]_{-\pi}^{\pi} = -\frac{1}{4}[1-1] = 0$$

Thus $\sin t$ and $\cos t$ are orthogonal functions in the inner product space in $[-\pi, \pi]$

Example 2: Consider the inner product space R^4 with the standard inner product. If vectors $u = (3, 2, K, -5)$ and $v = (1, K, 7, 3)$ are orthogonal, find the value of K.

Solution: It is given that u and v are orthogonal vectors in R^4.

$\therefore \quad \langle u, v \rangle = 0$

$\Rightarrow \quad 3 \cdot 1 + 2 \cdot K + K \cdot 7 + (-5) \cdot 3 = 0$

$\Rightarrow \quad 9K - 12 = 0 \qquad \Rightarrow K = \dfrac{4}{3}$

Example 3: Consider the vector space $R^{2 \times 3}$ of all 2×3 matrices with the inner product defined by $\langle A, B \rangle = tr(B^T A)$.

If $A = \begin{bmatrix} -2 & a & 3 \\ 1 & 0 & -2 \end{bmatrix}$ and $B = \begin{bmatrix} -4 & 3 & a \\ 5 & 7 & 2 \end{bmatrix}$ are matrices in $R^{2 \times 3}$ such that A is orthogonal to B, find a.

Solution: It is given that A is orthogonal to B.

$$\therefore \quad \langle A, B \rangle = 0$$

$$\Rightarrow \qquad\qquad tr(B^T A) = 0$$

$$\Rightarrow \qquad\qquad \sum_{i=1}^{3} (B^T A)_{ii} = 0$$

$$\Rightarrow \quad \sum_{i=1}^{3} \left(\sum_{r=1}^{3} (B^t)_{ir} ; (A)_{ri} \right) = 0$$

$$\Rightarrow \qquad \sum_{i=1}^{3} (\sum_{r=1}^{3} b_{ir} a_{ri}) = 0$$

$\Rightarrow$ Sum of the products of corresponding elements of A and $B = 0$

$\Rightarrow 8 + 3a + 3a + 5 + 0 - 4 = 0 \Rightarrow 6a - 9 = 0$

$$\Rightarrow \qquad a = \frac{9}{6} = \frac{3}{2}$$

Example 4: Two vectors u and v in an inner product space are orthogonal iff

$$\| u + v \|^2 = \| u \|^2 + \| v \|^2$$

Interpret the result geometrically.

Solution: We have

$$\| u + v \|^2 = \| u \|^2 + \| v \|^2$$

$\Leftrightarrow \quad \langle u + v, u + v \rangle = \langle u, u \rangle + \langle v, v \rangle$

$\Leftrightarrow \quad \langle u, u \rangle + \langle u, v \rangle + \langle v, u \rangle + \langle v, v \rangle = \langle u, u \rangle + \langle v, v \rangle$

$\Leftrightarrow \quad 2\langle u, v \rangle = 0$

$\qquad \langle u, v \rangle = 0v$

$\Leftrightarrow \quad u$ is orthogonal to v.

In geometrical interpretation, if vectors u and v are sides AB and AC of a triangle ABC, then vectors $u + v$ represents its third side BC.

$$u \perp v \Leftrightarrow \| u + v \|^2 = \| u \|^2 + \| v \|^2$$

can be interpreted geometrically as follow:

$$\Delta ABC \text{ is right angle triangle as } BC^2 = AB^2 + AC^2$$

Example 5: If u and v are vectors in an inner product space, then $u + v$ is orthogonal to $u - v$ if and only if $\|u\| = \|v\|$. Interpret the result geometrically.

Solution: $u + v$ is orthogonal to $u - v$.

$\Leftrightarrow \qquad\qquad\qquad \langle u + v, u - v \rangle = 0$

$\Rightarrow \quad \langle u, u \rangle + \langle u, -v \rangle + \langle v, u \rangle + \langle v, -v \rangle = 0$

$\Rightarrow \qquad \langle u, u \rangle - \langle u, v \rangle + \langle v, u \rangle - \langle v, v \rangle = 0$

$\Rightarrow \qquad\qquad\qquad \|u\|^2 - \|v\|^2 = 0$

$\Rightarrow \qquad\qquad\qquad\qquad \|u\|^2 = \|v\|^2$

$\Rightarrow \qquad\qquad\qquad\qquad \|u\| = \|v\|$

If two vectors u and v are adjacent sides AB and AC respectively of a parallelogram $ABCD$, then vectors $u + v$ and $u - v$ respresents its diagonals AC and BD respectively.

$\therefore \quad \langle u + v, u - v \rangle = 0 \Leftrightarrow \|u\| = \|u\|$

$\Rightarrow \quad AC \perp BD \Leftrightarrow AB = AD$

i.e. if diagonals of a parallelogram are perpendicular, then it is a rhombus.

Example 6: Find a non-zero vector u in R^3 that is orthogonal to the vectors $v_1 = (1, 1, 2)$, $v_2 = (2, 1, 3)$ and $v_3 = (1, 2, 3)$ in R^3 with standard inner product.

Solution: Let $u = (x, y, z)$ be the required vector.

Then $\langle u, v_1 \rangle = 0$, $\langle u, v_2 \rangle = 0$ and $\langle u, v_3 \rangle = 0$

$\Rightarrow x + y + 2z = 0$

$2x + y + 3z = 0$

$x + 2y + 3z = 0$

This is a homogeneous system of equations having non-trivial solution as the coefficient matrix is singular.

In matrix form the system can be written as

$$\begin{bmatrix} 1 & 1 & 2 \\ 2 & 1 & 3 \\ 1 & 2 & 3 \end{bmatrix} \begin{bmatrix} x \\ y \\ z \end{bmatrix} = \begin{bmatrix} 0 \\ 0 \\ 0 \end{bmatrix} \quad \begin{matrix} R_2 \to R_2 - 2R_1 \\ R_3 \to R_3 - R_1 \end{matrix} \quad \begin{bmatrix} 1 & 1 & 2 \\ 0 & 1 & 1 \\ 0 & 1 & 1 \end{bmatrix} \begin{bmatrix} x \\ y \\ z \end{bmatrix} = \begin{bmatrix} 0 \\ 0 \\ 0 \end{bmatrix} \quad R_3 - R_3 + R_2$$

$$\Rightarrow \begin{bmatrix} 1 & 1 & 2 \\ 0 & 1 & 1 \\ 0 & 0 & 0 \end{bmatrix} \begin{bmatrix} x \\ y \\ z \end{bmatrix} = \begin{bmatrix} 0 \\ 0 \\ 0 \end{bmatrix}$$

Thus, the given system is equivalent to $x + y + 2z = 0$, $-y - z = 0$

Here, only one variable is free. Taking $z = t$.

We obtain $x = -t$, $y = -t$, $z = t$

Thus $u = (-t, -t, t)$, $t \in R$ give vectors orthogonal to given vectors.

Putting $t = 1$, we get $(-1, -1, 1)$ as a vector orthogonal to v_1 v_2 and v_3.

Example 7: Find a non-zero vector orthogonal to the vectors $v_1 = (1, 2, 1)$ and $v_2 = (4, 5, 2)$ in inner product space R^3 with standard inner product.

Solution: Let $u = (x, y, z) \rightarrow R^3$ be the required vector. Then

$$\langle u, v_1 \rangle = 0 \text{ and } \langle u, v_2 \rangle = 0$$

$$x + 2y + z = 0 \text{ and } 4x + 5y + 2z = 0$$

$$\Rightarrow \quad x + 2y + z = 0 \text{ and } 2x + y = 0$$

(multiply first equation by 2 and sub. from second equation)

This system has only one free variable (x or y). Putting $x = 1$ in second equation, we get $z = 3$.

Thus, $u = (1, -2, 3)$ is a required vector orthogonal to v_1 and v_2.

7.6 ORTHOGONAL SETS

In this section, we shall extend the concept of orthogonality of vectors to orthogonality of sets.

Definition: Let V be an inner product space. A set S of non-zero vectors in V is called an orthogonal set, if each pair of vectors in S is a pair of orthogonal vectors.

i.e. $\langle u, v \rangle = 0$ for all $u, v \in S$, $u \neq v$.

Theorem 1: (Pythagoras) Let V be an inner product space and $\{v_1, v_2, ..., v_n\}$ be an orthogonal set of vectors in V. Then

$$\| v_1 + v_2 + ... + v_n \|^2 = \| v_1 \|^2 + \| v_2 \|^2 + ... + \| v_n \|^2$$

Proof: We have

$$\| v_1 + v_2 + ... + v_n \|^2 = \langle v_1 + v_2 + ... + v_n, v_1 + v_2 + ... + v_n \rangle$$

$$= \langle v_1, v_1 \rangle + \langle v_2, v_2 \rangle + ... + \langle v_n, v_n \rangle + 2 \sum_{i=1}^{n} \sum_{j=1}^{n} \langle v_i v_j \rangle$$

$$= \| v_1 \|^2 + \| v_2 \|^2 + ... + \| v_n \|^2 + 2 \times 0 \qquad [\because \langle v_i, v_j \rangle = 0 \ \forall \ i, j]$$

$$= \| v_1 \|^2 + \| v_2 \|^2 + ... + \| v_n \|^2$$

7.7 ORTHOGONAL BASIS

Let V be an inner product space. An orthogonal set of vectors in V is called an orthogonal basis of V if it is a basis of V.

An orthogonal set of vectors in an inner product space is linearly independent. Therefore, if V is an n dimensional inner product space and S is an orthogonal set consisting of non-zero vectors of V, then S forms an orthogonal basis of V.

Theorem 2: Let V be an inner product space and $\{v_1, v_2, ..., v_n\}$ be an orthogonal basis for V. Then for any u and v

$$u = \frac{\langle u, v_1 \rangle}{\langle v_1, v_1 \rangle} v_1 + \frac{\langle u, v_2 \rangle}{\langle v_2, v_2 \rangle} v_2 + ... + \frac{\langle u, v_n \rangle}{\langle v_n, v_n \rangle} v_n$$

i.e. $$u = \sum_{i=1}^{n} \frac{\langle u, v_i \rangle}{\| v_i \|^2} v_i$$

Proof: Since $\{v_1, v_2, ..., v_n\}$ is a basis for V and $u \in V$. Therefore, there exists

scalars $\lambda_1, \lambda_2, ..., \lambda_n \in R$ such that $u = \sum_{i=1}^{n} \lambda_i v_i$

Now, proceed as in the previous theorem.

Note: In the above theorem $\dfrac{\langle u, v_1 \rangle}{\| v_1 \|^2}, \dfrac{\langle u, v_2 \rangle}{\| v_2 \|^2}, ..., \dfrac{\langle u, v_n \rangle}{\| v_n \|^2}$ are known as the co-

ordinates of u relative to basis S.

Example 1: Let S be the set of vectors $v_1 = (1, 2, 1)$, $v_2 = (2, 1, -4)$ and $v_3 = (3, -2, 1)$ in the inner product space R^3 with standard inner product.

(i) Show that S is orthogonal and is the basis of R^3.

(ii) Find the coordinates of vectors $(7, 1, 9)$ relative to the basis S.

Solution:

(i) We have

$$\langle v_1, v_2 \rangle = 1 \times 2 + 2 \times 1 + 1 \times -4 = 0$$

$$\langle v_2, v_3 \rangle = 2 \times 3 + 1 \times -2 + -4 \times 1 = 0$$

and $\langle v_1, v_3 \rangle = 1 \times 3 + 2 \times -2 + 1 \times 1 = 0$

Thus, S is orthogonal and hence linearly independent. Since dim R^3, therefore, every linearly independent set of three vectors in R^3 forms basis of R^3. Hence S is a basis of R^3.

(ii) Let $u = (7, 1, 9)$. Then the coordinates of u relative to

$S = \{v_1, v_2, v_3\}$ are $\dfrac{\langle u, v_1 \rangle}{\| v_1 \|^2}, \dfrac{\langle u, v_2 \rangle}{\| v_2 \|^2}, \dfrac{\langle u, v_3 \rangle}{\| v_3 \|^2}$.

We have

$\langle u, v_1 \rangle = 7 \times 1 + 1 \times 2 + 1 \times 9 = 18$

$\langle u, v_2 \rangle = 7 \times 2 + 1 \times 1 + 9 \times -4 = -21$

$\langle u, v_3 \rangle = 7 \times 3 + 1 \times -2 + 9 \times 1 = 28$

$\| v_1 \|^2 = \langle v_1, v_1 \rangle = 1 + 4 + 1 = 6$

$$\|v_2\|^2 = \langle v_2, v_2 \rangle = 4 + 1 + 16 = 21$$
$$\|v_3\|^2 = \langle v_3, v_3 \rangle = 9 + 4 + 1 = 14$$

Thus, the coordinates of u relative to S are $\dfrac{18}{6}, \dfrac{-21}{21}, \dfrac{28}{14}$ or $3, -1, 2$

Hence $(7, 1, 9) = 3v_1 - v_2 + 2v_3$.

Example 2: Consider the inner product space R^4 with standard inner product.

Let $S = \{v_1, v_2, v_3, v_4\}$ be a subset of R^4, where $v_1 = (1, 1, 0, -1)$, $v_2 = (1, 2, 1, 3)$, $v_3 = (1, 1, -9, 2)$ and $v_4 = (16, -13, 1, 3)$.

(i) Show that S is orthogonal and a basis of R^4

(ii) Find the coordinates of an arbitrary vector $u = (a, b, c, d)$ in R^4 relative to the basis S.

Solution:

(i) We have

$$\langle v_1, v_2 \rangle = 1 \times 1 + 1 \times 2 + 0 \times 1 + (-1) \times 3 = 0$$
$$\langle v_1, v_3 \rangle = 1 \times 1 + 1 \times 1 + 0 \times 9 + (-1) \times 2 = 0$$
$$\langle v_1, v_4 \rangle = 1 \times 16 + 1 \times -13 + 0 \times 1 + (-1) \times 3 = 0$$
$$\langle v_2, v_3 \rangle = 1 \times 1 + 2 \times 1 + 1 \times -9 + 3 \times 2 = 0$$
$$\langle v_2, v_4 \rangle = 1 \times 16 + 2 \times -13 + 1 \times 1 + 3 \times 3 = 0$$
$$\langle v_3, v_4 \rangle = 1 \times 16 + 1 \times -13 + (-9) \times 1 + 2 \times 3 = 0$$

Thus, S is orthogonal and hence it is linearly independent. Consequently, S is a basis of R^4 as any four linearly independent vectors form of R^4.

(ii) The coordinates of u relative to the basis S are

$$\frac{\langle u, v_1 \rangle}{\|v_1\|^2} = \frac{a + b - d}{3}, \quad \frac{\langle u, v_2 \rangle}{\|v_2\|^2} = \frac{a + 2b + c + 3d}{15}$$

$$\frac{\langle u, v_3 \rangle}{\|v_3\|^2} = \frac{a + b - 9c + 2d}{87}, \quad \frac{\langle u, v_4 \rangle}{\|v_4\|^2} = \frac{16a - 13b + c + 3d}{435}$$

Example 3: Let $v_1 = (1, -2, 3, 4)$ and $v_2 = (3, -5, 7, 8)$ be two vectors in the inner product space R^4. Find a basis of the subspace S of R^4 that is orthogonal to v_1 and v_2.

Solution: We have

$$S = \{u = (x, y, z, t) \in R^4 : \langle u, v_1 \rangle = 0 \text{ and } \langle u, v_2 \rangle = 0\}$$

Now,

$$\langle u, v_1 \rangle = 0 \text{ and } \langle u, v_2 \rangle = 0$$

$\Rightarrow x - 2y + 3z + 4t = 0$ and $3x - 5y + 7z + 8t = 0$

$\Rightarrow x - 2y + 3z + 4t = 0$ and $x - y + z = 0$ [on eliminating t]

This system of equations has two free variables. Putting $x = 1$, $y = 2$ in $x - y + z = 0$, we get $z = 1$ and also substituting $x = 1$, $y = 2$, $z = 1$ in $x - 2y + 3z + 4t = 0$ we get $t = 0$.

$\therefore$ $u_1 = (1, 2, 1, 0) \in S$

Putting $x = 4$, $y = 4$ in $x - y + z = 0$ we get $z = 0$

Substituting these values in $x - 2y + 3z + 4t = 0$, we get

$$u_2 = (4, 4, 0, 1) \in S.$$

Thus $u_1 = (1, 2, 1, 0)$ and $u_2 = (4, 4, 0, 1)$ from a basis of R^4.

Example 4: Let S be the subspace of inner product space R^4 and orthogonal to the vectors $v_1 = (1, 1, 2, 2)$ and $v_2 = (0, 1, 2, -1)$. Find an orthogonal basis of S.

Solution: We have

$$S = \{u \in R^4 : \langle u, v_1 \rangle = 0, \langle u, v_2 \rangle = 0\}$$

Let $u = (x, y, z, t) \in S$. Then

$\langle u, v_1 \rangle = 0$ and $\langle u, v_2 \rangle = 0$

$\Rightarrow x + y + 2z + 2t = 0$ and $y + 2z - t = 0$

$\Rightarrow x + y + 2z + 2t = 0$ and $x + 3t = 0$

                 [on subtracting second equation from first]

Clearly, there are two free variables. Second equation has one free variable, say t. Consequently first equation also has free variable, say z, let us take z and t as free variables.

Now,

       $z = 1$, $t = 0 \Rightarrow x = 0$ and $y = -2$

$\therefore$ $u = (0, -2, 1, 0) \in S$.

Now, we have to find one more vector u_2 (say) in S, which is orthogonal to u_1 and u_1, u_2 are linearly independent.

Let $u_2 = (a, b, c, d)$. Then,

$\langle u_2, v_1 \rangle = 0$, $\langle u_2, v_2 \rangle = 0$

Now $\langle u_2, v_1 \rangle = 0$ and $\langle u_2, v_2 \rangle = 0$

$\Rightarrow a + b + 2c + 2d = 0$ and $a + 3d = 0$

            [proceeding as above in $\langle u_1, v_1 \rangle = 0$, $\langle u_1, v_2 \rangle = 0$]

$\langle u_2, v_1 \rangle = 0 \Rightarrow -2b + c = 0$

Thus, we have

       $a + b + 2c + 2d = 0$, $a + 3d = 0$ and $-2b + c = 0$

$\Rightarrow$ $a = -3d, b = \dfrac{d}{5}, c = \dfrac{2d}{5}$ [putting $d = 5$]

$\Rightarrow \qquad a = -15, b = 1, c = 2, d = 5$

$\therefore \qquad u_2 = (-15, 1, 2, 5)$

Hence u_1, u_2 from an orthogonal basis of S.

7.8 PROJECTIONS

In this section, we extend to discuss the concept of projection similar to geometry.

Projection of a Vector

Let V be an inner product space. The projection of a vector v along a non-zero vector w is the scalar multiple cw of w such that $v - cw$ is orthogonal to w.

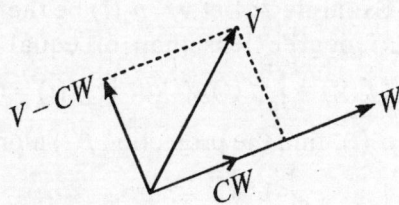

Now,

$\qquad cw$ is the projection of vector v on vector w.

$\Rightarrow v - cw$ is orthogonal to w

$\Rightarrow \langle v - cw, w \rangle = 0$

$\Rightarrow \langle v, w \rangle - c\langle w, w \rangle = 0$

$\Rightarrow c = \dfrac{\langle v, w \rangle}{\langle w, w \rangle}$

The projection of vector v along a non-zero vector w is denoted by $\langle v, w \rangle$

Thus, proj $\langle v, w \rangle = c = \dfrac{\langle v, w \rangle}{\langle w, w \rangle} w$

The scalar $c = \dfrac{\langle v, w \rangle}{\langle w, w \rangle}$ is called the component of v and w or the **Fouries Coefficients** of v with respcet to w.

Note: In three dimensional geometry the projection vector of vector $\overrightarrow{v}$ along a vector $\overrightarrow{w}$ is defined an $\dfrac{\overrightarrow{v} \cdot \overrightarrow{w}}{|\overrightarrow{w}|^2} \overrightarrow{w}$ which is same as what we have defined above.

Example 1: Find the projection of vector $v = (1, -2, 3, -4)$ along a vector $w = (1, 2, 1, 2)$ in the inner product space R^4 with standard inner product.

Solution: We have,

Projection of vector v along vector $w = \dfrac{\langle v, w \rangle}{\langle w, w \rangle} w$

It is given that $v = (1, -2, 3, -4)$ and $w = (1, 2, 1, 2)$
$\langle v, w \rangle = 1 - 4 + 3 - 8 = -8$ and $\langle w, w \rangle = 1 + 4 + 1 + 4 = 10$

$\therefore$ Projection of v along $w = \dfrac{\langle v, w \rangle}{\langle w, w \rangle} w = \dfrac{-8}{10}(1, 2, 1, 2)$

$$= \dfrac{-4}{5}, \dfrac{-8}{5}, \dfrac{-4}{5}, \dfrac{-8}{5}$$

Example 2: Let $v = p_2(t)$ be the inner product space of all polynomials of degree less than or equal to 2 with inner product defined by $\langle f, g \rangle = \int_0^1 f(t)g(t)dt$. If $f(t) = t^2$ and $g(t) = t + 3$ are two polynomials in $p_2(t)$, find the projection $f(t)$ along $g(t)$.

Solution: Required projection $= \dfrac{\langle f, g \rangle}{\langle g, g \rangle} g$

$$\langle f, g \rangle = \int_0^1 f(t)g(t)dt = \int_0^1 t^2(t+3)\,dt = \dfrac{5}{4}$$

$$\langle g, g \rangle = \int_0^1 g(t)g(t)dt = \int_0^1 (t+3)^2 dt = \dfrac{37}{3}$$

$\therefore$ Required projection $= \dfrac{\dfrac{5}{4}}{\dfrac{37}{3}}(t+3) = \dfrac{15}{148}(t+3)$

Example 3: In the inner product space $R^{2 \times 2}$ of all 2×2 matrices over R with inner product defined by $\langle A, B \rangle = tr\,(B^T A)$, find the projection of

$$A = \begin{bmatrix} 1 & 2 \\ 3 & 4 \end{bmatrix} \text{ along } B = \begin{bmatrix} 1 & 1 \\ 5 & 5 \end{bmatrix}$$

Solution: Required projection $\dfrac{\langle A, B \rangle}{\langle B, B \rangle} B$

Now

$$\langle A, B \rangle = tr\,(B^T A) = tr\left(\begin{bmatrix} 1 & 5 \\ 1 & 5 \end{bmatrix}\begin{bmatrix} 1 & 2 \\ 3 & 4 \end{bmatrix} \right) = tr \begin{bmatrix} 16 & 22 \\ 16 & 22 \end{bmatrix} = 38$$

$$\langle B, B \rangle = tr\,(B^T B) = tr\left(\begin{bmatrix} 1 & 5 \\ 1 & 5 \end{bmatrix}\begin{bmatrix} 1 & 1 \\ 5 & 5 \end{bmatrix} \right) = tr \begin{bmatrix} 26 & 26 \\ 26 & 26 \end{bmatrix} = 52$$

$$\therefore \quad \text{Required projection} = \frac{\langle A, B \rangle}{\langle B, B \rangle} B$$

$$= \frac{38}{52} \begin{bmatrix} 1 & 1 \\ 5 & 5 \end{bmatrix} = \frac{19}{26} \begin{bmatrix} 1 & 1 \\ 5 & 5 \end{bmatrix}$$

Example 4: Let S be the subspace of the inner product space R^4 spanned by the vectors $v_1 = (1, 1, 1, 1)$ and $v_2 = (-1, 0, 1, 0)$. Find the projection of vector $u = (1, 2, 5, 7)$ onto S.

Solution: Clearly, v_1 and v_2 are orthogonal vectors and so they form an orthogonal basis for S. Proj $(v, s) = \dfrac{\langle u, v_1 \rangle}{\langle v_1 v_1 \rangle} v_1 + \dfrac{\langle u, v_2 \rangle}{\langle v_2 v_2 \rangle} v_2$

$$\text{Proj } (v, s) = \frac{15}{4} v_1 + \frac{4}{2} v_2 = 4v_2 + 2v_2$$

$$= \frac{15}{4} (1, 1, 1, 1) + 2 (-1, 0, 1, 0)$$

$$\Rightarrow \text{Proj } (v, s) = \frac{1}{4} (7, 15, 23, 15)$$

Example 5: Consider the inner product space $p(t)$ of all polynomials with the inner product $\langle f, g \rangle = \int_0^1 f(t)g(t)dt$. Let S be a subspace of $p(t)$ spanned by the set $\{1, 2t - 1, 6t^2 - 6t + 1\}$. Find the projection of $f(t) = t^3$ onto S.

Solution: Clearly, $\{1, 2t - 1, 6t^2 - 6t + 1\}$ is an orthogonal set.

Let $f_1 = 1, f_2 = 2t - 1, f_3 = 6t^2 - 6t + 1$

Then

$$\text{proj} (f, s) = \frac{\langle f, f_1 \rangle}{\langle f_1, f_1 \rangle} f_1 + \frac{\langle f, f_2 \rangle}{\langle f_2, f_2 \rangle} f_2 + \frac{\langle f, f_3 \rangle}{\langle f_3, f_3 \rangle} f_3$$

Now

$$\langle f_1, f_1 \rangle = \int_0^1 1 dt = 1, \quad \langle f_2, f_2 \rangle = \int_0^1 (2t - 1)^2 \, dt = \frac{1}{3}$$

$$\langle f_3, f_3 \rangle = \int_0^1 (6t^2 - 6t + 1)^2 \, dt = \frac{1}{5}$$

$$\langle f, f_1 \rangle = \int_0^1 t^3 dt = \frac{1}{4}, \quad \langle f, f_2 \rangle = \int_0^1 t^3 (2t - 1) dt = \frac{3}{20}$$

$$\langle f, f_3 \rangle = \int_0^1 t^3 \left(6t^2 - 6t + 1 \right) dt = \frac{1}{20}$$

$$\therefore \quad \text{proj}(f, S) = \frac{1}{4} + \frac{9}{20}(2t - 1) + \frac{5}{20}\left(6t^2 - 6t + 1\right)$$

$$= \frac{3}{2}t^2 - \frac{3}{5}t + \frac{1}{20}$$

7.9 GRAM-SCHMIDT ORTHOGONALIZATION PROCESS

Let V be a finite dimensional inner product space. Then V being a finite dimension vector space, as a basis $B = \{v_1, v_2, ..., v_n\}$(say). This basis can be used to construct an orthogonal basis of V and form an ordinary basis for V and this process is known as the Gram-Schmidt orthogonalized process. The following theorem explain the construction process.

Theorem 1: (Gram-Schmidt orthogonalized process.) Every finite dimensional inner product space has an orthogonal basis.

Proof: Let V be a non-dimensional inner product space. Then V being a finite dimensional vector space, as a basis $B = \{v_1, v_2, ..., v_n\}$ be an ordinary basis for V. We shall now use this basis for V as follows:

Let $\quad w_1 = v_1$

$$w_2 = v_2 - \frac{\langle v_2, w_1 \rangle}{\langle w_1, w_1 \rangle} w_1$$

$$w_3 = v_3 - \frac{\langle v_3, w_1 \rangle}{\langle w_1, w_1 \rangle} w_1 - \frac{\langle v_3, w_2 \rangle}{\langle w_2, w_2 \rangle} w_2$$

$$w_4 = v_4 - \frac{\langle v_4, w_1 \rangle}{\langle w_1, w_1 \rangle} w_1 - \frac{\langle v_4, w_2 \rangle}{\langle w_2, w_2 \rangle} w_2 - \frac{\langle v_4, w_3 \rangle}{\langle w_3, w_3 \rangle} w_3$$

$$w_n = v_n - \frac{\langle v_n, w_1 \rangle}{\langle w_1, w_1 \rangle} w_1 - \frac{\langle v_n, w_2 \rangle}{\langle w_2, w_2 \rangle} w_2 - ... - \frac{\langle v_n, w_{n-1} \rangle}{\langle w_{n-1}, w_{n-1} \rangle} w_{n-1}$$

Then, $w_1, w_2, w_3, ..., w_n$ are given by

$w_k = v_k - c_{k1}w_1 - c_{k2}w_2 - c_{k3}w_3 - ... - c_{k-1}w_{k-1}$ for $k = 1, 2, 3, ...$ We shall now show that $\{w_1, w_2, ..., w_n\}$ is an orthogonal set. For this it is sufficient to show that each w_i is orthogonal to its preceding vectors $w_1, w_2, ..., w_{i-1}$.

Let $p(k)$ be the statement: Vector w_k is orthogonal to its preceding vectors $w_1, w_2, ..., w_{k-1}$.

We have

$$\langle w_2, w_1 \rangle = \langle v_2 - c_{21}w_1, w_1 \rangle$$

$$= \langle v_2, w_1 \rangle - \langle c_{21}w_1, w_1 \rangle$$

$$= \langle v_2, w_1 \rangle - c_{21} \langle w_1, w_1 \rangle$$

$$\Rightarrow \langle w_2, w_1 \rangle = \langle v_2, w_1 \rangle - \langle v_2, w_1 \rangle \qquad \left[\because c_{21} = \frac{\langle v_2, w_1 \rangle}{\langle w_1, w_1 \rangle} \right]$$

Let $p(k)$ be true. Then each of $w_1, w_2, ..., w_{k-1}$ is orthogonal to w_k.

Now, $w_{k+1} = v_{k+1} - c_{k+11} w_1 - c_{k+12} w_2 - ... - c_{k+1k} w_k$.

For any $i = 1, 2, ..., k$, we have

$$\langle w_{k+1}, w_i \rangle = \left\langle v_{k+1} - \sum_{r=1}^{k} c_{k+1r} w_r, w_i \right\rangle = \langle v_{k+1}, w_i \rangle - \sum_{r=1}^{k} c_{k+1r} \langle w_r, w_i \rangle$$

$$= \langle v_{k+1}, w_i \rangle - c_{k+1i} \langle w_i, w_i \rangle$$

$$\Rightarrow \langle w_{k+1}, w_i \rangle = \langle v_{k+1}, w_i \rangle - \langle w_{k+1}, w_i \rangle = 0$$

$\Rightarrow w_{k+1}$ is orthogonal to each of the vectors $w_1, w_2, ..., w_k$.

$\therefore \ p(k+1)$ is true.

Hence, by induction $\{w_1, w_2, ..., w_n\}$ is an orthogonal set of vectors in V. But every orthogonal set of vectors in an inner product space is linearly independent. So $\{w_1, w_2, ..., w_n\}$ is an orthogonal basis for V.

Let $\quad u_i = \dfrac{w_i}{\| w_i \|}, i = 1, 2, ..., n$

Then $\langle u_i, u_i \rangle = \left\langle \dfrac{w_i}{\| w_i \|}, \dfrac{w_i}{\| w_i \|} \right\rangle = \dfrac{1}{\| w_i \|^2} \langle w_i, w_i \rangle = 1$

$$\text{for all } i = 1, 2, ..., n$$

and $\quad \langle u_i, u_j \rangle = \left\langle \dfrac{w_i}{\| w_i \|}, \dfrac{w_j}{\| w_j \|} \right\rangle = \dfrac{1}{\| w_i \| \| w_j \|} \langle w_i, w_j \rangle = 0$

$$\text{for all } i, j = 1, 2, ..., n, \ i \ne j$$

Hence $\{u_1, u_2, ..., u_n\}$ is an orthogonal basis for V.

Example 1: Apply Gram-Schmidt orthogonalization process to the basis $B = \{(1, 0, 1), (1, 0, -1), (0, 3, 4)\}$ of the inner product space R^3 to find an orthogonal basis of R^3.

Solution: Let $v_1 = (1, 0, 1)$, $v_2 = (1, 0, -1)$ and $v_3 = (0, 3, 4)$. Further let $w_1 = v_1 = (1, 0, 1)$

$$[\because \langle v_2, w_1 \rangle = 0]$$

$$w_2 = v_2 - \frac{\langle v_2, w_1 \rangle}{\langle w_1, w_1 \rangle} w_1 = v_2 - 0 = v_2 = (1, 0, -1)$$

$$w_3 = v_3 - \frac{\langle v_3, w_1 \rangle}{\langle w_1, w_1 \rangle} w_1 - \frac{\langle v_3, w_2 \rangle}{\langle w_2, w_2 \rangle} w_2$$

$$w_3 = v_3 - \frac{4}{2} v_1 + \frac{4}{2} v_2$$

$$= v_3 - 2v_1 + 2v_2$$

$$w_3 = (0,3,4) + (-2,0,-2) + (2,0,-2) = (0,3,0)$$

Thus $\{w_1, w_2, w_3\}$ is an orthogonal basis of R^3.

In order to obtain an orthonormal basis of R^3, let us normalize w_1, w_2, w_3. We have

$$\| w_1 \|^2 = 2, \quad \| w_2 \|^2 = 2 \text{ and } \| w_3 \|^2 = 9$$

Let $u_i = \frac{w_i}{\| w_i \|}, i = 1, 2, 3.$

Then $u_1 = \left(\frac{1}{\sqrt{2}}, 0, \frac{1}{\sqrt{2}} \right)$, $u_2 = \left(\frac{1}{\sqrt{2}}, 0, \frac{-1}{\sqrt{2}} \right)$, $u_3 = (0,1,0)$

form an orthonormal basis for R^3.

Example 2: Let $V = p_3(t)$ be the vector space of all polynomials $f(t)$ of degree less than or equal to 3 with inner product defined by

$$\langle f, g \rangle = \int_{-1}^{1} f(t)g(t)dt.$$

Solution: Apply Gram-Schmidt orthogonalization process to find an orthogonal basis with integral coefficients and an orthonormal basis from the basis $\{1, t, t^2, t^3\}$.

Proof: Let $f_0 = 1, f_1 = t, f_2 = t^2, f_3 = t^3$ form the given basis. Then,

$$\langle f_0, f_0 \rangle = \int_{-1}^{1} 1 dt = 2, \quad \langle f_1, f_1 \rangle = \int_{-1}^{1} t^2 dt = \frac{2}{3}$$

$$\langle f_2, f_2 \rangle = \int_{-1}^{1} t^4 dt = \frac{2}{5}, \quad \langle f_3, f_3 \rangle = \int_{-1}^{1} t^6 dt = \frac{2}{7}$$

$$\langle f_0, f_1 \rangle = \int_{-1}^{1} t dt = 0, \quad \langle f_0, f_2 \rangle = \int_{-1}^{1} t^2 dt = \frac{2}{3}$$

$$\langle f_0, f_3 \rangle = \int_{-1}^{1} t^3 dt = 0, \quad \langle f_1, f_2 \rangle = \int_{-1}^{1} t^3 dt = 0$$

$$\langle f_1, f_3 \rangle = \int_{-1}^{1} t^4 dt = \frac{2}{5}, \quad \langle f_2, f_3 \rangle = \int_{-1}^{1} t^5 dt = 0$$

Let $g_0 = f_0 = 1$

$$g_1 = f_1 - \frac{\langle f_1, f_0 \rangle}{\langle f_0, f_0 \rangle} f_0 = t - 0 = t$$

$$g_2 = f_2 - \frac{\langle f_2, f_0 \rangle}{\langle f_0, f_0 \rangle} f_0 - \frac{\langle f_2, f_1 \rangle}{\langle f_1, f_1 \rangle} f_1 = t^2 - \frac{2}{3} \times \frac{1}{2} = t^2 - \frac{1}{3}$$

$$g_3 = f_3 - \frac{\langle f_3, f_0 \rangle}{\langle f_0, f_0 \rangle} f_0 - \frac{\langle f_3, f_1 \rangle}{\langle f_1, f_1 \rangle} f_1 - \frac{\langle f_3, f_2 \rangle}{\langle f_2, f_2 \rangle} f_2$$

$$= t^3 - \frac{2}{5} \times \frac{3}{2} \times t - 0 = t^3 - \frac{3}{5} t$$

Thus $\left\{ g_0 = 1, g_1 = t, g_2 = t^2 - \frac{1}{3}, g_3 = t^3 - \frac{3}{5} t \right\}$ is an orthogonal basis of

V. Multiplying g_2 by 3 and g_3 by 5, we obtain

$\left\{ \varnothing_0(t) = 1, \varnothing_1(t) = t, \varnothing_2(t) = 3t^2 - 1, \varnothing_3(t) = 5t^2 - 3t \right\}$ as an orthogonal basis with interchanged coefficients.

Now

$$\| \varnothing_0(t) \|^2 = \langle 1, 1 \rangle = \int_{-1}^{1} 1 \, dt = 2 \Rightarrow \| \varnothing_0(t) \| = \sqrt{2}$$

$$\| \varnothing_1(t) \|^2 = \langle t, t \rangle = \int_{-1}^{1} t^2 dt = \frac{2}{3} \Rightarrow \| \varnothing_1(t) \| = \sqrt{\frac{2}{3}}$$

$$\| \varnothing_2(t) \|^2 = \langle 3t^2 - 1, 3t^2 - 1 \rangle = \int_{-1}^{1} \left(3t^2 - 1 \right)^2 dt = \frac{8}{5} \Rightarrow \| \varnothing_2(t) \| = 2\sqrt{\frac{2}{5}}$$

$$\| \varnothing_3(t) \|^2 = \langle 5t^2 - 3t, 5t^2 - 3t \rangle = \int_{-1}^{1} \left(5t^2 - 3t \right)^2 dt = \frac{8}{7} \Rightarrow \| \varnothing_3(t) \| = 2\sqrt{\frac{2}{7}}$$

Hence, an orthogonal basis of $p_3(t)$ is

$$\left\{ \frac{1}{\sqrt{2}}, \sqrt{\frac{3}{2}} t, \frac{1}{2} \sqrt{\frac{5}{2}} \left(3t^2 - 1 \right), \frac{1}{2} \sqrt{\frac{7}{2}} \left(5t^2 - 3t \right) \right\}$$

Example 3: Let S be the subspace of an inner product space R^4 spanned by the vectors $v_1 = (1, 1, 1, 1)$, $v_2 = (1, 2, 4, 5)$, $v_3 = (1, -3, -4, -2)$ in R^4. Apply the Gram-Schmidt orthogonalization process to find an orthogonal basis and then an orthonormal basis of S.

Solution: We observe that the vectors v_1, v_2, v_3 form a linearly independent set. So $\{v_1, v_2, v_3\}$ is a basis for S. In order to orthogonalize this basis, let us define:

$$w_1 = v_1$$

$$w_2 = v_2 - \frac{\langle v_2, w_1 \rangle}{\langle w_1, w_1 \rangle} w_1 = v_2 - \frac{12}{4} v_1 = v_2 - 3v_1 = (-2, -1, 1, 2)$$

$$w_3 = v_3 - \frac{\langle v_3, w_1 \rangle}{\langle w_1, w_1 \rangle} w_1 - \frac{\langle v_3, w_2 \rangle}{\langle w_2, w_2 \rangle} w_2 = v_3 + \frac{8}{4} v_1 + \frac{7}{10} w_2 = \left(\frac{8}{5}, \frac{-17}{10}, \frac{-13}{10}, \frac{7}{5} \right)$$

Thus $\{w_1, w_2, w_3\}$ form an orthogonal basis of S.

Now,

$$\| w_1 \|^2 = \langle w_1, w_1 \rangle = 4, \quad \| w_2 \|^2 = \langle w_2, w_2 \rangle = 10$$

$$\| w_3 \|^2 = \langle w_3, w_3 \rangle = 910$$

Let $\quad u_i = \dfrac{w_i}{\| w_i \|}, i = 1, 2, 3.$ Then

$$\left\{ \begin{aligned} u_1 &= \left(\frac{1}{2}, \frac{1}{2}, \frac{1}{2}, \frac{1}{2} \right), u_2 = \left(\frac{-2}{\sqrt{10}}, \frac{-1}{\sqrt{10}}, \frac{1}{\sqrt{10}}, \frac{2}{\sqrt{10}} \right), \\ u_3 &= \left(\frac{16}{\sqrt{910}}, \frac{-17}{\sqrt{910}}, \frac{-13}{\sqrt{910}}, \frac{14}{\sqrt{910}} \right) \end{aligned} \right\}$$

is an orthogonal basis of S.

Example 4: Let S be the subspace of R^4 spanned by the vectors $v_1 = (1, 1, 1, 1)$, $v_2 = (1, -1, 2, 2)$, $v_3 = (1, 2, -3, -4)$. Apply the Gram-Schmidt orthogonalization process to find an orthogonal basis and then an orthonormal basis of S and hence find the projection of $v = (1, 2, -3, 4)$ onto S.

Solution: Let $w_1 = v_1 = (1, 1, 1, 1)$

$$w_2 = v_2 - \frac{\langle v_2, w_1 \rangle}{\langle w_1, w_1 \rangle} w_1 = v_2 - \frac{\langle v_2, v_1 \rangle}{\langle v_1, v_1 \rangle} v_1 = v_2 - v_1 = (0, -2, 1, 1)$$

$$w_3 = v_3 - \frac{\langle v_3, w_1 \rangle}{\langle w_1, w_1 \rangle} w_1 - \frac{\langle v_3, w_2 \rangle}{\langle w_2, w_2 \rangle} w_2 = v_3 + w_1 + \frac{11}{6} w_2$$

$$= \left(2, \frac{-2}{3}, \frac{-1}{6}, \frac{-7}{6} \right)$$

Let $\qquad w_3 = 6w_3 = (12, -4, -1, -7)$

Clearly $\{w_1, w_2, w_3\}$ form an orthogonal basis of S.

$$\therefore \text{ Proj}(v, S) = \frac{\langle v_1, w_1 \rangle}{\langle w_1, w_1 \rangle} w_1 + \frac{\langle v_1, w_2 \rangle}{\langle w_2, w_2 \rangle} w_2 + \frac{\langle v_1, w_3 \rangle}{\langle w_3, w_3 \rangle} w_3$$

$$\Rightarrow \text{Proj}(v, S) = w_1 - \frac{1}{2} w_2 - \frac{1}{10} w_3 = \left(\frac{-1}{5}, \frac{12}{5}, \frac{3}{5}, \frac{6}{5} \right)$$

7.10 *QR*-FACTORIZATION OF MATRICES

If an $m \times n$ matrix A has linearly independent columns $x_1, x_2, ..., x_n$, then Gram-Schmidt process is applied to $x_1, x_2, ..., x_n$ to factorise A.

The *QR*-Factorization

If A is an $m \times n$ matrix with linearly independent columns, then A can be factorized as $A = QR$, where Q is an $m \times n$ matrix whose columns form an orthogonal basis for column A and R is an $m \times n$ upper triangular invertible matrix with positive entries on its diagonal.

The columns of A form a basis $\{x_1, x_2, ..., x_n\}$ for col A. Construct an orthogonal basis $\{u_1, u_2, ..., u_n\}$ for $w = $ col A. This basis may be constructed by Gram-Schmidt process. Let

$$Q = \{u_1, u_2, ..., u_n\}$$

Example 1: Find QR factorization of $A = \begin{bmatrix} 1 & 0 & 0 \\ 1 & 1 & 0 \\ 1 & 1 & 1 \\ 1 & 1 & 1 \end{bmatrix}$

Solution: The columns of A are the vectors, x_1, x_2, x_3.

Let $x_1 = \begin{bmatrix} 1 \\ 1 \\ 1 \\ 1 \end{bmatrix}, x_2 = \begin{bmatrix} 0 \\ 1 \\ 1 \\ 1 \end{bmatrix}, x_3 = \begin{bmatrix} 0 \\ 0 \\ 1 \\ 1 \end{bmatrix}.$

By Gram-Schmidit process

Step 1: Let $v_1 = x_1$ and $w_1 = \text{span}\{x_1\} = \text{span}\{v_1\}$

Step 2: Let v_2 be the vector produced by subtracting from x_2 its projection onto the subspace w_1.

i.e. $\quad v_2 = x_2 - \dfrac{\langle x_2, v_1 \rangle}{\langle v_1, v_1 \rangle} v_1$

$$v_2 = \begin{bmatrix} 0 \\ 1 \\ 1 \\ 1 \end{bmatrix} - \frac{3}{4} \begin{bmatrix} 1 \\ 1 \\ 1 \\ 1 \end{bmatrix} = \begin{bmatrix} -\dfrac{3}{4} \\ \dfrac{1}{4} \\ \dfrac{1}{4} \\ \dfrac{1}{4} \end{bmatrix} = \begin{bmatrix} -3 \\ 1 \\ 1 \\ 1 \end{bmatrix}$$

$$v_3 = x_3 - \frac{\langle x_3, v_1 \rangle}{\langle v_1, v_1 \rangle} v_1 + \frac{\langle x_3, v_2 \rangle}{\langle v_2, v_2 \rangle} v_2$$

$$v_3 = \begin{bmatrix} 0 \\ 1 \\ 1 \\ 1 \end{bmatrix} - \frac{2}{4} \begin{bmatrix} 1 \\ 1 \\ 1 \\ 1 \end{bmatrix} + \frac{2}{12} \begin{bmatrix} -3 \\ 1 \\ 1 \\ 1 \end{bmatrix} = \begin{bmatrix} 0 \\ -\dfrac{2}{3} \\ \dfrac{1}{3} \\ \dfrac{1}{3} \end{bmatrix} = \begin{bmatrix} 0 \\ -2 \\ 1 \\ 1 \end{bmatrix}$$

$$\therefore \quad v_1 = \begin{bmatrix} 1 \\ 1 \\ 1 \\ 1 \end{bmatrix}, v_2 = \begin{bmatrix} -3 \\ 1 \\ 1 \\ 1 \end{bmatrix}, v_3 = \begin{bmatrix} 0 \\ -2 \\ 1 \\ 1 \end{bmatrix}$$

Then normalize the three vectors to obtain u_1, u_2, u_3 and list these vectors as the column of Q.

$$Q = \begin{bmatrix} \dfrac{1}{2} & \dfrac{-3}{\sqrt{2}} & \dfrac{-2}{\sqrt{6}} \\ \dfrac{1}{2} & \dfrac{1}{\sqrt{12}} & \dfrac{1}{\sqrt{6}} \\ \dfrac{1}{2} & \dfrac{1}{\sqrt{12}} & \dfrac{1}{\sqrt{6}} \\ \dfrac{1}{2} & \dfrac{1}{\sqrt{12}} & \dfrac{1}{\sqrt{6}} \end{bmatrix}$$

By constructing the first column of Q are an orthonormal basis of span$\{x_1, x_2, ..., x_n\}$.

∴ $A = QR$ for some R.

To find R:

Observe that $Q^T Q = I$ because the columns of Q are orthonormal.

Hence $Q^T A = Q^T (QR) = IR = R$

$$\therefore R = \begin{bmatrix} \dfrac{1}{2} & \dfrac{1}{2} & \dfrac{1}{2} & \dfrac{1}{2} \\ \dfrac{-3}{\sqrt{12}} & \dfrac{1}{\sqrt{12}} & \dfrac{1}{\sqrt{12}} & \dfrac{1}{\sqrt{12}} \\ \dfrac{-2}{\sqrt{6}} & \dfrac{1}{\sqrt{6}} & \dfrac{1}{\sqrt{6}} & \dfrac{1}{\sqrt{6}} \end{bmatrix} \begin{bmatrix} 1 & 0 & 0 \\ 1 & 1 & 0 \\ 1 & 1 & 1 \\ 1 & 1 & 1 \end{bmatrix}$$

$$R = \begin{bmatrix} 2 & \dfrac{3}{2} & 1 \\ 0 & \dfrac{3}{\sqrt{12}} & -\dfrac{2}{\sqrt{12}} \\ 0 & 0 & \dfrac{2}{\sqrt{16}} \end{bmatrix}$$

7.11 LEAST-SQUARES PROBLEMS

If A is an $m \times n$ matrix and B is in R^m, a least-square solution of $Ax = B$ is an x in R^n such that $\| B - Ax \| \leq \| B - A^T x \| \, \forall x$ in R^n. $Ax = B$ satisfies the equation $A^T Ax = A^T B$.

Example 1: Find a least-square solution of the inconsistent system $Ax = B$ for

$$A = \begin{bmatrix} 4 & 0 \\ 0 & 2 \\ 1 & 1 \end{bmatrix}, B = \begin{bmatrix} 2 \\ 0 \\ 11 \end{bmatrix}$$

Solution:

To use $A^T Ax = A^T B$

$$A^T A = \begin{bmatrix} 4 & 0 & 1 \\ 0 & 2 & 1 \end{bmatrix} \begin{bmatrix} 4 & 0 \\ 0 & 2 \\ 1 & 1 \end{bmatrix} = \begin{bmatrix} 17 & 1 \\ 1 & 5 \end{bmatrix}$$

$$A^T B = \begin{bmatrix} 4 & 0 & 1 \\ 0 & 2 & 1 \end{bmatrix} \begin{bmatrix} 2 \\ 0 \\ 11 \end{bmatrix} = \begin{bmatrix} 19 \\ 11 \end{bmatrix}$$

Then the equation $A^T Ax = A^T B$ becomes

$$\begin{bmatrix} 17 & 1 \\ 1 & 5 \end{bmatrix} \begin{bmatrix} x_1 \\ x_2 \end{bmatrix} = \begin{bmatrix} 19 \\ 11 \end{bmatrix} \quad A = \begin{bmatrix} a_{11} & a_{12} \\ b_{21} & b_{22} \end{bmatrix}$$

$$\text{Adj}(A) = \begin{bmatrix} b_{21} & -b_{21} \\ a_{12} & +a_{11} \end{bmatrix}$$

Row operations can be used to solve this system but since $A^T A$ is invertible and 2×2, compute

$$\left(A^T A \right)^{-1} = \frac{1}{84} \begin{bmatrix} 5 & -1 \\ -1 & 17 \end{bmatrix}$$

and then to solve $A^T Ax = A^T B$ as

$$x = \left(A^T A \right)^{-1} A^T B$$

$$= \frac{1}{84} \begin{bmatrix} 5 & -1 \\ -1 & 17 \end{bmatrix} \begin{bmatrix} 19 \\ 11 \end{bmatrix} = \frac{1}{84} \begin{bmatrix} 84 \\ 168 \end{bmatrix} = \begin{bmatrix} 1 \\ 2 \end{bmatrix}$$

Example 2: Find a least-square solution of $Ax = B$ for

$$A = \begin{bmatrix} 1 & 1 & 0 & 0 \\ 1 & 1 & 0 & 0 \\ 1 & 0 & 1 & 0 \\ 1 & 0 & 1 & 0 \\ 1 & 0 & 0 & 1 \\ 1 & 0 & 0 & 1 \end{bmatrix}, \quad B = \begin{bmatrix} -3 \\ -1 \\ 0 \\ 2 \\ 5 \\ 1 \end{bmatrix}$$

Solution: Compute

$$A^T A = \begin{bmatrix} 1 & 1 & 1 & 1 & 1 & 1 \\ 1 & 1 & 0 & 0 & 0 & 0 \\ 0 & 0 & 1 & 1 & 0 & 0 \\ 0 & 0 & 0 & 0 & 1 & 1 \end{bmatrix} \begin{bmatrix} 1 & 1 & 0 & 0 \\ 1 & 1 & 0 & 0 \\ 1 & 0 & 1 & 0 \\ 1 & 0 & 1 & 0 \\ 1 & 0 & 0 & 1 \\ 1 & 0 & 0 & 1 \end{bmatrix} = \begin{bmatrix} 6 & 2 & 2 & 2 \\ 2 & 2 & 0 & 0 \\ 2 & 0 & 2 & 0 \\ 2 & 0 & 0 & 2 \end{bmatrix}$$

$$A^T B = \begin{bmatrix} 1 & 1 & 1 & 1 & 1 & 1 \\ 1 & 1 & 0 & 0 & 0 & 0 \\ 0 & 0 & 1 & 1 & 0 & 0 \\ 0 & 0 & 0 & 0 & 1 & 1 \end{bmatrix} \begin{bmatrix} -3 \\ -1 \\ 0 \\ 2 \\ 5 \\ 1 \end{bmatrix} = \begin{bmatrix} 4 \\ -4 \\ 2 \\ 6 \end{bmatrix}$$

The augmented matrix for $A^T Ax = A^T B$ is

$$\begin{bmatrix} 6 & 2 & 2 & 2 & 4 \\ 2 & 2 & 0 & 0 & -4 \\ 2 & 0 & 2 & 0 & 2 \\ 2 & 0 & 0 & 2 & 6 \end{bmatrix} \approx \begin{bmatrix} 1 & 0 & 0 & 1 & 3 \\ 0 & 1 & 0 & -1 & -5 \\ 0 & 0 & 1 & -1 & -2 \\ 0 & 0 & 0 & 0 & 0 \end{bmatrix}$$

The general solution is $x_1 = 3 - x_4$, $x_2 = -5 + x_4$, $x_3 = -2 + x_4$ and x_4 is free variable. So the general least square solution of $Ax = B$ has the form

$$x = \begin{bmatrix} 3 \\ -5 \\ -2 \\ 0 \end{bmatrix} + x_4 \begin{bmatrix} -1 \\ 1 \\ 1 \\ 1 \end{bmatrix}$$

Example 3: Given A and B in Example 1, determine the least-square error in the least square solution of $Ax = B$.

Solution: From Example 1,

$$B = \begin{bmatrix} 2 \\ 0 \\ 11 \end{bmatrix} \text{ and } Ax = \begin{bmatrix} 4 & 0 \\ 0 & 2 \\ 1 & 1 \end{bmatrix} \begin{bmatrix} 1 \\ 2 \end{bmatrix} = \begin{bmatrix} 4 \\ 4 \\ 3 \end{bmatrix}$$

Hence

$$B - Ax = \begin{bmatrix} 2 \\ 0 \\ 11 \end{bmatrix} - \begin{bmatrix} 4 \\ 4 \\ 3 \end{bmatrix} = \begin{bmatrix} -2 \\ -4 \\ 8 \end{bmatrix}$$

and $\quad \| B - Ax \| = \sqrt{(-2)^2 + (-4)^2 + 8^2} = \sqrt{84}$

The least-square error is $\sqrt{84}$. For any x in R^2, the distance between B and the vector Ax is at least $\sqrt{84}$.

Example 4: Find the least-square solution of $Ax = B$ for

$$A = \begin{bmatrix} 1 & 3 & 5 \\ 1 & 1 & 0 \\ 1 & 1 & 2 \\ 1 & 3 & 3 \end{bmatrix}, \quad B = \begin{bmatrix} 3 \\ 5 \\ 7 \\ -3 \end{bmatrix}$$

Solution: The QR factorization of A

$$A = QR = \begin{bmatrix} \dfrac{1}{2} & \dfrac{1}{2} & \dfrac{1}{2} \\[6pt] \dfrac{1}{2} & -\dfrac{1}{2} & -\dfrac{1}{2} \\[6pt] \dfrac{1}{2} & -\dfrac{1}{2} & \dfrac{1}{2} \\[6pt] \dfrac{1}{2} & \dfrac{1}{2} & -\dfrac{1}{2} \end{bmatrix} \begin{bmatrix} 2 & 4 & 5 \\ 0 & 2 & 3 \\ 0 & 0 & 2 \end{bmatrix}$$

Then

$$Q^T B = \begin{bmatrix} \dfrac{1}{2} & \dfrac{1}{2} & \dfrac{1}{2} & \dfrac{1}{2} \\[6pt] \dfrac{1}{2} & -\dfrac{1}{2} & -\dfrac{1}{2} & \dfrac{1}{2} \\[6pt] \dfrac{1}{2} & -\dfrac{1}{2} & \dfrac{1}{2} & -\dfrac{1}{2} \end{bmatrix} \begin{bmatrix} 3 \\ 5 \\ 7 \\ -3 \end{bmatrix} = \begin{bmatrix} 6 \\ -6 \\ 4 \end{bmatrix}$$

The least-square solution 'x' satisfies $Rx = Q^T B$,

i.e.

$$\begin{bmatrix} 2 & 4 & 5 \\ 0 & 2 & 3 \\ 0 & 0 & 2 \end{bmatrix} \begin{bmatrix} x_1 \\ x_2 \\ x_3 \end{bmatrix} = \begin{bmatrix} 6 \\ -6 \\ 4 \end{bmatrix}$$

This equation is solved easily and yield

$$x = \begin{bmatrix} 10 \\ -6 \\ 2 \end{bmatrix}$$

Example 5: Find QR factorization of the matrix

$$\begin{bmatrix} 1 & 2 & 5 \\ -1 & 1 & -5 \\ -1 & 4 & -3 \\ 1 & -4 & 7 \\ 1 & 2 & 1 \end{bmatrix}$$

Solution:

Let
$$x_1 = \begin{bmatrix} 1 \\ -1 \\ -1 \\ 1 \\ 1 \end{bmatrix} \quad x_2 = \begin{bmatrix} 2 \\ 1 \\ 4 \\ -4 \\ 2 \end{bmatrix} \quad x_3 = \begin{bmatrix} 5 \\ -4 \\ -3 \\ 7 \\ 1 \end{bmatrix}$$

Step 1: Let $v_1 = x_1$ and $w_1 = \text{span}\{x_1\} = \text{span}\{v_1\}$

$$v_1 = x_1 = \begin{bmatrix} 1 \\ -1 \\ -1 \\ 1 \\ 1 \end{bmatrix}$$

Step 2: Let v_2 be the vectors produced by subtracting from x_2 in the subspace w_1, i.e.

$$v_2 = x_2 - \frac{\langle x_2, v_1 \rangle}{\langle v_1, v_1 \rangle} v_1$$

$$= \begin{bmatrix} 2 \\ 1 \\ 4 \\ -4 \\ 2 \end{bmatrix} - \frac{2-1-4-4+2}{1+1+1+1+1} \begin{bmatrix} 1 \\ -1 \\ -1 \\ 1 \\ 1 \end{bmatrix} = \begin{bmatrix} 2 \\ 1 \\ 4 \\ -4 \\ 2 \end{bmatrix}$$

$$v_2 = \begin{bmatrix} 1 \\ -1 \\ -1 \\ 1 \\ 1 \end{bmatrix} + \begin{bmatrix} 2 \\ -1 \\ 4 \\ -4 \\ 2 \end{bmatrix} = \begin{bmatrix} 3 \\ 0 \\ 3 \\ -3 \\ 3 \end{bmatrix}$$

$$v_3 = x_3 - \frac{\langle x_3, v_1 \rangle}{\langle v_1, v_1 \rangle} v_1 - \frac{\langle x_3, v_2 \rangle}{\langle v_2, v_2 \rangle} v_2$$

$$\langle x_3, v_1 \rangle = 5 + 4 + 3 + 7 + 1 = 20$$
$$\langle v_1, v_1 \rangle = 5$$
$$\langle x_3, v_2 \rangle = 15 + 0 - 9 - 21 + 3 = -12$$
$$\langle v_2, v_2 \rangle = 9 + 0 + 9 + 9 + 9 = 36$$

$$v_3 = \begin{bmatrix} 5 \\ -4 \\ -3 \\ 7 \\ 1 \end{bmatrix} - \frac{20}{5} \begin{bmatrix} 1 \\ -1 \\ -1 \\ 1 \\ 1 \end{bmatrix} + \frac{12}{36} \begin{bmatrix} 3 \\ 0 \\ 3 \\ -3 \\ 3 \end{bmatrix}$$

$$v_3 = \begin{bmatrix} 5-4+1 \\ -4+4+0 \\ -3+4+1 \\ 7-4-1 \\ 1-4+1 \end{bmatrix} = \begin{bmatrix} 2 \\ 0 \\ 2 \\ 2 \\ -2 \end{bmatrix}$$

$$Q = \begin{bmatrix} \dfrac{1}{\sqrt{5}} & \dfrac{3}{6} & \dfrac{2}{4} \\[2mm] -\dfrac{1}{5} & 0 & 0 \\[2mm] -\dfrac{1}{5} & \dfrac{+3}{6} & \dfrac{2}{4} \\[2mm] \dfrac{1}{5} & \dfrac{-3}{6} & \dfrac{2}{4} \\[2mm] \dfrac{1}{5} & \dfrac{3}{6} & \dfrac{-2}{4} \end{bmatrix} = \begin{bmatrix} \dfrac{1}{\sqrt{5}} & \dfrac{1}{2} & \dfrac{1}{2} \\[2mm] -\dfrac{1}{\sqrt{5}} & 0 & 0 \\[2mm] -\dfrac{1}{\sqrt{5}} & \dfrac{1}{2} & \dfrac{1}{2} \\[2mm] \dfrac{1}{\sqrt{5}} & -\dfrac{1}{2} & \dfrac{1}{2} \\[2mm] \dfrac{1}{\sqrt{5}} & \dfrac{1}{2} & -\dfrac{1}{2} \end{bmatrix}$$

$$R = Q^T A$$

$$= \begin{bmatrix} \dfrac{1}{\sqrt{5}} & \dfrac{-1}{\sqrt{5}} & \dfrac{-1}{\sqrt{5}} & \dfrac{1}{\sqrt{5}} & \dfrac{1}{\sqrt{5}} \\[2mm] \dfrac{1}{2} & 0 & \dfrac{1}{2} & -\dfrac{1}{2} & \dfrac{1}{2} \\[2mm] \dfrac{1}{2} & 0 & \dfrac{1}{\sqrt{5}} & \dfrac{1}{\sqrt{5}} & -\dfrac{1}{\sqrt{5}} \end{bmatrix} \begin{bmatrix} 1 & 2 & 5 \\ -1 & 1 & -4 \\ -1 & 4 & -3 \\ 1 & -4 & 7 \\ 1 & 2 & 1 \end{bmatrix}$$

$$= \begin{bmatrix} \dfrac{1}{\sqrt{5}}+\dfrac{1}{\sqrt{5}}+\dfrac{1}{\sqrt{5}}+\dfrac{1}{\sqrt{5}}+\dfrac{1}{\sqrt{5}} & \dfrac{2}{\sqrt{5}}-\dfrac{1}{\sqrt{5}}-\dfrac{4}{\sqrt{5}}-\dfrac{4}{\sqrt{5}}+\dfrac{2}{\sqrt{5}} & \dfrac{5}{\sqrt{5}}+\dfrac{4}{\sqrt{5}}+\dfrac{3}{\sqrt{5}}+\dfrac{7}{\sqrt{5}}+\dfrac{1}{\sqrt{5}} \\[3mm] \dfrac{1}{2}+0-\dfrac{1}{2}-\dfrac{1}{2}+\dfrac{1}{2} & 1+0+2+2+1 & \dfrac{5}{2}+0-\dfrac{3}{2}-\dfrac{7}{2}+\dfrac{1}{2} \\[3mm] \dfrac{1}{\sqrt{5}}+0-\dfrac{1}{\sqrt{5}}+\dfrac{1}{\sqrt{5}}-\dfrac{1}{\sqrt{5}} & \dfrac{2}{\sqrt{5}}+0-\dfrac{4}{\sqrt{5}}+\dfrac{4}{\sqrt{5}}-\dfrac{2}{\sqrt{5}} & \dfrac{5}{\sqrt{5}}+0-\dfrac{4}{\sqrt{5}}-\dfrac{3}{\sqrt{5}}-\dfrac{1}{\sqrt{5}} \end{bmatrix}$$

$$= \begin{bmatrix} \dfrac{5}{\sqrt{5}} & \dfrac{5}{\sqrt{5}} & \dfrac{20}{\sqrt{5}} \\[2mm] 0 & 6 & -2 \\[2mm] 0 & 0 & -\dfrac{3}{\sqrt{5}} \end{bmatrix} = R$$

EXERCISE

1. Find QR factorization of the matrix

$$A = \begin{bmatrix} 1 & 1 & -1 \\ 1 & 2 & 1 \\ 1 & 2 & -1 \end{bmatrix}$$

Ans. $Q = \begin{bmatrix} \dfrac{-1}{\sqrt{3}} & \sqrt{\dfrac{2}{3}} & 0 \\[2mm] \dfrac{-1}{\sqrt{3}} & \dfrac{1}{\sqrt{6}} & \dfrac{-1}{\sqrt{2}} \\[2mm] \dfrac{-1}{\sqrt{3}} & \dfrac{-1}{\sqrt{6}} & \dfrac{1}{\sqrt{2}} \end{bmatrix}$, $R = \begin{bmatrix} -\sqrt{3} & \dfrac{5\sqrt{3}}{3} & \dfrac{\sqrt{3}}{3} \\[2mm] 0 & -\sqrt{\dfrac{2}{3}} & -\sqrt{\dfrac{2}{3}} \\[2mm] 0 & 0 & -\sqrt{2} \end{bmatrix}$

2. Compute the QR decomposition of

$$A = \begin{bmatrix} 0 & 0 \\ 1 & 3 \\ 0 & 2 \end{bmatrix}$$

Ans. $A = \begin{bmatrix} 1 & 3 \\ 0 & 2 \\ 0 & 0 \end{bmatrix}$ and $Q = \begin{bmatrix} 0 & 0 & -1 \\ 1 & 0 & 0 \\ 0 & 1 & 0 \end{bmatrix}$

3. Find QR decomposition for the matrix

$$A = \begin{bmatrix} 0 & 1 & 1 \\ 1 & 1 & 2 \\ 0 & 0 & 3 \end{bmatrix}$$

Ans. $Q = \begin{bmatrix} 0 & 1 & 0 \\ 1 & 0 & 0 \\ 0 & 0 & 1 \end{bmatrix}$, $R = \begin{bmatrix} 1 & 1 & 2 \\ 0 & 1 & 1 \\ 0 & 0 & 3 \end{bmatrix}$

4. Find QR decomposition of

$$A = \begin{bmatrix} 1 & 0 & -1 \\ 1 & 0 & -3 \\ 0 & 1 & 1 \\ 0 & -1 & 1 \end{bmatrix}$$

Ans. $Q = \begin{bmatrix} \dfrac{1}{\sqrt{2}} & 0 & \dfrac{1}{2} \\[2mm] \dfrac{1}{\sqrt{2}} & 0 & \dfrac{-1}{2} \\[2mm] 0 & \dfrac{1}{\sqrt{2}} & \dfrac{1}{2} \\[2mm] 0 & -\dfrac{1}{\sqrt{2}} & \dfrac{1}{2} \end{bmatrix}$ and $R = \begin{bmatrix} \sqrt{2} & 0 & -2\sqrt{2} \\ 0 & \sqrt{2} & 0 \\ 0 & 0 & 2 \end{bmatrix}$

5. Find QR decomposition of $A = \begin{bmatrix} 1 & 0 \\ 1 & 1 \\ 0 & 1 \end{bmatrix}$

Ans. $Q = \begin{bmatrix} \dfrac{1}{\sqrt{2}} & \dfrac{1}{\sqrt{6}} \\[2mm] \dfrac{1}{\sqrt{2}} & \dfrac{1}{\sqrt{6}} \\[2mm] 0 & \sqrt{\dfrac{2}{3}} \end{bmatrix}$, $R = \begin{bmatrix} \dfrac{2}{\sqrt{2}} & \dfrac{1}{\sqrt{2}} \\[2mm] 0 & \sqrt{\dfrac{2}{3}} + \sqrt{\dfrac{1}{6}} \end{bmatrix}$.

8

Standard Euclidean Inner Product

8.1 INTRODUCTION

If you go back to the Euclidean n-space, we first introduced the concept of vectors and also introduced something called as a dot product. However, in this chapter, where we are dealing with the general vector space, we are yet to introduce anything even remotely like the dot product. It is time to do that. However, this chapter is about vector spaces in general. Here is the definition of this more general idea.

Definition 1: Suppose u, v and w are all vectors in vector space U and c is any scalar. An **inner product** on the vector space U is a function that associates with each pair of vectors in U, say u and v, real number denoted by $\{u, v\}$ that satisfies the following axioms.

(i) $\langle u, v \rangle = \langle v, u \rangle$

(ii) $\langle u + v, w \rangle = \langle u, w \rangle + \langle v, w \rangle$

(iii) $\langle cu, v \rangle = c \langle u, v \rangle$

(iv) $\langle u, u \rangle \geq 0$ and $\langle u, u \rangle = 0$ if and only if $u = 0$

A vector space along with an inner product is called an **inner product space**.

Example 1: The Euclidean inner product as defined in the Euclidean n-space section is an inner product.

Given two vectors in R^n, $u = (u_1, u_2, ..., u_n)$ and $v = (v_1, v_2, ..., v_n)$, the Euclidean inner product is defined to be

$$\langle u, v \rangle = u.v = u_1 v_1 + u_2 v_2 + ... + u_n v_n$$

Therefore, R^n is an inner product space.

Here are some more examples of inner products.

$$\langle u, v \rangle = w_1 u_1 v_1 + w_2 u_2 v_2 + ... + w_n u_n v_n = \langle v, u \rangle$$

Example 2: Suppose that $u = (u_1, u_2, ..., u_n)$ and $v = (v_1, v_2, ..., v_n)$ are two vectors in R^n and that $w_1, w_2, ..., w_n$ are **positive** real numbers (called **weights**), then the weighted Euclidean inner product is defined to be

$$\langle u, v \rangle = w_1 u_1 v_1 + w_2 u_2 v_2 + ... + w_n u_n v_n$$

So suppose that u, v and w are all vectors in R^n and that c is a scalar. First, we know that real numbers commute with multiplication. So, the first axiom is satisfied.

To show the second axiom is satisfied, we just need to run through the definition as follows,

$$\langle u+v,a \rangle = w_1(u_1+v_1)a_1 + w_2(u_2+v_2)a_2 + ... + w_n(u_n+v_n)a_n$$

$$= (w_1u_1a_1 + w_2u_2a_2 + ... + w_nu_na_n) + (w_1v_1a_1 + w_2v_2a_2 + ... + w_nv_na_n)$$

$$= \langle u,a \rangle + \langle v,a \rangle$$

and the second axiom is satisfied.

Here is the work for the third axiom.

$$\langle u+v,a \rangle = w_1(u_1+v_1)a_1 + w_2(u_2+v_2)a_2 + ... + w_n(u_n+v_n)a_n$$

$$= (w_1u_1a_1 + w_2u_2a_2 + ... + w_nu_na_n) + (w_1v_1a_1 + w_2v_2a_2 + ... + w_nv_na_n)$$

$\langle u,u \rangle = 0$ and so the fourth axiom is also satisfied.

Example 3: Suppose that $A = \begin{bmatrix} a_1 & a_3 \\ a_2 & a_4 \end{bmatrix}$ and $B = \begin{bmatrix} b_1 & b_3 \\ b_2 & b_4 \end{bmatrix}$ are two matrices in M_{22}. An inner product on M_{22} can be defined as

$$\langle A,B \rangle = tr(A^TB)$$

where $tr(C)$ is the trace of the matrix C.

$$tr(A^TB) = tr(B^TA) = a_1b_1 + a_2b_2 + a_3b_3 + a_4b_4$$

Example 4: Suppose that $f = f(x)$ and $g = g(x)$ are two continuous functions on the interval $[a,b]$. In other words, they are in the vector space $C[a,b]$. An inner product on $C[a,b]$ can be defined as,

$$\langle f,g \rangle = \int_a^b f(x)g(x)dx$$

Showing that this is an inner product is fairly simple. Suppose that f, g and h are continuous functions in $C[a, b]$ and that c is any scalar.

Here is the work showing that the first axiom is satisfied.

$$\langle f,g \rangle = \int_a^b f(x)g(x)dx = \int_a^b g(x)f(x)dx = \langle g,f \rangle$$

The second axiom is just as simple,

$$\langle f+g,h \rangle = \int_a^b (f(x)+g(x))h(x)dx$$

$$= \int_a^b f(x)h(x)dx + \int_a^b g(x)h(x)dx = \langle f,h \rangle + \langle g,h \rangle$$

Here is the third axiom,

$$\langle cf,g\rangle = \int_a^b cf(x)g(x)dx = c\int_a^b f(x)g(x)dx = c\langle f,g\rangle$$

First, we will start with the following,

$$\langle f,f\rangle = \int_a^b f(x)f(x)dx = \int_a^b f^2(x)dx$$

Now, if you integrate a continuous function which is greater than or equal to zero, then the integral must also be greater than or equal to zero. Hence,

$$\langle f,f\rangle \geq 0$$

Next, if $f = 0$, then clearly we have $\langle f,f\rangle = 0$. If we have

$$\langle f,f\rangle = \int_a^b f^2(x)dx = 0\,,\text{ then we must also have } f = 0.$$

Example 5: Suppose that $f = f(x)$ and $g = g(x)$ are two vectors in $C[a,b]$ and further suppose that $w(x) > 0$ is a continuous function called a weight inner product on $C[a,b]$ can be defined as,

$$\langle f,g\rangle = \int_a^b f(x)g(x)w(x)dx$$

Definition 2: Suppose that U is an inner product space. The **norm** or **length** of a vector u in U is defined to be

$$\| u \| = \langle u,u\rangle^{\frac{1}{2}}$$

Definition 3: Suppose that U is an inner product space and that u and v are two vectors in U. The distance between u and v, denoted by $d(u,v)$ is defined to be

$$d(u,v) = \| u - v \|$$

Example 6: For each of the following compute $\langle u,v\rangle$, $\| u \|$ and $d(u, v)$ for the given pair of vectors and inner product.

(i) $u = (2,-1, 4)$ and $v = (3, 2, 0)$ in R^3 with the standard Euclidean inner product.

(ii) $u = (2,-1, 4)$ and $v = (3, 2, 0)$ in R^3 with the weighted Euclidean inner product using the weights $w_1 = 2$, $w_2 = 6$, $w_3 = \dfrac{1}{5}$.

(iii) $u = x$ and $v = x^2$ in $C[0, 1]$ using the inner product.

Solution:

(i) $u = (2,-1,4)$ and $v = (3, 2, 0)$ in R^3 with the standard Euclidean inner product.

$$\langle u,v\rangle = (2)(3) + (-1)(2) + (4)(0) = 4$$

$$\| u \| = \langle u,u \rangle^{\frac{1}{2}} = \sqrt{(2)^2 + (-1)^2 + (4^2)} = \sqrt{21}$$

$$d(u,v) = \| u - v \| = \| (-1,-3,4) \| = \sqrt{(-1)^2 + (-3)^2 + (4)^2} = \sqrt{26}$$

(ii) $u = (2, -1, 4)$ and $v = (3, 2, 0)$ in R^3 with the weighted Euclidean inner product using the weights $w_1 = 2$, $w_2 = 6$, $w_3 = \dfrac{1}{5}$.

$$\langle u,v,w \rangle = (2)(3)(2) + (-1)(2)(6) + (4)(0)\left(\frac{1}{5}\right) = 0$$

$$\| u \| = \langle u,v \rangle^{\frac{1}{2}} = \sqrt{(2)^2(2) + (-1)^2(6) + (4^2)\left(\frac{1}{5}\right)} = \sqrt{\frac{86}{5}} = \sqrt{17.2}$$

$$d(u,v) = \| u - v \| = \| (-1,-3,4) \| = \sqrt{(1-1)^2(2) + (-3)^2(6) + (4)^2\left(\frac{1}{5}\right)}$$

$$= \sqrt{\frac{296}{5}}$$

(iii) $u = x$ and $v = x^2$ in $C[0, 1]$ using the inner product.

$$\langle u,v \rangle = \int_0^1 x(x^2)dx = \int_0^1 x^3 dx = \frac{1}{4}\left|x^4\right|_0^1 = \frac{1}{4}$$

$$\| u \| = \langle u,u \rangle^{\frac{1}{2}} = \sqrt{\int_0^1 x(x)dx} = \sqrt{\int_0^1 x^2 dx} = \sqrt{\frac{1}{3}\left|x^3\right|_0^1} = \frac{1}{\sqrt{3}}$$

$$d(u,v) = \| u - v \| = \| x - x^2 \| = \sqrt{\int_0^1 (x - x^2)^2 \, dx} = \sqrt{\frac{1}{5}x^5 - \frac{1}{2}x^4 + \frac{1}{3}x^3}\Big|_0^1$$

$$= \frac{1}{\sqrt{30}}$$

Theorem 1: Suppose u, v and w are vectors in an inner product space and c is any scalar. Then

(i) $\langle u, v + w \rangle = \langle u,v \rangle + \langle u,w \rangle$

(ii) $\langle u - v, w \rangle = \langle u,w \rangle - \langle v,w \rangle$

(iii) $\langle u, v - w \rangle = \langle u,v \rangle - \langle u,w \rangle$

(iv) $\langle cu,v \rangle = c\langle u,v \rangle$

(v) $\langle u,0 \rangle = \langle 0,u \rangle = 0$

Theorem 2: Cauchy-Schwarz Inequality: Suppose u and v are two vectors in an inner product space, then

$$|\langle u, v \rangle| \le \| u \| \, \| v \|$$

Theorem 3: Suppose u and v are two vectors in an inner product space and c is a scalar, then

  (i) $\| u \| \ge 0$

  (ii) $\| u \| = 0$ if and only if $u = v$

  (iii) $\| cu \| = |c| \, \| u \|$

  (iv) $\| u + v \| \le \| u \| + \| v \|$ (usually called the Triangle Inequality.)

Theorem 4: Suppose u, v and w are vectors in an inner product space. Then

  (i) $d(u, v) \ge 0$

  (ii) $d(u, v) = 0$ if and only if $u = v$

  (iii) $d(u, v) = d(v, u)$

  (iv) $d(u, v) \le d(u, w) + d(w, v)$ (usually called the Triangle Inequality.)

Definition 4: Suppose that u and v are two vectors in an inner product space. They are said to be orthogonal if $\langle u, v \rangle = 0$.

Example 7: The two vectors $u = (2, -1, 4)$ and $v = (3, 2, 0)$ in R^3 are not orthogonal with respect to the standard Euclidean inner product but are orthogonal with respect to the weighted Euclidean inner product with weights $w_1 = 2$, $w_2 = 6$ and $w_3 = \dfrac{1}{5}$.

We saw the computations for these back in Example 6.

Theorem 5: Suppose that u and v are two orthogonal vectors in an inner product space, then

$$\| u + v \|^2 = \| u \|^2 + \| v \|^2$$

Definition 5: Suppose that W is a subspace of an inner product space U. We say that a vector u from U is orthogonal to W, if it is orthogonal to every vector in W. The set of all vectors that are orthogonal to W is called the orthogonal complement of W and is denoted by W^1.

We say that W and W^1 are orthogonal complements.

Theorem 6: Suppose W is a subspace of an inner product space U. Then

  (i) W^1 is a subspace of U.

  (ii) Only the zero vector $\mathbf{0}$ is common to both W and W^1.

  (iii) $(W^1)^1 = W$. In other words, the orthogonal complement of W^1 is W.

Theorem 7: If A is an $n \times m$ matrix, then
  (i) The null space of A and the row space of A are orthogonal complements in R^m with respect to the standard Euclidean inner product.
  (ii) The null space of A^T and the column space of A are orthogonal complements in R^n with respect to the standard Euclidean inner product.

8.2 ORTHONORMAL BASIS

Definition 1: Suppose that S is a set of vectors in an inner product space.
  (i) If each pair of distinct vectors from S are orthogonal, then we call S is an **orthogonal set.**
  (ii) If S is an orthogonal set and each of the vectors in S also has a norm of 1, then we call S is an **orthonormal set.**

Example 1: Given the three vectors $v_1 = (2,0,-1)$, $v_2 = (0,-1,0)$ and $v_3 = (2,0,4)$ in R^3, answer each of the following.
  (i) Show that they form an orthogonal set under the standard Euclidean inner product for R^3 but not an orthonormal set.
  (ii) Turn them into a set of vectors that will form an orthonormal set of vectors under the standard Euclidean inner product for R^3.

Solution:
  (i) To show that they form an orthogonal set under the standard Euclidean inner product for R^3 but not an orthonormal set, compute the inner product of all the possible pairs and show that they are all zero.

$$\langle v_1, v_2 \rangle = (2)(0) + (0)(-1) + (-1)(0) = 0$$

$$\langle v_1, v_3 \rangle = (2)(2) + (0)(0) + (-1)(4) = 0$$

$$\langle v_2, v_3 \rangle = (0)(2) + (-1)(0) + (0)(4) = 0$$

$$\| v_1 \| = \sqrt{(2)^2 + (0)^2 + (-1)^2} = \sqrt{5}$$

$$\| v_2 \| = \sqrt{(0)^2 + (-1)^2 + (0)^2} = 1$$

$$\| v_3 \| = \sqrt{(2)^2 + (0)^2 + (4)^2}$$
$$= \sqrt{20}$$
$$= 2\sqrt{5}$$

So, only one of them has a norm of 1, therefore, they are not orthonormal set of vectors.

(ii)
$$\frac{1}{\|\,v\,\|}v$$

This new vector will have a norm of 1. So, we can turn each of the vectors above into a set of vectors with norm 1.

$$u_1 = \frac{1}{\|\,v_1\,\|}v_1 = \frac{1}{\sqrt{5}}(2,0,-1) = \left(\frac{2}{\sqrt{5}},0,-\frac{1}{\sqrt{5}}\right)$$

$$u_2 = \frac{1}{\|\,v_2\,\|}v_2 = \frac{1}{1}(0,-1,0) = (0,-1,0)$$

$$u_3 = \frac{1}{\|\,v_3\,\|}v_3 = \frac{1}{2\sqrt{5}}(2,0,4) = \left(\frac{1}{\sqrt{5}},0,\frac{2}{\sqrt{5}}\right)$$

All that remains to show is that this new set of vectors is still orthogonal. Verify that

$$\langle u_1,u_2\rangle = \langle u_1,u_3\rangle = \langle u_2,u_3\rangle = 0$$

and so we have turned the three vectors into a set of vectors that form an orthonormal set.

We have the following orthogonal sets.

Theorem 1: Suppose $S = \{v_1,v_2,...,v_n\}$ is an orthogonal set of non-zero vectors in an inner product space, then S is also a set of linearly independent vectors.

Proof: Note that we need the vectors to be non-zero vectors because the zero vector could be in a set of orthogonal vectors and yet we know that, if a set includes the zero vector it will be linearly dependent.

So, that these vectors are linearly independent (since we have excluded the zero vector) let us form the equation, $c_1v_1 + c_2v_2 + ... + c_nv_n = 0$ and we will need to show that only the scalars $c_1 = 0$, $c_2 = 0$, ..., $c_n = 0$

In fact, we can do this in a single step. All we need to do is take the inner product of both sides with respect to v_i, $i = 1, 2,..., n$ and then use the properties of inner products to rearrange.

$$\langle c_1v_1 + c_2v_2 + ... + c_nv_n, v_i\rangle = \langle 0,v_i\rangle$$

$$\langle c_1v_1,v_i\rangle + \langle c_2v_2,v_i\rangle + ... + \langle c_nv_n,v_i\rangle = 0$$

$$c_1\langle v_1,v_i\rangle + c_2\langle v_2,v_i\rangle + ... + c_n\langle v_n,v_i\rangle = 0$$

Now, we know the vectors in S are orthogonal.

Therfore $\langle v_i,v_j\rangle = 0$ if $i \neq j$ and so this reduces to

$$c_i\langle v_i,v_i\rangle = 0$$

Since we know that the vectors are all non-zero, we have $\langle v_i, v_i \rangle > 0$ and so the only way that this can be zero is $c_i = 0$. We have shown that, we must have $c_1 = 0$, $c_2 = 0,...,c_n = 0$ and so these vectors are linearly independent.

Definition 2: Suppose that $S = \{u_1, u_2,...,u_n\}$ is a basis for an inner product space.

(i) If S is an orthogonal set, then we call S is an orthogonal basis.

(ii) If S is an orthonormal set, then we call S is an orthonormal basis.

Theorem 2: Suppose that $S = \{v_1, v_2,...,v_n\}$ is an orthogonal basis for an inner product space and that u is any vector from the inner product space, then

$$u = \frac{\langle u, v_1 \rangle}{\| v_1 \|^2} v_1 + \frac{\langle u, v_2 \rangle}{\| v_2 \|^2} v_2 + ... + \frac{\langle u, v_n \rangle}{\| v_n \|^2} v_n$$

If S is an orthonormal basis, then

$$u = \langle u, v_1 \rangle v_1 + \langle u, v_2 \rangle v_2 + ... + \langle u, v_n \rangle v_n$$

Proof: We will just show that the first formula holds. Once we show that, the second will follow directly from the fact that all the vectors in an orthonormal set have a norm of 1.

So, given u, we need to find scalars $c_1, c_2,...,c$ so that

$$u = c_1 v_1 + c_2 v_2 + ... + c_n v_n$$

To find these scalars simply take the inner product of both sides with respect to v_i, $i = 1, 2,...,n$.

$$\langle u, v_i \rangle = \langle c_1 v_1 + c_2 v_2 + ... + c_n v_n, v_i \rangle$$
$$= c_1 \langle v_1, v_i \rangle + c_2 \langle v_2, v_i \rangle + ... + c_n \langle v_n, v_i \rangle$$

Now, since we have an orthogonal basis, we know that $\langle v_i, v_j \rangle = 0$ if $i \neq j$ and so, this reduces to

$$\langle u, v_i \rangle = c_i \langle v_i, v_i \rangle$$

Also, because u_i is a basis vector, we know that it is not the zero vector and so, we also know that $\langle v_i, v_i \rangle > 0$. This gives

$$c_i = \frac{\langle u, v_i \rangle}{\langle v_i, v_i \rangle}$$

However, from the definition of the norm, we can also write this as

$$c_i = \frac{\langle u, v_i \rangle}{\| v_i \|^2}$$

Example 2: Given that $v_1 = (2, -1, 0)$, $v_2 = (1, 0, -1)$ and $v_3 = (3, 7, -1)$ is a basis of R^3 and assuming that the standard Euclidean inner product, construct an orthogonal basis for R^3.

Solution:

Apply the Gram-Schmidt process a couple of times. The first step is easy.

$$u_1 = v_1 = (2, -1, 0)$$

Here is the formula for the second vector in our orthogonal basis.

$$u_2 = v_2 - \frac{\langle v_2, u_1 \rangle}{\| u_1 \|^2} u_1$$

and here is all the quantities that we need.

$$\langle v_2, u_1 \rangle = 2 \quad \| u_1 \|^2 = 5$$

The second vector is

$$u_2 = (1, 0, -1) - \frac{2}{5}(2, -1, 0) = \left(\frac{1}{5}, \frac{2}{5}, -1 \right)$$

The formula for the third (and final vector) is

$$u_3 = v_3 - \frac{\langle v_3, u_1 \rangle}{\| u_1 \|^2} u_1 - \frac{\langle v_3, u_2 \rangle}{\| u_2 \|^2} u_2$$

and here are the quantities that we need for this step.

$$\langle v_3, u_1 \rangle = -1, \quad \langle v_3, u_2 \rangle = \frac{22}{5}, \quad \| u_1 \|^2 = 5, \quad \| u_2 \|^2 = \frac{6}{5}$$

The third vector is

$$u_3 = (3, 7, -1) - \frac{-1}{5}(2, -1, 0) - \frac{\frac{22}{5}}{\frac{6}{5}}\left(\frac{1}{5}, \frac{2}{5}, -1 \right) = \left(\frac{8}{3}, \frac{16}{3}, \frac{8}{3} \right)$$

So, the orthogonal basis that we have constructed is

$$u_1 = (2, -1, 0) \text{ and } u_2\left(\frac{1}{5}, \frac{2}{5}, -1 \right) \text{ and } u_3 = \left(\frac{8}{3}, \frac{16}{3}, \frac{8}{3} \right)$$

You should verify that it, in fact, forms an orthogonal set.

Example 3: Given that $v_1 = (2, -1, 0)$, $v_2 = (1, 0, -1)$ and $v_3 = (3, 7, -1)$ is a basis of R^3 and assuming that the standard Euclidean inner product, construct an orthonormal basis for R^3 to verify orthogonal set (as the example above).

Solution:

$$\|u_1\| = \sqrt{5}, \quad \|u_2\| = \frac{\sqrt{30}}{5} \text{ and } \|u_3\| = \frac{8\sqrt{6}}{3} \quad \text{(Example 2)}$$

Note that, in order to eliminate as many square root as possible we rationalized the denominators of the fractions here.

Dividing by the norms gives the following set of vectors.

$$u_1 = \left(\frac{2}{\sqrt{5}}, -\frac{1}{\sqrt{5}}, 0\right), \; u_2 = \left(\frac{1}{\sqrt{30}}, \frac{2}{\sqrt{30}}, -\frac{5}{\sqrt{30}}\right) \text{ and } u_3 = \left(\frac{1}{\sqrt{6}}, \frac{2}{\sqrt{6}}, \frac{5}{\sqrt{6}}\right)$$

The first new vector will be

$$u_1 = \frac{1}{\|v_1\|} v_1 = \frac{1}{\sqrt{5}}(2, -1, 0) = \left(\frac{2}{\sqrt{5}}, -\frac{1}{\sqrt{5}}, 0\right)$$

Now, to get second vector, we first need to compute

$$w = v_2 - \frac{\langle v_2, u_1 \rangle}{\|u_1\|^2} u_1 = v_2 - \langle v_2, u_1 \rangle u_1$$

$$\langle v_2, u_1 \rangle = \frac{2}{\sqrt{5}}$$

Here, is the new orthogonal vector

$$w = (1, 0, -1) - \frac{2}{\sqrt{5}}\left(\frac{2}{\sqrt{5}}, -\frac{1}{\sqrt{5}}, 0\right) = \left(\frac{1}{5}, \frac{2}{5}, -1\right)$$

$$u_2 = \frac{1}{\|w\|} w = \frac{5}{\sqrt{30}}\left(\frac{1}{5}, \frac{2}{5}, -1\right) = \left(\frac{1}{\sqrt{30}}, \frac{2}{\sqrt{30}}, -\frac{5}{\sqrt{30}}\right)$$

Finally, for the third orthogonal vector the formula will be

$$w = v_3 - \langle v_3, u_1 \rangle u_1 - \langle v_3, u_2 \rangle u_2$$

$$\langle v_3, u_1 \rangle = -\frac{1}{\sqrt{5}} \quad \langle v_3, u_2 \rangle = \frac{22}{\sqrt{30}}$$

The orthogonal vector is then

$$w = (3, 7, -1) - \left(-\frac{1}{\sqrt{5}}\right)\left(\frac{2}{\sqrt{5}}, -\frac{1}{\sqrt{5}}, 0\right) - \frac{22}{\sqrt{30}}\left(\frac{1}{\sqrt{30}}, \frac{2}{\sqrt{30}}, -\frac{5}{\sqrt{30}}\right)$$

$$= \left(\frac{8}{3}, \frac{16}{3}, \frac{8}{3}\right)$$

Here is the final step to get our third orthonormal vector for this problem.

$$u_3 = \frac{1}{\|w\|} w = \frac{3}{8\sqrt{6}}\left(\frac{8}{3}, \frac{16}{3}, \frac{8}{3}\right) = \left(\frac{1}{\sqrt{6}}, \frac{2}{\sqrt{6}}, \frac{1}{\sqrt{6}}\right)$$

Example 4: Given that $v_1 = (1, 1, 1, 1)$, $v_2 = (1, 1, 1, 0)$, $v_3 = (1, 1, 0, 0)$ and $v_4 = (1, 0, 0, 0)$ is a basis of R^4 and assuming that we are working with the standard Euclidean inner product, construct an orthonormal basis for R^4.

Solution:

The first vector is

$$u_1 = v_1 = (1, 1, 1, 1)$$

Here the inner product and norm we need for the second vector

$$\langle v_2, u_1 \rangle = 3 \qquad \| u_1 \|^2 = 4$$

The second orthogonal vector is

$$u_2 = (1, 1, 1, 0) - \frac{3}{4}(1, 1, 1, 1) = \left(\frac{1}{4}, \frac{1}{4}, \frac{1}{4}, -\frac{3}{4} \right)$$

For the third vector, we need the following inner products and norms

$$\langle v_3, u_1 \rangle = 2, \quad \langle v_3, u_2 \rangle = \frac{1}{2}, \quad \| u_1 \|^2 = 4, \quad \| u_2 \|^2 = \frac{3}{4}$$

and the third orthogonal vector is

$$u_3 = (1, 1, 0, 0) - \frac{2}{4}(1, 1, 1, 1) - \frac{\frac{1}{2}}{\frac{3}{4}}\left(\frac{1}{4}, \frac{1}{4}, \frac{1}{4}, -\frac{3}{4} \right) = \left(\frac{1}{3}, \frac{1}{3}, -\frac{2}{3}, 0 \right)$$

Finally, for the fourth orthogonal vector

$$\langle v_4, u_1 \rangle = 1, \qquad \langle v_4, u_2 \rangle = \frac{1}{4}, \qquad \langle v_4, u_3 \rangle = \frac{1}{3}$$

$$\| u_1 \|^2 = 4, \qquad \| u_2 \|^2 = \frac{3}{4}, \qquad \| u_3 \|^2 = \frac{2}{3}$$

and the fourth vector in our new orthogonal basis is

$$u_4 = (1, 0, 0, 0) - \frac{1}{4}(1, 1, 1, 1) - \frac{\frac{1}{4}}{\frac{3}{4}}\left(\frac{1}{4}, \frac{1}{4}, \frac{1}{4}, -\frac{3}{4} \right) - \frac{\frac{1}{3}}{\frac{2}{3}}\left(\frac{1}{3}, \frac{1}{3}, -\frac{2}{3}, 0 \right)$$

$$= \left(\frac{1}{2}, -\frac{1}{2}, 0, 0 \right)$$

The orthogonal basis are

$$u_1 = (1, 1, 1, 1), \ u_2 = \left(\frac{1}{4}, \frac{1}{4}, \frac{1}{4}, -\frac{3}{4} \right), \ u_3 = \left(\frac{1}{3}, \frac{1}{3}, -\frac{2}{3}, 0 \right) \text{ and}$$

$$u_4 = \left(\frac{1}{2}, -\frac{1}{2}, 0, 0\right)$$

Next, we need their norms, so we can turn this set into an orthonormal basis.

$$\| u_1 \| = 2, \quad \| u_2 \| = \frac{\sqrt{3}}{2}, \quad \| u_3 \| = \frac{\sqrt{6}}{3} \text{ and } \| u_4 \| = \frac{\sqrt{2}}{2}$$

The orthonormal basis is

$$w_1 = \frac{1}{\| u_1 \|} u_1 = \left(\frac{1}{2}, \frac{1}{2}, \frac{1}{2}, \frac{1}{2}\right)$$

$$w_2 = \frac{1}{\| u_2 \|} u_2 = \left(\frac{1}{2\sqrt{3}}, \frac{1}{2\sqrt{3}}, \frac{1}{2\sqrt{3}}, -\frac{1}{2\sqrt{3}}\right)$$

$$w_3 = \frac{1}{\| u_3 \|} u_3 = \left(\frac{1}{\sqrt{6}}, \frac{1}{\sqrt{6}}, -\frac{2}{\sqrt{6}}, 0\right)$$

$$w_4 = \frac{1}{\| u_4 \|} u_4 = \left(\frac{1}{\sqrt{2}}, -\frac{1}{\sqrt{2}}, 0, 0\right)$$

8.3 LEAST SQUARES

In this section, we are going to take a look at an important application of orthogonal projections to inconsistent systems of equations. Recall that a system is called inconsistent if there are no solutions to the system.

Example 1: Find the equation of the line that runs through the four points $(1, -1)$, $(4, 11)$, $(-1, -9)$ and $(-2, -13)$.

Solution:

The values of m and b for which the line $y = mx + b$ will run through the four points given above give the following system of equations.

$$m + b = -1$$
$$4m + b = 11$$
$$-m + b = -9$$
$$-2m + b = -13$$

The corresponding matrix form of this system is

$$\begin{bmatrix} 1 & 1 \\ 4 & 1 \\ -1 & 1 \\ -2 & 1 \end{bmatrix} \begin{bmatrix} m \\ b \end{bmatrix} = \begin{bmatrix} -1 \\ 11 \\ -9 \\ -13 \end{bmatrix}$$

By solving this system (either the matrix form or the equations) gives us the solution

$$m = 4, \quad b = -5$$

So, the line $y = 4x - 5$ will run through the four points given above. Note that this makes a consistent system.

Example 2: Use least squares to find the equation of the line that will best approximate the points $(-3, 70)$, $(1, 21)$, $(-7, 110)$ and $(5, -35)$.

Solution:

The system of equations that we need to solve

$$AX = B$$

$$\begin{bmatrix} -3 & 1 \\ 1 & 1 \\ -7 & 1 \\ 5 & 1 \end{bmatrix} \begin{bmatrix} m \\ b \end{bmatrix} = \begin{bmatrix} 70 \\ 21 \\ 110 \\ -35 \end{bmatrix}$$

So, we have

$$A^T B = \begin{bmatrix} -22 \\ 0 \\ -21 \end{bmatrix} \quad B = \begin{bmatrix} 70 \\ 21 \\ 110 \\ -35 \end{bmatrix}$$

The normal system that we need to solve is then

$$\begin{bmatrix} -3 & 1 & -7 & 5 \\ 1 & 1 & 1 & 1 \end{bmatrix} \begin{bmatrix} -3 & 1 \\ 1 & 1 \\ -7 & 1 \\ 5 & 1 \end{bmatrix} \begin{bmatrix} m \\ b \end{bmatrix} = \begin{bmatrix} -3 & 1 & -7 & 5 \\ 1 & 1 & 1 & 1 \end{bmatrix} \begin{bmatrix} 70 \\ 21 \\ 110 \\ -35 \end{bmatrix}$$

$$\begin{bmatrix} 84 & -4 \\ -4 & 4 \end{bmatrix} \begin{bmatrix} m \\ b \end{bmatrix} = \begin{bmatrix} -1134 \\ 166 \end{bmatrix}$$

This is a fairly simple system to solve. We get,

$$m = -\frac{121}{10} = -12.1, \quad b = \frac{147}{5} = 29.4$$

So the line that best approximates all the points above is given by

$$y = -12.1x + 29.4$$

Example 3: Find the least squares solution to the following system of equations.

$$\begin{bmatrix} 2 & -1 & 1 \\ 1 & -5 & 2 \\ -3 & 1 & -4 \\ 1 & -1 & 1 \end{bmatrix} \begin{bmatrix} x_1 \\ x_2 \\ x_3 \end{bmatrix} = \begin{bmatrix} -4 \\ 2 \\ 5 \\ -1 \end{bmatrix}$$

Solution:

$$A = \begin{bmatrix} 2 & -1 & 1 \\ 1 & -5 & 2 \\ -3 & 1 & -4 \\ 1 & -1 & 1 \end{bmatrix} \quad A^T = \begin{bmatrix} 2 & 1 & -3 & 1 \\ -1 & -5 & 1 & -1 \\ 1 & 2 & -4 & 1 \end{bmatrix}$$

$$B = \begin{bmatrix} -4 \\ 2 \\ 5 \\ -1 \end{bmatrix} \quad A^T A = \begin{bmatrix} 15 & -11 & 17 \\ -11 & 28 & -16 \\ 17 & -16 & 22 \end{bmatrix} \quad A^T B = \begin{bmatrix} -22 \\ 0 \\ -21 \end{bmatrix}$$

The normal system is

$$\begin{bmatrix} 15 & -11 & 17 \\ -11 & 28 & -16 \\ 17 & -16 & 22 \end{bmatrix} \begin{bmatrix} x_1 \\ x_2 \\ x_3 \end{bmatrix} = \begin{bmatrix} -22 \\ 0 \\ -21 \end{bmatrix}$$

$$x_1 = -\frac{18}{7}, \quad x_2 = -\frac{151}{210}, \quad x_3 = \frac{107}{210}$$

In vector form, the least squares solution is then

$$\bar{x} = \begin{bmatrix} -\dfrac{18}{7} \\ -\dfrac{151}{210} \\ \dfrac{107}{210} \end{bmatrix}$$

Example 4: Compute the error in the solution of Example 2.

Solution:

First, the line that we found using least squares is

$$y = -12.1x + 29.4$$

$$\bar{\varepsilon}_1 = 70 - \left(-12.1(-3) + 29.4\right) = 4.3$$

$$\bar{\varepsilon}_2 = 21 - \left(-12.1(1) + 29.4\right) = 3.7$$

$$\bar{\varepsilon}_3 = 110 - \left(-12.1(-7) + 29.4\right) = -4.1$$

$$\bar{\varepsilon}_4 = -35 - \left(-12.1(5) + 29.4\right) = -3.9$$

$$\bar{\varepsilon} = \begin{bmatrix} 70 \\ 21 \\ 110 \\ -35 \end{bmatrix} - \begin{bmatrix} -3 & 1 \\ 1 & 1 \\ -7 & 1 \\ 5 & 1 \end{bmatrix} \begin{bmatrix} -12.1 \\ 29.4 \end{bmatrix} = \begin{bmatrix} 4.3 \\ 3.7 \\ -4.1 \\ -3.9 \end{bmatrix}$$

The square of the error and the error is then

$$\|\bar{\varepsilon}\|^2 = (4.3)^2 + (3.7)^2 + (-4.1)^2 + (-3.9)^2 = 64.2$$

$$\Rightarrow \quad \|\bar{\varepsilon}\| = \sqrt{64.2} = 8.0125$$

8.4 *QR*-DECOMPOSITION

In this section, we are going to look at a way to "decompose" or "factorise" an $n \times m$ matrix as follows.

Theorem 1: Suppose that A is an $n \times m$ matrix with linearly independent columns. Then A can be factored as

$$A = QR$$

where Q is an $n \times m$ matrix with orthonormal columns and R is an invertible $m \times m$ upper triangular matrix.

Proof: This will consist of actually constructing Q and R and showing that they, in fact, do multiply to give A.

Suppose that we perform the Gram-Schmidt process on these vectors and arrive at a set of orthonormal vectors $u_1, u_2,..., u_m$. Next define Q to be the $n \times m$ matrix whose columns are $u_1, u_2,..., u_m$ and so Q will be a matrix with orthonormal columns. We can then write A and Q as

$$A = \begin{bmatrix} c_1 | c_2 | \cdots | c_m \end{bmatrix} \quad Q = \begin{bmatrix} u_1 | u_2 | \cdots | u_m \end{bmatrix}$$

Next, each of the c_i's are in span $\{u_1, u_2,..., u_m\}$. We know from theorem 2 of the previous section that we can write each c_i as a linear combination of $u_1, u_2,..., u_m$ in the following manner.

$$c_1 = \langle c_1, u_1 \rangle u_1 + \langle c_1, u_2 \rangle u_2 + ... + \langle c_1, u_m \rangle u_m$$

$$c_2 = \langle c_2, u_1 \rangle u_1 + \langle c_2, u_2 \rangle u_2 + ... + \langle c_2, u_m \rangle u_m$$

$$\vdots$$

$$c_m = \langle c_m, u_1 \rangle u_1 + \langle c_m, u_2 \rangle u_2 + ... + \langle c_m, u_m \rangle u_m$$

Next, define R to be the $m \times m$ matrix defined as

$$R = \begin{bmatrix} \langle c_1, u_1 \rangle & \langle c_2, u_1 \rangle & \cdots & \langle c_m, u_1 \rangle \\ \langle c_1, u_2 \rangle & \langle c_2, u_2 \rangle & \cdots & \langle c_m, u_2 \rangle \\ \vdots & \vdots & \ddots & \vdots \\ \langle c_1, u_m \rangle & \langle c_2, u_m \rangle & \cdots & \langle c_m, u_m \rangle \end{bmatrix}$$

Now, let us examine the product QR.

$$QR = \begin{bmatrix} u_1 | u_2 | \cdots | u_m \end{bmatrix} \begin{bmatrix} \langle c_1, u_1 \rangle & \langle c_2, u_1 \rangle & \cdots & \langle c_m, u_1 \rangle \\ \langle c_1, u_2 \rangle & \langle c_2, u_2 \rangle & \cdots & \langle c_m, u_2 \rangle \\ \vdots & \vdots & \ddots & \vdots \\ \langle c_1, u_m \rangle & \langle c_2, u_m \rangle & \cdots & \langle c_m, u_m \rangle \end{bmatrix}$$

From the section on matrix arithmetic, we know that the jth column of this product is simply Q times the jth column of R. However, if you work through a couple of these, you will see that when we multiply Q with the jth column of R, we arrive at the formula for c_j. In other words,

$$QR = \begin{bmatrix} u_1 | u_2 | \cdots | u_m \end{bmatrix} \begin{bmatrix} \langle c_1, u_1 \rangle & \langle c_2, u_1 \rangle & \cdots & \langle c_m, u_1 \rangle \\ \langle c_1, u_2 \rangle & \langle c_2, u_2 \rangle & \cdots & \langle c_m, u_2 \rangle \\ \vdots & \vdots & \ddots & \vdots \\ \langle c_1, u_m \rangle & \langle c_2, u_m \rangle & \cdots & \langle c_m, u_m \rangle \end{bmatrix}$$

$$= \begin{bmatrix} c_1 | c_2 | \cdots | c_m \end{bmatrix}$$
$$= A$$

So, we can factorise A as a product of Q and R has the correct form. Now all that we need to do is to show that R is an invertible upper triangular matrix. First, from the Gram-Schmidt process, we know that u_k is orthogonal to $c_1, c_2, \ldots, c_{k-1}$. This means that, all the inner products below the main diagonal must be zero, since, they are all of the form $\langle c_i, u_j \rangle$ with $i < j$.

Now, we know from Theorem 2 from the special matrices that a triangular matrix will be invertible if the main diagonal entries, $\langle c_i, u_j \rangle$, are non-zero. This is fairly easy to show. Here is the general formula for u_i from the Gram-Schmidt process.

$$u'_i = c_i = \langle c_i, u_1 \rangle u_1 - \langle c_i, u_2 \rangle u_2 - \ldots - \langle c_i, u_{i-j} \rangle u_{i-j} \rightarrow u_i = \frac{u'_i}{\left\| u'_i \right\|}$$

Recall that, we are assuming the orthonormal u_i's, so the norms are not needed in the formula for

$u_1, u_2,..., u_{i-1}$. Note that, we also know that $\left\| u_i' \right\| \neq 0$.

Now, solving this for c_i and using $u_i' = \left\| u_i' \right\| u_i$ gives

$$c_i = u_i' + \left\langle c_i, u_1 \right\rangle u_1 + \left\langle c_i, u_2 \right\rangle u_2 + ... + \left\langle c_i, u_{i-1} \right\rangle u_{i-1}$$

$$= \left\| u_i' \right\| u_i + \left\langle c_i, u_1 \right\rangle u_1 + \left\langle c_i, u_2 \right\rangle u_2 + ... + \left\langle c_i, u_{i-1} \right\rangle u_{i-1}$$

$$\left\langle c_i, u_i \right\rangle = \left\langle \left\| u_i' \right\| u_i + \left\langle c_i, u_1 \right\rangle u_1 + \left\langle c_i, u_2 \right\rangle u_2 + ... + \left\langle c_i, u_{i-1} \right\rangle u_{i-1}, u_i \right\rangle$$

$$\left\langle \left\| u_i' \right\| u_i, u_i \right\rangle + \left\langle c_i, u_1 \right\rangle \left\langle u_1, u_i \right\rangle + \left\langle c_i, u_2 \right\rangle \left\langle u_2, u_i \right\rangle + ... + \left\langle c_i, u_{i-1} \right\rangle \left\langle u_{i-1}, u_i \right\rangle$$

$$= \left\| u_i' \right\| \left\langle u_i, u_i \right\rangle + \left\langle c_i, u_1 \right\rangle \left\langle u_1, u_i \right\rangle + \left\langle c_i, u_2 \right\rangle \left\langle u_2, u_i \right\rangle + ... + \left\langle c_i, u_{i-1} \right\rangle \left\langle u_{i-1}, u_i \right\rangle$$

However, the u_i's are an orthonormal basis vectors and so we know that

$$\left\langle u_j, u_i \right\rangle = 0 \quad j = 1, 2, ..., i-1 \quad \left\langle u_i, u_i \right\rangle \neq 0$$

Using these, we see that the diagonal entries are nothing more than,

$$\left\langle c_i, u_i \right\rangle = \left\| u_i' \right\|, \quad \left\langle u_i, u_i \right\rangle \neq 0$$

So the diagonal entries of R are non-zero and hence R must be invertible.

Example 1: Find the QR-decomposition for the matrix

$$A = \begin{bmatrix} 2 & 1 & 3 \\ -1 & 0 & 7 \\ 0 & -1 & -1 \end{bmatrix}$$

Solution:

The columns from A are

$$c_1 = \begin{bmatrix} 2 \\ -1 \\ 0 \end{bmatrix} \quad c_2 = \begin{bmatrix} 1 \\ 0 \\ -1 \end{bmatrix} \quad c_3 = \begin{bmatrix} 3 \\ 7 \\ -1 \end{bmatrix}$$

We performed Gram-Schmidt process on these vectors. So the orthonormal vectors that we will use for Q are

$$u_1 = \begin{bmatrix} \dfrac{2}{\sqrt{5}} \\ -\dfrac{1}{\sqrt{5}} \\ 0 \end{bmatrix} \qquad u_2 = \begin{bmatrix} \dfrac{1}{\sqrt{30}} \\ \dfrac{7}{\sqrt{30}} \\ -\dfrac{5}{\sqrt{30}} \end{bmatrix} \qquad u_3 = \begin{bmatrix} \dfrac{1}{\sqrt{6}} \\ \dfrac{2}{\sqrt{6}} \\ \dfrac{1}{\sqrt{6}} \end{bmatrix}$$

and the matrix Q is

$$Q = \begin{bmatrix} \dfrac{2}{\sqrt{5}} & \dfrac{1}{\sqrt{30}} & \dfrac{1}{\sqrt{6}} \\ -\dfrac{1}{\sqrt{5}} & \dfrac{7}{\sqrt{30}} & \dfrac{2}{\sqrt{6}} \\ 0 & -\dfrac{5}{\sqrt{30}} & \dfrac{1}{\sqrt{6}} \end{bmatrix}$$

The matrix R is

$$R = \begin{bmatrix} \langle c_1,u_1 \rangle & \langle c_2,u_1 \rangle & \langle c_3,u_1 \rangle \\ 0 & \langle c_2,u_2 \rangle & \langle c_3,u_2 \rangle \\ 0 & 0 & \langle c_3,u_3 \rangle \end{bmatrix} = \begin{bmatrix} \sqrt{5} & \dfrac{2}{\sqrt{5}} & -\dfrac{1}{\sqrt{5}} \\ 0 & \dfrac{6}{\sqrt{30}} & \dfrac{22}{\sqrt{30}} \\ 0 & 0 & \dfrac{16}{\sqrt{6}} \end{bmatrix}$$

So the *QR*-decomposition for this matrix is

$$\begin{bmatrix} 2 & 1 & 3 \\ -1 & 0 & 7 \\ 0 & -1 & -1 \end{bmatrix} = \begin{bmatrix} \dfrac{2}{\sqrt{5}} & \dfrac{1}{\sqrt{30}} & \dfrac{1}{\sqrt{6}} \\ -\dfrac{1}{\sqrt{5}} & \dfrac{7}{\sqrt{30}} & \dfrac{2}{\sqrt{6}} \\ 0 & -\dfrac{5}{\sqrt{30}} & \dfrac{1}{\sqrt{6}} \end{bmatrix} \begin{bmatrix} \sqrt{5} & \dfrac{2}{\sqrt{5}} & -\dfrac{1}{\sqrt{5}} \\ 0 & \dfrac{6}{\sqrt{30}} & \dfrac{22}{\sqrt{30}} \\ 0 & 0 & \dfrac{16}{\sqrt{6}} \end{bmatrix}$$

Example 2: Find the least squares solution to the following system of equations.

$$\begin{bmatrix} 2 & -1 & 1 \\ 1 & -5 & 2 \\ -3 & 1 & -4 \\ 1 & -1 & 1 \end{bmatrix} \begin{bmatrix} x_1 \\ x_2 \\ x_3 \end{bmatrix} = \begin{bmatrix} -4 \\ 2 \\ 5 \\ -1 \end{bmatrix}$$

Solution:

Here are the columns of A.

$$c_1 = \begin{bmatrix} 2 \\ 1 \\ -3 \\ 1 \end{bmatrix} \qquad c_2 = \begin{bmatrix} -1 \\ -5 \\ 1 \\ -1 \end{bmatrix} \qquad c_3 = \begin{bmatrix} 1 \\ 2 \\ -4 \\ 1 \end{bmatrix}$$

Now, we need to perform Gram-Schmidt process on these to get a set of orthonormal vectors. The first step is

$$u_1 = c_1 = \begin{bmatrix} 2 \\ 1 \\ -3 \\ 1 \end{bmatrix}$$

Here is the inner product and norm for the second step.

$$\langle c_2, u_1 \rangle = -11 \qquad \|u_1\|^2 = 15$$

The second vector is then

$$u_2 = c_2 - \frac{\langle c_2, u_1 \rangle}{\|u_1\|^2} u_1 = \begin{bmatrix} -1 \\ -5 \\ 1 \\ -1 \end{bmatrix} - \frac{-11}{15} \begin{bmatrix} 2 \\ 1 \\ -3 \\ 1 \end{bmatrix} = \begin{bmatrix} \dfrac{7}{15} \\[4pt] -\dfrac{64}{15} \\[4pt] -\dfrac{6}{5} \\[4pt] -\dfrac{4}{15} \end{bmatrix}$$

The final step will require the following inner products and norms

$$\langle c_3, u_1 \rangle = 17 \qquad \langle c_3, u_2 \rangle = -\frac{53}{15} \qquad \|u_1\|^2 = 15 \qquad \|u_2\|^2 = \frac{299}{15}$$

The third and final orthogonal vector is then

$$u_3 = c_3 - \frac{\langle c_3, u_1 \rangle}{\|u_1\|^2} u_1 - \frac{\langle c_3, u_2 \rangle}{\|u_2\|^2} u_2$$

$$
= \begin{bmatrix} 1 \\ 2 \\ -4 \\ 1 \end{bmatrix} - \frac{17}{15} \begin{bmatrix} 2 \\ 1 \\ -3 \\ 1 \end{bmatrix} - \frac{53}{15} \begin{bmatrix} \dfrac{7}{15} \\[4pt] \dfrac{64}{15} \\[4pt] \dfrac{299}{15} \\[4pt] \dfrac{6}{5} \\[4pt] \dfrac{4}{15} \end{bmatrix} = \begin{bmatrix} -\dfrac{354}{299} \\[4pt] \dfrac{33}{299} \\[4pt] \dfrac{243}{299} \\[4pt] -\dfrac{243}{299} \\[4pt] -\dfrac{54}{299} \end{bmatrix}
$$

If we divide each of them by their norms, we will get the orthonormal vectors that we need for the decomposition. The norms are

$$
\|u_1\| = \sqrt{15}, \quad \|u_2\| = \frac{\sqrt{4485}}{15} \quad \text{and} \quad \|u_3\| = \frac{3\sqrt{20930}}{299}
$$

The orthonormal vectors are

$$
w_1 = \begin{bmatrix} \dfrac{2}{\sqrt{15}} \\[6pt] \dfrac{1}{\sqrt{15}} \\[6pt] -\dfrac{3}{\sqrt{15}} \\[6pt] \dfrac{1}{\sqrt{15}} \end{bmatrix}, \quad w_2 = \begin{bmatrix} \dfrac{7}{\sqrt{4485}} \\[6pt] -\dfrac{64}{\sqrt{4485}} \\[6pt] -\dfrac{18}{\sqrt{4485}} \\[6pt] -\dfrac{4}{\sqrt{4485}} \end{bmatrix} \quad \text{and} \quad w_3 = \begin{bmatrix} -\dfrac{118}{\sqrt{20930}} \\[6pt] \dfrac{11}{\sqrt{20930}} \\[6pt] -\dfrac{81}{\sqrt{20930}} \\[6pt] -\dfrac{18}{\sqrt{20930}} \end{bmatrix}
$$

$$
Q = \begin{bmatrix} \dfrac{2}{\sqrt{15}} & \dfrac{7}{\sqrt{4485}} & -\dfrac{118}{\sqrt{20930}} \\[8pt] \dfrac{1}{\sqrt{15}} & -\dfrac{64}{\sqrt{4485}} & \dfrac{11}{\sqrt{20930}} \\[8pt] -\dfrac{3}{\sqrt{15}} & -\dfrac{18}{\sqrt{4485}} & -\dfrac{81}{\sqrt{20930}} \\[8pt] \dfrac{1}{\sqrt{15}} & -\dfrac{4}{\sqrt{4485}} & -\dfrac{18}{\sqrt{20930}} \end{bmatrix}
$$

Finally R is given by

$$R = \begin{bmatrix} \langle c_1,u_1 \rangle & \langle c_2,u_1 \rangle & \langle c_3,u_1 \rangle \\ 0 & \langle c_2,u_2 \rangle & \langle c_3,u_2 \rangle \\ 0 & 0 & \langle c_3,u_3 \rangle \end{bmatrix} = \begin{bmatrix} \sqrt{15} & -\dfrac{11}{\sqrt{15}} & \dfrac{17}{\sqrt{15}} \\ 0 & \dfrac{299}{\sqrt{4485}} & -\dfrac{53}{\sqrt{4485}} \\ 0 & 0 & \dfrac{210}{\sqrt{20930}} \end{bmatrix}$$

We can now proceed with the least squares process. First, we need Q^T.

$$Q^T = \begin{bmatrix} \dfrac{2}{\sqrt{15}} & \dfrac{1}{\sqrt{15}} & -\dfrac{3}{\sqrt{15}} & \dfrac{1}{\sqrt{15}} \\ \dfrac{7}{\sqrt{4485}} & -\dfrac{64}{\sqrt{4485}} & -\dfrac{18}{\sqrt{4485}} & -\dfrac{4}{\sqrt{4485}} \\ -\dfrac{118}{\sqrt{20930}} & \dfrac{11}{\sqrt{20930}} & -\dfrac{81}{\sqrt{20930}} & \dfrac{18}{\sqrt{20930}} \end{bmatrix}$$

The normal system can then be written as

$$\begin{bmatrix} \sqrt{15} & -\dfrac{11}{\sqrt{15}} & \dfrac{17}{\sqrt{15}} \\ 0 & \dfrac{299}{\sqrt{4485}} & -\dfrac{53}{\sqrt{4485}} \\ 0 & 0 & \dfrac{210}{\sqrt{20930}} \end{bmatrix} \begin{bmatrix} x_1 \\ x_2 \\ x_3 \end{bmatrix} =$$

$$\begin{bmatrix} \dfrac{2}{\sqrt{15}} & \dfrac{1}{\sqrt{15}} & -\dfrac{3}{\sqrt{15}} & \dfrac{1}{\sqrt{15}} \\ \dfrac{7}{\sqrt{4485}} & -\dfrac{64}{\sqrt{4485}} & -\dfrac{18}{\sqrt{4485}} & -\dfrac{4}{\sqrt{4485}} \\ -\dfrac{118}{\sqrt{20930}} & \dfrac{11}{\sqrt{20930}} & -\dfrac{81}{\sqrt{20930}} & -\dfrac{18}{\sqrt{20930}} \end{bmatrix} \begin{bmatrix} -4 \\ 2 \\ 5 \\ -1 \end{bmatrix}$$

$$\begin{bmatrix} \sqrt{15} & -\dfrac{11}{\sqrt{15}} & \dfrac{17}{\sqrt{15}} \\ 0 & \dfrac{299}{\sqrt{4485}} & -\dfrac{53}{\sqrt{4485}} \\ 0 & 0 & \dfrac{210}{\sqrt{20930}} \end{bmatrix} \begin{bmatrix} x_1 \\ x_2 \\ x_3 \end{bmatrix} = \begin{bmatrix} -\dfrac{22}{\sqrt{15}} \\ -\dfrac{242}{\sqrt{4485}} \\ \dfrac{107}{\sqrt{20930}} \end{bmatrix}$$

This corresponds to the following system of equations.

$$\sqrt{15}x_1 - \frac{11}{\sqrt{15}}x_2 + \frac{17}{\sqrt{15}}x_3 = -\frac{22}{\sqrt{15}} \quad \Rightarrow \quad x_1 = -\frac{18}{7}$$

$$-\frac{299}{\sqrt{4485}}x_2 - \frac{53}{\sqrt{4485}}x_3 = -\frac{242}{\sqrt{4485}} \quad \Rightarrow \quad x_2 = -\frac{151}{210}$$

$$\frac{210}{\sqrt{20930}}x_3 = \frac{107}{\sqrt{20930}} \quad \Rightarrow \quad x_3 = \frac{107}{210}$$

These are the same values that we received in the previous section.

8.5 EIGENVALUES AND EIGENVECTORS

Introduction

In this section, we will be looking at special situations, where given a square matrix A and a vector x, the product Ax will be the same as the scalar multiplication λx for some scalar λ. This idea has important applications in many areas of mathematics and science.

We will also have a quick review of determinants, since they will be required in order to do the work in the eigenvalues and eigenvectors. We will also take a look at an application that uses eigenvalues.

Definition 1: If $A = \begin{bmatrix} a_{11} & a_{12} \\ a_{21} & a_{22} \end{bmatrix}$, then the determinant of A is

$$\det(A) = \begin{vmatrix} a_{11} & a_{12} \\ a_{21} & a_{22} \end{vmatrix} = a_{11}a_{22} - a_{12}a_{21}$$

Definition 2: If $A = \begin{bmatrix} a_{11} & a_{12} & a_{13} \\ a_{21} & a_{22} & a_{23} \\ a_{31} & a_{32} & a_{33} \end{bmatrix}$, then the determinant of A is

$$\det(A) = \begin{vmatrix} a_{11} & a_{12} & a_{13} \\ a_{21} & a_{22} & a_{23} \\ a_{31} & a_{32} & a_{33} \end{vmatrix}$$

$$= a_{11}a_{22}a_{33} + a_{12}a_{23}a_{31} + a_{13}a_{21}a_{32} - a_{12}a_{21}a_{33} - a_{11}a_{23}a_{32} - a_{13}a_{22}a_{31}$$

As noted in the introduction of this chapter, we are going to start with a square matrix A and try to determine vector x and scalar λ so that we will have $Ax = \lambda x$.

In other words, this happens when multiplying x by the matrix A will be equivalent to multiplying x by the scalar λ. This will not be possible for all vectors x nor will it be possible for all scalars λ.

Definition 3: Suppose that A is an $n \times n$ matrix. Also suppose that x is a non-zero vector from R^n and that λ is any scalar (this can be zero) so that

$$Ax = \lambda x$$

We call x is an eigenvector of A and λ is an eigenvalue of A.

We will often call x is the eigenvector corresponding to or associated with λ and we will often call λ is the eigenvalue corresponding to or associated with x.

Example 1: Compute the determinant of each of the following matrices.

(i) $A = \begin{bmatrix} 3 & 2 \\ -9 & 5 \end{bmatrix}$

(ii) $B = \begin{bmatrix} 3 & -5 & 4 \\ -2 & -1 & 8 \\ -11 & 1 & 7 \end{bmatrix}$

(iii) $C = \begin{bmatrix} 2 & -6 & 2 \\ 2 & -8 & 3 \\ -3 & 1 & 1 \end{bmatrix}$

Solution:

(i) $A = \begin{bmatrix} 3 & 2 \\ -9 & 5 \end{bmatrix}$

$\det(A) = (3)(5)-(2)(-9) = 33$

(ii) $B = \begin{bmatrix} 3 & -5 & 4 \\ -2 & -1 & 8 \\ -11 & 1 & 7 \end{bmatrix}$

$\det(B) = \begin{vmatrix} 3 & -5 & 4 \\ -2 & -1 & 8 \\ -11 & 1 & 7 \end{vmatrix}$

$\det(B) = (3)(-1)(7) + (5)(8)(-11) + (4)(-2)(1)-(5)(-2)(7)-(3)(8)(1)-$
$$(-4)(-1)(-11) = -467$$

(iii) $C = \begin{bmatrix} 2 & -6 & 2 \\ 2 & -8 & 3 \\ -3 & 1 & 1 \end{bmatrix}$

$$\det(C) = \begin{vmatrix} 2 & -6 & 2 \\ 2 & -8 & 3 \\ -3 & 1 & 1 \end{vmatrix}$$

$$= (2)(-8)(1) + (-6)(3)(-3) + (2)(2)(1) - (-6)(2)(1) -$$
$$(2)(3)(1) - (2)(-8)(-3) = 0$$

Definition 4: Suppose A is a square matrix.

(i) If $\det(A) = 0$, we call A is a **singular** matrix.

(ii) If $\det(A) \neq 0$, we call A is a **non-singular** matrix.

So, in Example 1 above, both A and B are non-singular, while C is singular.

Theorem 1: Suppose that A is an $n \times n$ triangular matrix with diagonal entries $a_{11}, a_{22}, ..., a_{nn}$. The determinant of A is

$$\det(A) = a_{11}a_{22}...a_{nn}$$

Example 2: Compute the determinant of each of the following matrices.

$$A = \begin{bmatrix} 5 & 0 & 0 \\ 0 & -3 & 0 \\ 0 & 0 & 4 \end{bmatrix} \quad B = \begin{bmatrix} 6 & 0 \\ 2 & -1 \end{bmatrix} \quad C = \begin{bmatrix} 10 & 5 & 1 & 3 \\ 0 & 0 & -4 & 9 \\ 0 & 0 & 6 & 4 \\ 0 & 0 & 0 & 5 \end{bmatrix}$$

Solution:

Determinants are

$$\det(A) = (5)(-3)(4) = -60$$
$$\det(B) = (6)(-1) = -6$$
$$\det(C) = (10)(0)(6)(5) = 0$$

Definition 5: If A is a square matrix, then the **minor** of a_{ij}, denoted by M_{ij}, is the determinant of the submatrix that results from removing the ith row and jth column of A.

Definition 6: If A is a square matrix, then the **cofactor** of a_{ij}, denoted by C_{ij}, is the number $(-1)^{i+j} M_{ij}$.

Example 3: For the following matrix, compute the cofactors C_{12}, C_{24} and C_{32}.

$$A = \begin{bmatrix} 4 & 0 & 10 & 4 \\ -1 & 2 & 3 & 9 \\ 5 & -5 & -1 & 6 \\ 3 & 7 & 1 & -2 \end{bmatrix}$$

Solution:

In order to compute the cofactors, we first need the minor associated with each cofactor. Remember that in order to compute the minor, we remove the ith row and jth column of A.

So, to compute M_{12} (which we will need for C_{12}), we need to compute the determinant of the matrix, we get by removing the 1st row and 2nd column of A.

$$\Rightarrow M_{12} = \begin{vmatrix} -1 & 3 & 9 \\ 5 & -1 & 6 \\ 3 & 1 & -2 \end{vmatrix} = 160$$

Verify the determinant computation. Now we can get the cofactor.

$$C_{12} = (-1)^{1+2} M_{12} = (-1)^3 (160) = -160$$

Let us now move onto the second cofactor. Here is the work for the minor.

Now, $\qquad M_{24} = \begin{vmatrix} 4 & 0 & 10 \\ 5 & -5 & -1 \\ 3 & 7 & 1 \end{vmatrix} = 508$

The cofactor in this case is

$$C_{24} = (-1)^{2+4} M_{24} = (-1)^6 (508) = 508$$

$$\Rightarrow M_{32} = \begin{vmatrix} 4 & 10 & 4 \\ -1 & 3 & 9 \\ 3 & 1 & -2 \end{vmatrix} = 150$$

$$C_{32} = (-1)^{3+2} M_{32} = (-1)^5 (150) = -150$$

$$\begin{bmatrix} + & - & + & - & \cdots \\ - & + & - & + & \cdots \\ + & - & + & - & \cdots \\ - & + & - & + & \cdots \\ \vdots & \vdots & \vdots & \vdots & \ddots \end{bmatrix}$$

To use the table for the cofactor C_{ij}, we simply go to the ith row and jth column in the table above and if there is a " + " there we leave the minor alone and if there is a "−" there we will take a "−1" onto the appropriate minor. So, for C_{34} we go to the 3rd row and 4th column and see that we have a minus sign and so we know that $C_{34} = -M_{34}$.

Theorem 2: If A is an $n \times n$ matrix,

(i) Choose any row, say row i, then
$$\det (A) = a_{i1}C_{i2} + a_{i2}C_{2j} + \ldots + a_{in}C_{in}$$

(ii) Choose any column, say column j, then,
$$\det (A) = a_{1j}C_{1j} + a_{2j}C_{2j} + \ldots + a_{nj}C_{nj}$$

Example 4: For the following matrix, compute the determinant using the given cofactor expansions.

$$A = \begin{bmatrix} 4 & 2 & 1 \\ -2 & -6 & 3 \\ -7 & 5 & 0 \end{bmatrix}$$

(i) Expand along the first row.

(ii) Expand along the third row.

(iii) Expand along the second column

Solution:

(i) Expand along the first row.

Here is the cofactor expansion in terms of symbols for this part.
$$\det (A) = a_1 C_1 + a_{12}C_{12} + a_{13}C_{13}$$

Here is the work for this expansion.

$$\det(A) = (4)(+1)\begin{vmatrix} -6 & 3 \\ 5 & 0 \end{vmatrix} + (2)(-1)\begin{vmatrix} -2 & 3 \\ -7 & 0 \end{vmatrix} + (1)(+1)\begin{vmatrix} -2 & -6 \\ -7 & 5 \end{vmatrix}$$

$$= 4(-15) - 2(21) + (1)(-52) = -154$$

Verify 2×2 determinant computations.

(ii) Expand along the third row.

We will do this one without the explanations.
$$\det (A) = a_{31}C_{31} + a_{32}C_{32} + a_{33}C_{33}$$

$$(-7)(+1)\begin{bmatrix} 2 & 1 \\ -6 & 3 \end{bmatrix} + (5)(-1)\begin{bmatrix} 4 & 1 \\ -2 & 3 \end{bmatrix} + (0)(+1)\begin{vmatrix} 4 & 2 \\ -2 & -6 \end{vmatrix}$$

$$= -7(12) - 5(14) + (0)(-20)$$

$$= -154$$

(iii) Expand along the second column.

$$\det(A) = a_{12}C_{12} + a_{22}C_{22} + a_{32}C_{32}$$

$$(2)(-1)\begin{vmatrix} -2 & 3 \\ -7 & 0 \end{vmatrix} + (-6)(+1)\begin{vmatrix} 4 & 1 \\ -7 & 0 \end{vmatrix} + (5)(+1)\begin{vmatrix} 4 & 1 \\ -2 & 3 \end{vmatrix}$$

$$= -2(21) - 6(7) - 5(14) = -154$$

Again same as the first two as we expected.

Example 5: Suppose $A = \begin{bmatrix} 6 & 16 \\ -1 & -4 \end{bmatrix}$, then $x = \begin{bmatrix} -8 \\ 1 \end{bmatrix}$ is an eigenvector with corresponding eigenvalue 4.

$$Ax = \begin{bmatrix} 6 & 16 \\ -1 & -4 \end{bmatrix}\begin{bmatrix} -8 \\ 1 \end{bmatrix} = \begin{bmatrix} -32 \\ 4 \end{bmatrix} = 4\begin{bmatrix} -8 \\ 1 \end{bmatrix} = \lambda x$$

Let us start with $Ax = \lambda x$ and rewrite it as follows

$$Ax = \lambda Ix$$
$$\lambda Ix - Ax = 0$$
$$(\lambda I - A)x = 0$$

Now, if λ is going to be an eigenvalue of A, this system must have a non-zero solution x, since we know that eigenvectors associated with λ cannot be the zero vector so $\det(\lambda I - A) = 0$

So, eigenvalues will be scalars λ for which the matrix $\lambda I - A$ will be singular, i.e. $\det(\lambda I - A) = 0$. Let us get a couple of more definitions out of the eigenvalues and then we will work out some examples of finding eigenvalues.

Definition 7: Suppose A is an $n \times n$ matrix, then $\det(\lambda I - A) = 0$ is called the characteristic equation of A. When computed, it will be an nth degree polynomial in this form,

$$p(\lambda) = \lambda^n + c_{n-1}\lambda^{n-1} + \ldots + c_1\lambda + c_0$$

called the characteristic polynomial of A.

Definition 8: Suppose A is an $n \times n$ matrix and that $\lambda_1, \lambda_2, \ldots, \lambda_n$ is the complete list of all the eigenvalues of A including repeats. If λ occurs exactly once in this list, then we call λ a simple eigenvalue. If λ occurs $k \geq 2$ times in the list, we say that λ has multiplicity of k.

Example 6: Find all the eigenvalues for the given matrices.

(i) $A = \begin{bmatrix} 6 & 16 \\ -1 & -4 \end{bmatrix}$

(ii) $A = \begin{bmatrix} -4 & 2 \\ 3 & -5 \end{bmatrix}$

(iii) $A = \begin{bmatrix} 7 & -1 \\ 4 & 3 \end{bmatrix}$

Solution:

(i) $A = \begin{bmatrix} 6 & 16 \\ -1 & -4 \end{bmatrix}$

We will do this one with a little more detail than we will do the other two.

$$\lambda I - A = \begin{bmatrix} \lambda & 0 \\ 0 & \lambda \end{bmatrix} - \begin{bmatrix} 6 & 16 \\ -1 & -4 \end{bmatrix} = \begin{bmatrix} \lambda - 6 & -16 \\ 1 & \lambda + 4 \end{bmatrix}$$

Next, we need the determinant of this matrix which gives us the characteristic polynomial.

$$\det(\lambda I - A) = (\lambda - 6)(\lambda + 4) - (-16) = \lambda^2 - 2\lambda - 8$$

Now, set this equal to zero and solve for the eigenvalues.

$$\lambda^2 - 2\lambda - 8 = (\lambda - 4)(\lambda + 2) = 0 \Rightarrow \lambda_1 = -2, \lambda_2 = 4$$

So, we have two eigenvalues and since they occur only once in the list, they are both simple eigenvalues.

(ii) $A = \begin{bmatrix} -4 & 2 \\ 3 & -5 \end{bmatrix}$

Here is the matrix $\lambda I - A$ and its characteristic polynomial.

$$\lambda I - A = \begin{bmatrix} \lambda + 4 & -2 \\ -3 & \lambda + 5 \end{bmatrix} \qquad \det(\lambda I - A) = \lambda^2 + 9\lambda + 14$$

Now, set the characteristic polynomial equal to zero and solve for the eigenvalues.

$$\lambda^2 + 9\lambda + 14 = (\lambda + 7)(\lambda + 2) = 0 \Rightarrow \lambda_1 = -7, \lambda_2 = -2$$

Again, we get two simple eigenvalues.

(iii) $A = \begin{bmatrix} 7 & -1 \\ 4 & 3 \end{bmatrix}$

Here, is the matrix $\lambda I - A$ and its characteristic polynomial.

$$\lambda I - A = \begin{bmatrix} \lambda - 7 & 1 \\ -4 & \lambda - 3 \end{bmatrix} \qquad \det(\lambda I - A) = \lambda^2 - 10\lambda + 25$$

Now, set the characteristic polynomial equal to zero and solve for the eigenvalues.

$$\lambda_2 - 10\lambda + 25 = (\lambda - 5)^2 = 0 \implies \lambda_{1,2} = 5$$

Example 7: Find all the eigenvalues for the given matrices.

(i) $A = \begin{bmatrix} 4 & 0 & 1 \\ -1 & -6 & -2 \\ 5 & 0 & 0 \end{bmatrix}$

(ii) $A = \begin{bmatrix} 6 & 3 & -8 \\ 0 & -2 & 0 \\ 1 & 0 & -3 \end{bmatrix}$

(iii) $A = \begin{bmatrix} 0 & 1 & 1 \\ 1 & 0 & 1 \\ 1 & 1 & 0 \end{bmatrix}$

(iv) $A = \begin{bmatrix} 4 & 0 & -1 \\ 0 & 3 & 0 \\ 1 & 0 & 2 \end{bmatrix}$

Solution:

(i) $A = \begin{bmatrix} 4 & 0 & 1 \\ -1 & -6 & -2 \\ 5 & 0 & 0 \end{bmatrix}$

$$\lambda I - A = \begin{bmatrix} \lambda & 0 & 0 \\ 0 & \lambda & 0 \\ 0 & 0 & \lambda \end{bmatrix} - \begin{bmatrix} 4 & 0 & 1 \\ -1 & -6 & -2 \\ 5 & 0 & 0 \end{bmatrix} = \begin{bmatrix} \lambda - 4 & 0 & -1 \\ 1 & \lambda + 6 & 2 \\ -5 & 0 & \lambda \end{bmatrix}$$

$$\det(\lambda I - A) = \begin{vmatrix} \lambda - 4 & 0 & -1 \\ 1 & \lambda + 6 & 2 \\ -5 & 0 & \lambda \end{vmatrix}$$

$$= \lambda(\lambda - 4)(\lambda + 6) - 5(\lambda + 6)$$

$$= \lambda^3 + 2\lambda^2 - 29\lambda - 30$$
$$\Rightarrow \lambda^3 + 2\lambda^2 - 29\lambda - 30 = 0$$
$$(\lambda + 1)(\lambda + 6)(\lambda - 5) = 0$$
$$\Rightarrow \lambda_1 = -1, \lambda_2 = -6, \lambda_3 = 5$$

So this matrix has three simple eigenvalues.

(ii) $\quad A = \begin{bmatrix} 6 & 3 & -8 \\ 0 & -2 & 0 \\ 1 & 0 & -3 \end{bmatrix}$

Here is $\lambda I - A$ and the characteristic polynomial for this matrix.

$$\lambda I - A = \begin{bmatrix} \lambda - 6 & -3 & 8 \\ 0 & \lambda + 2 & 0 \\ -1 & 0 & \lambda + 3 \end{bmatrix} \quad \det(\lambda I - A) = \lambda^3 - \lambda^2 - 16\lambda - 20 = 0$$

$$(\lambda + 2)^2 (\lambda - 5) = 0 \Rightarrow \lambda_{1,2} = -2, \lambda_3 = 5$$

So, we have one double eigenvalue and one simple eigenvalue.

(iii) $A = \begin{bmatrix} 0 & 1 & 1 \\ 1 & 0 & 1 \\ 1 & 1 & 0 \end{bmatrix}$

Here is $\lambda I - A$ and the characteristic polynomial for this matrix.

$$\lambda I - A = \begin{bmatrix} \lambda & -1 & -1 \\ -1 & \lambda & -1 \\ -1 & -1 & \lambda \end{bmatrix}$$

$$\det(\lambda I - A) = \lambda^3 - 3\lambda - 2$$

$$\lambda^3 - 3\lambda - 2 = (\lambda + 1)^2 (\lambda - 2) = 0$$

So we can see that we have got two eigenvalues $\lambda_{1,2} = -1$ (a multiplicity 2 eigenvalue) and $\lambda_3 = 2$ (a simple eigenvalue).

(iv) $A = \begin{bmatrix} 4 & 0 & -1 \\ 0 & 3 & 0 \\ 1 & 0 & 2 \end{bmatrix}$

Here is $\lambda I - A$ and the characteristic polynomial for this matrix.

$$\lambda I - A = \begin{bmatrix} \lambda - 4 & 0 & 1 \\ 0 & \lambda - 3 & 0 \\ -1 & 0 & \lambda - 2 \end{bmatrix}$$

$$\det(\lambda I - A) = \lambda^3 - 9\lambda^2 + 27\lambda - 27 = 0$$

$$\therefore \lambda_{1,2,3} = 3$$

Theorem 3: Suppose A is an $n \times n$ triangular matrix. Then the eigenvalues will be the diagonal entries, $a_{11}, a_{22},..., a_{nn}$.

Proof: We will give the proof for an upper triangular matrix, and leave it to you to verify the proof for a lower triangular and a diagonal matrix.

$$A = \begin{bmatrix} a_{11} & a_{12} & \cdots & a_{1n} \\ 0 & a_{22} & \cdots & a_{2n} \\ \vdots & \vdots & \ddots & \vdots \\ 0 & 0 & \cdots & a_{nn} \end{bmatrix}$$

Now, we can write down $\lambda I - A$.

$$\lambda I - A = \begin{bmatrix} \lambda - a_{11} & -a_{12} & \cdots & -a_{1n} \\ 0 & \lambda - a_{22} & \cdots & -a_{2n} \\ \vdots & \vdots & \ddots & \vdots \\ 0 & 0 & \cdots & \lambda - a_{nn} \end{bmatrix}$$

$$\det(\lambda I - A) = (\lambda - a_{11})(\lambda - a_{22})\cdots(\lambda - a_{nn})$$

Setting this equal to zero and solving gives the eigenvalues as

$$\lambda_1 = a_{11}, \quad \lambda_2 = a_{22} \ ... \ \lambda_n = a_{nn}$$

Example 8: Find the eigenvalues of the following matrix.

$$A = \begin{bmatrix} 6 & 0 & 0 & 0 & 0 \\ 9 & -4 & 0 & 0 & 0 \\ -2 & 0 & 11 & 0 & 0 \\ 1 & -1 & 3 & 0 & 0 \\ 0 & 1 & -7 & 4 & 8 \end{bmatrix}$$

Solution:
Since this is a lower triangular matrix, we can use the previous theorem to write down the eigenvalues. It will simply be the main diagonal entries.

The eigenvalues are

$$\lambda_1 = 6, \; \lambda_2 = -4, \; \lambda_3 = 11, \; \lambda_4 = 0, \; \lambda_5 = 8$$

Definition 9: The set of all solutions to $(\lambda I - A)x = 0$ is called the eigen space of A corresponding to λ.

Example 9: For each of the following matrices, determine the eigenvectors corresponding to each eigenvalue and determine a basis for the eigenspace of the matrix corresponding to each eigenvalue.

(i) $A = \begin{bmatrix} 6 & 16 \\ -1 & -4 \end{bmatrix}$

(ii) $A = \begin{bmatrix} 7 & -1 \\ 4 & 3 \end{bmatrix}$

Solution:

$$(\lambda I - A)x = 0$$

(i) $A = \begin{bmatrix} 6 & 16 \\ -1 & -4 \end{bmatrix}$

We know that the eigenvalues for this matrix are $\lambda_1 = -2$ and $\lambda_2 = 4$. Let us first find the eigenvector(s) and eigenspace for $\lambda_1 = -2$. Referring to Example 5 for the formula for $\lambda_1 = -2$ into this, we can see that the system we need to solve is

$$\begin{bmatrix} -8 & -16 \\ 1 & 2 \end{bmatrix} \begin{bmatrix} x_1 \\ x_2 \end{bmatrix} = \begin{bmatrix} 0 \\ 0 \end{bmatrix}$$

Verify that the solution to this system is

$$x_1 = -2t, \qquad x_2 = t$$

Therefore, the general eigenvector corresponding to $\lambda_1 = -2$ is of the form

$$x = \begin{bmatrix} -2t \\ t \end{bmatrix} = t \begin{bmatrix} -2 \\ 1 \end{bmatrix}$$

The eigenspace is all vectors of this form and so we can see that a basis for the eigenspace corresponding $\lambda_1 = -2$ is

$$v_1 = \begin{bmatrix} -2 \\ 1 \end{bmatrix}$$

Let us find the eigenvector(s) and eigenspace for $\lambda_2 = 4$. Put $\lambda_2 = 4$

in the formula for $(\lambda I - A)$ from Example 5 which gives the following system, we need to solve

$$\begin{bmatrix} -2 & -16 \\ 1 & 8 \end{bmatrix}\begin{bmatrix} x_1 \\ x_2 \end{bmatrix} = \begin{bmatrix} 0 \\ 0 \end{bmatrix}$$

The solution to this system is $x_1 = -8t$, $x_2 = t$

The general eigenvector and a basis for the eigenspace corresponding to $\lambda_2 = 4$ is

$$x = \begin{bmatrix} -8t \\ t \end{bmatrix} = t\begin{bmatrix} -8 \\ 1 \end{bmatrix} \text{ and } v_2 = \begin{bmatrix} -8 \\ 1 \end{bmatrix}$$

$$\lambda_1 = -2, \quad v_1 = \begin{bmatrix} -2 \\ 1 \end{bmatrix}, \quad \lambda_2 = 4, \quad v_2 = \begin{bmatrix} -8 \\ 1 \end{bmatrix}$$

Note that, these eigenvectors are linearly independent vectors.

(ii)
$$A = \begin{bmatrix} 7 & -1 \\ 4 & 3 \end{bmatrix}$$

From Example 6, we know that $\lambda_{1,2} = 5$ is a double eigenvalue and so there will be a single eigenspace to compute for this matrix. Using the formula for $\lambda I - A$ from Example 6 and let $\lambda_{1,2} = 5$ into this gives the following system that we will solve for the eigenvector and eigen space.

$$\begin{bmatrix} -2 & 1 \\ -4 & 2 \end{bmatrix}\begin{bmatrix} x_1 \\ x_2 \end{bmatrix} = \begin{bmatrix} 0 \\ 0 \end{bmatrix}$$

The solution to this system is $x_1 = \begin{bmatrix} \dfrac{1}{2}t \end{bmatrix}$ and $x_2 = t$.

The general eigenvector and a basis for the eigenspace corresponding $\lambda_{1,2} = 5$ is

$$x = \begin{bmatrix} \dfrac{1}{2}t \\ t \end{bmatrix} = t\begin{bmatrix} \dfrac{1}{2} \\ 1 \end{bmatrix} \text{ and } v_1 = \begin{bmatrix} \dfrac{1}{2} \\ 1 \end{bmatrix}$$

Example 10: Find eigenvalues and eigenvectors of

(i) $A = \begin{bmatrix} 4 & 0 & 1 \\ -1 & -6 & -2 \\ 5 & 0 & 0 \end{bmatrix}$

The eigenvalues for this matrix are (Example 7) $\lambda_1 = -1$, $\lambda_2 = -6$ and $\lambda_3 = 5$

So we will have three eigenspaces.

Starting with $\lambda_1 = -1$, we will need to find the solution to the following system

$$\begin{bmatrix} -5 & 0 & -1 \\ 1 & 5 & 2 \\ -5 & 0 & -1 \end{bmatrix} \begin{bmatrix} x_1 \\ x_2 \\ x_3 \end{bmatrix} = \begin{bmatrix} 0 \\ 0 \\ 0 \end{bmatrix} \Rightarrow x_1 = -\frac{1}{5}t, \ x_2 = -\frac{9}{25}t \text{ and } x_3 = t$$

The general eigenvector and a basis for the eigenspace corresponding to $\lambda_1 = -1$ is,

$$x = \begin{bmatrix} -\dfrac{1}{5}t \\ -\dfrac{9}{25}t \\ t \end{bmatrix} = t \begin{bmatrix} -\dfrac{1}{5} \\ -\dfrac{9}{25} \\ 1 \end{bmatrix} \text{ and } v_1 = \begin{bmatrix} -\dfrac{1}{5} \\ -\dfrac{9}{25} \\ 1 \end{bmatrix}$$

Now, let us take a look at $\lambda_2 = -6$. Here is the system, we need to solve,

$$\begin{bmatrix} -10 & 0 & -1 \\ 1 & 0 & 2 \\ -5 & 0 & -6 \end{bmatrix} \begin{bmatrix} x_1 \\ x_2 \\ x_3 \end{bmatrix} = \begin{bmatrix} 0 \\ 0 \\ 0 \end{bmatrix} \Rightarrow x_1 = 0, \ x_2 = t \text{ and } x_3 = 0$$

Here, is the general eigenvector and a basis for the eigenspace corresponding to $\lambda_2 = -6$.

$$x = \begin{bmatrix} 0 \\ t \\ 0 \end{bmatrix} = t \begin{bmatrix} 0 \\ 1 \\ 0 \end{bmatrix} \text{ and } v_2 = \begin{bmatrix} 0 \\ 1 \\ 0 \end{bmatrix}$$

Finally, here is the system for $\lambda_3 = 5$.

$$\begin{bmatrix} 1 & 0 & -1 \\ 1 & 11 & 2 \\ -5 & 0 & 5 \end{bmatrix} \begin{bmatrix} x_1 \\ x_2 \\ x_3 \end{bmatrix} = \begin{bmatrix} 0 \\ 0 \\ 0 \end{bmatrix} \Rightarrow x_1 = t, \ x_2 = -\frac{3}{11}t \text{ and } x_3 = t$$

The general eigenvector and a basis for the eigenspace corresponding $\lambda_3 = 5$ is then

$$x = \begin{bmatrix} t \\ -\dfrac{3}{11}t \\ t \end{bmatrix} = t\begin{bmatrix} 1 \\ -\dfrac{3}{11} \\ 1 \end{bmatrix} \text{ and } v_3 = \begin{bmatrix} 1 \\ -\dfrac{3}{11} \\ 1 \end{bmatrix}$$

$$\lambda_1 = -1 \text{ and } v_1 = \begin{bmatrix} -\dfrac{1}{5} \\ -\dfrac{9}{25} \\ 1 \end{bmatrix}, \ \lambda_2 = -6 \text{ and } v_2 = \begin{bmatrix} 0 \\ 1 \\ 0 \end{bmatrix}, \lambda_3 = 5 \text{ and } v_3 = \begin{bmatrix} 1 \\ -\dfrac{3}{11} \\ 1 \end{bmatrix}$$

Verify that these three vectors are linearly independent vectors.

(ii)
$$A = \begin{bmatrix} 6 & 3 & -8 \\ 0 & -2 & 0 \\ 1 & 0 & -3 \end{bmatrix}$$

The eigenvalues for this matrix are (Example 7) $\lambda_{1,2} = -2$ and $\lambda_3 = 5$ So, it looks like, we will have two eigenspaces to find for this matrix. We will start with $\lambda_{1,2} = -2$. Here is the system that we need to solve and its solution.

$$\begin{bmatrix} -8 & -3 & 8 \\ 0 & 0 & 0 \\ -1 & 0 & 1 \end{bmatrix}\begin{bmatrix} x_1 \\ x_2 \\ x_3 \end{bmatrix} = \begin{bmatrix} 0 \\ 0 \\ 0 \end{bmatrix}$$

$$x_1 = 8t, \quad x_2 = 0 \text{ and } x_3 = t$$

The general eigenvector and a basis for the eigenspace corresponding to $\lambda_{1,2} = -2$ is then

$$x = \begin{bmatrix} t \\ 0 \\ t \end{bmatrix} = t\begin{bmatrix} 1 \\ 0 \\ 1 \end{bmatrix} \text{ and } v_1 = \begin{bmatrix} 1 \\ 0 \\ 1 \end{bmatrix}$$

Note that, even though we have a double eigenvalue, we get a single basis vector here.

Next, the system for $\lambda_3 = 5$ that we need to solve and its solution is,

$$\begin{bmatrix} -1 & -3 & 8 \\ 0 & 7 & 0 \\ -1 & 0 & 8 \end{bmatrix} \begin{bmatrix} x_1 \\ x_2 \\ x_3 \end{bmatrix} = \begin{bmatrix} 0 \\ 0 \\ 0 \end{bmatrix} , \quad x_1 = 8t, \ x_2 = 0 \text{ and } x_3 = t$$

The general eigenvector and a basis for the eigenspace corresponding to $\lambda_3 = 5$ is,

$$x = \begin{bmatrix} 8t \\ 0 \\ t \end{bmatrix} = t \begin{bmatrix} 8 \\ 0 \\ 1 \end{bmatrix} \text{ and } v_2 = \begin{bmatrix} 8 \\ 0 \\ 1 \end{bmatrix}$$

A set of eigenvalue/eigenvector pairs for this matrix is,

$$\lambda_{1,2} = -2 \text{ and } v_1 = \begin{bmatrix} 1 \\ 0 \\ 1 \end{bmatrix}, \ \lambda_3 = 5 \ v_2 = \begin{bmatrix} 8 \\ 0 \\ 1 \end{bmatrix}$$

(iii)
$$A = \begin{bmatrix} 0 & 1 & 1 \\ 1 & 0 & 1 \\ 1 & 1 & 0 \end{bmatrix}$$

As with the previous part, we have got two eigenvalues (Example 7), $\lambda_{1,2} = -1$ and $\lambda_3 = 2$ and so we will again have two eigen spaces to find.

We will start with $\lambda_{1,2} = -1$. Here is the system we need to solve,

$$\begin{bmatrix} -1 & -1 & -1 \\ -1 & -1 & -1 \\ -1 & -1 & -1 \end{bmatrix} \begin{bmatrix} x_1 \\ x_2 \\ x_3 \end{bmatrix} = \begin{bmatrix} 0 \\ 0 \\ 0 \end{bmatrix} \Rightarrow x_1 = -s-t, \ x_2 = s \text{ and } x_3 = t$$

The general eigenvector corresponding to $\lambda_{1,2} = -1$ is

$$x = \begin{bmatrix} -s-t \\ s \\ t \end{bmatrix} = t \begin{bmatrix} -1 \\ 0 \\ 1 \end{bmatrix} + s \begin{bmatrix} -1 \\ 1 \\ 0 \end{bmatrix}$$

Now, the eigenspace by the two vectors above and since they are linearly independent, we can see that a basis for the eigenspace corresponding to $\lambda_{1,2} = -1$ is,

$$v_1 = \begin{bmatrix} -1 \\ 0 \\ 1 \end{bmatrix}$$

$$v_2 = \begin{bmatrix} -1 \\ 1 \\ 0 \end{bmatrix}$$

Here is the system for $\lambda_3 = 2$ that we need to solve,

$$v_2 = \begin{bmatrix} 0 \\ 1 \\ 0 \end{bmatrix}$$

$x_1 = t$, $x_2 = t$ and $x_3 = t$

The general eigenvector and a basis for the eigenspace corresponding to $\lambda_3 = 2$ is,

$$x = \begin{bmatrix} t \\ t \\ t \end{bmatrix} = t \begin{bmatrix} 1 \\ 1 \\ 1 \end{bmatrix} \quad \text{and} \quad v_3 = \begin{bmatrix} 1 \\ 1 \\ 1 \end{bmatrix}$$

$$\lambda_1 = -1 \text{ and } v_1 = \begin{bmatrix} -1 \\ 0 \\ 1 \end{bmatrix}, \ \lambda_2 = -1 \text{ and } v_2 = \begin{bmatrix} -1 \\ 1 \\ 0 \end{bmatrix}, \ \lambda_3 = 2 \text{ and } v_3 = \begin{bmatrix} 1 \\ 1 \\ 1 \end{bmatrix}$$

Note that we listed the eigenvalue of "−1" twice, once for each eigen vector. You should verify that these are all linearly independent.

(iv) $A = \begin{bmatrix} 4 & 0 & -1 \\ 0 & 3 & 0 \\ 1 & 0 & 2 \end{bmatrix}$

In this case, we had a single eigenvalue (Example 7), $\lambda_{1,\,2,\,3} = 3$, so we will have a single eigenspace to find. Here is the system and its solution for this eigenvalue.

$$\begin{bmatrix} -1 & 0 & 1 \\ 0 & 0 & 0 \\ -1 & 0 & 1 \end{bmatrix} \begin{bmatrix} x_1 \\ x_2 \\ x_3 \end{bmatrix} = \begin{bmatrix} 0 \\ 0 \\ 0 \end{bmatrix} \Rightarrow x_1 = t, \ x_2 = 8, \ x_3 = t$$

The general eigenvector corresponding $\lambda_{1,2,3} = 3$ is then,

$$x = \begin{bmatrix} t \\ s \\ t \end{bmatrix} = t \begin{bmatrix} 1 \\ 0 \\ 1 \end{bmatrix} + s \begin{bmatrix} 0 \\ 1 \\ 0 \end{bmatrix}$$

As with the previous example, we can see that the eigenspace is spanned by the two vectors above and since they are linearly independent, we can see that a basis for the eigenspace corresponding to $\lambda_{1,2,3} = 3$ is

$$v_1 = \begin{bmatrix} 1 \\ 0 \\ 1 \end{bmatrix}$$

$$v_2 = \begin{bmatrix} 0 \\ 1 \\ 0 \end{bmatrix}$$

Note that the two vectors above would also make a nice pair of eigenvectors for the single.

9

Diagonalization

9.1 INTRODUCTION

An $n \times n$ matrix with n distinct equivalence is diagonalizable, if and only if A has n linearly independent eigenvectors.

In fact $A = PDP^{-1}$, where D is a diagonal matrix, iff the columns of P are n linearly independent eigenvectors of A. In this case, the diagonal entries of D are equivalence of A that corresponds to the eigenvectors in P.

If the eigenvectors are linearly independent, then P is invertible and $AP = PD \Rightarrow A = PDP^{-1}$.

9.2 REDUCTION TO DIAGONAL FORM

Theorem 1: If a square matrix A of order n has n linearly independent eigenvectors, then a matrix P can be found, such that $P^{-1}AP$ is a diagonal matrix.

Proof: Let A be a square matrix of order 3. Let $\lambda_1, \lambda_2, \lambda_3$ be its eigenvalues and

$$X_1 = \begin{bmatrix} x_1 \\ y_1 \\ z_1 \end{bmatrix}, \ X_2 = \begin{bmatrix} x_2 \\ y_2 \\ z_2 \end{bmatrix} \text{ and } X_3 = \begin{bmatrix} x_3 \\ y_3 \\ z_3 \end{bmatrix} \text{ be the corresponding eigen-}$$

vectors.

Denoting the square matrix $[X_1 \ X_2 \ X_3] = \begin{bmatrix} x_1 & x_2 & x_3 \\ y_1 & y_2 & y_3 \\ z_1 & z_2 & z_3 \end{bmatrix}$ by P, we have

$$AP = A[X_1 \ X_2 \ X_3] = [AX_1 \ AX_2 \ AX_3] = [\lambda_1 X_1, \lambda_2 X_2, \lambda_3 X_3]$$

$$= \begin{bmatrix} \lambda_1 x_1 & \lambda_2 x_2 & \lambda_3 x_3 \\ \lambda_1 y_1 & \lambda_2 y_2 & \lambda_3 y_3 \\ \lambda_1 z_1 & \lambda_2 z_2 & \lambda_3 z_3 \end{bmatrix}$$

$$= \begin{bmatrix} x_1 & x_2 & x_3 \\ y_1 & y_2 & y_3 \\ z_1 & z_2 & z_3 \end{bmatrix} \begin{bmatrix} \lambda_1 & 0 & 0 \\ 0 & \lambda_2 & 0 \\ 0 & 0 & \lambda_3 \end{bmatrix}$$

$$= PD$$

329

where D is the diagonal matrix.

$\therefore P^7AP = P^7PD = D$, which proves the theorem.

Note:

1. The matrix P which diagonalises A is called the modal matrix of A and the resulting diagonal matrix D is known as the spectral matrix of A.
2. The diagonal matrix has the eigenvalues of A as its diagonal elements.
3. The matrix P, which diagonalise A, constitutes the eigenvectors of A.

9.3 SIMILARITY OF MATRICES

A square matrix $\widehat{A}$ of order n is called similar to a square matrix A of order n if $\widehat{A} = P^{-1}AP$ for some non-singular $n \times n$ matrix P.

This transformation of a matrix A by a non-singular matrix P to $\widehat{A}$ is called a similarity transformation.

9.4 POWERS OF A MATRIX

Diagonalisation of a matrix is quite useful for obtaining powers of a matrix.

Let A be the square matrix. Then a non-singular matrix P can be found, such that

$$D = P^{-1}AP$$

$$D^n = (P^{-1}AP)(P^{-1}AP) = P^{-1}A^2P \qquad [\because PP^{-1} = I]$$

Similarly, $D^3 = P^{-1}A^3P$ and in general, $D^n = P^{-1}A^nP$ \qquad ...(1)

To obtain A^n, premultiply Eq. (1) by P and post-multiply by P^{-1}.

Then $\qquad D^nP^{-1} = PP^{-1}A^nPP^{-1} = A^n$

which gives A^n.

Thus $\qquad\qquad\qquad A^n = PD^nP^{-1}$

where $\qquad\qquad\qquad D^n = \begin{bmatrix} \lambda_1^n & 0 & 0 \\ 0 & \lambda_2^n & 0 \\ 0 & 0 & \lambda_3^n \end{bmatrix}$

Working Procedure

1. Find the eigenvalues of the square matrix A.
2. Find the corresponding eigenvectors and write the modal matrix P.
3. Find the diagonal matrix D from $D = P^{-1}DP$.
4. Obtain A^n from $A^n = PDP^{-1}$.

9.5 REDUCTION OF QUADRATIC FORM TO CANONICAL FORM

A homogeneous expression of the second degree in any number of variables

is called a quadratic form. For instance, if $A = \begin{bmatrix} a & h & g \\ h & b & f \\ g & f & c \end{bmatrix}$, $X = \begin{bmatrix} x \\ y \\ z \end{bmatrix}$ and

$X^1 = [xyz]$, then

$$X^1AX = ax^2 + by^2 + cz^2 + 2fyz + 2gzx + 2hyx \qquad ...(2)$$

which is a quadratic form.

Let λ_1, λ_2, λ_3 be the eigenvalues of the matrix A and

$$X_1 = \begin{bmatrix} x_1 \\ y_1 \\ z_1 \end{bmatrix}, \quad X_2 = \begin{bmatrix} x_2 \\ y_2 \\ z_2 \end{bmatrix}, \quad X_3 = \begin{bmatrix} x_3 \\ y_3 \\ z_3 \end{bmatrix}$$

be its corresponding eigenvectors in the normalized form (i.e. each element is divided by square root of sum of the squares of all three elements in the eigenvector).

Then $\qquad P^{-1}AP = \begin{bmatrix} \lambda_1 & 0 & 0 \\ 0 & \lambda_2 & 0 \\ 0 & 0 & \lambda_3 \end{bmatrix}$

where $\qquad P = \begin{bmatrix} x_1 & x_2 & x_3 \\ y_1 & y_2 & y_3 \\ z_1 & z_2 & z_3 \end{bmatrix}$

Hence the quadratic form (2) is reduced to a canonical form (or sum of squares form or principal axes form)

$$\lambda_1 x^2 + \lambda_2 y^2 + \lambda_3 z^2$$

and P is the matrix of transformation which is an orthogonal matrix.

Note:

Congruent (or orthogonal) transformation: The diagonal matrix D and the matrix A are called congruent matrices and the above method of reduction is called congruent (or orthogonal) transformation.

Index: The number of positive terms in canonical form of a quadratic form is known as the index of the form.

Signature: Signature of the quadratic form is the difference between the positive terms and negative terms in its canonical form.

9.6 NATURE OF QUADRATIC FORM

A real quadratic form $X'AX$ in n variables is said to be
  (i) Positive definite: If all the eigenvalues of $A > 0$.
  (ii) Negative definite: If all the eigenvalues of $A < 0$.
  (iii) Positive semidefinite: If all the eigenvalues of $A \leq 0$ and at least one eigenvalue $= 0$.
  (iv) Indefinite: If some of the eigenvalues of A are +ve and others –ve.

Example 1: Find a matrix P, which transforms the matrix $A = \begin{bmatrix} 1 & 1 & 3 \\ 1 & 5 & 1 \\ 3 & 1 & 1 \end{bmatrix}$

to diagonal form. Hence calculate A^4.

Solution: The characteristic equation is

$$|A - \lambda I| = \begin{vmatrix} 1-\lambda & 1 & 3 \\ 1 & 5-\lambda & 1 \\ 3 & 1 & 1-\lambda \end{vmatrix} = \lambda^3 - 7\lambda^2 + 36 = 0$$

$\therefore$ The eigenvalues of A are $\lambda = -2, 3, 6$ and the eigenvectors are $(-1, 0, 1)$, $(1, -1, 1)$ and $(1, 2, 1)$. Writing these eigenvectors as the three columns, the required transformation matrix (modal matrix) is

$$P = \begin{bmatrix} -1 & 1 & 1 \\ 0 & -1 & 2 \\ 1 & 1 & 1 \end{bmatrix}$$

To find P^{-1},

$$P = \begin{vmatrix} -1 & 1 & 1 \\ 0 & -1 & 2 \\ 1 & 1 & 1 \end{vmatrix} = \begin{vmatrix} a_1 & b_1 & c_1 \\ a_2 & b_2 & c_2 \\ a_3 & b_3 & c_3 \end{vmatrix} \text{(say)}$$

$A_1 = -3, B_1 = 2, C_1 = 1, A_2 = 0, B_2 = -2, C_2 = 2, A_3 = 3, B_3 = 2, C_3 = 1.$

Also $\qquad |P| = a_1 A_1 + b_1 B_1 + c_1 C_1 = 6$

$$P^{-1} = \frac{1}{|P|} \begin{bmatrix} A_1 & A_2 & A_3 \\ B_1 & B_2 & B_3 \\ C_1 & C_2 & C_3 \end{bmatrix}$$

$$= \frac{1}{6} \begin{bmatrix} -3 & 0 & 3 \\ 2 & -2 & 2 \\ 1 & 2 & 1 \end{bmatrix}$$

Thus

$$D = P^{-1}AP = \begin{bmatrix} -2 & 0 & 0 \\ 0 & 3 & 0 \\ 0 & 0 & 6 \end{bmatrix}$$

$$D^4 = \begin{bmatrix} (-2)^4 & 0 & 0 \\ 0 & 3^4 & 0 \\ 0 & 0 & 6^4 \end{bmatrix} = \begin{bmatrix} 16 & 0 & 0 \\ 0 & 81 & 0 \\ 0 & 0 & 1296 \end{bmatrix}$$

Hence $A^4 = PD^4P^{-1}$

$$= \frac{1}{6} \begin{bmatrix} -1 & 1 & 1 \\ 0 & -1 & 2 \\ 1 & 1 & 1 \end{bmatrix} \begin{bmatrix} 16 & 0 & 0 \\ 0 & 81 & 0 \\ 0 & 0 & 1296 \end{bmatrix} \begin{bmatrix} -3 & 0 & 3 \\ 2 & -2 & 2 \\ 1 & 2 & 1 \end{bmatrix}$$

$$= \begin{bmatrix} -1 & 1 & 1 \\ 0 & -1 & 2 \\ 1 & 1 & 1 \end{bmatrix} \begin{bmatrix} -8 & 0 & 8 \\ 27 & -27 & 27 \\ 216 & 512 & 216 \end{bmatrix}$$

$$= \begin{bmatrix} 251 & 485 & 235 \\ 485 & 1051 & 485 \\ 235 & 485 & 251 \end{bmatrix}$$

Example 2: Reduce the quadratic form $3x^2 + 5y^2 + 3z^2 - 2yz + 2zx - 2xy$ to the canonical form. Also specify the matrix of transformation.

Solution: The matrix of the given quadratic form is

$$A = \begin{bmatrix} 3 & -1 & 1 \\ -1 & 5 & -1 \\ 1 & -1 & 3 \end{bmatrix}$$

Its characteristic equation is $|A - \lambda I| = 0$

i.e.

$$\begin{vmatrix} 3-\lambda & -1 & 1 \\ -1 & 5-\lambda & -1 \\ 1 & -1 & 3-\lambda \end{vmatrix} = 0$$

which gives $\lambda = 2, 3, 6$ as its eigenvalues. Hence the given quadratic form reduces to the canonical form as

$$\lambda_1 x^2 + \lambda_2 y^2 + \lambda_3 z^2, \quad \text{i.e.} \quad 2x^2 + 3y^2 + 6z^2$$

To find the matrix of transformation from $[A - \lambda I]X = 0$, we obtain the equations

$$(3 - \lambda)x - y + z = 0, \quad -x + (5 - \lambda)y - z = 0, \quad x - y + (3 - \lambda)z = 0$$

Now corresponding to $\lambda = 2$, the eigenvector is $(1, 0, -1)$ and its normalised form is $\left(\dfrac{1}{\sqrt{2}}, 0, -\dfrac{1}{\sqrt{2}} \right)$.

Similarly, corresponding to $\lambda = 3$, the eigenvector is $(1, 1, 1)$ and its normalised form is $\left(\dfrac{1}{\sqrt{3}}, \dfrac{1}{\sqrt{3}}, \dfrac{1}{\sqrt{3}} \right)$.

Finally, corresponding to $\lambda = 6$, the eigenvector is $(1, -2, 1)$ and its normalised form is $\left(\dfrac{1}{\sqrt{6}}, \dfrac{-2}{\sqrt{6}}, \dfrac{1}{\sqrt{6}} \right)$.

Hence the matrix of transformation is

$$P = \begin{bmatrix} \dfrac{1}{\sqrt{2}} & \dfrac{1}{\sqrt{3}} & \dfrac{1}{\sqrt{6}} \\[2mm] 0 & \dfrac{1}{\sqrt{3}} & \dfrac{-2}{\sqrt{6}} \\[2mm] \dfrac{-1}{\sqrt{2}} & \dfrac{1}{\sqrt{3}} & \dfrac{1}{\sqrt{6}} \end{bmatrix}$$

Note: Index of the quadratic form $= 3$. Its signature is also 3.

Example 3: Find the nature of the following quadratic forms:

(i) $x^2 + 5y^2 + z^2 + 2xy + 2yz + 6zx$

(ii) $3x^2 + 5y^2 + 3z^2 - 2yz + 2yz - 2xy$

Solution: (i) The matrix of the quadratic form is

$$A = \begin{bmatrix} 1 & 1 & 3 \\ 1 & 5 & 1 \\ 3 & 1 & 1 \end{bmatrix}$$

The eigenvalues of A are $(-2, 3, 6)$ (by using Example 1)

Two of these eigenvalues being positive and one being negative, the given quadratic form is indefinite.

(ii) The matrix of the quadratic form is

$$A = \begin{bmatrix} 3 & -1 & 1 \\ -1 & 5 & -1 \\ 1 & -1 & 3 \end{bmatrix}$$

The eigenvalues of A are 2, 3, 6. (by using Example 2)
All these eigenvalues being positive, the given quadratic form is positive definite.

Example 4: Diagonalize the following matrix, if possible

$$A = \begin{bmatrix} 1 & 3 & 3 \\ -3 & -5 & -3 \\ 3 & 3 & 1 \end{bmatrix}$$

Find an invertible matrix P and a diagonal matrix D such that $A = PDP^{-1}$.

Solution:

To find $\quad |A - \lambda I| = 0$

$\Rightarrow \quad -\lambda^3 - 3\lambda^2 + 4 = 0$

$\Rightarrow -(\lambda - 1)(\lambda + 2)^2 = 0$

$\therefore$ The eigenvalues are $\lambda = 1, -2, -2$.
The linearly independent eigenvectors of A:

Basis for $\lambda = 1$; $V_1 = \begin{bmatrix} 1 \\ -1 \\ 1 \end{bmatrix}$

Basis for $\lambda = -2$; $V_2 = \begin{bmatrix} -1 \\ 1 \\ 0 \end{bmatrix}$ and $V_3 = \begin{bmatrix} -1 \\ 0 \\ 1 \end{bmatrix}$

$\therefore \{V_1, V_2, V_3\}$ is a linearly independent set.

$$\therefore \quad P = [V_1\ V_2\ V_3] = \begin{bmatrix} 1 & -1 & -1 \\ -1 & 1 & 0 \\ 1 & 0 & 1 \end{bmatrix}$$

$$\therefore \quad D = \begin{bmatrix} 1 & 0 & 0 \\ 0 & -2 & 0 \\ 0 & 0 & -2 \end{bmatrix}$$

Verify that $AP = PD$, i.e. $A = PDP^{-1}$

$$AP = \begin{bmatrix} 1 & 3 & 3 \\ -3 & -5 & -3 \\ 3 & 3 & 1 \end{bmatrix} \begin{bmatrix} 1 & -1 & -1 \\ -1 & 1 & 0 \\ 1 & 0 & 1 \end{bmatrix} = \begin{bmatrix} 1 & 2 & 2 \\ -1 & -2 & 0 \\ 1 & 0 & -2 \end{bmatrix}$$

$$PD = \begin{bmatrix} 1 & -1 & -1 \\ -1 & 1 & 0 \\ 1 & 0 & 1 \end{bmatrix} \begin{bmatrix} 1 & 0 & 0 \\ 0 & -2 & 0 \\ 0 & 0 & -2 \end{bmatrix} = \begin{bmatrix} 1 & 2 & 2 \\ -1 & -2 & 0 \\ 1 & 0 & -2 \end{bmatrix}$$

Hence verified.

Example 5: Verify that the following matrix is orthogonal or not.

$$A = \begin{bmatrix} 3 & -2 & 4 \\ -2 & 6 & 2 \\ 4 & 2 & 3 \end{bmatrix}$$

Solution:

The characteristic equation is $|A - \lambda I| = 0$

$$-\lambda^3 + 12\lambda^2 - 21\lambda - 98 = 0$$

$$\Rightarrow \qquad -(\lambda - 7)^2 (\lambda + 2) = 0$$

$$\lambda = 7, 7, -2$$

The calculation produce bases for the eigenspaces

$$\lambda = 7, \ V_1 = \begin{bmatrix} 1 \\ 0 \\ 1 \end{bmatrix}, \ V_2 = \begin{bmatrix} -\dfrac{1}{2} \\ 1 \\ 0 \end{bmatrix} \quad \lambda = -2, \ V_3 = \begin{bmatrix} -1 \\ -\dfrac{1}{2} \\ 1 \end{bmatrix}$$

Although, V_1 and V_2 are linearly independent, they are not orthogonal.

9.7 QUADRATIC FORMS

Diagonalization of Symmetric Matrix

A symmetric matrix is a matrix A, such that, $A^T = A$. A matrix A is said to be orthogonally diagonalizable, if there is an orthogonal matrix P(so $P^{-1} = P^T$) and a diagonal matrix D, such that $A = PDP^T = PDP^{-1}$

An orthogonally diagonalizable matrix A with orthonormal eigenvectors $u_1, u_2, ..., u_n$ can be written as $A = \lambda_1 u_1 u_1^T + ... + \lambda_n u_n u_n^T$.

This representation of A is called a spectoral decomposition of A. Further, each matrix $u_j u_j^T$ is a projection matrix.

Example:

Symmetric:
$$\begin{bmatrix} 1 & 0 \\ 0 & -2 \end{bmatrix}, \begin{bmatrix} 0 & 2 & 0 \\ 2 & 3 & 8 \\ 0 & 8 & -3 \end{bmatrix}, \begin{bmatrix} a & b & c \\ b & d & e \\ c & e & f \end{bmatrix}$$

Non-symmetric:
$$\begin{bmatrix} 1 & -3 \\ 3 & 0 \end{bmatrix}, \begin{bmatrix} 1 & -4 & 0 \\ -6 & 1 & -4 \\ 0 & -6 & 1 \end{bmatrix}, \begin{bmatrix} 5 & 4 & 3 & 2 \\ 4 & 3 & 2 & 1 \\ 3 & 2 & 1 & 0 \end{bmatrix}$$

Theorem 1: If A is an $n \times n$ symmetric matrix, then the eigenvectors of A associated with distinct equivalence are orthogonal.

Proof:

Let
$$u_1 = \begin{bmatrix} a_1 \\ a_2 \\ . \\ . \\ . \\ a_n \end{bmatrix} \text{ and } u_2 = \begin{bmatrix} b_1 \\ b_2 \\ . \\ . \\ . \\ b_n \end{bmatrix}$$

be eigenvectors of A associated with distinct equivalence λ_1 and λ_2 respectively,

i.e. $Ax_1 = \lambda_1 x_1$ and $Ax_2 = \lambda_2 x_2$

Thus $x_1^T Ax_2 = x_1^T (Ax_2) = x_1^T \lambda_2 x_2 = \lambda_2 x_1^T x_2$

and $x_1^T (Ax_2) = (x_1^T A^T) x_2 = (Ax_1)^T x_2$

$$= (\lambda_1 x_1)^T x_2$$
$$= \lambda_1 x_1^T x_2$$

$\therefore \quad x_1^T Ax_2 = \lambda_2 x_1^T x_2 = \lambda_1 x_1^T x_2$

such that $\lambda_1 \neq \lambda_2, x_1^T x_2 = 0$

Example 1:

Let
$$A = \begin{bmatrix} 0 & 0 & -2 \\ 0 & -2 & 0 \\ -2 & 0 & 3 \end{bmatrix}$$

A is symmetric matrix.

∴ The characteristic eq. is

$$|A - \lambda I| = 0$$

$$\Rightarrow \quad \begin{vmatrix} -\lambda & 0 & -2 \\ 0 & -2-\lambda & 0 \\ -2 & 0 & 3-\lambda \end{vmatrix} = 0$$

$$-\lambda\left[(-2-\lambda)(3-\lambda) - 0\right] - 0 - 2\left[0 + 2(-2-\lambda)\right] = 0$$

$$-\lambda\left(-6 + 2\lambda - 3\lambda + \lambda^2\right) - 4(-2-\lambda) = 0$$

$$-\lambda\left(\lambda^2 - \lambda - 6\right) + 8 + 4\lambda = 0$$

$$-\lambda^3 + \lambda^2 + 6\lambda + 4\lambda + 8 = 0$$

$$-\lambda^3 + \lambda^2 + 10\lambda + 8 = 0$$

$$+\lambda^3 - \lambda^2 - 10\lambda - 8 = 0$$

$$(\lambda + 2)(\lambda^2 - 3\lambda - 4) = 0$$

$$(\lambda + 2)(\lambda - 4)(\lambda + 1) = 0$$

∴ The equivalence of A are $-2, 4, -1$, i.e. $\lambda = -2, 4, -1$.
The eigenvectors associated with these eigenvalues are

$$\lambda_1 = -2, \quad x_1 = \begin{bmatrix} 0 \\ 1 \\ 0 \end{bmatrix}, \quad \lambda_2 = 4, \quad x_2 = \begin{bmatrix} -1 \\ 0 \\ 2 \end{bmatrix}$$

and $\quad \lambda_3 = -1, \quad x_3 = \begin{bmatrix} 2 \\ 0 \\ 1 \end{bmatrix}$

Thus,

x_1, x_2, x_3 are orthogonal.

Very important result:

If A is an $n \times n$ symmetric matrix, then there exists an orthogonal matrix P such that

$$D = P^{-1}AP = P^T AP,$$

where $\text{Col}_1(P), \text{Col}_2(P), ..., \text{Col}_n(P)$ are n linearly independent eigenvectors of A and the diagonal elements of D are the eigenvalues of A associated with these eigenvectors.

Example 2:

Let $\quad A = \begin{bmatrix} 0 & 2 & 2 \\ 2 & 0 & 2 \\ 2 & 2 & 0 \end{bmatrix}$

Find an orthogonal matrix P and diagonal matrix D such that $D = P^T A P$.

Solution: We need to find orthonormal eigenvectors of A and the associated eigenvalues first.

∴ The characteristic equation is

$$|A - \lambda I| = 0$$

$$|\lambda I - A| = \begin{vmatrix} \lambda & -2 & -2 \\ -2 & \lambda & -2 \\ -2 & -2 & \lambda \end{vmatrix} = 0$$

$$\Rightarrow \quad (\lambda + 2)^2 (\lambda - 4) = 0$$

Thus $\lambda = -2, -2, 4$.

Case 1: As $\lambda = -2$, solve for the homogeneous system

$$(-2I - A) X = 0$$

$$\Rightarrow \quad \begin{bmatrix} -2 & -2 & -2 \\ -2 & -2 & -2 \\ -2 & -2 & -2 \end{bmatrix} X$$

$$= \begin{bmatrix} -2 & 0 & 0 \\ 0 & -2 & 0 \\ 0 & 0 & -2 \end{bmatrix} - \begin{bmatrix} 0 & 2 & 2 \\ 2 & 0 & 2 \\ 2 & 2 & 0 \end{bmatrix}$$

∴ The eigenvectors are

$$t \begin{bmatrix} -1 \\ 1 \\ 0 \end{bmatrix} + s \begin{bmatrix} -1 \\ 0 \\ 1 \end{bmatrix}, \text{ where } t, s \in R, \ t \neq 0 \text{ or } s \neq 0$$

$$\Rightarrow \quad V_1 = \begin{bmatrix} -1 \\ 1 \\ 0 \end{bmatrix}, \ V_2 = \begin{bmatrix} -1 \\ 0 \\ 1 \end{bmatrix} \text{ are two eigenvectors of } A$$

However, the two eigenvectors are not orthogonal, we can obtain two orthonormal eigenvectors via. Gram-Schmidt process.

The orthogonal eigenvectors are

$$V_1^* = V_1 = \begin{bmatrix} -1 \\ 1 \\ 0 \end{bmatrix}$$

$$V_2^* = V_2 - \frac{\langle V_2 V_1^* \rangle}{\langle V_1^* V_1^* \rangle} V_1^* = \begin{bmatrix} -\dfrac{1}{2} \\ -\dfrac{1}{2} \\ 1 \end{bmatrix} = \begin{bmatrix} -1 \\ -1 \\ 2 \end{bmatrix}$$

Standardizing these two eigenvectors results in

$$W_1 = \frac{V_1^*}{\| V_1^* \|} = \begin{bmatrix} -\dfrac{1}{\sqrt{2}} \\ \dfrac{1}{\sqrt{2}} \\ 0 \end{bmatrix}$$

$$W_2 = \frac{V_2^*}{\| V_2^* \|} = \begin{bmatrix} -\dfrac{1}{\sqrt{6}} \\ -\dfrac{1}{\sqrt{6}} \\ \dfrac{2}{\sqrt{6}} \end{bmatrix}$$

Case 2: As $\lambda = 4$, solve for the homogeneous system

$$(4I - A)X = 0$$

The eigenvectors are

$$r \begin{bmatrix} 1 \\ 1 \\ 1 \end{bmatrix}, \ r \in R, \ r \neq 0$$

$\Rightarrow \qquad V_3 = \begin{bmatrix} 1 \\ 1 \\ 1 \end{bmatrix}$ is an eigenvector of A.

Standardizing the eigenvector results in

$$W_3 = \frac{V_3}{\| V_3 \|} = \begin{bmatrix} \dfrac{1}{\sqrt{3}} \\ \dfrac{1}{\sqrt{3}} \\ \dfrac{1}{\sqrt{3}} \end{bmatrix}$$

$$P = \begin{bmatrix} W_1 & W_2 & W_3 \end{bmatrix} = \begin{bmatrix} -\dfrac{1}{\sqrt{2}} & -\dfrac{1}{\sqrt{6}} & \dfrac{1}{\sqrt{3}} \\ \dfrac{1}{\sqrt{2}} & -\dfrac{1}{\sqrt{6}} & \dfrac{1}{\sqrt{3}} \\ 0 & \dfrac{2}{\sqrt{6}} & \dfrac{1}{\sqrt{3}} \end{bmatrix}$$

$$D = \begin{bmatrix} -2 & 0 & 0 \\ 0 & -2 & 0 \\ 0 & 0 & 4 \end{bmatrix}$$

and $\quad D = P^T A P$

Example 3: Diagonalize the matrix $A = \begin{bmatrix} 6 & -2 & -1 \\ -2 & 6 & -1 \\ -1 & -1 & 5 \end{bmatrix}$

Solution: The characteristic equation of A is

$$|A - \lambda I| = 0$$

$$\begin{vmatrix} 6-\lambda & -2 & -1 \\ -2 & 6-\lambda & -1 \\ -1 & -1 & 5-\lambda \end{vmatrix} = 0$$

$$(6-\lambda)\big[(6-\lambda)(5-\lambda)-1\big] + 2\big[-2(5-\lambda)-1\big] - 1\big[2+6-\lambda\big] = 1$$

$$(6-\lambda)\big[30-6\lambda-5\lambda+\lambda^2-1\big] + 2\big[-10+2\lambda-1\big] - 1\big[8-\lambda\big] = 0$$

$$(6-\lambda)\big(\lambda^2-11\lambda+29\big) + 2\big(2\lambda-11\big) - 1\big(8-\lambda\big) = 0$$

$$6\lambda^2 - 66\lambda + 174 - \lambda^3 + 11\lambda^2 - 29\lambda + 4\lambda - 22 - 8 + \lambda = 0$$

$$-\lambda^3 + 17\lambda^2 - 90\lambda + 144 = 0$$

$$(\lambda-8)(\lambda-6)(\lambda-3) = 0$$

$\therefore$ The eigenvalues are $\lambda = 8, 6, 3$.
To calculate the eigenspaces:

$$\lambda = 8, \ V_1 = \begin{bmatrix} -1 \\ 1 \\ 0 \end{bmatrix}, \quad \lambda = 6, \ V_2 = \begin{bmatrix} -1 \\ -1 \\ 2 \end{bmatrix} \text{ and } \lambda = 3, \ V_3 = \begin{bmatrix} 1 \\ 1 \\ 1 \end{bmatrix}$$

We can normalize V_1, V_2, V_3 to produce the unit eigenvectors.

$$u_1 = \begin{bmatrix} -\dfrac{1}{\sqrt{2}} \\ \dfrac{1}{\sqrt{2}} \\ 0 \end{bmatrix}, \quad u_2 = \begin{bmatrix} -\dfrac{1}{\sqrt{6}} \\ -\dfrac{1}{\sqrt{6}} \\ \dfrac{2}{\sqrt{6}} \end{bmatrix}, \quad u_3 = \begin{bmatrix} \dfrac{1}{\sqrt{3}} \\ \dfrac{1}{\sqrt{3}} \\ \dfrac{1}{\sqrt{3}} \end{bmatrix}$$

Let $P = \begin{bmatrix} -\dfrac{1}{\sqrt{2}} & -\dfrac{1}{\sqrt{6}} & \dfrac{1}{\sqrt{3}} \\ \dfrac{1}{\sqrt{2}} & -\dfrac{1}{\sqrt{6}} & \dfrac{1}{\sqrt{3}} \\ 0 & \dfrac{2}{\sqrt{6}} & \dfrac{1}{\sqrt{3}} \end{bmatrix}$ and $D = \begin{bmatrix} 8 & 0 & 0 \\ 0 & 6 & 0 \\ 0 & 0 & 3 \end{bmatrix}$

Then $A = PDP^{-1}$ as usual. Since P is square and has orthonormal columns, P is an orthogonal matrix and P^{-1} is simply P^T.

Theorem 2: If A is symmetric, then any two eigenvectors forming different eigenspace are orthogonal.

Proof: Let V_1 and V_2 be eigenvectors that corresponds to distinct eigenvalues, say λ_1 and λ_2. To show that $V_1 V_2 = 0$

Compute

$$\lambda_1 V_1 V_2 = \left(\lambda_1 V_1\right)^T V_2 = \left(A V_1\right)^T V_2 \quad \text{(since } V_1 \text{ is an eigenvector)}$$
$$= \left(V_1^T A^T\right) V_2$$
$$= V_1^T \left(A V_2\right) \quad \left(A^T = A\right)$$
$$= V_1^T \left(\lambda_2 V_2\right) \text{ (since } V_2 \text{ is an eigenvector of } A = \lambda_2)$$
$$\lambda_1 V_1 V_2 = \lambda_2 V_1 V_2$$

Hence $\quad \left(\lambda_1 - \lambda_2\right) V_1 V_2 = 0$

But $\lambda_1 - \lambda_2 \neq 0$, so $V_1 V_2 = 0$

Example 4: Diagonalize $A = \begin{bmatrix} 0 & 0 & -2 \\ 0 & -2 & 0 \\ -2 & 0 & 3 \end{bmatrix}$

Solution: A is symmetric matrix, then the characteristic equation is

$$|A - \lambda I| = 0$$
$$\Rightarrow \quad \lambda^3 - \lambda^2 - 10\lambda - 8 = 0$$
$$(\lambda + 2)(\lambda - 4)(\lambda + 1) = 0$$

$\therefore$ The eigenvalues of A are $-2, 4, -1$. Then eigenvectors associated with these eigenvalues are

$$\lambda_1 = -2, \ x_1 = \begin{bmatrix} 0 \\ 1 \\ 0 \end{bmatrix}, \ \lambda_2 = 4, \ x_2 = \begin{bmatrix} -1 \\ 0 \\ 2 \end{bmatrix} \text{ and } \lambda_3 = -1, \ x_3 = \begin{bmatrix} 2 \\ 0 \\ 1 \end{bmatrix}$$

Then x_1, x_2, x_3 are orthogonal.

Example 5: Let $A = \begin{bmatrix} 0 & 2 & 2 \\ 2 & 0 & 2 \\ 2 & 2 & 0 \end{bmatrix}$

Find an orthogonal matrix P and a diagonal matrix D such that $D = P^{-1}AP$.

Solution: We need to find orthonormal eigenvectors of A and the associated eigenvalues first.

$\therefore$ The characteristic equation is

$$|A - \lambda I| = 0$$

$$\Rightarrow \quad (\lambda + 2)^2 (\lambda - 2) = 0$$

Thus $\lambda = -2, -2, 4$ (eigenvalues)

As $\lambda = -2$, solve for the homogeneous system

$$[A + \lambda I] X = 0$$

$$\begin{bmatrix} 0 & 2 & 2 \\ 2 & 0 & 2 \\ 2 & 2 & 0 \end{bmatrix} + \begin{bmatrix} -2 & 0 & 0 \\ 0 & -2 & 0 \\ 0 & 0 & -2 \end{bmatrix} \begin{bmatrix} x \\ y \\ z \end{bmatrix} = \begin{bmatrix} 0 \\ 0 \\ 0 \end{bmatrix}$$

$$-2x + 2y + 2z = 0$$
$$2x - 2y + 2z = 0$$
$$2x + 2y - 2z = 0$$

$\therefore$ The eigenvectors are

$$x \begin{bmatrix} -1 \\ 1 \\ 0 \end{bmatrix} + y \begin{bmatrix} -1 \\ 0 \\ 1 \end{bmatrix}, \ x, y \in R, \ x \neq 0, \ y \neq 0$$

$$\Rightarrow \quad V_1 = \begin{bmatrix} -1 \\ 1 \\ 0 \end{bmatrix}, \ V_2 = \begin{bmatrix} -1 \\ 0 \\ 1 \end{bmatrix} \text{ as two eigenvectors of '}A\text{'}$$

However, the two eigenvectors are not orthogonal eigenvectors.
Apply Gram-Schmidt process.
The orthogonal eigenvectors are

$$V_1 = V_1^* = \begin{bmatrix} -1 \\ 1 \\ 0 \end{bmatrix}$$

$$V_2 = V_2^* - \frac{\langle V_2 V_1 \rangle}{\langle V_1 V_1 \rangle} V_1 = \begin{bmatrix} -\dfrac{1}{2} \\ \dfrac{1}{2} \\ 0 \end{bmatrix}$$

Standardizing these two eigenvectors result in

$$W_1 = \frac{V_1^*}{\| V_1^* \|} = \begin{bmatrix} -\dfrac{1}{\sqrt{2}} \\ \dfrac{1}{\sqrt{2}} \\ 0 \end{bmatrix}$$

$$W_2 = \frac{V_2}{\| V_2 \|} = \begin{bmatrix} \dfrac{-1}{\sqrt{2}} \\ 0 \\ \dfrac{1}{\sqrt{2}} \end{bmatrix}$$

As $\qquad \lambda = 4,$
$$[A - 4I] X = 0$$
The eigenvectors are

$$z \begin{bmatrix} 1 \\ 1 \\ 1 \end{bmatrix}, \; z \in R, \; z \neq 0$$

$$\Rightarrow \quad V_3 = \begin{bmatrix} 1 \\ 1 \\ 1 \end{bmatrix} \text{ is an eigenvector of } A.$$

Standardizing the eigenvector results in

$$W_3 = \frac{V_3}{\|V_3\|} = \begin{bmatrix} \dfrac{1}{\sqrt{3}} \\ \dfrac{1}{\sqrt{3}} \\ \dfrac{1}{\sqrt{3}} \end{bmatrix}$$

$$P = [W_1 \ W_2 \ W_3] = \begin{bmatrix} -\dfrac{1}{\sqrt{2}} & -\dfrac{1}{\sqrt{2}} & \dfrac{1}{\sqrt{3}} \\ \dfrac{1}{\sqrt{2}} & 0 & \dfrac{1}{\sqrt{3}} \\ 0 & \dfrac{1}{\sqrt{2}} & \dfrac{1}{\sqrt{3}} \end{bmatrix}$$

$$D = \begin{bmatrix} -2 & 0 & 0 \\ 0 & -2 & 0 \\ 0 & 0 & 4 \end{bmatrix}$$

$$D = P^{-1}AP$$

Example 6: Let $X = \begin{bmatrix} x_1 \\ x_2 \end{bmatrix}$. Compute $X^T A X$ for the following matrix

$A = \begin{bmatrix} 4 & 0 \\ 0 & 3 \end{bmatrix}$.

Solution: $x^T A x = [x_1 \ x_2] \begin{bmatrix} 4 & 0 \\ 0 & 3 \end{bmatrix} \begin{bmatrix} x_1 \\ x_2 \end{bmatrix} = [x_1 \ x_2] \begin{bmatrix} 4x_1 \\ 3x_2 \end{bmatrix} = 4x_1^2 + 3x_2^2$

Example 7: Find the matrix of the quadratic form $q = x^2 - 6xy + 2y^2$.

Solution: The two variables x, y can be treated as x_1 and x_2.

$$a_{11} = 1, \ a_{22} = 3, \ a_{12} = -\frac{6}{2} = -3 = a_{21}$$

$\therefore$ The matrix A of $q = \begin{bmatrix} 1 & -3 \\ -3 & 3 \end{bmatrix}$, $q = \begin{bmatrix} a_{11} & a_{12} \\ a_{21} & a_{22} \end{bmatrix}$

$$X = \begin{bmatrix} x \\ y \end{bmatrix}, \text{ thus } q = X^1 A X$$

$$q = \begin{bmatrix} x & y \end{bmatrix} \begin{bmatrix} 1 & -3 \\ -3 & 3 \end{bmatrix} \begin{bmatrix} x \\ y \end{bmatrix}$$

Example 8: Obtain the matrix of the quadratic form
$$q = ax^2 + 2hxy + by^2 + 2fyz + 2gzx + ez^2$$
and write in a matrix form.

Solution:

The variables are $x = x_1, y = x_2, z = x_3$

$$a_{11} = a, \quad a_{22} = b, \quad a_{33} = e$$

$$a_{12} = a_{21} = \frac{2h}{2} = h, \quad a_{23} = \frac{2f}{2} = f = a_{32}$$

$$a_{31} = a_{13} = \frac{2g}{2} = g$$

$$\therefore \text{ The matrix } A \text{ of } q = \begin{bmatrix} a & h & g \\ h & b & f \\ g & f & e \end{bmatrix}$$

Let $X = \begin{bmatrix} x \\ y \\ z \end{bmatrix}$

Then $q = X^T AX$

$$= \begin{bmatrix} x & y & z \end{bmatrix} \begin{bmatrix} a & h & g \\ h & b & f \\ g & f & e \end{bmatrix} \begin{bmatrix} x \\ y \\ z \end{bmatrix}$$

Example 9: For x in R^3, let $Q(x) = 5x_1^2 + 3x_2^2 + 2x_3^2 - x_1 x_2 + 8x_2 x_3$

Solution: $Q(x) = \begin{bmatrix} 5 & -\dfrac{1}{2} & 0 \\ -\dfrac{1}{2} & 3 & 4 \\ 0 & 4 & 2 \end{bmatrix}$

$$Q = X^T AX$$

Example 10: Write the quadratic form 'q' in variables x_1, x_2, x_3 with

$$A = \begin{bmatrix} 1 & -1 & 2 \\ -1 & 2 & 3 \\ 2 & 3 & 4 \end{bmatrix} \text{ as its matrix.}$$

Solution: $q = X^T A X$

where $X = \begin{bmatrix} x_1 \\ x_2 \\ x_3 \end{bmatrix}$

$$q = [x_1 \ x_2 \ x_3] \begin{bmatrix} 1 & -1 & 2 \\ -1 & 2 & 3 \\ 2 & 3 & 4 \end{bmatrix} \begin{bmatrix} x_1 \\ x_2 \\ x_3 \end{bmatrix}$$

$$= (x_1 - x_2 + 2x_3)(-x_1 + 2x_2 + 3x_3)(2x_1 + 3x_2 + 4x_3) \begin{bmatrix} x_1 \\ x_2 \\ x_3 \end{bmatrix}$$

$$= x_1(x_1 - x_2 + 2x_3) + x_2(-x_1 + 2x_2 + 3x_3) + x_3(2x_1 + 3x_2 + 4x_3)$$

$$= x_1^2 + 2x_2^2 + 4x_3^2 - 2x_1x_2 + 6x_2x_3 + 4x_3x_1$$

Example 11: Discuss the nature of the following quadratic forms.

(i) $x_1^2 + x_2^2 + x_3^2 + x_1x_2 + x_2x_3 + x_3x_1$

Solution: (i) The matrix A of the given quadratic form is given by

$$A = \begin{bmatrix} 1 & \dfrac{1}{2} & \dfrac{1}{2} \\ \dfrac{1}{2} & 1 & \dfrac{1}{2} \\ \dfrac{1}{2} & \dfrac{1}{2} & 1 \end{bmatrix}$$

$M_1 = |1| = 1 > 0$

$$M_2 = \begin{vmatrix} 1 & \dfrac{1}{2} \\ \dfrac{1}{2} & 1 \end{vmatrix} = 1 - \dfrac{1}{4} = \dfrac{3}{4} > 0$$

$$M_3 = |A| = \dfrac{1}{2} > 0$$

$\therefore$ The quadratic form is positive definite.

(ii) $10x^2 + 2y^2 + 5z^2 + 6yz - 10zx - 4xy$

Solution:

$$A = \begin{bmatrix} 10 & -2 & -5 \\ -2 & 2 & 3 \\ -5 & 3 & 5 \end{bmatrix}$$

$M_1 = |10| = 10 > 0$

$M_2 = \begin{vmatrix} 10 & -2 \\ -2 & 2 \end{vmatrix} = 20 - 2 = 16 > 0$

$M_3 = |A| = 0$

The quadratic form is positive semidefinite.

(iii) $X^1 \begin{bmatrix} 1 & 2 & 3 \\ 2 & 4 & 8 \\ 2 & 8 & 4 \end{bmatrix} X$

Solution:

$M_1 = |1| = 1 > 0$

$M_2 = \begin{vmatrix} 1 & 2 \\ 2 & 4 \end{vmatrix} = 4 - 4 = 0$

$M_3 = |A| = -8 > 0$

$\therefore$ The quadratic form is indefinite.

(iv) $3x_1^2 + 5x_2^2 + 3x_3^2 - 2x_2x_3 + 2x_3x_1 - 2x_1x_2$

Solution:

$$A = \begin{bmatrix} 3 & -1 & 1 \\ -1 & 5 & -1 \\ 1 & -1 & 3 \end{bmatrix}$$

$M_1 = |3| = 3 > 0$

$M_2 = \begin{vmatrix} 3 & -1 \\ -1 & 5 \end{vmatrix} = 15 - 1 = 14 > 0$

$M_3 = |A| = 36 > 0$

$\therefore$ The quadratic form is positive definite.

(v) $-3x_1^2 - 3x_2^2 - 7x_3^2 - 6x_1x_2 - 6x_2x_3 - 6x_3x_1$

Solution:

$$A = \begin{bmatrix} -3 & -3 & -3 \\ -3 & -3 & -3 \\ -3 & -3 & -7 \end{bmatrix}$$

$$M_1 = |-3| = 3 > 0$$

$$M_2 = \begin{vmatrix} -3 & -3 \\ -3 & -3 \end{vmatrix} = 0$$

$$M_3 = |A| = 0$$

$\therefore$ The quadratic form is negative definite.

(vi) $-4x^2 - 2y^2 - 13z^2 - 4xy - 8yz - 4xz$

Solution:

$$A = \begin{bmatrix} -4 & -2 & -2 \\ -2 & -2 & -4 \\ -2 & -4 & -13 \end{bmatrix}$$

$$M_1 = |-4| = 4 > 0$$

$$M_2 = \begin{vmatrix} -4 & -2 \\ -2 & 2 \end{vmatrix} = 8 - 4 = 4 > 0$$

$$M_3 = |A| = -12 < 0$$

$\therefore$ The quadratic form is negative definite.

EXERCISE

1. Let $A = \begin{bmatrix} -4 & -6 \\ 3 & 5 \end{bmatrix}$

Find the non-singular matrix P and the diagonal matrix D such that $D = P^{-1}AP$ and find A^n, n is any positive integer.

Ans. $P = \begin{bmatrix} -1 & -2 \\ 1 & 1 \end{bmatrix}$, $P = \begin{bmatrix} 2 & 0 \\ 0 & -1 \end{bmatrix}$ and $D^n = \begin{bmatrix} 2^n & 0 \\ 0 & (-1)^n \end{bmatrix}$

$$= (P^{-1}AP)(P^{-1}AP)\ldots(P^{-1}AP) = P^{-1}A^nP$$

$$= \begin{bmatrix} -[2^n + 2(-1)^{n+1}] & -[2^{n+1} + 2(-1)^{n+1}] \\ 2^n + (-1)^{n+1} & 2^{n+1} + (-1)^{n+1} \end{bmatrix}$$

2. Diagonalize the matrix

$$A = \begin{bmatrix} 2 & -2 & 1 \\ -1 & 3 & -1 \\ 2 & -4 & 3 \end{bmatrix}$$

Ans. $P = \begin{bmatrix} 2 & -1 & 1 \\ 1 & 0 & -1 \\ 0 & 1 & 2 \end{bmatrix}$, $D = \begin{bmatrix} 1 & 0 & 0 \\ 0 & 1 & 0 \\ 0 & 0 & 6 \end{bmatrix}$, $P = \begin{bmatrix} \dfrac{1}{5} & \dfrac{3}{5} & \dfrac{1}{5} \\ \dfrac{-2}{5} & \dfrac{4}{5} & \dfrac{3}{5} \\ \dfrac{1}{5} & \dfrac{-2}{5} & \dfrac{1}{5} \end{bmatrix}$

3. The matrix A has eigenvalues 1, 2 and -1 with corresponding eigenvectors $(1, 1, 0)$, $(1, 2, 1)$ and $(0, 1, 2)$. Find A and compute A^5.

Ans. $D = \begin{bmatrix} 1 & 0 & 0 \\ 0 & 2 & 0 \\ 0 & 0 & -1 \end{bmatrix}$, $P = \begin{bmatrix} 1 & 1 & 0 \\ 1 & 2 & 1 \\ 0 & 1 & 2 \end{bmatrix}$, $P^{-1} = \begin{bmatrix} 3 & -2 & 1 \\ -2 & 2 & -1 \\ 1 & -1 & 1 \end{bmatrix}$

$$A = PDP^{-1} = \begin{bmatrix} -1 & 2 & -1 \\ -6 & 7 & -4 \\ -6 & 6 & -4 \end{bmatrix}, \quad A^5 = \begin{bmatrix} -61 & 62 & -31 \\ -126 & 127 & -64 \\ -66 & 66 & -34 \end{bmatrix}$$

4. Find the maximum and minimum values of $Q(\vec{x}) = 9x_1^2 + 4x_2^2 + 3x_3^2$ subject to the constraint $x^T \vec{x} x = 1$.

Ans. 9, 3, $Q(\vec{x}) = 3$ and $\vec{x} = (0, 0, 1)$

5. If $A = \begin{bmatrix} \dfrac{-1}{2} & \dfrac{-\sqrt{3}}{2} & 0 \\ -\dfrac{\sqrt{3}}{2} & \dfrac{1}{2} & 0 \\ 0 & 0 & 0 \end{bmatrix}$ and $P = \begin{bmatrix} \dfrac{1}{2} & \dfrac{\sqrt{3}}{2} & 0 \\ \dfrac{-\sqrt{3}}{2} & \dfrac{1}{2} & 0 \\ 0 & 0 & 1 \end{bmatrix}$,

show that $P^{-1}AP$ is a diagonal matrix.

6. Show that the linear transformation $H = \begin{bmatrix} \cos\theta & \sin\theta \\ -\sin\theta & \cos\theta \end{bmatrix}$, where

$\theta = \dfrac{1}{2}\tan^{-1}\dfrac{2h}{a-b}$ changes the matrix to the diagonal form

$D = HCH^T$.

7. By diagonalising the matrix $A = \begin{bmatrix} -1 & 3 \\ -2 & 4 \end{bmatrix}$ find A^4.

Ans. $\begin{bmatrix} -29 & 45 \\ -30 & 46 \end{bmatrix}$

8. Diagonalise the matrix

(i) $\begin{bmatrix} -1 & 2 & -2 \\ 1 & 2 & 1 \\ -1 & -1 & 0 \end{bmatrix}$ (ii) $\begin{bmatrix} 1 & 0 & -1 \\ 1 & 2 & 1 \\ 2 & 2 & 3 \end{bmatrix}$

Ans. (i) $\begin{bmatrix} 1 & 0 & 0 \\ 0 & \sqrt{5} & 0 \\ 0 & 0 & -\sqrt{5} \end{bmatrix}$ (ii) $\begin{bmatrix} 1 & 0 & 0 \\ 0 & 2 & 0 \\ 0 & 0 & 3 \end{bmatrix}$

9. Find the eigenvector of the matrix $\begin{bmatrix} 6 & -2 & 2 \\ -2 & 3 & -1 \\ 2 & -1 & 3 \end{bmatrix}$ and hence reduce

$6x^2 + 3y^2 + 3z^2 - 2yz + 4zx - 4xy$ to a "sum of squares".

Ans. $(1, 1, -1), (1, 1, -1), (2, -1, 1), 4x^2 + y^2 + z^2$.

10. Reduce the quadratic form $2xy + 2yz + 2zx$ into canonical form.

Ans. $x^2 + y^2 - 2z^2$.

11. Find the eigenvalues, eigenvectors and the modal of the matrix

$\begin{bmatrix} 1 & 0 & 0 \\ 0 & 3 & -1 \\ 0 & -1 & 3 \end{bmatrix}$. Reduce the quadratic form $x_1^2 + 3x_2^2 + 3x_3^2 - 2x_2x_3$ to

a canonical form.

Ans. 1, 2, 4; (1, 0, 0), (0, 1, 1), (0, 1, −1); $\begin{bmatrix} 1 & 0 & 0 \\ 0 & 1 & 1 \\ 0 & 1 & -1 \end{bmatrix}$, $x_1^2 + 2x_2^2 + 4x_3^2$

12. Reduce the following quadratic forms into a "sum of squares" by an orthogonal transformation and give the matrix of transformation. Also state the nature of each of these.

(i) $3x_1^2 + 3x_2^2 + 3x_3^2 + 2x_1x_2 + 2x_1x_3 - 2x_2x_3$

(ii) $8x^2 + 7y^2 + 3z^2 - 12xy - 8yz + 4zx$

Ans. (i) $x_1^2 + 4x_2^2 + 4x_3^2$, $\begin{bmatrix} \dfrac{-1}{\sqrt{3}} & 0 & \dfrac{2}{\sqrt{6}} \\[2mm] \dfrac{1}{\sqrt{3}} & \dfrac{1}{\sqrt{2}} & \dfrac{1}{\sqrt{6}} \\[2mm] \dfrac{1}{\sqrt{3}} & \dfrac{-1}{\sqrt{2}} & \dfrac{1}{\sqrt{6}} \end{bmatrix}$, positive definite.

(ii) $3y^2 + 15z^2$, $\begin{bmatrix} \dfrac{1}{3} & \dfrac{2}{3} & \dfrac{2}{3} \\[2mm] \dfrac{2}{3} & \dfrac{1}{3} & \dfrac{-2}{3} \\[2mm] \dfrac{2}{3} & \dfrac{-2}{3} & \dfrac{1}{3} \end{bmatrix}$, positive semidefinite.

13. Show that the form $5x_1^2 + 26x_2^2 + 10x_3^2 + 4x_2x_3 + 14x_3x_1 + 6x_1x_2$ is a positive semidefinite and find a non-zero set of values of x_1, x_2, x_3 which make the form zero.

10 Elementary Canonical Forms

10.1 INTRODUCTION

To study a linear operator T on the finite-dimensional space V, by decomposing T into a direct sum of operators, which are in some elements.

This is done through the characteristic values and vectors of T in certain special cases, i.e. when the minimal polynomial for T factor over the scalar field F into a product of distinct minimal polynomials of degree 1.

10.2 THE PRIMARY DECOMPOSITION THEOREM

Theorem 1: Let T be a linear operator on the finite-dimensional vector space V over the field F. Let P be the minimal polynomial for T,

$$P = P_i^{r_1} \dots P_k^{r_1}$$

where the P_i are distinct irreducible minimal polynomials over F and the r_1 are positive integers.

Let W_i be the null space of $P_i(T)r_1$, $i = 1, \dots, k$

Then

(i) $V_1 W_1 \oplus \dots \oplus V_k W_k$

(ii) Each W_i is invariant under T

(iii) If T_i is the operator induced on W_i by T_i, then the minimal polynomial for T_i is $P_i^{r_1}$

Proof: We have to find a polynomial h_i such that $h_i(T)$ is the identity on W_i and is zero on the other W_i and so that $h_e(T) + \dots + h_k(T) = I$, etc.

For each t, let $f_i = \dfrac{P}{P_j^{r_1}} = \underset{j \neq i}{\pi} \, P_j^{r_1}$

Since $p_1, \dots, p_k$ are distinct prime polynomials, the polynomials $f_1, \dots, f_i$ are relatively prime. Thus, there are polynomials $g_1, \dots, g_k$ such that

$$\sum_{i=1}^{x} f_i g_i = 1$$

If $i = f$, then $f_i f_i$ is divisible by the polynomial P, because $f_i f_i$ contains each $P_m^{r_m}$ as a factor.

353

We have to show $n_i = f_i g_i$.

Let $E_i = h_i(T) = f_i(T)g_i(T)$ since $h_e + ... + h_k = 1$ and P divides $f_i f_i$ for $i \neq j$, we have

$$E_i + ... + E_k = 1$$
$$E_i E_j = 0, \text{ if } i \neq j$$

Thus the E_i's are projections which correspond to some direct-sum decomposition of the space V.

If α is in the change of E_i, then $\alpha = \alpha_1, \alpha_2, ...$ and so on.

$$P_i(T)^{r_1} \alpha = P_i(T)^{r_1} E_i \alpha$$
$$= P_i(T)^{r_1} f_i(T) g_i(T) \alpha = 0$$

is the minimal polynomial P.

Corollary: If $E_1, ..., E_k$ are the projections associated with the primary decomposition of T, then each E_i is a polynomial in T, and accordingly if a linear operator U commute with T, then U commutes with each of the E_i, i.e. each subspace W_i is invariant under U.

The minimal polynomial for T is a product of first degree polynomials, i.e. the case for which each p_i is of the form $p_i = x - c_i$.

Now the large of E_i the null space W_i of $(T - C_i I)^{r_i}$.

Put $\qquad D = C_1 E_1 + ... + C_k E_k$

D is a diagonalizable operator which we call diagonalizable part of T. $N = T - D$, now

$$T = TE_1 + ... + TE_k$$
$$D = C_1 E_1 + ... + C_k E_k$$

So

$$N = (T - C_1 I) E_1 + ... + (T - C_k I) E_k$$

Then, $\qquad N_2 = (T - C_1 I) E_1 + ... + C_k E_k$

and in general

$$N_r = (T - C_1 I)r\, E_1 + ... + (T - C_k I)r\, E_k$$

When $r \geq n$ for each ; $N_r = 0$ because the operator $(T - C_i I)r$ is the large of E_i.

Definition: Let N be a linear operator on the vector space V. We say that N is nilpotent if there is some positive integer r such that $N^r = 0$.

Theorem 2: Let T be a linear operator on the finite-dimensional vector space V over the field F. Suppose that for the minimal polynomial, there is a diagonalizable operator D on V and a nilpotent operator N on V such that

(i) $T = D + N$

(ii) $DN = ND$

The diagonalizable operator D and the nilpotent operator N are uniquely determined by (i) and (ii) and each of them is a polynomial in T.

Proof: We have just observed that we can write $T = D + N$, where D is diagonalizable and N is nilpotent and where D and N not only commute but are polynomials in T. Now suppose that, we also have $T = D' + N'$ where D' is diagonalizable and N' is nilpotent then $D'N' = N'D'$.

We shall prove that $D = D'$ and $N = N'$.

Since D' and N' commute with one another $T = D' + N'$, we see that D' and N' commute with T. Thus D' and N' commute with any polynomial in T; hence they commute with D and N.

Now, $D + N = D' + N'$ and all four of these operators commute with one another.

Since D and D' are both diagonalizable and they commute, they are simultaneously diagonalizable and $D - D'$ is diagonalizable. Since N and N' are both nilpotent and they commute, the operator $(N' - N)$ is nilpotent using the fact that N and N' commute.

$$(N' - N)^r = \sum_{j=0}^{r} \binom{r}{j}(N')^{r-1}(-N)^i$$

and so, when r is sufficiently large, every term in this expression for $(N' - N)^r$ will be 0.

Corollary: Let V be the finite-dimensional vector space over an algebraically closed field F, e.g. the field of complex numbers. Then every linear operator T and V can be written as the sum of a diagonalizable operator D and a nilpotent operator N, which commute. These operators D and N are unique and each is a polynomial in T.

From these results, we see that study of linear operators on vector spaces over an algebraically closed field is essentially reduced to the study of nilpotent operators. For vector spaces over non-algebraically closed fields, we still need to find some substitute for characteristic values and vectors.

10.3 JORDAN CANONICAL FORM

An operator 'T' can be put into Jordan canonical form, if its characteristic and minimal polynomials field into linear polynomials.

This is always true if 'K' is the complex field. In any case, they can always internal the base field k to field in which the characteristic and minimum polynomial do factor into linear factors. In a broad sense, every operation has a Jordan canonical form. Every matrix is similar to a matrix in Jordan canonical form.

Let the matrix T_i is ordered basis which will be the direct sum of matrices

$$\begin{bmatrix} c & 0 & \cdots & 0 & 0 \\ 2 & c & \cdots & 0 & 0 \\ \vdots & \vdots & & \vdots & \vdots \\ 0 & 0 & & 2 & c \end{bmatrix}$$

each with c_i. Furthermore, the size of these matrices decrease as one reads from left to right. A matrix of the form is called an **"elementary Jordan matrix with characteristic value"**.

Let us now put all these bases for the W_i together, we obtained an ordered basis for V. Let us describe the matrix A of T in the ordered basis. The matrix A is the direct form

$$A = \begin{bmatrix} A_1 & 0 & \cdots & 0 \\ 0 & A_2 & \cdots & 0 \\ \vdots & \vdots & & \vdots \\ 0 & 0 & \cdots & A_k \end{bmatrix}$$

of matrices $A_1, \ldots, A_k$. Each A_i is of the form

$$A_i = \begin{bmatrix} J_1^{(f)} & 0 & \cdots & 0 \\ 0 & J_2^{(f)} & \cdots & 0 \\ \vdots & \vdots & & \vdots \\ 0 & 0 & \cdots & J_{n_i}^{(f)} \end{bmatrix}$$

where each $J_1^{(f)}$ is an elementary Jordan matrix with characteristic value c_i. Also within each A_i, the size of the matrices $J_1^{(f)}$ decreases as J increases. An $n \times n$ matrix A which satisfies all the conditions described above is said to be in "Jordan form".

Theorem: Let $T : V \to V'$ be a linear operator whose characteristic and minimum polynomials are respectively

$$\Delta(f) = (t - \lambda_1)^{n_1}, \ldots, (t - \lambda_r)^{n_r} \quad \text{and} \quad m(f) = (t - \lambda_1)^{m_1}, \ldots, (t - \lambda_r)^{m_r},$$

where the λ_i are distinct scalars. Then T has a block diagonal matrix representation J whose diagonal entries are of the form

$$J_{ij} = \begin{bmatrix} \lambda_i & 1 & 0 & \cdots & 0 & 0 \\ 0 & \lambda_i & 1 & \cdots & 0 & 0 \\ \cdots & \cdots & \cdots & \cdots & \cdots & \cdots \\ 0 & 0 & 0 & \cdots & \lambda_i & i \\ 0 & 0 & 0 & \cdots & 0 & \lambda_i \end{bmatrix}$$

For each λ_i, the corresponding blocks J_{ij} have the following properties.

(i) There is at least one J_{ij} of order m_i, all other are of order $\leq m_i$.

(ii) The sum of the orders of the J_{ij} is n_i.

(iii) The number of J_{ij} equals the geometric multiplicity of $\lambda_i 1 + N$.

(iv) The number of J_{ij} of each possible order is uniquely determined by T.

The matrix J appearing in the above theorem is called the Jordan canonical form of the operator T. A diagonal block J_{ij} is called a Jordan block belonging to the eigenvalue λ_i. Observe that

$$\begin{bmatrix} \lambda_i & 1 & 0 & \dots & 0 & 0 \\ 0 & \lambda_i & 1 & \dots & 0 & 0 \\ \dots & \dots & \dots & \dots & \dots & \dots \\ 0 & 0 & 0 & \dots & \lambda_i & i \\ 0 & 0 & 0 & \dots & 0 & \lambda_i \end{bmatrix} =$$

$$\begin{bmatrix} \lambda_i & 0 & \dots & 0 & 0 \\ 0 & \lambda_i & \dots & 0 & 0 \\ \dots & \dots & \dots & \dots & \dots \\ \dots & \dots & \dots & \dots & \dots \\ 0 & 0 & \dots & \lambda_i & 0 \\ 0 & 0 & \dots & 0 & \lambda_i \end{bmatrix} + \begin{bmatrix} 0 & 1 & 0 & \dots & 0 & 0 \\ 0 & 0 & 1 & \dots & 0 & 0 \\ \dots & \dots & \dots & \dots & \dots & \dots \\ 0 & 0 & 0 & \dots & 0 & 1 \\ 0 & 0 & 0 & \dots & 0 & 1 \\ 0 & 0 & 0 & \dots & 0 & 0 \end{bmatrix}$$

That is $J_{ij} = \lambda_i 1 + N$

where N is nilpotent block appearing in theorem of nilpotent operators. In fact the above theorem shows that 'T' can be decomposed into operator, each the sum of a scalar and a nilpotent operator.

WORKED EXAMPLES

Example 1: Suppose J is a linear operator on c^2, the characteristic polynomial for T is either $(x - c_1)(x - c_2)$, where c_1 and c_2 are distinct complex numbers $(x - c)^2$. T is diagonalizable and is represented in the

basis of $\begin{bmatrix} c_1 & 0 \\ 0 & c_2 \end{bmatrix}$.

In the latter case, the minimal polynomial for T may be $(x - c)$ in which case $T = CI$ or may be $(x - c)^2$ in which case is represented in some ordered basis by the matrix.

$$\begin{bmatrix} c & 0 \\ 1 & c \end{bmatrix}$$

Thus, every 2×2 matrix over the field of complex numbers is similar to a matrix of one of the two types displayed above, possibly with $c_1 = c_2$.

Example 2: Let A be the complex 3×3 matrix

$$A = \begin{bmatrix} 2 & 0 & 0 \\ a & 2 & 0 \\ b & c & -1 \end{bmatrix}$$

The characteristic polynomial for A is obviously $(x - 2)^2$. Either this is the minimal polynomial, in which case 'A' is similar to

$$\begin{bmatrix} 2 & 0 & 0 \\ 1 & 2 & 0 \\ 0 & 0 & -1 \end{bmatrix}$$

or the minimal polynomial is $(x - 2)(x + 1)$ in which case A is similar to

$$\begin{bmatrix} 2 & 0 & 0 \\ 0 & 2 & 0 \end{bmatrix}$$

Now, $(A - 2I)(A + I) = \begin{bmatrix} 0 & 0 & 0 \\ 3a & 0 & 0 \\ ac & 0 & 0 \end{bmatrix}$ and this A is similar to a diagonal

matrix and $a = 0$.

Example 3: Let $A = \begin{bmatrix} 2 & 0 & 0 & 0 \\ 1 & 2 & 0 & 0 \\ 0 & 0 & 2 & 0 \\ 0 & 0 & a & 2 \end{bmatrix}$

The characteristic polynomial for A is $(x - 2)^4$. Since A is the direct sum of two 2×2 matrices, it is clear that the minimal polynomial for A is $(x - 2)^4$. Now if $a = 0$ or $a = 1$, then the matrix A is in Jordan form.

Notice that the two matrices obtained for $a = 0$ and $a = 1$ have the same characteristic polynomial and the same minimal polynomial but are not similar because for the first matrix the solution space of $(A - 2I)$ has dimension 3 while for the second matrix it has dimension 2.

Example 4: Linear differential equations with constant coefficient provide a nice illustration of the Jordan form. Let $a_0, \ldots, a_{n-1}$ be complex numbers and let V be the space of all n times differential functions f on an interval of the real time which satisfy the differential equation,

$$a_n \frac{d^n f}{dx^n} + a_{n-1}\frac{d^{n-1}f}{dx^{n-1}} + \dots + a_1 \frac{df}{dx} + a_0 f = 0$$

Let D be the differential operator. Then V is invariant under D because V is the null space of $p(D)$
where,

$$p = a_n x^n + \dots + a_1 x + a_0$$

What is the Jordan form for the differential operator on V?

Let $c_i, \dots, c_k$ be the distinct complex roots of p.

$$p_2 (x - c_1)^{r_1} \dots (x - c_k)^{r_k}$$

Let V_i be the null space of $(D - c_i I)^{r_i}$ that is the set of solutions to the differential equation.

$$(D - c_i I)^{r_i} f = 0$$

Then, we noted in primary decomposition theorem that

$$V = V_i + \dots + V_k$$

Let the differential equation $Df = cf$ is vascular multiple of exponential function $f(x) = e^{cx}$.

$\therefore$ The operator N has a cyclic vector. A good choice for a cyclic vector is $g = x^{r-1}h$

$$g(x) = x^{r-1}e^{ax}$$

This gives $N_g = (r-1)x^{r-2h}$

$$N_g^{r-1} = (r-1)! h$$

This shows that the Jordan form for D is the direct sum of k and elementary Jordan matrices.

19.4 INTERACTIVE ESTIMATES FOR "EIGENVALUES"

The power method: The power method to an $n \times n$ matrix A with a strictly dominant eigenvalue λ_i, which means that λ_1 must be larger in absolute value than the all other eigenvalues. In this case, the power method produces a scalar sequence that approaches λ_1 and a vector sequence that approaches a corresponding eigenvector.

Assume for simplicity that A is diagonalizable and R^n has a basis for eigenvectors $V_1, \dots, V_n$. So, there corresponding eigenvalues $\lambda_1, \dots, \lambda_n$ decreases in size.

i.e.
$$|\lambda_1| \geq |\lambda_2| \geq |\lambda_3| \geq \dots \geq |\lambda_n| \qquad \dots (1)$$

X in R^n is written as $X = c_i V_i + \dots + c_n V_n$, then

$$A^k x = c_1 (\lambda_1)^k V_1 + c_2 (\lambda_2)^k V_2 + \ldots + c_n (\lambda_n)^k V_n \ (k = 1, 2 \ldots)$$

Assume $c_1 \neq 0$, then decoding by $(\lambda_1)^k$

$$\frac{1}{(\lambda_1)^k} A^k x = c_1 V_1 + c_2 \left(\frac{\lambda_2}{\lambda_1}\right)^k V_2 + \ldots + c_n \left(\frac{\lambda_n}{\lambda_1}\right)^k V_n (k = 1, 2 \ldots) \quad \ldots (2)$$

From Eq. (2), the fractions $\dfrac{\lambda_2}{\lambda_1}, \ldots, \dfrac{\lambda_n}{\lambda_1}$ are all less than 1 in magnitude hence,

$$(\lambda_1)^k A^k x \rightarrow c_i V_i \ \text{as} \ k \rightarrow \infty \quad \ldots (3)$$

Example 1: Let $A = \begin{bmatrix} 1.8 & 0.8 \\ 0.2 & 1.2 \end{bmatrix}$, $V_1 = \begin{bmatrix} 4 \\ 1 \end{bmatrix}$ and $x = \begin{bmatrix} 0.5 \\ 1 \end{bmatrix}$, then A has the

eigenvalues 2 and 3, and the eigenspace for $V_1 = 2$ is the line through 0 and v_i for $k = 0, \ldots, 8$. Compute $A^k x$ and construct the line through 0 and $A^k x$. What happens as k increases?

Solution: $A = \begin{bmatrix} 1.8 & 0.8 \\ 0.2 & 1.2 \end{bmatrix}$ $x = \begin{bmatrix} -0.5 \\ 1 \end{bmatrix}$

$$Ax = \begin{bmatrix} 1.8 & 0.8 \\ 0.2 & 1.2 \end{bmatrix} \begin{bmatrix} -0.5 \\ 1 \end{bmatrix} = \begin{bmatrix} -0.1 \\ 1.1 \end{bmatrix}$$

$$A^2 x = A(Ax) = \begin{bmatrix} 1.8 & 0.8 \\ 0.2 & 1.2 \end{bmatrix} \begin{bmatrix} -0.1 \\ 1.1 \end{bmatrix} = \begin{bmatrix} -0.7 \\ 1.3 \end{bmatrix}$$

$$A^3 x = A(A^2 x) = \begin{bmatrix} 1.8 & 0.8 \\ 0.2 & 1.2 \end{bmatrix} \begin{bmatrix} -0.7 \\ 1.3 \end{bmatrix} = \begin{bmatrix} 2.3 \\ 4.7 \end{bmatrix}$$

$$A^4 x = A(A^3 x) = \begin{bmatrix} 1.8 & 0.8 \\ 0.2 & 1.2 \end{bmatrix} \begin{bmatrix} 2.3 \\ 4.7 \end{bmatrix} = \begin{bmatrix} 5.5 \\ 2.5 \end{bmatrix}$$

$$A^5 x = A(A^4 x) = \begin{bmatrix} 1.8 & 0.8 \\ 0.2 & 1.2 \end{bmatrix} \begin{bmatrix} 5.5 \\ 2.5 \end{bmatrix} = \begin{bmatrix} 11.9 \\ 4.1 \end{bmatrix}$$

$$A^6 x = A(A^5 x) = \begin{bmatrix} 1.8 & 0.8 \\ 0.2 & 1.2 \end{bmatrix} \begin{bmatrix} 11.9 \\ 4.1 \end{bmatrix} = \begin{bmatrix} 24.7 \\ 7.3 \end{bmatrix}$$

$$A^7 x = A(A^6 x) = \begin{bmatrix} 1.8 & 0.8 \\ 0.2 & 1.2 \end{bmatrix} \begin{bmatrix} 24.7 \\ 7.3 \end{bmatrix} = \begin{bmatrix} 50.3 \\ 13.7 \end{bmatrix}$$

$$A^8 x = A(A^7 x) = \begin{bmatrix} 1.8 & 0.8 \\ 0.2 & 1.2 \end{bmatrix} \begin{bmatrix} 50.3 \\ 13.7 \end{bmatrix} = \begin{bmatrix} 101.5 \\ 26.5 \end{bmatrix}$$

The direction is determined by x, Ax, A^2x, ..., A^8x.

The lines seems to be approaching the line representing the equation space spanned by V_1, and it is determined by V_1 goes to zero as $k \to \infty$.

Example 2: Apply the power method to $A = \begin{bmatrix} 6 & 5 \\ 1 & 2 \end{bmatrix}$ with $X_0 = \begin{bmatrix} 0 \\ 1 \end{bmatrix}$. Stop corresponding under vector of A.

Solution: $AX_0 = \begin{bmatrix} 6 & 5 \\ 1 & 2 \end{bmatrix}\begin{bmatrix} 0 \\ 1 \end{bmatrix} = \begin{bmatrix} 5 \\ 2 \end{bmatrix}$, $\mu = 5$

Scale AX_0 by $1/\mu_0$ to get X_1, compute AX_1, and identify the target only in AX_1

$$X_1 = \frac{1}{\mu_0} AX_0 = \frac{1}{5}\begin{pmatrix} 5 \\ 2 \end{pmatrix} = \begin{bmatrix} 1 \\ 0.4 \end{bmatrix}$$

$$AX_1 = \begin{bmatrix} 6 & 5 \\ 1 & 2 \end{bmatrix}\begin{bmatrix} 1 \\ 0.4 \end{bmatrix} = \begin{bmatrix} 8 \\ 1.8 \end{bmatrix}, \quad \mu_1 = 8$$

Scale AX_1 by $1/\mu_1$ to get X_2. Compute AX_2 and identify the largest only in AX_2.

$$X_2 = \frac{1}{\mu_1} AX_1 = \frac{1}{8}\begin{bmatrix} 8 \\ 1.8 \end{bmatrix} = \begin{bmatrix} 1 \\ 0.225 \end{bmatrix}$$

$$AX_2 = \begin{bmatrix} 6 & 5 \\ 1 & 2 \end{bmatrix}\begin{bmatrix} 1 \\ 0.225 \end{bmatrix} = \begin{bmatrix} 7.125 \\ 1.450 \end{bmatrix}, \quad \mu_2 = 7.125$$

Scale AX_2 by $1/\mu_2$ to get X_3 and so on.

k	0	1	2	3	4	5
r_k	$\begin{bmatrix} 0 \\ 1 \end{bmatrix}$	$\begin{bmatrix} 1 \\ 0.4 \end{bmatrix}$	$\begin{bmatrix} 1 \\ 0.225 \end{bmatrix}$	$\begin{bmatrix} 1 \\ 0.2035 \end{bmatrix}$	$\begin{bmatrix} -1 \\ 0.2005 \end{bmatrix}$	$\begin{bmatrix} -1 \\ 0.20007 \end{bmatrix}$
AX_k	$\begin{bmatrix} 5 \\ 2 \end{bmatrix}$	$\begin{bmatrix} 8 \\ 1.8 \end{bmatrix}$	$\begin{bmatrix} 7.125 \\ 1.430 \end{bmatrix}$	$\begin{bmatrix} 7.0175 \\ 1.4070 \end{bmatrix}$	$\begin{bmatrix} 7.0025 \\ 1.4010 \end{bmatrix}$	$\begin{bmatrix} 7.00036 \\ 1.40014 \end{bmatrix}$

From the above table, it strongly suggests that $\{x_k\}$ approaches $(1, 2)$ and $\{r_k\}$ approaches to 7.

$\therefore$ $(1, 2)$ is an eigenvector and 7 is dominating eigenvalue.

10.5 CHARACTERISTIC VALUES

Definition 1: Let V be a vector space over the field F and let T be a linear operator on V.

A characteristic value of T is a scalar c in F, such that there is a non-zero vector α in V with $T\alpha = c\alpha$.

If c is a characteristic value of T, then

(i) Any α, such that, $T\alpha = c\alpha$ is called a characteristic vector of T associated with characteristic value C.

(ii) The collection of all α such that $T\alpha = c\alpha$ is called the characteristic space associated with c.

Theorem 1: Let T be a linear operator on a finite dimensional space V and let c be a scalar. The following are equivalent.

(i) c is a characteristic value of T.

(ii) The operator $(T - cI)$ is singular.

(iii) $\det (T - cI) = 0$.

Definition 2: If A is an $n \times n$ matrix over the field F, a characteristic value of A in F is a scalar c in F such that the matrix $(A - cI)$ is singular.

The characteristic values of A in F are just the scalar c in F such that $f(c) = 0$

$\therefore f$ is the characteristic polynomial of A.

Therefore the matrices have the same characteristic polynomial.

Proof: If $\qquad B = P^{-1} AP$, then

$$\det (XI - B) = \det (XI - P^{-1} AP)$$
$$= \det (P^{-1} (XI - A) P)$$
$$= \det P^{-1} . \det (XI - A). \det P$$

Example 1: Let T be the linear operator on R^2, which represent the standard ordered basis by the matrix

$$A = \begin{bmatrix} 0 & -1 \\ 1 & 0 \end{bmatrix}$$

Solution: The characteristic polynomial for T is

$$\det (XI - A) = \begin{vmatrix} x & 1 \\ -i & x \end{vmatrix} = x^2 + 1$$

This polynomial has no real roots. T has no characteristic values.

Example 2: If A is real (3×3) matrix,

then $\qquad \begin{bmatrix} 3 & 1 & -1 \\ 3 & 2 & -1 \\ 2 & 2 & 0 \end{bmatrix}$

Solution: Then the characteristic polynomial is

$$\begin{vmatrix} x-3 & 1 & -1 \\ -2 & x-2 & 1 \\ -2 & -2 & x \end{vmatrix} = x^3 - 5x^2 + 8 - 4 = (x-1)(x-i)$$

$\therefore$ Characteristic values of A are 1 and 2

$$A - I = \begin{bmatrix} 2 & 1 & 1 \\ 2 & 1 & -1 \\ 2 & 2 & -1 \end{bmatrix}$$

$$A - 2I = \begin{bmatrix} 1 & 1 & -1 \\ 2 & 0 & -1 \\ 2 & 2 & -2 \end{bmatrix}$$

Evident that $A - 2I$ also has rank 2, so that, the space of characteristic vector, associated with the characteristic value 2 has dimension 1.
$\therefore T\alpha = 2\alpha$ only, if α is a scalar multiple of $\alpha = (1, 1, 2)$

Example 3: Let T be a linear operator on the finite-dimensional space V. We say that, T is diagonalizable if there is a basis for V of each vector, which is 2 characteristic vector of T.

Solution: Let T be a diagonalizable linear operator.

Let $c_1,..., c_k$ be the distinct characteristic values of T represented by a diagonal matrix, which has its diagonal matrices of the scalars c_i each. If c_i is repeated d_i times, then the matrix has the form

$$[T]_B = \begin{bmatrix} c_1 I_1 & 0 & ... & 0 \\ 0 & c_2 I_2 & ... & 0 \\ \vdots & \vdots & & \vdots \\ 0 & ... & ... & c_k I_k \end{bmatrix}$$

I is the $d_j \times d_i$ identity matrix

$$f = (x - c_1)^{d_1},...,(x - c_k)^{d_k}$$

Linear factors of the characteristic polynomial.

Lemma: Let T be a linear operator on the finite dimensional space V. Let $c_i,..., c_k$ be the distinct characteristic values of T and let W_i be the space of characteristic value c_i. If $W = W_1 +...+ W_k$, then

$$\dim W = \dim W_1 +...+ \dim W_k.$$

If B_1 is an ordered basis for W_i, then $B = B(B_i,...,B_k)$ is an ordered basis for W.

Theorem 2: Let T be a linear operator on a finite dimensional space V. Let $c_1,..., c_k$ be the distinct characteristic values of T and let W_i be the null space of $(T - C_i I)$. The following are equivalent.

(i) T is diagonalizable

(ii) The characteristic polynomial for T is

$$f = (X - C_1)^{d_i},..., (X - Ck)^{d_k} \text{ and}$$

$$\dim W_i = d_i \text{ where } i = 1, 2,..., k$$

(iii) $\dim W_1 + ... + \dim W_k = \dim V.$

10.6 ANNIHILATING POLYNOMIAL

Suppose T is a linear operator on a finite dimensional vector space over the field F and $f(x)$ is a polynomial over F, if $f(T) = 0$ then we say that, the polynomial $f(x)$ annihilates (reduces) the linear operator T.

Similarly, suppose A is a square matrix of order n over a field F and $F(1)$ is a polynomial over F. If $f(A) = 0$, then we say that the polynomial $f(x)$ annihilates the matrix A.

Minimal Polynomial: A polynomial in x over a field F is called a minimal polynomial if the coefficients of the highest power of x in it is unity.

$x^3 - 2x^2 + \dfrac{5}{7}x + 5$ is minimal polynomial of degree 3 over the field of rational numbers.

Minimal polynomial: Suppose T is a linear operators on an N dimensional vector space $V(F)$. The minimal polynomial of lowest degree over the field F that annihilates T is called the minimal polynomial of T. Also, if $f(x)$ is the minimal polynomial of T, the equation $f(x) = 0$ is called minimal equation of the linear operator T.

We can define the minimal polynomial of a matrix. Suppose A is a square matrix of order n over the field F. The minimal polynomial of lowest degree over the field F that annihilate A is called minimal polynomial of A.

Theorem 1: The minimal polynomial $m(t)$ of a matrix divides every polynomial that A as a zero in particular $m(t)$ divides the characteristic polynomial $f(t)$ of A.

Theorem 2: The characteristic polynomial $f(t)$ and minimal polynomial $m(t)$ of a matrix A have the same irreducible factors.

Theorem 3: If a is a scalar and larger value of matrix A, if and only if A is a root of the minimal polynomial of A.

WORKED EXAMPLES

Example 1: Find the minimal polynomial of $A = \begin{bmatrix} 2 & 2 & -5 \\ 3 & 7 & -15 \\ 1 & 2 & -4 \end{bmatrix}$.

Solution : The characterstic polynomial $|A - \lambda I| = 0$

$$= \begin{bmatrix} 2-\lambda & 2 & -5 \\ 3 & 7-\lambda & -15 \\ 1 & 2 & -4-\lambda \end{bmatrix}$$

$(2-\lambda)\big[(7-\lambda)(-4-\lambda)+30\big] - 2\big[3(-4-\lambda)+15\big] - 5\big[6-(7-\lambda)\big] = 0$

$(2-\lambda)\big[-28+4\lambda-7\lambda+\lambda^2+30\big] - 2\big[-12-3\lambda+15\big] - 5\big[6-7+\lambda\big] = 0$

$(2-\lambda)\big[\lambda^2-3\lambda+2\big] - 6\lambda-6+5-5\lambda = 0$

$$2\lambda^2 - \lambda^3 - 6\lambda + 3\lambda^2 + 4 - 2\lambda - 7\lambda - 17 = 0$$
$$-\lambda^3 + 5\lambda^2 - 22\lambda + 1 = 0$$
$$\lambda^3 - 5\lambda^2 + 7\lambda - 3 = 0 \qquad \dots(1)$$

$$f(t) = t^3 - 5t^2 + 7t - 3$$
$$f(t) = (t-1)^2 (t-3)$$

Minimal polynomial $m(t)$ must divide $f(t)$ and also each irreducible factor of $f(t)$ and $(t-1)$ and $(t-3)$ are $m(t)$ is exactly one that, such that

$$g(t) = (t-1)(t-3)$$
$$h(t) = (t-1)^2 (t-3)$$

By Cayley-Hamilton theorem are
$$H(A) = f(A) = 0$$
Hence, we need to test that
$$g(A) = (A - I)(A - 3I)$$

$$= \begin{bmatrix} 1 & 2 & -5 \\ 3 & 6 & -15 \\ 1 & 2 & -5 \end{bmatrix} \begin{bmatrix} -1 & 2 & -5 \\ 3 & 4 & -15 \\ 1 & 2 & -7 \end{bmatrix}$$

$$= \begin{bmatrix} -0 & 0 & -5-30+35 \\ -3+18-15 & 6+24-30 & -15+60-05 \\ -1+6-5 & 2+8-10 & -5-30-35 \end{bmatrix} = \begin{bmatrix} 0 & 0 & 0 \\ 0 & 0 & 0 \\ 0 & 0 & 0 \end{bmatrix}$$

$$g(t) = m(t) = (t-1)(t-3) = t^2 - 4t + 3$$

is the minimal polynomial.

Example 2: Find the numeral polynomial $m(t)$ of A.

$$A = \begin{bmatrix} 4 & -2 & 2 \\ 6 & -3 & 4 \\ 3 & -2 & 3 \end{bmatrix}$$

Solution:
$$|A - \lambda I| = 0$$

$$\begin{vmatrix} 4-\lambda & -2 & 2 \\ 6 & -3-\lambda & 4 \\ 3 & -2 & 3-\lambda \end{vmatrix} = 0$$

$$(4-\lambda)[(-3-\lambda)(3-\lambda)+8] + 2[18-6\lambda-12] + 2[-12+9+3\lambda] = 0$$

$$(4-\lambda)[-9-3\lambda+3\lambda+\lambda^2+8] + 12 - 12\lambda + 6\lambda - 6 = 0$$

$$(4-\lambda)[\lambda^2 - 1] + 6 - 6\lambda = 0$$

$$4\lambda^2 - \lambda^3 - 4 + \lambda + 6 - 6\lambda = 0$$

$$-\lambda^3 + 4\lambda^2 - 5\lambda + 2 = 0$$

$$\lambda^3 - 4\lambda^2 + 5\lambda - 2 = 0$$

$$t^3 - 4t^2 + 5t - 2 = 0$$

$$f(t) = (t-1)^2(t-2)$$

$$m(t) = (t-1)(t-2) \text{ or } (t-1)^2(t-2)$$

$$= (A-I)(A-2I)$$

$$= \begin{bmatrix} 3 & -2 & 2 \\ 6 & -4 & 4 \\ 3 & -2 & 2 \end{bmatrix} \begin{bmatrix} 2 & -2 & 2 \\ 6 & -5 & 4 \\ 3 & -2 & 1 \end{bmatrix}$$

$$= \begin{bmatrix} 6-12+6 & -6+10-4 & 6-8+2 \\ 12-24+12 & -12+20-8 & 12-16+4 \\ 6-12+6 & -6+10-4 & 6-8+2 \end{bmatrix} = \begin{bmatrix} 0 & 0 & 0 \\ 0 & 0 & 0 \\ 0 & 0 & 0 \end{bmatrix}$$

So minimal polynomial of $m(t) = (t-1)(t-2)$.

Example 3: Find the minimal polynomial of the matrix

$$A = \begin{bmatrix} 3 & -2 & 2 \\ 4 & -4 & 6 \\ 2 & -3 & 5 \end{bmatrix}$$

Solution:

$$|A - \lambda I| = \begin{vmatrix} 3-\lambda & -2 & 2 \\ 4 & -4-\lambda & 6 \\ 2 & -3 & 5-\lambda \end{vmatrix} = 0$$

$$(3-\lambda)[(-4-\lambda)(5-\lambda)+18] +$$
$$2[4(5-\lambda)-12+2[-12-2(-4-\lambda)]] = 0$$

$$(3-\lambda)[-20-5\lambda+4\lambda+\lambda^2+18] +$$
$$2[20-4\lambda-12]+2[-12+8+2\lambda] = 0$$

$$(3-\lambda)[\lambda^2-\lambda-2]+2[-4\lambda-8]+2[2\lambda-4] = 0$$

$$3\lambda^2-\lambda^3-3\lambda+\lambda^2+2\lambda-6-8\lambda-16+4\lambda-8 = 0$$

$$\lambda^3-4\lambda^2+5\lambda-2 = 0$$

$$f(t) = t^3-4t^2+5t-2 = (t-1)^2(t-2)$$

$$g(t) = (t-1)(t-2)$$
$$h(t) = (t-1)^2(t-2)$$
$$g(A) = (A-I)(A-2I)$$

$$= \begin{bmatrix} 2 & -2 & 2 \\ 4 & -5 & 6 \\ 2 & -3 & 4 \end{bmatrix} \begin{bmatrix} 1 & -2 & 2 \\ 4 & -6 & 6 \\ 2 & -3 & 3 \end{bmatrix} \neq 0$$

$$m(t) \neq g(t)$$

$m(t) = h(t) = (t-2)(t-2)^2$ is the minimal polynomial.

Example 4: Find the minimal polynomial of $A = \begin{bmatrix} 5 & 1 \\ 3 & 7 \end{bmatrix}$.

Solution:

$$|A - \lambda I| = 0$$

$$\begin{vmatrix} 5-\lambda & 1 \\ 3 & 7-\lambda \end{vmatrix} = 0$$

$$(5-\lambda)(7-\lambda) - 3 = 0$$
$$35 - 7\lambda - 5\lambda + \lambda^2 - 3 = 0$$
$$35 - 12\lambda + \lambda^2 - 3 = 0$$
$$\lambda^2 - 12\lambda + 32 = 0$$
$$f(t) = t^2 - 12t + 32$$
$$= (t-4)(t-8) \text{ is the minimal polynomial.}$$

10.7 DIRECT SUM DECOMPOSITION

A vector space v is termed the direct sum of subspaces $w_1, ..., w_r$, written

$$v = w_1 \oplus w_2 + ... + \oplus w_r$$

if every vector $v \in V$ can be written uniquely in the form

$$v = w_1 + w_2 + ... + w_r$$

Suppose $w_1, w_2, ..., w_r$ are subspaces of v, and suppose,

$$B_1 = \left\{ w_{11} + w_{12} + ... + w_{1n_1} \right\}$$

$$B_r = \left\{ w_{r1} + w_{r2} + ... + w_{rn_1} \right\}$$

are bases of $w_1, w_2, ..., w_r$, respectively, then v is the direct sum of the w_i if and only if the union $B = B_1 \cup ... \cup B_r$ is a basis of v, $T : v \to v$ is linear and v is the direct sum of T-invariant subspaces $w_1, w_2, ..., w_r$.

$$v = w_1 \oplus \ldots \oplus w_r \text{ and } T(w_i) \subseteq w_i$$

Let T_i denote the restriction of T to w_i, then T is said to be decomposable into the operator T_i or T is said to be the direct sum of T_i, written $T = T_1 \oplus \ldots \oplus T_r$. Also, the subspaces $w_1, \ldots, w_r$ are said to reduce T or to form a T-invariant direct-sum decomposition of v.

Consider, the special case, where two subspaces u and w reduce an operator $T : v \to v$, say $\dim u = 2$ and $\dim w = 2$ and suppose $\{u_1, u_2\}$ and $\{w_1, w_2, w_3\}$ are back of u and w respectively. If T_1 and T_2 denote the restrictions of T to u and w respectively, then

$$T_1(u_1) = a_{11}u_1 + a_{12}u_2$$
$$T_2(u_2) = a_{21}u_1 + a_{22}u_2$$
$$T_2(w_1) = b_{11}w_1 + b_{12}w_2 + b_{13}w_3$$
$$T_2(w_2) = b_{21}w_1 + b_{22}w_2 + b_{23}w_3$$
$$T_2(w_3) = b_{31}w_1 + b_{32}w_2 + b_{33}w_3$$

Accordingly, the following matrices A, B, M are the matrix representation of T_1, T_2, T_3 respectively.

$$A = \begin{bmatrix} a_{11} & a_{21} \\ a_{12} & a_{22} \end{bmatrix} \text{ and } B = \begin{bmatrix} b_{11} & b_{21} & b_{31} \\ b_{12} & b_{22} & b_{32} \\ b_{13} & b_{23} & b_{33} \end{bmatrix}$$

$$M = \begin{bmatrix} A & 0 \\ 0 & B \end{bmatrix}$$

The block diagonal matrix M results from the fact that $\{u_1, u_2, w_1, w_2, w_3\}$ is a basis of v.

Theorem: (Generalised)

Suppose $T : v \to v$ is linear and suppose v is the direct sum of T-invariant subspaces, say $w_1, \ldots, w_r$. If M is a matrix representation of the restriction of T to w_i, then T can be represented by the block diagonal matrix

$$M = \text{diag}\left(A_1, A_2, \ldots, A_r\right)$$

invariant directsum decompositions. Suppose w_1, w_2, ..., w_r are subspaces of v with respective bases

$$B_1 = \{w_{11} + w_{12} + \ldots + w_{1n_1}\}$$
$$B_r = \{w_{r1} + w_{r2} + \ldots + w_{rn_1}\}$$

Then, v is the direct sum of the w_i, if and only if, the union $B = v_i B_i$ is a basis of v. Suppose B is a basis of v.

$$v = a_{11}w_{11} + \ldots + a_{1n_1} w_{1n_2} + \ldots + a_{r1}w_{r1} + \ldots + a_{rn}w_{rn}$$

$$= w_1 + w_2 + \ldots + w_r$$
$$v = w_1 + w_2' + \ldots + w_r'$$

Since $\{w_{i1}, \ldots, w_i n_i\}$ is a basis of w_i,

$$w_i' = b_{i1} w_{i1} + \ldots + b_{ini} w_{ini} \text{ and so on}$$

$$v = b_{11} w_{11} + \ldots + b_{1n1} w_{in1} + \ldots + b_{ri} w_{r1} + \ldots + b_{ru} w_{rnr}$$

Since B is a basis of v, hence $w_i = w_i'$ and so, the sum for v is unique. Accordingly v is the direct sum of the w_i.

Conversely, suppose v is the direct sum of the w_i, then for any $v \in V$

$v = w_i + \ldots + w_n$, where $w_i \in W_i$. Since $\{w_{ij}\}$ is a basis of w_{ig}, each w_i is a linear combination of the w_{ij} and so v is a linear combination of the elements of B. Thus B spans v. We now show that B is linearly independent, suppose

$$a_{11} w_{11} + \ldots + a_{1n_i} w_{in_i} + \ldots + a_{r1} w_{r1} + \ldots + a_{rn_r} w_r n_r = 0$$

$a_{i1} w_{i1} + \ldots + a_{in_i} w_{in_i} \in w_i$, we have also that $0 = 0 + 0 \ldots 0 \in w$ and since, such a sum for 0 is unique

$$a_{i1} w_{i1} + \ldots + a_{in_i} w_{in_i} = 0 \text{ for } i = 1, \ldots, r$$

Suppose $T : V \to V$ is linear and suppose $T = T_1 \oplus T_2$ with respect to a T-invariant direct sum decomposition $V = U \oplus W$.
Show that

(i) $m(t)$ is the least common multiple of $m_1(t)$ and $m_2(t)$, where $m(t)$, $m_1(t)$, $m_2(t)$ all the minimum polynomials of T, T_1, T_2.

(ii) $D(t) = D_1$ (t) $D_2(t)$, where $D(t)$, $D_1(t)$, $D_2(t)$ are the characteristic polynomials of T, T_1, T_2 respectively.

(iii) Each of $m_1(T)$ and $m_2(T)$ divides $m(T)$. Now suppose $f(T)$ is a multiple of both $m_1(T)$ and $m_2(T)$, then $f(T_1)(u) = 0$ and $f(T_2)(w) = 0$. Let $v \in \underline{V}$, then $v = u + w$ with $u \in U$ and $w \in W$. Now $f(T) v = f(T)u + f(T)w = f(T_1)u + f(T_2)w = 0 \times 0 = 0$,

That is, T is a zero of $f(T)$ and $m(T)$ divides $f(T)$ and so, $m(T)$ is the least common multiple of $m_1(T)$ and $m_2(T)$.

(iv) T has a matrix representation $M = \begin{bmatrix} A & 0 \\ 0 & B \end{bmatrix}$, where A and B are

matrix representations of T_1 and T_2 respectively. Then, as required

$$D(t) = |tI - M| = \begin{vmatrix} tI - A & 0 \\ 0 & tI - B \end{vmatrix} = |tI - A||tI - B|$$

$$= \Delta_1(t), \Delta_2(t)$$

10.8 SINGULAR VALUE DECOMPOSITION

Introduction

A special factorization $A = QDP^{-1}$ or $A = QDP^{+1}$ is called the singular value decomposition.

The singular value decomposition is based on the ordinary decomposition. The absolute values of the eigenvalues of a symmetric matrix A.

If $$Ax = \lambda x \quad \text{and} \quad \|x\| = 1$$

then $$\| Ax \| = \| \lambda x \| = |\lambda| \, \| x \| = |\lambda| \qquad \ldots(1)$$

If λ_1 is the eigenvalue corresponding to unit eigenvector v_1, i.e. the length of Ax is maximized.

When $$x = V \text{ and } \| AV_1 \| = |\lambda_1| \qquad \text{[being equation (1)]}$$

The decomposition of A involves an $m \times n$ "diagonal" matrix Σ of the form

$$\Sigma = \begin{bmatrix} D & 0 \\ 0 & 0 \end{bmatrix} \qquad \ldots(2)$$

Let A be an $m \times n$ matrix with rank r. Then there exists an $m \times n$ matrix Σ as in Eq. (2) for which the diagonal entries in D are the first singular values of $A, \sigma \geq \sigma_2 \geq \ldots \geq \sigma_n > 0$ and there exist an $m \times m$ orthogonal matrix U and an $n \times n$ orthogonal matrix V, such that

$$A = U \Sigma V^T$$

Any factorization $A = U \Sigma V^T$, with U and V orthogonal, Σ as in equation(2) and positive diagonal entries in 'D' is called a **singular value decomposition** (SVD) of A.

Where $$U = \begin{bmatrix} u_1, u_2, \ldots, u_m \end{bmatrix}$$

$$u_1 = \frac{1}{\| AV_1 \|} AV_1 = \frac{1}{T_1} AV_1, \text{ where } T_1 = \| AV_1 \| \text{ and}$$

$$u_2 = \frac{1}{\| AV_2 \|} AV_2 = \frac{1}{T_2} AV_2 \text{ and so on } T_2 = \| AV_2 \|$$

$$V = \begin{bmatrix} V_1, V_2, \ldots \end{bmatrix} \text{ are eigenvectors}$$

$$\Sigma = \begin{bmatrix} T_1 & 0 & \cdots \\ 0 & T_2 & \cdots \\ 0 & 0 & T_2 \cdots \end{bmatrix}$$

$$U\Sigma = \begin{bmatrix} T_1 u_1, \ldots, T_r u_r \end{bmatrix}$$

$$U\Sigma = AV$$

Since V is an orthogonal matrix

$$U\Sigma V^T = AVV^T = A$$

Example 1: Find a singular value decomposition $A = \begin{bmatrix} 4 & 11 & 4 \\ 8 & 7 & -2 \end{bmatrix}$.

Solution:

First compute $A^T A = \begin{bmatrix} 4 & 8 \\ 11 & 7 \\ 4 & -2 \end{bmatrix} \begin{bmatrix} 4 & 11 & 4 \\ 8 & 7 & -2 \end{bmatrix}$

$$A^T A = \begin{bmatrix} 80 & 100 & 40 \\ 100 & 170 & 140 \\ 40 & 140 & 200 \end{bmatrix}$$

The eigenvalues of $A^T A$ are

$$\left| A^T A - \lambda I \right| = 0$$

$$\begin{vmatrix} 80-\lambda & 100 & 40 \\ 100 & 170-\lambda & 140 \\ 40 & 140 & 200-\lambda \end{vmatrix} = 0$$

$$(80-\lambda)\left[(170-\lambda)(200-\lambda)-19600\right]-100\left[100(200-\lambda)-5600\right]$$
$$+40\left[14000-40(170-\lambda)\right]=0$$

$$(80-\lambda)\left[340000-170\lambda-300\lambda+\lambda^2-19600\right]-100\left[20000-100\lambda-5600\right]=0$$

$$(80-\lambda)\left[\lambda^2-370\lambda+14400\right]-100\left[-100\lambda+14400\right]+40(40\lambda-7200)=0$$

$$80\lambda^2-29600\lambda+115200 = 0$$

$$\begin{bmatrix} 8 & 10 & 4 \\ 10 & 17 & 14 \\ 4 & 14 & 20 \end{bmatrix} \begin{bmatrix} 8-\lambda & 10 & 4 \\ 10 & 17-\lambda & 14 \\ 4 & 14 & 20-\lambda \end{bmatrix} = 0$$

$$(8-\lambda)\left[(17-\lambda)(20-\lambda)196\right]-10\left[10(20-\lambda)-56\right]+4\left[140-4(17\lambda)\right]=0$$

$$(8-\lambda)\left[340-17\lambda-20\lambda+\lambda^2-196\right]-10\left[200-10\lambda-56\right]+4\left[140-68+4\lambda\right]=0$$

$$(8-\lambda)\left[\lambda^2-37\lambda+144\right]-10\left[-10\lambda+144\right]+4\left[4\lambda+72\right]=0$$

$$8\lambda^2-296\lambda+1152-\lambda^3+37\lambda^2-144\lambda+100\lambda-1440+16\lambda+288=0$$

$$-\lambda^3+45\lambda^2-324\lambda=0$$

$$\lambda^3-45\lambda^2+324\lambda=0$$

$$\lambda\left(\lambda^2-45\lambda+324\right)=0$$

$$\lambda(\lambda-36)(\lambda-9)=0$$

$$\lambda=0, \ \lambda=36, \ \lambda=9$$

$$\lambda_1 = 0, \ \lambda_2 = 360, \ \lambda_3 = 90$$
$$\lambda_1 = 360, \ \lambda_2 = 90, \ \lambda_3 = 0$$

Corresponding to unit eigenvectors are the eigenvalues

let $\lambda_1 = 360$

$$\begin{bmatrix} 80-360 & 100 & 40 \\ 100 & 170-360 & 140 \\ 40 & 140 & 200-360 \end{bmatrix} \begin{bmatrix} 1 \\ 1 \\ 1 \end{bmatrix} = 0$$

$$\begin{bmatrix} -280 & 100 & 40 \\ 100 & -190 & 140 \\ 40 & 140 & -160 \end{bmatrix} \begin{bmatrix} 1 \\ 1 \\ 1 \end{bmatrix} = 0$$

$$-28x + 10y + 4z = 0$$
$$10x - 19y + 14z = 0$$
$$4x + 14y - 16z = 0$$

$$\frac{x}{\begin{vmatrix} 10 & 4 \\ -19 & 14 \end{vmatrix}} = \frac{-y}{\begin{vmatrix} -28 & 4 \\ 10 & 14 \end{vmatrix}} = \frac{z}{\begin{vmatrix} -28 & 10 \\ 10 & -19 \end{vmatrix}}$$

$$\frac{x}{140+76} = \frac{-y}{-392-40} = \frac{z}{532-100}$$

$$\frac{x}{216} = \frac{-y}{-432} = \frac{z}{432} = \frac{x}{1} = \frac{-y}{2} = \frac{z}{2}$$

$\therefore$ Eigenvectors are $\begin{bmatrix} 1 \\ 2 \\ 2 \end{bmatrix}$

Let $\quad \lambda_2 = 90$, eigenvectors are $\begin{bmatrix} -2 \\ -1 \\ 2 \end{bmatrix}$

Let $\lambda_3 = 0$, eigenvectors are $\begin{bmatrix} -2 \\ -2 \\ 1 \end{bmatrix}$

$$V_1 = \begin{bmatrix} 1/3 \\ 2/3 \\ 2/3 \end{bmatrix}, \quad V_2 = \begin{bmatrix} -2/3 \\ -1/3 \\ 2/3 \end{bmatrix}, \quad V_3 = \begin{bmatrix} -2/3 \\ -2/3 \\ 1/3 \end{bmatrix}$$

The first maximum value of $\|AX\|^2 = 360$

$\therefore$ The vector AV_1

$$AV_1 = \begin{bmatrix} 4 & 11 & 14 \\ 8 & 7 & -2 \end{bmatrix} \begin{bmatrix} 1/3 \\ 2/3 \\ 2/3 \end{bmatrix} = \begin{bmatrix} 18 \\ 6 \end{bmatrix}$$

For $|X| = 1$, the maximum of $\|AX\|$ is $\|AV\|$

$$A = \|AX\| = \|AV_1\| = \sqrt{360} = 6\sqrt{10}$$

The second singular value of A is the maximum of $\|AX\|$ all unit vectors

$$AV_2 = \begin{bmatrix} 4 & 11 & 14 \\ 8 & 7 & -2 \end{bmatrix} \begin{bmatrix} -2/3 \\ -1/3 \\ 2/3 \end{bmatrix} = \begin{bmatrix} 3 \\ -9 \end{bmatrix}$$

$\|AV_2\| = \sqrt{90} = 3\sqrt{10}$ and $\|AV_3\| = 0$

Arrange the eigenvalues of $A^T A$ in decreasing order, i.e. 360, 90, 0
Construct V:

i.e. $V = \begin{bmatrix} V_1 & V_2 & V_3 \end{bmatrix} = \begin{bmatrix} 1/3 & -2/3 & -2/3 \\ 2/3 & -1/3 & -2/3 \\ 2/3 & 2/3 & 1/3 \end{bmatrix}$

The square roots of the eigenvalues are the singular values.

$$T_1 = 6\sqrt{10}, \quad T_2 = 3\sqrt{10}, \quad T_3 = 0$$

The matrix is the same size as A with D in the upper left corner and with 0's elsewhere

$$D = \begin{bmatrix} 6\sqrt{10} & 0 \\ 0 & 3\sqrt{10} \end{bmatrix}$$

$$\Sigma = \begin{bmatrix} D & O \end{bmatrix} = \begin{bmatrix} 6\sqrt{10} & 0 & 0 \\ 0 & 3\sqrt{10} & 0 \end{bmatrix}$$

To construct
  $\|AV_1\| = T_1, \quad \|AV_2\| = T_2$

$$u_1 = \frac{1}{T_1} AV_1 = \frac{1}{6\sqrt{10}} \begin{bmatrix} 18 \\ 6 \end{bmatrix} = \begin{bmatrix} 3/\sqrt{10} \\ 1/\sqrt{10} \end{bmatrix}$$

$$u_2 = \frac{1}{T_2} AV_2 = \frac{1}{3\sqrt{10}} \begin{bmatrix} 3 \\ -9 \end{bmatrix} = \begin{bmatrix} 1/\sqrt{10} \\ -3/\sqrt{10} \end{bmatrix}$$

$$U = \begin{bmatrix} u_1, & u_2 \end{bmatrix} = \begin{bmatrix} 3/\sqrt{10} & 1/\sqrt{10} \\ 1/\sqrt{10} & -3/\sqrt{10} \end{bmatrix}$$

$\therefore$ The singular value decomposition of A is

  $A = U \Sigma V^T$

$$A = \begin{bmatrix} 3/\sqrt{10} & 1/\sqrt{10} \\ 1/\sqrt{10} & -3/\sqrt{10} \end{bmatrix} \begin{bmatrix} 6\sqrt{10} & 0 & 0 \\ 0 & 3\sqrt{10} & 0 \end{bmatrix} \begin{bmatrix} 1/3 & 2/3 & 2/3 \\ -2/3 & -1/3 & 2/3 \\ -2/3 & -2/3 & 1/3 \end{bmatrix}$$

Example 2: Find the singular value decomposition of $A = \begin{bmatrix} 1 & -1 \\ -2 & 2 \\ 2 & -2 \end{bmatrix}$

Solution: Compute $A^T A = \begin{bmatrix} 1 & -2 & 2 \\ -1 & 2 & -2 \end{bmatrix} \begin{bmatrix} 1 & -1 \\ -2 & 2 \\ 2 & -2 \end{bmatrix}$

$$A^T A = \begin{bmatrix} 9 & -9 \\ -9 & 9 \end{bmatrix}$$

$\therefore$ The eigenvalues of $A^T A$ by

$$|A^T A - \lambda I| = 0$$

$$\begin{vmatrix} 9 - \lambda & -9 \\ -9 & 9 - \lambda \end{vmatrix} = 0$$

$$(9 - \lambda)^2 - 81 = 0$$

$$\cancel{81} + \lambda^2 - 18\lambda - \cancel{81} = 0$$

$$\lambda^2 - 18\lambda = 0$$

$$\lambda(\lambda - 18) = 0$$

$$\lambda = 0, \quad \lambda - 18 = 0$$

$\therefore$ The eigenvalues are 18 and 0 corresponding to unit eigenvectors

$$V_1 = \begin{bmatrix} 1/\sqrt{2} \\ -1/\sqrt{2} \end{bmatrix}, \quad V_2 = \begin{bmatrix} 1/\sqrt{2} \\ 1/\sqrt{2} \end{bmatrix}$$

$\therefore$ There unit vectors form the columns of V.

$$V = \begin{bmatrix} V_1 & V_2 \end{bmatrix} = \begin{bmatrix} 1/\sqrt{2} & 1/\sqrt{2} \\ -1/\sqrt{2} & 1/\sqrt{2} \end{bmatrix}$$

The singular values are $T_1 = \sqrt{18} = 3\sqrt{2}$ and $T_2 = 0$.

Since, there is only one non-zero singular vector, the matrix D may be written as a singular number,

i.e. $\qquad\qquad D = 3\sqrt{2}$

The matrix Σ is same size in A with 'D' in its upper left corner.

$$\Sigma = T_1 = \sqrt{18} = \begin{bmatrix} D & 0 \\ 0 & 0 \\ 0 & 0 \end{bmatrix} = \begin{bmatrix} 3\sqrt{2} & 0 \\ 0 & 0 \\ 0 & 0 \end{bmatrix}$$

To construct U, first construct AV_1 and AV_2.

$$AV_1 = \begin{bmatrix} 2/\sqrt{2} \\ -4/\sqrt{2} \\ 4/\sqrt{2} \end{bmatrix}, \quad AV_2 = \begin{bmatrix} 0 \\ 0 \\ 0 \end{bmatrix}$$

$\therefore \| AV_1 \| = T_1 = 3\sqrt{2}$ and $\| AV_2 \| = T_2 = 0$

$$U_1 = V_1 = \frac{1}{3\sqrt{2}} \quad AV_1 = \begin{bmatrix} 1/3 \\ -2/3 \\ 2/3 \end{bmatrix}$$

The after columns of U are found by the set $\{U\}$ to an orthogonal basis for R^3.

In this case, we need two orthogonal unit vectors u_2 and u_3 that are orthogonal to u_1.

Each vector must satisfy $u_1^T x = 0$

which is equivalent to the equation $x_1 - 2x_2 + 2x_3 = 0$

Case 1:

$$x_1 = 2x_2 - 2x_3, \qquad +2x_2 = +(2x_3 + x_1), \qquad 2x_3 = (2x_2 - x_1)$$
$$2x_2 = 2x_3 + x_1$$

$$\ldots(1) \qquad\qquad \ldots(2) \qquad\qquad \ldots(3)$$

$x_3 = 0$

$2x_2 = x_1, \qquad x_2 = k, \qquad x_1 = 2k, \qquad x_3 = 0$

$2x_2 = 0 + x_1 \Rightarrow 2x_2 = 2k \qquad\qquad x_2 = k$

where $k = 1$, $x_1 = 2$, $x_2 = 1$, $x_3 = 0$

$$w_1 = \begin{bmatrix} 2 \\ 1 \\ 0 \end{bmatrix}, \quad w_1 = \begin{bmatrix} 2k \\ k \\ 0 \end{bmatrix}$$

Case 2: Put $x_2 = 0$

$x_1 = -2x_3, \quad x_3 = k$

$x_1 = -2k, \quad x_2 = 0, \quad x_3 = k$

$$w_2 = \begin{bmatrix} -2k \\ 0 \\ k \end{bmatrix}, \text{ where } k = 1$$

$$w_1 = \begin{bmatrix} 2 \\ 1 \\ 0 \end{bmatrix}, \quad w_2 = \begin{bmatrix} -2 \\ 0 \\ 1 \end{bmatrix}$$

By normalization of w_1, w_2 are

$$u_2 = \begin{bmatrix} 2/\sqrt{5} \\ 1/\sqrt{5} \\ 0 \end{bmatrix}, \quad u_3 = \begin{bmatrix} -2/\sqrt{5} \\ 0 \\ 1/\sqrt{5} \end{bmatrix}$$

Finally set $U = [u_1, u_2, u_3] = \begin{bmatrix} 1/3 & 2/\sqrt{5} & -2/\sqrt{5} \\ -2/3 & 1/\sqrt{5} & 0 \\ 2/3 & 0 & 1/\sqrt{5} \end{bmatrix}$

$$A = \begin{bmatrix} 1 & -1 \\ -2 & 2 \\ 2 & -2 \end{bmatrix} = U\Sigma V^T$$

$$= \begin{bmatrix} 1/3 & 2/\sqrt{5} & -2/\sqrt{5} \\ -2/3 & 1/\sqrt{5} & 0 \\ 2/3 & 0 & 1/\sqrt{5} \end{bmatrix} \begin{bmatrix} 3\sqrt{2} & 0 \\ 0 & 0 \\ 0 & 0 \end{bmatrix} \begin{bmatrix} 1/\sqrt{2} & -1/\sqrt{2} \\ 1/\sqrt{2} & 1/\sqrt{2} \end{bmatrix}$$

EXERCISE

Find the singular value decomposition of the matrix and verify that $A = U\Sigma V^T$.

(i) $\begin{bmatrix} -3 & 1 \\ 6 & -2 \\ 6 & -2 \end{bmatrix}$ (ii) $\begin{bmatrix} 1 & 1 \\ 0 & 1 \\ -1 & 1 \end{bmatrix}$ (iii) $\begin{bmatrix} 2 & 3 \\ 0 & 2 \end{bmatrix}$

Modules

11.1 INTRODUCTION

Previously we have dealt with the algebraic structures consisting of a non-void set with one or two binary operations satisfying certain axioms. Our aim will be to study algebraic structures that consist of two non-void sets, a ring and other abelian group, and a mapping associating with each ordered pair, consisting of an element of the ring and an element of the abelian group to a unique element of the abelian group. This chapter deals with modules while vector space has been studied in the previous chapter.

11.2 DEFINITION AND EXAMPLES

Left-module

An algebraic structure $(M, R, \oplus, \odot)$ consisting of a non-void set M, a ring R, a binary operation $\oplus$ on M and an external mapping $\odot : R \times M \to M$ associating each $r \in R$, $a \in M$ to a unique element $r \odot a \in M$ is said to be a left R-module or simply a left module over ring R, if the following axioms are satisfied:

Axiom-1: $(M, \oplus)$ is an abelian group.

Axiom-2: For all $a, b \in M$ and $r, s \in R$, we have,

(i) $r \odot (a \oplus b) = r \odot a \oplus r \odot b$

(ii) $(r + s) \odot a = r \odot a \oplus s \odot a$

(iii) $(r \odot s) \odot a = r \odot (s \odot a)$

The elements of the ring R are called **scalars** and the mapping $\odot : R \times M \to M$ is called **scalar multiplication.**

In the above definition, if we replace $\odot : R \times M \to M$ by $M \times R \to M$ such that the analogues of axiom-2 (i)–(iii) hold, then the algebraic structure $(M, R, \oplus, \odot)$ is called a right R-module or simply a right module over ring R.

In the above definition, the symbol '+' has been used for addition in the ring R and the symbol '·' has been used for multiplication in R.

Remark 1: In modules, we will be dealing with two types of zeros (additive identities) (i) zero element of the additive abelian group M and (ii) zero element of the ring R. In order to avoid any confusion, we shall be using the symbol 0 to denote the zero element of ring R and the symbol 0_M to denote the zero element of the abelian group M. The zero element 0 of ring R is also known as the **scalar zero.**

Remark 2: Since $(M, \oplus)$ is an abelian group, for any $a, b, c \in M$, we have

(i) $\left.\begin{array}{l} a \oplus b = a \oplus c \Rightarrow b = c \\ b \oplus a = c \oplus a \Rightarrow b = c \end{array}\right\}$ (cancellation laws)

(ii) $a \oplus b = 0_M \Rightarrow b = -a$ and $a = -b$

(iii) $-(-a) = a$

(iv) $a \oplus b = a \Rightarrow b = 0_M$

(v) $-(a \oplus b) = (-a) \oplus (-b)$

(vi) 0_M is unique

(vii) For each $a \in M, -a \in M$ is unique

We shall say that M is a left (right) R-module or M is a left (right) R-module. Thus, whenever we say that M is a left (right) module over the ring R or M is a left (right) R-module, it always mean that $(M, \oplus)$ is an abelian group and $\odot : R \times M \to M(\odot : M \times R \to M)$ is a mapping such that axiom-2 (i) – (iii) are satisfied.

Remark 3: We shall use the same symbol '+' for addition in the abelian group M and addition in the ring R. Similarly, the scalar multiplication $\odot$ and the multiplication in R will be denoted by the same symbol '×'.

We have talked about left and right R-modules. Now a natural question arises. Is it necessary to distinguish between right and left modules? Suppose M is a left R-module. Cannot we make M into a right R-module by defining $ar = ra$ for all $a \in M$ and $r \in R$? The answer is that we can if R is a commutative ring as shown in the following lemma. If R is not a commutative ring on a left R-module, M cannot be made into a right R-module.

Lemma: Let M be a left R-module over a commutative ring R. Then M is also a right R-module and vice versa.

Proof: Since M is a left R-module for each $a \in M$ and $r \in R$, $r \cdot a$ is a uniquely defined element of M, such that for all $a, b \in M$ and all $r, s \in R$

(i) $r \cdot (a + b) = r \cdot a + r \cdot b$

(ii) $(r + s) \cdot a = r \cdot a + s \cdot a$

(iii) $(r \cdot s) \cdot a = r \cdot (s \cdot a)$

Define $a \cdot r = r \cdot a$ for all $a \in M$ and all $r \in R$.

For any $a, b \in M$ and $r, s \in R$, we observe the following properties:

(i) $(a + b) \cdot r = r \cdot (a + b)$

$\Rightarrow (a + b) \cdot r = r \cdot a + r \cdot b$

$\Rightarrow (a + b) \cdot r = a \cdot r + b \cdot r$

(ii) $a \cdot (r + s) = (r + s) \cdot a$

$\Rightarrow a \cdot (r + s) = r \cdot a + s \cdot a$

$\Rightarrow a \cdot (r + s) = a \cdot r + a \cdot s$

(iii) $a \cdot (r \cdot s) = (r \cdot s) \cdot a$

$\Rightarrow a \cdot (r \cdot s) = s \cdot (r \cdot a)$ [by commutativity of multiplication on R]

$\Rightarrow a \cdot (r \cdot s) = s \cdot (a \cdot r)$

$\Rightarrow a \cdot (r \cdot s) = (a \cdot r) \cdot s$

Thus, M is an additive abelian group such that for each $a \in M$ and $r \in R$, $a \cdot r$ is a uniquely defined element of M and properties (i) – (iii) are satisfied.

Hence M is a right R-module over ring R.

Proceeding in the similar manner we can show that if M is a right R-module, then it is left R-module also.

Remark 4: In future, we shall write *ar* for $a \cdot r$

Remark 5: As proved in the above lemma that in case of a commutative ring R, every left R-module is a right R-module and every right R-module is a left R-module. Thus in this case, we are justified in referring simply to R-modules and using either left or right notation. However, if R is not a commutative ring, we must be careful to make the distinction between left and right R-modules. Note that left and right R-modules in case of a non-commutative ring are different structures. They cannot be identified or considered the same.

Remark 6: In future, unless stated otherwise, all R-modules are left R-modules.

Unitary Module: Let R be a ring with unity. An R-module M is called a **unitary module** if $Ia = a$ for all $a \in M$.

Every additive abelian group is a unitary Z-module as Z is a ring with unity.

WORKED EXAMPLES

Example 1: Every ring is a module over its any subring.

Solution: Let R be a ring and S be an arbitrary subring of R. Since R is an additive abelian group, therefore, axiom-1 holds.

Taking multiplication in R as scalar multiplication, we find that the axiom-2(i) to axiom-2(iii) are respectively, the left distributive, right distributive and associative laws.

Hence R is a module over its subring S.

Since S is an arbitrary subring of ring R, therefore, every ring is a module over its any subring.

Remark 7: The converse of this example is not true, i.e. a subring is not necessarily a module over the ring. For example, the ring Z of integers is not a module over the ring Q of rational numbers because the multiplication of a rational number and an integer is not always an integer.

Example 2: Every ring is a module over itself.

Solution: Since every ring is a subring of itself, therefore the result follows from Example 1.

Remark 8: In order to test whether a given non-void set M forms a module over a ring R, we must proceed as follows:

(i) Define a binary operation on M.

(ii) Define scalar multiplication on M, which associates each scalar in R and each element in M to a unique element in M.

(iii) Define equality of elements in M.

(iv) Check whether axiom-1 and axiom-2 are satisfied relative to the binary operation on M and scalar multiplication thus defined.

Example 3: Every additive abelian group is a module over the ring Z of integers.

Solution: Let M be an additive abelian group. In order to give a module structure to M over the ring Z of integers, we define scalar multiplication on M as follows:

Scalar multiplication on M: For any $n \in Z$ and $a \in M$, we define

$$na = \begin{cases} \underset{(n\text{-times})}{a+a+...+a} & , \text{ if } n > 0 \\ 0 & , \text{ if } n = 0 \\ \underset{(n\text{-times})}{(-a)+(-a)+...+(-a)} & , \text{ if } n < 0 \end{cases}$$

Clearly $na \in M$ for all $a \in M$ and for all $n \in Z$

Since A is an additive abelian group, therefore, addition on M is defined. Thus, addition and scalar multiplication on M are defined. So, it remains to verify the axiom-2 (i) to axiom-2 (iii).

Axiom-2: For $a, b \in M$ and $m, n \in Z$, we have

(i) If $n > 0$, then

$$n(a+b) = \underset{n\text{-times}}{(a+b)+(a+b)+...+(a+b)}$$

[by def. of scalar multiplication]

$$= \underset{n\text{-times}}{(a+a+...+a)} + \underset{n\text{-times}}{(b+b+...+b)}$$

[by comm. and assoc. of addition on M]

$$= na + nb \qquad \text{[by def. of scalar multiplication]}$$

(ii) If $n = 0$, then

$$n(a+b) = 0$$

$\Rightarrow n(a+b) = 0+0 = na+nb$

(iii) If $n < 0$, then

$$n(a+b) = \{-(a+b)\} + \{-(a+b)\} + ... + \{-(a+b)\}$$
$$\underbrace{}_{n\text{-times}}$$
[by def. of scalar multiplication]

$$= \underbrace{(-a-b)+(-a-b)+...+(-a-b)}_{n\text{-times}}$$
[∵ + is commutative on M]

$$= \underbrace{\{(-a)+(-a)+...+(-a)\}}_{|n|\text{-times}} + \underbrace{\{(-b)+(-b)+...+(-b)\}}_{|n|\text{-times}}$$

$$\begin{bmatrix} \text{by commutativity} \\ \text{and associativity} \\ \text{of addition on } M \end{bmatrix}$$

$$= |n|(-a) + |n|(-b)$$

$$= (-n)(-a) + (-n)(-b) \qquad [\because n<0 \therefore |n| = -n]$$

$$= na + nb \qquad \text{[by def. of scalar multiplication]}$$

Thus, $n(a+b) = na+nb$ for all $n \in Z$

Similarly, we can show that axiom-2(ii) and axiom-2(iii) are true.

Hence M is a module over Z or M is a Z-module.

Remark 9: In the above example, we have proved that every additive abelian group is a Z-module. In fact every abelian group M can be regarded as a Z-module, if we define $na = an$ for $a \in M$ and $n \in Z$.

Remark 10: Since every cyclic group is abelian, therefore, every cyclic group can also be considered as a Z-module.

Example 4: Let R be a ring and let I be a left ideal of R. Then, I is an R-module.

Solution: Since I is a left ideal of R, therefore, I is an additive abelian group. We define scalar multiplication on I as follows:

Scalar multiplication on I: For any $r \in R$ and $a \in I$, let ra be the ordinary product of these elements as elements of R. Since I is a left ideal of R, therefore $ra \in I$, for all $r \in R$ and $a \in I$.

In order to prove that I is an R-module, we have to verify axiom-2(i) to axiom-2(iii).

Axiom-2: For any $a, b \in I$ and $r, s \in R$, we have

(i) $r(a+b) = ra+rb$ by left distributivity of multiplication on R over addition on R.

(ii) $(r+s)a = ra+sa$ by right distributivity of multiplication on R over addition on R.

(iii) $(rs)a = r(sa)$ follows from associativity of multiplication on R. Hence I is an R-module.

Remark 11: Since every ideal is a left ideal, therefore, every ideal of a ring R is an R-module.

Example 5: Let R be a ring, then the set $R[x]$ of all polynomials over the ring R in indeterminate x is an R-module.

Solution: In order to give a module structure to $R[x]$, we define addition, scalar multiplication and equality in $R[x]$ as follows:

Addition on $R[x]$: If $f(x) = \sum_i a_i x^i$, $g(x) = \sum_i b_i x^i \in R[x]$, then

$$f(x) + g(x) = \sum_i (a_i + b_i)x^i$$

Clearly, $f(x) + g(x) \in R[x]$ because $a_i + b_i \in R$ for all i.

Scalar multiplication on $R[x]$: For any $\lambda \in R$

$f(x) = \sum_i a_i x^i \in R[x], \lambda f(x)$ is defined as the polynomial $\sum_i (\lambda a_i)x^i$

i.e. $\lambda f(x) = \sum_i (\lambda a_i)x^i$.

Obviously, $\lambda f(x) \in R[x]$ as $\lambda a_i \in R$ for all i.

Equality of two elements of $R[x]$: For any

$$f(x) = \sum_i a_i x^i, \quad g(x) = \sum_i b_i x^i \in R[x],$$

we define

$$f(x) = g(x) \Leftrightarrow a_i = b_i \text{ for all } i.$$

Now we shall verify axiom-1 and axiom-2.

Axiom-1: $R[x]$ is an abelian group under addition defined above:

Associativity: If $f(x) = \sum_i a_i x^i$, $g(x) = \sum_i b_i x^i, h(x) = \sum_i c_i x^i \in R[x]$, then

$$\{f(x) + g(x)\} + h(x) = \left(\sum_i (a_i + b_i)x^i\right) + \sum_i c_i x^i$$

$$= \sum_i \{(a_i + b_i) + c_i\}x^i$$

$$= \sum_i \{a_i + (b_i + c_i)\}x^i$$

[by associativity of addition on R]

$$= \sum_i a_i x^i + \sum_i (b_i + c_i)x^i$$

$$= f(x) + \{g(x) + h(x)\}$$

So, addition is associative on $R[x]$.

Commutativity: If $f(x) = \sum_i a_i x^i$, $g(x) = \sum_i b_i x^i \in R[x]$,
then

$$f(x) + g(x) = \sum_i (a_i + b_i)x^i = \sum_i (b_i + a_i)x^i$$

[by commutativity of addition on R]

$$\Rightarrow \quad f(x) + g(x) = g(x) + f(x)$$

So, addition is commutative on $R[x]$.

Existence of additive identity: Since $\hat{0}(x) = \sum_i 0 x^i \in R[x]$ is such that for

all $\qquad f(x) = \sum_i a_i x^i \in R[x]$

$$\hat{0}(x) + f(x) = \sum_i a_i x^i = f(x) \quad [\because 0 \text{ is the additive identity in } R]$$

Thus, $\hat{0}(x) + f(x) = f(x) = f(x) + \hat{0}(x)$ for all $f(x) \in R[x]$

$\therefore$ $\hat{0}(x)$ is identity element (zero) for addition on $R[x]$.

Existence of additive inverse: Let $f(x) = \sum_i a_i x^i$ be an arbitrary polynomial

in $R[x]$. Then, $-f(x) = \sum_i (-a_i)x^i \in R[x]$ such that

$$f(x) + \{-f(x)\} = \sum_i a_i x^i + \sum_i (-a_i)x^i = \sum_i \{a_i + (-a_i)\}x^i = \sum_i 0 x^i = \hat{0}(x)$$

Thus, for each $f(x) \in R[x]$, there exists $-f(x) \in R[x]$ such that

$$f(x) + \{-f(x)\} = \hat{0}(x) = \{f(x)\} - f(x)$$

$\therefore$ Each $f(x)$ has its additive inverse in $R[x]$.

Hence, $R[x]$ is an abelian group for addition.

Axiom-2: For any $f(x) = \sum_i a_i x^i, g(x) = \sum_i b_i x^i \in R[x]$ and $\lambda, \mu \in R$
we have,

(i) $\lambda\{f(x) + g(x)\} = \lambda\left\{\sum_i (a_i + b_i)x^i\right\}$

$$= \sum_i \lambda(a_i + b_i)x^i$$

$$= \sum_i (\lambda a_i + \lambda b_i)x^i$$

[by left distributivity of multiplication over addition]

$$= \sum_i (\lambda a_i)x^i + \sum_i (\lambda b_i)x^i = \lambda f(x) + \lambda g(x)$$

(ii) $(\lambda + \mu)f(x) = \sum_i (\lambda + \mu)a_i x^i$

$$= \sum_i (\lambda a_i + \mu a_i)x^i$$

[by right distributivity of multiplication over addition]

$$= \sum_i (\lambda a_i)x^i + \sum_i (\mu a_i)x^i$$

$$= \lambda f(x) + \mu f(x)$$

(iii) $(\lambda \mu)f(x) = \sum_i (\lambda \mu)a_i x^i$

$$= \sum_i \lambda(\mu a_i)x^i$$

[by associativity of multiplication on R]

$$= \lambda \sum_i (\mu a_i)x^i = \lambda\{\mu f(x)\}$$

(iv) $f(x) = \sum_i (Ia_i)x^i = \sum_i a_i x^i$ [$\because$ I is unity in R]

$$= f(x)$$

Hence, $R[x]$ is an R-module.

Remark 12: This example becomes trivial, if we consider R as a subring of $R[x]$.

Example 6: Let R be a ring, and let n be a positive integer. Then,

$$R^n = \{(a_1, a_2, ..., a_n) : a_i \in R \text{ for all } i \in n\} \text{ is an } R\text{-module.}$$

Solution: To give a module structure to R^n over ring R, we first define an additive binary operation on R^n, scalar multiplication on R^n and equality of any two elements of R^n as follows:

Addition on R^n: For any $x = (a_1, a_2, ..., a_n), y = (b_1, b_2, ..., b_n) \in R^n$, we define

$$x + y = (a_1 + b_1, a_2 + b_2, ..., a_n + b_n)$$

$$\Rightarrow x + y \in R^n \qquad [\because a_i + b_i \in R \text{ for all } i \in n]$$

Thus, addition is a binary operation on R^n.

Scalar multiplication on R^n: For any $x = (a_1, a_2, ..., a_n) \in R^n$ and $\lambda \in F$, we define

$$\lambda x = (\lambda a_1, \lambda a_2, ..., \lambda a_n)$$
$$\Rightarrow \lambda x \in R[x] \qquad\qquad [\because \lambda a_i \in R \text{ for all } i \in n].$$

Thus, scalar multiplication is defined as $R[x]$.

Equality of two elements of R^n: For any

$$x = (a_1, a_2, ..., a_n) \text{ and } y = (b_1, b_2, ..., b_n) \in R[x], \text{ we define}$$
$$x = y \Leftrightarrow a_i = b_i \text{ for all } i \in n$$

Thus, we have defined addition and scalar multiplication on $R[x]$ and equality of any two elements of $R[x]$. Let us now verify axiom-1 and axiom-2.

Axiom-1: R^n is an abelian group under addition

Associativity: For any

$$x = (a_1, a_2, ..., a_n), y = (b_1, b_2, ..., b_n), z = (c_1, c_2, ..., c_n) \in R^n, \text{ we have}$$
$$(x + y) + z = (a_1 + b_1, a_2 + b_2, ..., a_n + b_n) + (c_1, c_2, ..., c_n)$$
$$= ((a_1 + b_1) + c_1, (a_2 + b_2) + c_2, ..., (a_n + b_n) + c_n)$$
$$= (a_1 + (b_1 + c_1), a_2 + (b_2 + c_2), ..., a_n + (b_n + c_n))$$

[by associativity of addition on R]

$$= (a_1, a_2, ..., a_n) + (b_1 + c_1, b_2 + c_2, ..., b_n + c_n)$$
$$= x + (y + z)$$

So, addition is associative on R^n.

Commutativity: For any $x = (a_1, a_2, ..., a_n), y = (b_1, b_2, ..., b_n) \in R^n$, we have

$$x + y = (a_1 + b_1, a_2 + b_2, ..., a_n + b_n)$$
$$= (b_1 + a_1, b_2 + a_2, ..., b_n + a_n)$$

[by commutativity of addition on R]

$$\Rightarrow \qquad\qquad x + y = y + x$$

So, addition is commutative on R^n.

Existence of additive identity: Since $0 \in R$, therefore $0 = (0, 0, ..., 0) \in R^n$

such that for all $\quad x = (a_1, a_2, ..., a_n) \in R^n$, we have

$$x + 0 = (a_1, a_2, ..., a_n) + (0, 0, ..., 0)$$
$$= (a_1 + 0, ..., a_2 + 0, ..., a_n + 0)$$
$$\Rightarrow \qquad\qquad = (a_1, a_2, ..., a_n) = x \qquad [\because a_i + 0 = a_i \text{ for } i \in n]$$
$$\therefore \qquad\qquad x + 0 = x = 0 + x \text{ for all } x \in R^n$$

So, $0 = (0, 0, ..., 0)$ is the identity element for addition on R^n.

Existence of additive inverse: Let $x = (a_1, a_2, ..., a_n)$ be an arbitrary element of R^n. Then, $-x = (-a_1, -a_2, ..., -a_n) \in R^n$ such that

$$x + (-x) = (a_1 + (-a_1), a_2 + (-a_2), ..., a_n + (-a_n)) = (0, 0, ..., 0) = 0$$

Thus, for every $x = (a_1, a_2, ..., a_n) \in R^n$, there exists

$-x = (-a_1, -a_2, ..., -a_n) \in R^n$, such that $x + (-x) = 0 = (-x) + x$

So, every $x \in R^n$ has its additive inverse.

Hence, R^n is an abelian group under addition.

Axiom-2: For any $x = (a_1, a_2, ..., a_n), y = (b_1, b_2, ..., b_n) \in R^n$ and $\lambda, \mu \in R$, we have

(i) $\lambda(x + y) = \lambda(a_1 + b_1, a_2 + b_2, ..., a_n + b_n)$

$$= [\lambda(a_1 + b_1), \lambda(a_2 + b_2), ..., \lambda(a_n + b_n)]$$

$$= (\lambda a_1 + \lambda b_1, \lambda a_2 + \lambda b_2, ..., \lambda a_n + \lambda b_n)$$

[by left distributivity of multiplication over addition on R]

$$= (\lambda a_1, \lambda a_2, ..., \lambda a_n) + (\lambda b_n, \lambda b_n, ..., \lambda b_n)$$

$$= \lambda x + \lambda y$$

(ii) $(\lambda + \mu)x = ((\lambda + \mu)a_1, (\lambda + \mu)a_2, ..., (\lambda + \mu)a_n)$

$$= (\lambda a_1 + \mu a_1, \lambda a_2 + \mu a_2, ..., \lambda a_n + \mu a_n)$$

[By left distributivity of multiplication over addition on R]

$$= (\lambda a_1, \lambda a_2, ..., \lambda a_n) + (\mu a_1, \mu a_2, ..., \mu a_n) = \lambda x + \mu x$$

(iii) $(\lambda \mu)x = (\lambda \mu)a_1, (\lambda \mu)a_2, ..., (\lambda \mu)a_n)$

$$= [\lambda(\mu a_1), \lambda(\mu a_2), ..., \lambda(\mu a_n)]$$

[by associativity of multiplication on R]

$$= \lambda(\mu a_1, \mu a_2, ..., \mu a_n) = \lambda(\mu x)$$

Hence, R^n is R-module.

Example 7: Let R be a ring. Then the set $R^{m \times n}$ of all $m \times n$ matrices over R is a module over ring R.

Solution: In order to prove that, $R^{m \times n}$ is a module over ring R, we first define addition and scalar multiplication on $R^{m \times n}$ and also the equality of any two elements of $R^{m \times n}$ as follows:

Addition on $R^{m \times n}$: For any $A = [a_{ij}], B = [b_{ij}]$ in $R^{m \times n}$, we define

$A + B = [a_{ij} + b_{ij}]$, i.e. addition on $R^{m \times n}$ is addition of matrices.

Scalar multiplication on $R^{m \times n}$: For any $A = [a_{ij}] \in R^{m \times n}$, we define $rA = [ra_{ij}]$, i.e. scalar multiplication on $R^{m \times n}$ is usually scalar multiplication $R^{m \times n}$ of the matrix A by the element $r \in R$.

Equality of any two elements of $R^{m \times n}$: For any $A = [a_{ij}], B = [b_{ij}] \in R^{m \times n}$, we define

$$A = B \Leftrightarrow a_{ij} = b_{ij} \text{ for all } i \in m, j \in n$$

Thus, we have defined addition, scalar multiplication on $R^{m \times n}$ and equality of any two elements of $R^{m \times n}$. Now we have to verify axiom-1 and axiom-2.

Axiom-1: $R^{m \times n}$ is an abelian group under addition of matrices:

Associativity: For any $A = [a_{ij}], B = [b_{ij}], C = [c_{ij}] \in R^{m \times n}$, we have

$$\begin{aligned}
(A + B) + C &= [a_{ij} + b_{ij}] + [c_{ij}] \\
&= [(a_{ij} + b_{ij}) + c_{ij}] \\
&= [a_{ij} + (b_{ij} + c_{ij})] \text{ [by associativity of addition on } R] \\
&= [a_{ij}] + [b_{ij} + c_{ij}] \\
&= A + (B + C)
\end{aligned}$$

So, addition of matrices is associative on $R^{m \times n}$.

Existence of additive identity: The null matrix $O = [0]$ is the identity element for addition because

$$A + O = A = O + A \quad \text{for all } A \in R^{m \times n}$$

Existence of additive inverse: Let $A = [a_{ij}]$ be an arbitrary matrix over ring R. Then $-A = [-a_{ij}] \in R^{m \times n}$ such that

$$A + (-A) = [-a_{ij} + (-a_{ij})] = [0] = O = (-A) + A$$

Thus, each $A \in R^{m \times n}$ has its additive inverse $-A \in R^{m \times n}$.

So, every element in $R^{m \times n}$ has its additive inverse in $R^{m \times n}$.

Hence $R^{m \times n}$ is an abelian group under matrix addition.

Axiom-2: For any $A = [a_{ij}], B = [b_{ij}] \in R^{m \times n}$ and $\lambda, \mu \in R$, we have

(i) $\lambda(A + B) = [\lambda(a_{ij} + b_{ij})]$

$$= [\lambda(a_{ij} + b_{ij})]$$

[by left distributivity of multiplication over addition on R]

$$= [\lambda a_{ij}] + [\lambda b_{ij}]$$

$$= \lambda A + \lambda B$$

(ii) $(\lambda + \mu)A = [(\lambda + \mu)a_{ij}]$

$$= [\lambda a_{ij} + \mu a_{ij}]$$

[by right distributivity of multiplication over addition on R]

$$= [\lambda a_{ij}] + [\mu a_{ij}]$$

$$= \lambda A + \mu A$$

(iii) $\quad (\lambda\mu)A = [(\lambda\mu)a_{ij}]$

$\qquad\qquad = [\lambda(\mu a_{ij})]$ \qquad\qquad [by associativity of multiplication on R]

$\qquad\qquad = \lambda(\mu A)$

Hence $R^{m\times n}$ is a module over ring R.

Particular case: Taking $m = 1$ (or $n = 1$) the set of all $1 \times n$(or $m \times 1$) matrices, i.e. the set of all n (or m)-tuples, denoted by R^n (or R^m) is a module over ring R.

Example 8: Let X be a non-void set. Let R be a ring and let A be an R-module. Then the set $A^X = \{f : X \to A\}$ of all functions from X to A is an R-module under addition and scalar multiplication and A^X defined by

$$(f + g)(x) = f(x) + g(x)$$

and $(\lambda f)x = \lambda f(x)$ respectively, for all $f, g \in A^X$ and all $\lambda \in R$.

Solution: We define equality of any two elements of A^X as follows:

For any $f, g \in A^X$, we define

$f = g \Leftrightarrow f(x) = g(x)$ for all $x \in X$

Thus addition, scalar multiplication and equality of any two elements of A^X are defined.

We shall now verify axiom-1 and axiom-2.

Axiom-1: A^X is an abelian group under addition defined above:

Associativity: Let $f, g, h \in A^X$. Then

$\qquad [(f + g) + h](x) = (f + g)(x) + h(x)$

$\Rightarrow \quad [(f + g) + h](x) = [f(x) + g(x)] + h(x)$

$\Rightarrow \quad [(f + g) + h](x) = f(x) + [g(x) + h(x)]$

$\qquad\qquad\qquad\qquad$ [by associativity of addition on A]

$\Rightarrow \quad [(f + g) + h](x) = f(x) + (g + h)(x)$

$\Rightarrow \quad [(f + g) + h](x) = [f + (g + h)](x)$ for all $x \in X$

$\therefore \qquad\qquad (f + g) + h = f + (g + h)$

So, addition is associative on A^X.

Commutativity: For any $f, g \in A^X$

$\qquad (f + g)(x) = f(x) + g(x)$

$\qquad\qquad\qquad = g(x) + f(x)$ \quad [by commutativity of addition on A]

$\qquad (f + g)(x) = (g + f)(x)$ for all $x \in X$

$\therefore \qquad\qquad f + g = g + f$

So, addition is commutative on A^X.

Existence of additive identity: The function $\hat{0}(x) = 0_A \in A$ for all $x \in A$ is the additive identity because for any $f \in A^X$

$$(f + \hat{0})(x) = f(x) + \hat{0}(x) = f(x) + 0_A = f(x) = (\hat{0} + f)(x)$$

for all $x \in X$

$$\Rightarrow \quad f + \hat{0} = \hat{0} + f \text{ for all } f \in A^X$$

So, $\hat{0} : X \to A$ is the additive identity.

Existence of additive inverse: Let f be an arbitary function in A^X. Then a function $-f$ defined by $(-f)(x) = f(x)$ for all $x \in X$ is additive inverse of f because

$$\begin{aligned}
(f + (-f))(x) &= f(x) + (-f)(x) \\
&= f(x) - f(x) = 0_A \\
&= \hat{0}(x) = ((-f) + f)(x) \text{ for all } x \in X
\end{aligned}$$

Hence, A^X is an abelian group under addition.

Axiom-2: For any $f, g \in A^X$ and $\lambda, \mu \in R$, we have

(i) $\quad [\lambda(f + g)](x) = \lambda(f + g)(x)$

$$\begin{aligned}
\Rightarrow [\lambda(f + g)](x) &= \lambda[(f(x) + g(x)] \\
&= \lambda f(x) + \lambda g(x) \qquad \text{[by axiom-2 (i) in } A] \\
&= (\lambda f)(x) + (\lambda g)(x) \\
&= [\lambda f + \lambda g](x) \text{ for all } x \in X
\end{aligned}$$

$$\therefore \quad\quad \lambda(f + g) = \lambda f + \lambda g$$

(ii) $\quad [(\lambda + \mu)f](x) = (\lambda + \mu)f(x)$ $\qquad$ [by axiom-2 (ii) in A]

$$\begin{aligned}
\Rightarrow [(\lambda + \mu)f](x) &= \lambda f(x) + \mu f(x) \\
&= (\lambda f)(x) + (\mu f)(x) \\
&= [\lambda f + \mu f](x) \text{ for all } x \in X
\end{aligned}$$

$$\therefore \quad\quad (\lambda + \mu)f = \lambda f + \mu f$$

(iii) $\quad [(\lambda\mu)f](x) = (\lambda\mu)f(x)$

$$\begin{aligned}
\Rightarrow [(\lambda\mu)f](x) &= \lambda(\mu f(x)) \\
&= \lambda[(\mu f)(x)] \\
&= [\lambda(\mu f)](x) \text{ for all } x \in X
\end{aligned}$$

$$\therefore \quad\quad (\lambda\mu)f = \lambda(\mu f)$$

Hence, A^X is a module over the ring R.

Example 9: Let M_1 and M_2 be two R-modules. Then their cartesian product $M_1 \times M_2 = \{(a_1, a_2) : a_1 \in M_1, a_2 \in M_2\}$ is a module over ring R.

Solution: We define addition, scalar multiplication and equality in $M_1 \times M_2$. If $(a_1, a_2), (b_1, b_2) \in M_1 \times M_2$, then we define

$$(a_1, a_2) + (b_1, b_2) = (a_1 + b_1, a_2 + b_2)$$

Since $a_1 + b_1 \in M_1$ and $a_2 + b_2 \in M_2$, therefore

$$(a_1 + b_1, a_2 + b_2) \in M_1 \times M_2$$

So, addition is a binary operation on $M_1 \times M_2$.

Scalar multiplication: For any $(a_1, a_2) \in M_1 \times M_2$ and $\lambda \in R$, we define

$$\lambda(a_1, a_2) = (\lambda a_1, \lambda a_2)$$

Since M_1 and M_2 are modules over ring R, therefore $\lambda a_1 \in M_1$ and $\lambda a_2 \in M_2$.

Consequently, $\lambda(a_1, a_2) = (\lambda a_1, \lambda a_2) \in M_1 \times M_2$

Equality of any two elements of $M_1 \times M_2 : (a_1, a_2)$ and (b_1, b_2) in $M_1 \times M_2$, now it remains to verify axiom-1 and axiom-2.

Axiom-1: $M_1 \times M_2$ is an abelian group under addition:

Associativity: For any $(a_1, a_2), (b_1, b_2), (c_1, c_2) \in M_1 \times M_2$, we have

$$
\begin{aligned}
[(a_1, a_2) + (b_1, b_2)] + (c_1, c_2) &= (a_1 + b_1, a_2 + b_2) + (c_1, c_2) \\
&= ((a_1 + b_1) + c_1, (a_2 + b_2) + c_2) \\
&= (a_1 + (b_1 + c_1), a_2 + (b_2 + c_2)) \\
&= (a_1, a_2) + (b_1 + c_1, b_2 + c_2) \\
&= (a_1, a_2) + [(b_1, b_2) + (c_1, c_2)]
\end{aligned}
$$

So, addition is associative on $M_1 \times M_2$.

Commutativity: For $(a_1, a_2), (b_1, b_2) \in M_1 \times M_2$, we have

$$
\begin{aligned}
(a_1, a_2) + (b_1, b_2) &= (a_1 + b_1, a_2 + b_2) \\
&= (b_1 + a_1, b_2 + a_2) \\
&= (b_1, b_2) + (a_1, a_2)
\end{aligned}
$$

So, addition is commutative on $M_1 \times M_2$.

Existence of additive identity: If 0_{M_1} and 0_{M_2} are zeros in M_1 and M_2 respectively, then $\left(0_{M_1}, 0_{M_2}\right)$ is zero (additive identity) in $M_1 \times M_2$ because for any $(a_1, a_2) \in M_1 \times M_2$

$$
\begin{aligned}
(a_1, a_2) + \left(0_{M_1}, 0_{M_1}\right) &= \left(a_1 + 0_{M_1}, a_2 + 0_{M_2}\right) \\
&= (a_1, a_2) \\
&= \left(0_{M_1} + 0_{M_2}\right) + (a_1, a_2)
\end{aligned}
$$

[by commutativity of addition on $M_1 \times M_2$]

Existence of additive inverse: Let $(a_1, a_2) \in M_1 \times M_2$, then $(-a_1, -a_2)$ is its additive inverse because

$$(a_1, a_2) + (-a_1, -a_2) = (a_1 + (-a_1), a_2 + (-a_2))$$

$$= \left(0_{M_1}, 0_{M_2}\right)$$

$$= (-a_1, -a_2) + (a_1, a_2)$$

[by commutativity of addition of $M_1 \times M_2$]

Thus, each element in $M_1 \times M_2$ has its additive inverse.

Hence, $M_1 \times M_2$ is an abelian group under addition.

Axiom-2: For any $(a_1, a_2) \in M_1 \times M_2$ and $\lambda, \mu \in R$, we have

(i) $\quad \lambda[(a_1, a_2) + (b_1, b_2)] = \lambda(a_1 + b_1, a_2 + b_2)$

$$= (\lambda(a_1 + b_1), \lambda(a_2 + b_2))$$

$$= (\lambda a_1 + \lambda b_1, \lambda a_2 + \lambda b_2)$$

[axiom-2 (i) in M_1 and M_2]

$$= (\lambda a_1 + \lambda a_2), (\lambda b_1, \lambda b_2)$$

$$= (a_1, a_2) + \lambda(b_1, b_2)$$

(ii) $\quad (\lambda + a)(a_1, a_2) = ((\lambda + \mu)a_1, (\lambda + \mu)a_2$

$$= (\lambda a_1 + \mu a_1, \lambda a_2 + \mu a_2)$$

[by axiom-2(ii) in M_1 and M_2]

$$= (\lambda a_1, \lambda a_2) + (\mu a_1, \mu a_2)$$

$$= \lambda(a_1, a_2) + \mu(a_1, a_2)$$

(iii) $\quad (\lambda\mu)(a_1, a_2) = (\lambda\mu)a_1, (\lambda\mu)a_2)$

$$= (\lambda(\mu a_1), \lambda(\mu a_2)$$

[by axiom-2 (iii) in M_1 and M_2]

$$= \lambda(\mu a_1, \mu a_2)$$

$$= \lambda[\mu(a_1, a_2)]$$

Hence, $M_1 \times M_2$ is a module over ring R.

Remark: $M_1 \times M_2$ is called the direct product of the R-module M_1 and M_2.

Example 10: Let A be an R-module. Then for any $n \in N$ the set $A^n = \{f : n \to A\}$ is a module over ring R.

Solution: It is a particular case of Example 8, when X is replaced by $n = \{1, 2, ...\}$

EXERCISE

1. Let R be a ring and let S be the set of all sequences $< a_i >, a_i \in R$. Then show that S is an R-module under the addition and scalar multiplication defined as

$$< a_i > + < b_i > = < a_i + b_i >$$

$$\lambda < a_i > = < a_i >$$

where $\lambda, a_i, b_i \in R$

2. Let M be an additive abelian group. Show that there is only one way of making it a Z-module.
3. If R is a ring and M is an R-module, then prove that
$$n(ra) = r(na) \text{ for all } n \in Z, r \in R \text{ and } a \in M$$
4. Let R be a ring and let M be an R-module but not unique. Then show that there exists $a \neq 0$ such that $ra = 0_M$ for all $r \in R$.
5. Mark each of the following as true or false:
   (i) Every additive abelian group is a Z-module.
   (ii) Every abelian group is a Z-module.
   (iii) Every cyclic grop is a Z-module.

Answers

5. (i) T   (ii) T   (iii) T

11.3 ELEMENTARY PROPERTIES OF MODULES

Theorem 1: Let M be an R-module. For all $r \in R$ and all $a \in M$, we have
(i) $r0_M = 0_M$
(ii) $0a = 0_M$
(iii) $(-r)a = -(ra) = r(-a)$
(iv) If R is a ring with unity 1 and A is a unitary module over R, then
$$(-1)a = -a = 1(-a)$$
(v) If r is a unit and A is a unitary module over ring R, then
$$ra = 0_M \Rightarrow a = 0_M$$

Proof:

(i) For any $r \in R$, we have
$$r0_M = r(0_M + 0_M) \qquad\qquad (\because 0_M + 0_M = 0_M)$$
$$\Rightarrow \quad r0_M = r0_M + r0_M \qquad\qquad \text{[by axiom-2 (i)]}$$
$$\Rightarrow r0_M + 0_M = r0_M + r0_M \quad [\because 0_M \text{ is the additive identity in } M]$$
$$\Rightarrow \quad r0_M = 0_M \qquad\qquad \text{[by left cancellation law in } M]$$
Hence, $r0_M = 0_M$ for all $r \in R$

(ii) For any $a \in M$, we have
$$0a = (0+0)a \qquad\qquad [\because 0+0 = 0 \text{ in ring } R]$$
$$\Rightarrow \quad 0a = 0a + 0a \qquad\qquad \text{[by axiom-2 (ii)]}$$
$$\Rightarrow \quad 0a + 0_M = 0a + 0a \qquad [\because 0_M \text{ is the additive identity in } M]$$
$$\Rightarrow \quad 0a = 0_M \qquad\qquad \text{[by left cancellation law in } M]$$
Hence, $0a = 0_M$ for all $a \in M$.

(iii) For any $r \in R$, we have
$$r + (-r) = 0$$
$$\Rightarrow [r + (-r)]a = 0a \quad \text{for all } a \in M$$
$$\Rightarrow ra + (-r)a = 0a \quad \text{for all } a \in M \qquad\qquad \text{[by axiom-2 (ii) in } M]$$

$$= 0_M \text{ for all } a \in M \qquad \text{[by (ii)]}$$

$$\Rightarrow \qquad (-r)a = -(ra) \text{ for all } a \in M$$

Thus, $(-r)a = -(ra)$ for all $r \in R$

For any $a \in M$, we have

$$a + (-a) = 0_M$$

$$\Rightarrow r[a + (-a)] = r0_M \text{ for all } r \in R$$

$$\Rightarrow ra + r(-a) = r0_M \text{ for all } r \in R \qquad \text{[by axiom-2(i)]}$$

$$= 0_M \quad \text{ for all } r \in R \qquad \text{[By (i)]}$$

$$\Rightarrow \qquad r(-a) = (ra)$$

$$\therefore \qquad r(-a) = -(r) \text{ for all } r \in R \text{ and all } a \in M$$

(iv) Putting $r = 1$ in (iii), we get

$$(-1)a = (1a) = 1(-a)$$

$$\Rightarrow \qquad (-1)a = -a = 1(-a)$$

$$[\because M \text{ is unitary module } \therefore 1a = a \text{ for all } a \in M]$$

$$\therefore \qquad (-1)a = -a = 1(-a) \text{ for all } a \in M$$

(v) Since r is a unit, in R, therefore, $r^{-1} \in R$ such that $r^{-1}r = 1$

Now, $ra = 0_M$

$$\Rightarrow \qquad r^{-1}(ra) = r^{-1}0_M$$

$$\Rightarrow \qquad (r^{-1}r)a = r^{-1}0_M \qquad \text{[by axiom-2 (iii)]}$$

$$\Rightarrow \qquad (1)a = 0_M \qquad \text{[By (i)]}$$

$$\Rightarrow \qquad a = 0_M \qquad [\because M \text{ is a unitary module}]$$

Thus, if r is a unit and $ra = 0_M$, then $a = 0_M$

Remark: In future, we shall write $a - b$ for $a + (-b)$ for any $a, b \in M$.

Theorem 2: Let M be an R-module. Then for all $a, b \in M$ and $r, s \in R$, we have

(i) $r(a - b) = ra - rb$ (ii) $(r - s)a = ra - sa$

Proof:

(i) For any $r \in R$ and any $a, b \in M$, we have

$$r(a - b) = r(a + (-b))$$

$$= ra + r(-b) \qquad \text{[by axiom-2 (i)]}$$

$$= ra + (-(rb)) \qquad \text{[by theorem 1 (iii)]}$$

$$= ra - rb$$

(ii) For any $r, s \in R$ and $a \in M$, we have

$$(r - s)a = [r + (-s)]a$$

$$= ra + (-s)a \qquad \text{[by axiom-2(ii)]}$$

$$= ra + (-(sa)) \qquad \text{[theorem 1 (ii)]}$$

$$= ra - sa$$

$\therefore (r - s)a = ra - sa$ for all $r, s \in R$ **and all** $a \in M$.

11.4 SUBMODULES

Continuing the pattern of other algebraic structures, i.e. groups, rings, fields, etc. where we have studied subgroups, subrings, etc. we shall now define submodules.

Submodules

A non-void subset N of R-module M is called a R-submodule (or simply submodule) of M, if

(i) $a - b \in N$ for all $a, b \in N$

(ii) $ra \in N$ for all $a \in N$ and all $r \in R$

In other words, an R-module of M is a subgroup N of the additive abelian group $(M, +)$ such that $ra \in N$ for all $r \in R$ and all $a \in N$.

Clearly $\{\underline{0}\}$ and M itself are R-submodules of M. These two submodules are called *trivial (improper) R-submodules of M* and any other R-submodule of M is called a *non-trivial (proper) R-submodule of M*.

Remark: Note that if N is an R-submodule of M, then N is also an R module in its own right.

Irreducible Module

An R-module M is said to be an irreducible module if its only submodules are improper submodules.

WORKED EXAMPLES

Example 1: If M is an abelian group, then any subgroup of M is a Z-submodule of M.

Solution: Let N be a subgroup of an additive abelian group M. Then,

$$a - b \in N \text{ for all } a, b \in N$$

Since every subgroup of an abelian group is abelian, therefore, N is an additive abelian group. But we know that every abelian group is a Z-module. Therefore, N is a Z-module. Consequently, $na \in N$ for all $n \in Z$ and for all $a \in N$.

Hence, N is a Z-submodule of M.

Example 2: If M is an R-module and $a \in M$, then the set $Ra = \{ra : r \in R\}$ is an R-submodule of M.

Solution: Let x be an arbitrary element of Ra. Then $x = ra$ for some $r \in R$. Since M is an R-module

$$\therefore \qquad r \in R \text{ and } a \in M \Rightarrow ra \in M \Rightarrow x \in M$$

Thus $x \in Ra \Rightarrow x \in M$

So $\qquad Ra \subset M$

Now $\qquad 0 \in R \Rightarrow 0a \in Ra \Rightarrow 0_M \in Ra \Rightarrow Ra \neq \phi$

Thus, Ra is a non-void subset of M.

In order to prove that Ra is an R-submodule of M, it remains to prove that for any $x, y \in Ra$

$$x - y \in Ra \text{ and for any } r \in R, \ x \in Ra, \ rx \in Ra$$

Let $x, y \in Ra$. Then there exist $r_1, r_2 \in R$ such that

$$x = r_1 a, y = r_2 a$$
$$\Rightarrow \qquad x - y = r_1 a - r_2 a = (r_1 - r_2)a$$
$$\Rightarrow \qquad x - y \in Ra \qquad\qquad [\because r_1 - r_2 \in R]$$

Thus, $x - y \in Ra$ for all $x, y \in Ra$

For any $r \in R$, we have

$$rx = r(r_1 a) = (r r_1)a \qquad\qquad \text{[by axiom-2 (iii)]}$$
$$\Rightarrow \qquad rx \in Ra \qquad\qquad [\because r r_1 \in R]$$

Thus, $rx \in Ra$ for all $r \in R$ and all $x \in Ra$.

Hence, Ra is an R-submodule of M.

Example 3: Let x be an arbitrary element of N. Then the set $N = \{ra + na : r \in R, n \in Z\}$ is a submodule of M.

Solution: Let x be an arbitrary element of N. Then $x = r_1 a + n_1 a$ for some $r_1 \in R$ and $n_1 \in Z$ Now,

$$r_1 \in R, \ a \in M$$
$$\Rightarrow \quad r_1 a \in M \text{ and } n_1 a \in M$$
$$\qquad\qquad [\because M \text{ is an } R\text{-module and } (M, +) \text{ is a group}]$$
$$\Rightarrow \quad r_1 a + n_1 a \in M$$
$$\Rightarrow \quad x \in M$$

Thus, $x \in N \Rightarrow x \in M$

$$\therefore \qquad N \subset M$$

Since $0 \in R$ and $0 \in Z$, therefore $0a + 0a = 0_M + 0_M \in N$

$\therefore N$ is a non-void subset of M.

Let x, y be any two elements of N. Then there exist $r_1, r_2 \in R$ and $n_1, n_2 \in Z$ such that

$$x = r_1 a + n_1 a, \ y = r_2 a + n_2 a$$
$$\Rightarrow \quad x - y = (r_1 a + n_1 a) - (r_2 a + n_2 a)$$
$$= (r_1 - r_2)a + (n_1 - n_2)a$$
$$= r_3 a + n_3 a, \text{ where } r_3 = r_1 - r_2 \in R \text{ and } n_3 = n_1 - n_2 \in Z$$
$$\Rightarrow \quad x - y \in N$$
$$\therefore \qquad x - y \in N \text{ for all } x, y \in N$$

Let $r \in R$ and $x \in N$. Then

$$x \in N \Rightarrow x = r_1 a + n_1 a \text{ for some } r_1 \in R \text{ and } n_1 \in R$$

Case I: When $n_1 \geq 0$

In this case, we have

$$rx = r(r_1 a + n_1 a)$$
$$= r(r_1 a) + r(n_1 a) \qquad\qquad [\because M \text{ is an } R\text{-module}]$$

$$= (rn_1)a + r(a + a + \ldots + a)$$
$$\underbrace{\qquad\qquad}_{n_1\text{-times}}$$

$$= (rn_1)a + ra + ra + \ldots + ra$$

$$= \underbrace{(rr_1 + r + r + \ldots + r)a}_{n_1\text{-times}}$$

$$= n_1 a, \text{ where } n_1 = \underbrace{r + r + \ldots + r}_{n_1\text{-times}} \in R$$

$$\Rightarrow \qquad rx = n_1 a + 0_M, \text{ where } 0_M \in M$$
$$\Rightarrow \qquad rx = n_1 a + 0a, \text{ where } 0 \in Z$$
$$\Rightarrow \qquad rx \in N$$

Case II: When $n_1 < 0$

In this case, we have

$$\Rightarrow \qquad rx = r(n_1 a + n_1 a)$$
$$= r(n_1 a) + r(n_1 a) \qquad\qquad\qquad [\because M \text{ is an } R\text{-module}]$$
$$= r(n_1 a) + r\underbrace{\{(-a) + (-a) + \ldots + (-a)\}}_{|n_1|\text{-times}}$$

$$= (rn_1)a + \underbrace{r(-a) + r(-a) + \ldots + (-a)}_{|n_1|\text{-times}} \quad [\because M \text{ is an } R\text{-module}]$$

$$= (rn_1)a + \underbrace{(-r)a + (-r)a + \ldots + (-r)a}_{}$$

$$= \underbrace{\{rn_1 + (-r) + (-r) + \ldots + (-r)\}a}_{|n_1|\text{-times}}$$

$$= n_2 a, \text{ where } n_2 = rn_1 + (-r) + (-r) + \ldots + (-r) \in R$$
$$= n_2 0 + 0_M, \text{ where } 0_M \in M$$
$$= n_2 a + 0a, \text{ where } 0 \in Z \qquad\qquad [\because 0_M = 0a]$$

$$\Rightarrow \qquad rx \in Z$$
$$\therefore \qquad rx \in Z \text{ for all } r \in R \text{ and all } x \in N$$

Hence, N is an R-submodule of M.

11.5 FINITELY GENERATED SUBMODULE

Submodule Generated by a Subset

Let M be an R-module, and let S be a subset of M. An R-submodule N of M is called the **R-submodule** generted by S, if

(i) $S \subset N$

(ii) If K is an R-submodule of M such that $K \subset S$, then $K \supset N$

In other words, the smallest R-module M generated by a subset S of M is denoted by $[S]$. If $S = \{a_1, a_2, \ldots, a_n\}$ is a finite set, then the R-submodule of M generated by S is also written as $[a_1, a_2, \ldots, a_n]$.

Remark: Since the smallest R-submodule of an R-module M containing the void set is 0_M, therefore the R-module of M generated by the void set is 0_M.

Finitely Generated Module

An R-module M is called a finitely generated module if there exists a finite subset $\{a_1, a_2, ..., a_n\}$ of M such that $M = [a_1, a_2, ..., a_n]$

The elements $a_1, a_2, ..., a_n$ are said to generate M.

WORKED EXAMPLES

Example 1: Let R be a ring with unity 1. If M is an R-module such that $a \in M$, then $Ra = \{ra : r \in R\}$ is the R-submodule of M generated by $\{a\}$, that is, $Ra = [a]$.

Solution: Clearly, Ra is an R-submodule of M. In order to prove that Ra is the R-submodule of M generated by $\{a\}$, it is sufficient to prove that Ra is the smallest R-submodule of M containing a.

Since $1 \in R$, therefore $1a = a \in Ra$.

Let N be an R-module of M containing a and x be an arbitrary element of Ra. Then $x = ra$ for some $r \in R$.

Now, $a \in N$ and $r \in R$

$\Rightarrow ra \in N$ $[\because N$ is R-module in its own]

$\Rightarrow x \in N$

Thus, $x \in Ra \Rightarrow x \in N$

So, $Ra \subset N$

Thus, every R-submodule of M containing 'a' contains Ra.

Hence, R_a is the smallest submodule of M containing a, i.e. $Ra = [a]$.

Example 2: Let M be an R-module and $a \in M$. Then the set $N = \{ra + na : r \in R, mn \in Z\}$ is the R-submodule of M generated by a, i.e. $N = [a]$. Further, if R has unity 1, then $N = Ra$.

Solution: N is an R-submodule of M.

Now,

$\qquad 0 \in R$ and $1 \in Z$

$\Rightarrow 0a + 1a = 0 + a \in N$

$\Rightarrow a \in N$

$\Rightarrow N$ is an R-submodule of M containing a.

Let K be an R-submodule of M containing a. Then $ra \in K$ for all $r \in R$ $a \in K$

Also, $na \in K$ for all $n \in Z$ $[\because (K, +)$ is an abelian group]

$\therefore ra + na \in K$ for all $r \in R$ and all $n \in Z$.

$\Rightarrow N \subset K$

Thus, N is the smallest R-submodule of M containing $\{a\}$.

Hence $N = [a]$.

Now, let R be a ring with unity and let x be an arbitrary element of N. Then, $x = ra + na$ for some $r \in R$ and for some $n \in Z$.

Now two cases arise.

Case I: When $n \geq 0$.

In this case, we have
$$x = ra + na = ra + n(1a)$$
$$\Rightarrow \quad x = ra + (\underbrace{1a + 1a + \ldots 1a}_{n\text{-times}})$$
$$\Rightarrow \quad x = (r + \underbrace{1 + 1 + \ldots 1}_{n\text{-times}})a$$
$$\Rightarrow \quad x = n_1 a, \text{ where } n_1 = r + \underbrace{1 + 1 + \ldots + 1}_{n\text{-times}}$$
$$\Rightarrow \quad x \in Ra$$

Case II: When $n < 0$

In this case, we have
$$x = ra + na = ra + (\underbrace{(-a) + (-a) + \ldots + (-a)}_{|n|\text{-times}})$$
$$\Rightarrow \quad x = ra + \underbrace{(-1)a + (-1)a + \ldots + (-1)a}_{|n|\text{-times}}$$
$$\Rightarrow \quad x = (r + \underbrace{(-1) + (-1) + \ldots + (-1)}_{|n|\text{-times}})a$$
$$\Rightarrow \quad x = n_2 a, \text{ where } n_2 = r + \underbrace{(-1) + (-1) + \ldots + (-1)}_{|n|\text{-times}} \in R$$
$$\Rightarrow \quad x \in Ra$$

Thus, in either case, we have $x \in Ra$. So $N \subset Ra$. Obviously, $Ra \subset N$ Hence $N = Ra$.

11.6 ALGEBRA OF SUBMODULES

Theorem 1: The intersection of any two R-submodules of an R-module M is an R-submodule of M.

Proof: Let N_1 and N_2 be two R-submodules of an R-module M. Then,
$$0_M \in N_1, 0_M \in N_2 \text{ and } N_1 \subset M, N_2 \supset M$$
$$\Rightarrow 0_M \in N_1 \cap N_2 \text{ and } N_1 \cap N_2 \subset M$$
$$\Rightarrow N_1 \cap N_2 \text{ is a non-void subset of } M.$$

Let a, b, be any two arbitrary elements of $N_1 \cap N_2$. Then
$$a, b \in N \cap N_2$$

$\Rightarrow$ $a, b \in N_1$ and $a, b \in N_2$

$\Rightarrow$ $a - b \in N_1$ and $a - b \in N_2$ [$\because$ N_1 and N_2 are R-submodules of M]

$\Rightarrow$ $a - b \in N_1 \cap N_2$

Thus, $a - b \in N_1 \cap N_2$ for all $a, b \in N_1 \cap N_2$

Let r be an arbitrary element of R. Then

$\quad r \in R, \ a \in N_1 \cap N_2$

$\Rightarrow$ $r \in R, \ a \in N_1$ and $a \in N_2$

$\Rightarrow$ $r \in R, a \in N_1$ and $a \in N_2$

$\Rightarrow$ $ra \in N_1$ and $ra \in N_2$ [$\because$ N_1 and N_2 are R-submodules of M]

$\Rightarrow$ $ra \in N_1 \cap N_2$

Thus, $ra \in N_1 \cap N_2$ for all $r \in R$ and $a \in N_1 \cap N_2$.

Hence $N_1 \cap N_2$ is an R-submodule of M.

Theorem 2: The instruction of an arbitrary family of R-submodules of an R-module M is an R-module of M.

Proof: Let $\{N_i : i \in I\}$ be an arbitary family of R-submodules of an R-module M. Here I is the index set such that for each $i \in I$, N_i is an R-submodule of M.

N_i is an R-submodule of M for all $i \in I$.

$\Rightarrow$ $0_M \in N_i$ and $N_i \subset M$ for all $i \in I$

$\Rightarrow$ $0_M \in \underset{i \in I}{\cap} N_i \subset M$

$\Rightarrow$ $\underset{i \in I}{\cap} N_i$ is a non-void subset of M.

Let a, b be any two arbitrary elements in $\underset{i \in I}{\cap} N_i$. Then

$\quad a, b \in \underset{i \in I}{\cap} N_i$

$\Rightarrow$ $a, b \in N_i$ for all $i \in I$

$\Rightarrow$ $a - b \in N_i$ for all $i \in I$ [$\because$ N_i is an R-submodule of M]

$\Rightarrow$ $a - b \in \underset{i \in I}{\cap} N_i$

Thus, $a - b \in \underset{i \in I}{\cap} N_i$ for all $a, b \in \underset{i \in I}{\cap} N_i$.

Let r be an arbitrary element of R and $a \in \underset{i \in I}{\cap} N_i$. Then

$\quad r \in R, \ a \in \underset{i \in I}{\cap} N_i$

$\Rightarrow$ $r \in R$ and $a \in N_i$ for all $i \in I$

$\Rightarrow$ $ra \in N_i$ for all $i \in I$ [$\because$ N_i is an R-submodule of M for all $i \in I$]

$\Rightarrow$ $ra \in \underset{i \in I}{\cap} N_i$

Thus, $ra \in \bigcap_{i \in I} N_i$ for all $a \in \bigcap_{i \in I} N_i$ and $r \in R$.

Hence, $\bigcap_{i \in I} N_i$ is an R-submodule of M.

Theorem 3: The union of any two R-submodules of an R-module M is an R-submodule of M iff one is contained in the other.

Proof: Let N_1 and N_2 be two R-submodules of an R-module M. We have to prove that $N_1 \cup N_2$ is an R-submodule of M iff either $N_1 \cup N_2$ or $N_2 \cup N_1$.

If $N_1 \cup N_2$, then $N_1 \cup N_2 = N_2$, which is an R-submodule of M.

If $N_2 \cup N_1$, then $N_1 \cup N_2 = N_1$, which is an R-submodule of M.

Hence, in either case, $N_1 \cup N_2$ is an R-submodule of M.

Conversely, suppose that $N_1 \cup N_2$ is an R-submodule of M. Then we have to prove that either $N_1 \subset N_2$ or $N_2 \subset N_1$.

If possible, let $N_1 \not\subset N_2$ and $N_2 \not\subset N_1$. Then

$N_1 \not\subset N_2 \Rightarrow$ There exists $a \in N_1$ such that $a \notin N_2$

and $N_2 \not\subset N_1 \Rightarrow$ There exists $b \in N_2$ such that $b \notin N_1$.

Now,

$a \in N_1, b \in N_2 \Rightarrow a,b \in N_1 \cup N_2$

$\Rightarrow a-b \in N_1 \cup N_2$ $\qquad [\because N_1 \cup N_2$ is an R-submodule of $M]$

$\Rightarrow a-b \in N_1$ or $a-b \in N_2$

If $a-b \in N_1$, then

$\qquad a-(a-b) \in N_1 \qquad [\because a \in N_1$ and N_1 is an R-submodule of $M]$

$\Rightarrow b \in N_1$, which is a contradiciton. $\qquad [\because b \notin N_1]$

Again, if $a-b \in N_2$, then

$\qquad (a-b)+b \in N_2 \qquad [\because b \in N_2$ and N_2 is an R-submodule of $M]$

$\Rightarrow a \in N_2$, which is a contradiction. $\qquad [\because a \notin N_2]$

Since the contradictions arise by assuming that $N_1 \not\subset N_2$ and $N_2 \not\subset N_1$, hence, either $N_1 \subset N_2$ or $N_2 \subset N_1$.

Theorem 4: Let S be a subset of an R-module M. Then the intersection of the family of R-submodules of M containing S is the R-module generated by S.

Proof: Let $\{N_i : i \in I\}$ be the family of R-submodules of M containing S. Here I is the index set such that for each $i \in I$ there is an R-submodule of M containing S. By Theorem 2, $\bigcap_{i \in I} N_i$ is an R-module of M. Since $S \subset N_i$ for all $i \in I$, therefore $S \subset \bigcap_{i \in I} N_i$. Thus, $\bigcap_{i \in I} N_i$ is an R-submodule of M containing S.

Let K be an R-submodule of M containing S. Then K is one of the members of the family. Consequently, $\bigcap_{i \in I} N_i \subset K$.

Hence, $\bigcap_{i \in I} N_i$ is the smallest R-submodule of M containing S, i.e. $\bigcap_{i \in I} N_i = [S]$.

Sum of Submodules

Let N_1 and N_2 be two R-modules of an R-module M. Then their sum $N_1 + N_2$ is the set of all elements of the form $a_1 + a_2$, where $a_1 \in N_1$ and $a_2 \in N_2$,

i.e. $$N_1 + N_2 = \{a_1 + a_2 : a_1 \in N_1 \text{ and } a_2 \in N_2\}$$

Theorem 5: The sum of two R-submodules of an R-module is an R-submodule of M.

Proof: Let N_1 and N_2 be two R-submodules of an R-module M. Then by definition

$$N_1 + N_2 = \{a_1 + a_2 : a_1 \in N_1, a_2 \in N_2\}$$

Since N_1 and N_2 are R-submodules of M, therefore

$0_M \in N_1$, $0_M \in N_2$

$\Rightarrow 0_M + 0_M \in N_1 + N_2$

$\Rightarrow 0_M \in N_1 + N_2$

$\Rightarrow N_1 + N_2$ is non-void

Let x be an arbitrary element of $N_1 + N_2$. Then there exists $a_1 \in N_1, a_2 \in N_2$ such that $x = a_1 + a_2$.

Now,

$\quad a_1 \in N_1$ and $a_2 \in N_2$

$\Rightarrow a_1 \in M$ and $a_2 \in M$ $\qquad [\because N_1 \subset M, N_2 \subset M]$

$\Rightarrow a_1 + a_2 \in M$ $\qquad\qquad [\because (M, +) \text{ is a group}]$

$\Rightarrow x \in M$

$\therefore \ x \in N_1 + N_2$

$\Rightarrow x \in M$

$\Rightarrow N_1 + N_2 \subset M$.

So $N_1 + N_2$ is a non-void subset of M.

Let $x = a_1 + a_2, y = b_1 + b_2 \in N_1 + N_2$. Then $a_1, b_1 \in N_1$ and $a_2, b_2 \in N_2$.

$\therefore \quad x - y = (a_1 + a_2) - (b_1 + b_2)$

$\Rightarrow x - y = (a_1 - b_1) + (a_2 - b_2)$

$\qquad\qquad$ [using commutativity and associativity of addition on M]

Since N_1 and N_2 are R-submodules of M, therefore

$$a_1, b_1 \in N_1 \Rightarrow a_1 - b_1 \in N_1$$

and
$$a_2, b_2 \in N_2 \Rightarrow a_2 - b_2 \in N_2$$

$$\therefore (a_1 - b_1) + (a_2 - b_2) \in N_1 + N_2$$

$$\Rightarrow \quad x - y \in N_1 + N_2$$

So $\quad x - y \in N_1 + N_2$ for all $x, y \in N_1 + N_2$

Let r be an arbitrary element of R. Then

$$rx = r(a_1 + a_2) = ra_1 + ra_2$$

Since N_1 and N_2 are R-submodules of M, therefore

and
$$\left. \begin{array}{l} r \in Ra_1, a_1 \in N_1 \Rightarrow ra_1 \in N_1 \\ r \in Ra_2, a_2 \in N_2 \Rightarrow ra_2 \in N_2 \end{array} \right\} \Rightarrow rx = ra_1 + ra_2 \in N_1 + N_2$$

Thus, $rx \in N_1 + N_2$ for all $r \in R$ and all $x \in N_1 + N_2$.

Hence $N_1 + N_2$ is an R-module of M.

Theorem 6: Let N_1 and N_2 be R-submodules of an R-module M. Then $N_1 + N_2$ is the smallest R-submodule of M containing $N_1 \cup N_2$, that is, $N_1 + N_2 = [N_1 \cup N_2]$.

Proof: Clearly, $N_1 + N_2$ is an R-submodules of M.   [*see* Theorem 5]

Let x be an arbitrary element of $N_1 \cup N_2$. Then $x \in N_1$ or $x \in N_2$.

If $x \in N_1$, then $x = x + 0_M \in N_1 + N_2$, where $0_M \in N_2$

If $x \in N_2$, then $x = x + 0_M \in N_1 + N_2$, where $0_M \in N_1$

Thus, $x \in N_1 \cup N_2 \Rightarrow x \in N_1 + N_2$ $\therefore N_1 \cup N_2 \subset N_1 + N_2$

Let K be an R-submodule of M containing $N_1 \cup N_2$, then it contains $N_1 + N_2$. Hence, $N_1 + N_2$ is the smallest R-submodule of M containing $N_1 \cup N_2$.

Theorem 7: Let $N_1, N_2, ..., N_k$ be R-submodules of an R-module M. Then $N_1 + N_2 + ... + N_k = \{a_1 + a_2 + ... + a_k : a_i \in N_i, i = 1, ..., k\}$ is also an R-submodule of M.

Proof: For any a in a R-module M, we know that, Ra is an R-submodule of M. From above theorem, it follows that if $(a_1, a_2, ..., a_n)$ is a list of n elements in a R-module M, then $Ra_1 + Ra_2 + ... + Ra_n$ is an R-submodule of M.

Direct Sum of Submodules

An R-module M is said to be the direct sum of its two R-submodules N_1 and N_2 if each element $a \in M$ is uniquely expressed as $a = a_1 + a_2$, where $a \in N_1$ and $a \in N_2$. M is said to be the direct sum of its R-submodules N_1, N_2, ..., N_k if each element $a \in M$ can be expressed uniquely as

$$a = a_1 + a_2 + ... + a_k, \text{ where } a_1 \in N_i, \ i = 1, 2, ..., k$$

If M is the direct sum of its R-modules $N_1, N_2,..., N_k$, then we write

$$M = N_1 \oplus N_2 \oplus ... \oplus N_k$$

Theorem 8: Let $N_1, N_2,..., N_k$ be R-submodules of an R-module M. Then the following are equivalent.

(i) $M = N_1 \oplus N_2 \oplus ... \oplus N_k$

(ii) $\displaystyle\sum_{i=1}^{k} a_i = 0_M \Rightarrow a_i = 0_M$ for all $i \in \underline{k}$

(iii) $\displaystyle N_i \cap \sum_{\substack{j=1 \\ j \neq 1}}^{k} N_j = \{0_M\}, i \in \underline{k}$

Proof: In order to prove the equivalence of three statements, it is sufficient to show that (i) $\Rightarrow$ (ii) $\Rightarrow$ (iii) $\Rightarrow$ (i).

(i) $\Rightarrow$ (ii)

Let M be the direct sum of $N_1, N_2,..., N_k$ and let $\displaystyle\sum_{i=1}^{k} a_i = 0_M$

Since each element in M has a unique representation in terms of elements of $N_1, N_2,..., N_k$

$\therefore \quad \displaystyle\sum_{i=1}^{k} a_i = 0_M = 0_M + 0_M + ... + 0_M \Rightarrow a_i = 0_M$ for all $i \in \underline{k}$

(ii) $\Rightarrow$ (iii).

Let x be an arbitrary element of $\displaystyle N_i \cap \sum_{\substack{j=1 \\ j \neq 1}}^{k} N_j$. Then

$x \in N_i$ and $x \in \displaystyle\sum_{\substack{j=1 \\ j \neq 1}}^{k} N_j$

$\Rightarrow$ There exist elements $a_1 \in A_1, a_2 \in A_2,..., a_i \in A_i,..., a_k \in A_n$ such that $x = a_1 + a_2 + ... + a_{i-1} + a_{i+1} + ... + a_k$ and $x - a_i$.

$\Rightarrow a_i = a_1 + a_2 + ... + a_{i-1} + a_{i+1} + ... + a_k$

$\Rightarrow a_1 + a_2 + ... + a_{i-1} + (-a_1) + a_{i+1} + ... + a_k = 0_M$

$\Rightarrow a_1 = a_2 = ... = a_{i-1} = (-a_1) = a_{i+1} = ... = a_k = 0_M$ \quad [from (ii)]

$\Rightarrow x = 0_M$

Since x is an arbitrary element $x \in \sum_{\substack{j=1 \\ j\neq 1}}^{k} N_j$, therefore

$$x \in \sum_{\substack{j=1 \\ j\neq 1}}^{k} N_j \implies x = 0_M \text{ for all } i = 1, 2, ..., k$$

Hence, $N_i \cap \sum_{\substack{j=1 \\ j\neq 1}}^{k} N_j = \{0_M\}$ for all $i = 1, 2, ..., k$.

(iii) $\implies$ (i)

Let $N_i \cap \sum_{\substack{j=1 \\ j\neq 1}}^{k} N_j = \{0_M\}$ for all $i = 1, 2, ..., k$. Then we have to show that

each element in M has a unique representation in terms of elements in N_1, $N_2, ..., N_k$.

Let a be an arbitrary element of M such that

$$a = a_1 + a_2 + ... + a_k, a = b_1 + b_2 + ... + b_k, a_i, b_i \in N_i \text{ for } i = 1, 2, ..., k$$

Then

$$a_1 + a_2 + ... + a_k = b_1 + b_2 + ... + b_k$$

$$\implies (a_1 - b_1) + (a_2 - b_2) + ... + (a_k - b_k) = 0_M$$

[by commutativity and associativity of addition on A]

$$\implies a_i - b_i = -\sum_{\substack{j=1 \\ j\neq 1}}^{k} (a_j - b_j)$$

$$\implies a_i - b_i = -\sum_{\substack{j=1 \\ j\neq 1}}^{k} \{-(a_j - b_j)\}$$

$$\implies a_i - b_i = \sum_{\substack{j=1 \\ j\neq 1}}^{k} N_j \text{ for all } i = 1, 2, ..., k \quad [\because -(a_j - b_j) \in N_j \text{ for all } j]$$

$$\implies a_i - b_i = N_i \cap \sum_{\substack{j=1 \\ j\neq 1}}^{k} N_j \text{ for all } i = 1, 2, ..., k$$

$$[\because a_j - b_j \in N_i \text{ for all } i]$$

$\Rightarrow a_i - b_i = 0_M$ for $i = 1,2,...,k.$ $\qquad [\because N_i \cap \sum_{\substack{j=1 \\ j \neq 1}}^{k} N_j = \{\underline{0}\}$ for all $i]$

$\Rightarrow a_i = b_i$ for all $i = 1,2,...,k.$

Thus, $a \in M$ has a unique represenation. Hence M is the direct sum of $N_1, N_2, N_3,..., N_k$

Complement of a Submodule

Let M be an R-module and N_1 be an R-submodule of M. Then an R-submodule N_2 of M is said to be complement of N_1 if

$$M = N_1 \oplus N_2$$

Independent Submodules

Let $N_1, N_2,..., N_n$ be R-submodules of an R-module M. Then $N_1, N_2,...,N_n$ are said to be independent if

$$N_i \cap \sum_{\substack{j=1 \\ j \neq 1}}^{n} N_j = \{0_M\} \text{ for all } i = 1,2,...,n.$$

Theorem 9: Let $N_1, N_2,..., N_k$ be R-submodules of an R-module M such that $M = N_1 \oplus N_2 \oplus ... \oplus N_n$. Then the following are equivalent.

 (i) $M = N_1 \oplus N_2 \oplus ... \oplus N_n$

 (ii) $N_1, N_2,..., N_n$ are independent.

 (iii) For each $a_i \in N_i, \sum_{i=1}^{k} a_i = 0_M \Rightarrow a_i = 0_M$

Proof: *See* Theorem 8.

Theorem 10: Let R be a ring with unity 1 and M be an R-module. If M is generated by a set $\{a_1, a_2,..., a_n\}$, then $M = \{r_1 a_1 + r_2 a_2 + ... + r_n a_n : r_1 \in R\}$ that is, $M = Ra_1 + Ra_2 + ... + Ra_n = \sum_{i=1}^{n} Ra_i$

Proof: Since M is generated by the set $\{a_1, a_2,..., a_n\}$, therefore M is the smallest R-submodule of itself containing $\{a_1, a_2,..., a_n\}$. In order to prove the theorem, it is sufficient to prove that $\sum_{i=1}^{n} Ra_i = M$. Then

$m_1 = r_1 a_1 + ... + r_n a_n, \ m_2 = s_1 a_1 + ... + s_n a_n$ for some $r_i, s_i \in R$

$\therefore \ m_1 - m_2 = (r_1 a_1 + ... + r_n a_n) - (s_1 a_1 + ... + s_n a_n)$

$$\Rightarrow m_1 - m_2 = (r_1 - s_1)a_1 + \ldots + (r_n - s_n)a_n \in \sum_{i=1}^{n} Ra_i \quad [\because r_i - s_i \in R]$$

$$\Rightarrow m_1 - m_2 \in \sum_{i=1}^{n} Ra_i$$

Thus, $m_1 - m_2 \in \sum_{i=1}^{n} Ra_i$ for all $m_1, m_2 \in \sum_{i=1}^{n} Ra_i$

Let $m = \sum r_i a_i \in \sum_{i=1}^{n} Ra_i$ and $r \in R$.

Then

$$rm = r\left(\sum_{i=1}^{n} ra_i\right) = r(r_1 a_1 + \ldots + r_n a_n)$$

$$\Rightarrow rm = r(r_1 a) + \ldots + r(r_n a) = (rr_1)a + \ldots + (rr_n)a \in \sum_{i=1}^{n} Ra_i$$

Thus, $rm \in \sum_{i=1}^{n} Ra_i$ for all $r \in R$

Also, $a_i = 1a_1 = 0a_1 + 0a_2 + \ldots + 0a_{i-1} + 1a_{i+1} + \ldots + 0a_n \in \sum_{i=1}^{n} Ra_i$ for all

$i \in \underline{n}$

Hence, $\sum_{i=1}^{n} Ra_i$ is an R-submodule of M containing $\{a_1, a_2, \ldots, a_n\}$

Consequently, we have $M = \sum_{i=1}^{n} Ra_i$

Theorem 1: Let $\{N_i : i \in n\}$ be a family of R-submodules of an R-module M. Then $\sum_{i=1}^{n} N_i$ is the smallest R-submodule of M containing $\underset{i \in n}{\cup}$.

That is $\sum_{i=1}^{n} N_i = [\underset{i \in n}{\cup} N_i]$.

Proof: It is generalization of Theorem 6.

11.7 QUOTIENT MODULES

Like other algebraic structures, we also have quotient modules or factor modules. In this section, we will develop the structure of a quotient module and study some of its properties.

Let N be an R-submodule of an R-module M. Then N is additive subgroup of the additive abelian group M. Let M/N be the set of all left cosets (since M is an additive abelian group, therefore there is no distinction between left and right cosets of N in M and we may simply call cosets) of N in M, i.e.

$$M/N = \{a + N : a \in M\}$$

Our main objective in this section is to the set M/N with the structure of an R-module. For this purpose, we define addition and scalar multiplication on M/N as follows:

Addition on M/N: For any $a + N, b + N \in M / N$, we define

$$(a + N) + (b + N) = (a + b) + N$$

Scalar multipliction on M/N: If $a + N \in M / N$ and $r \in R$, then we define scalar multiplication on M/N as follows:

$$r(a + N) = ra + N$$

Equality of elements in M/N: Since N is an additive abelian subgroup of the additive abelian group M, therefore for any $a + N, b + N \in M / N$

$$a + N = b + N \Leftrightarrow a - b \in N$$

Thus, we have defined addition and scalar multiplication on M/N and also the equality of any two elements of M/N. Now, we shall establish that M/N possesses a module structure under addition and scalar multiplication defined above.

Theorem 1: Let N be an R-module of an R-module M. Then the set

$$M/N = \{a + N : a \in M\}$$

is an R-module for the addition and scalar multiplication defined as follows:

$$(a + N) + (b + N) = (a + b) + N \text{ and}$$
$$r(a + N) = ra + N \text{ for all } a + N, b + N \in M / N \text{ and for all } r \in R.$$

Proof: First of all we will show that, above rules for addition and scalar multiplication on M/N are well defined rules, i.e. are independent of the particular representative chosen to defined a coset.

Let $a + N = a' + N$ and $b + N = b' + N$, where $a, b, a', b' \in M$. Then

$$a + N = a' + N \Rightarrow a - a' \in N \text{ and } b + N = a - a' \in N \text{ and}$$
$$b + N = b' + N \Rightarrow b - b' \in N$$

Now,

$$a - a' \in N, \; b - b' \in N$$
$$\Rightarrow \quad (a - a') + (b - b') \in N \qquad\qquad [\because (N, +) \text{ is a group}]$$
$$\Rightarrow \quad (a + b) - (a' + b') \in N$$
$$\Rightarrow \quad (a + b) + N = (a' + b') + N \qquad [\because (N, +) \text{ is subgroup of } (M, +)]$$
$$\Rightarrow \quad (a + N) + (b + N) = (a' + N) + (b' + N)$$

Thus,

$$a + N = a' + N \text{ and } b + N = a' + N$$

$\Rightarrow \quad (a+N)+(b+N) = (a'+N)+(b'+N)$ for all $a,b,a',b'\in M$

So, above defined addition of M/N is well defined.

And

$$r\in R, a-a'\in N$$

$\Rightarrow \quad r(a-a')\in N$ $\qquad\qquad$ [$\because N$ is an R-submodule]

$\Rightarrow \quad ra-ra'\in N$

$\Rightarrow \quad ra+N = ra'+N$ $\qquad\qquad$ [$\because (N,+)$ is subgroup of $(M,+)$]

Therefore, scalar multiplication on M/N is well defined.

M/N is an abelian group under addition:

Associativity: For any $a+N, b+N, c+N \in M/N$, we have

$$\{(a+N)+(b+N)\}+(c+N) = \{(a+b)+N\}+(c+N)$$
$$= \{(a+b)+c\}+N$$
$$= \{(a+(b+c)\}+N$$
$$= (a+N)+(b+c)+N)$$
$$= (a+N)+\{(b+N)+(c+N)\}$$

So, addition is associative on M/N.

Commutativity: For any $a+N, b+N \in M/N$, we have

$(a+N)+(b+N) = (a+b)+N$

$\qquad\qquad = (b+a)+N$ $\qquad$ [by commutativity of addition on M]

$\qquad\qquad = (b+N)+(a+N)$

So, addition is commutative on M/N.

Existence of additive identity: Since $0_M \in M$, therefore

$$0_M + N = N \in M/N.$$

Now,

$(a+N)+(0_M + N) = (a+0_M)+N = (a+N)$ for all $a+N\in M/N$

$(a+N)+(0_M + N) = a+N = (0_M + N)+(a+N)$

for all $a+N \in M/N$

So, $0_M + N = N$. This is the identity element for addition on M/N.

Existence of additive inverse: Let $a+N$ be an arbitrary element in M/N. Then

$$a\in M \Rightarrow a\in M \Rightarrow (-a)+N \in M/N$$

Thus, for each $a+N\in M/N$ there exists $(-a)+N \in M/N$ such that

$(a+N)+((-a)+N = [a+(-a)]+N = 0_M + N = N$

$\Rightarrow \quad (a+N)+((-a)+N) = 0_M + N + ((-a)+N)+(a+N)$

$\qquad\qquad$ [by commutativity of addition on M/N]

So, each $a+N\in M/N$ has its additive inverse $(-a+N)\in M/N$

Hence M/N is an additive abelian group.

For any $a+N, b+N\in M/N$ and $r,s\in R$, we have

(i) $r[(a+N)+(b+N)] = r[(a+b)+N]$
$$= [r(a+b)]+N$$
$$= (ra+rb)+N \qquad \text{[by axiom-2 (i) in } M]$$
$$= (ra+N)+(rb+N) \text{ [by. def. of add. on } M/N]$$
$$= r(a+N)+r(b+N)$$
$$\text{[by def. of scalar mult. on } M/N]$$

(ii) $(r+s)(a+N) = (r+s)a+N \qquad \text{[by def. of scalar mult. on } M/N]$
$$= (ra+sa)+N \qquad \text{[by axiom-2 (ii) in } M]$$
$$= (ra+N)+(sa+N) \qquad \text{[by def. add.on } M/N]$$
$$= r(a+N)+s(a+N)$$
$$\text{[by def. of scalar mult. on } M/N]$$

(iii) $rs(a+N) = (rs)a+N$
$$= r(sa)+N \qquad \text{[by axiom-2(iii) in } M]$$
$$= r[sa+N]$$
$$= r[s(a+N)] \qquad \text{[by def. of scalar mult. on } M/N]$$
Hence M/N is an R-module.

Quotient Module

Let M be an R-module and N be an R-submodule of M. Then the set M/N $=\{a+N:a\in M\}$ is an R-module for the addition and scalar multiplication defined as follows:
$$(a+N)+(b+N) = (a+b)+N$$
$$r(a+N) = ra+N$$
for all $a+N, b+N \in M/N$ for all $r \in R$.

This R-module is called a quotient module (or a factor module) of M by N.

EXERCISE

1. Mark each of the following as true or false:
   (i) If M is an R-module over a ring R with unity 1, then
   $$(-1)a = -a = a(-1) \text{ for all } a \in M.$$
   (ii) Every module has exactly two submodules.
   (iii) Every module has at least two submodules.
   (iv) The union of two submodules of an R-module is a submodule.
2. Let M be an R-module. Then prove that
   $$n(ra) = r(na) \text{ for all } n \in Z, r \in R \text{ and } a \in M.$$
3. Show that a left (right) ideal I in a ring R is a left (right) R-module.
4. Let M be an R-module and $RM = \left\{ \sum_i r_i a_i : r_i \in R, a_i \in M \right\}$. Then prove that RM is an R-module of M.
5. Which of the following are R-submodules of R^3?

   (i) $\{(a_1,a_2,a_3): a_1 + a_2 + a_3 = 0\}$

   (ii) $\{(a_1,a_2,a_3): a_1 + a_2 + a_3 = 1\}$

   (iii) $\{(a_1,a_2,a_3): a_1 = 1\}$.

6. Let M be an R-module. Show that the set $\{r \in R : rM = \{0_M\}\}$ is a left ideal of R.

7. For any ring R, prove that an R-submodule of the R-module R is exactly the same thing as a left ideal of R.

8. Let R be a ring with unity and M be an R-module (not a unitary module). Then there exists $0_M \neq a \in M$ such that $r_a = 0_M$ for all $r \in R$.

9. Let A, B and C be R-modules of an R-module M such that $A \subset B$. Show that $A \cap B(B+C) = B + A \cap C$.

   Give an example of three R-modules A, B, C of an R-module M such that $A \cap B(B+C) \neq B + A \cap C$.

10. Let $A \oplus B$ and $C \oplus D$ be direct sums of submodules of M such that $A \oplus B$ $A \oplus B = C \oplus D$.

Answers

   1. (i) T (ii) F (iii) T (iv) F 5. (i)

11.8 R-HOMOMORPHISMS

After defining submodules and quotient modules, we now define homomorphisms from one module to another module. This is done only for modules over the same ring.

R-Homomorphism: Let M and N be R-modules. A mapping f from M to N is called an **R-homomorphism** (or an R-linear mapping or linear transformation) of M into N if

   (i) $f(a+b) = f(a) + f(b)$

   (ii) $f(ra) = rf(a)$ for all $a,b \in M$ and all $r \in R$.

   This definition stipulates that an R-homomorphism is a homomorphism of abelian groups.

   The set of all R-homomorphisms of an R-module M into an R-module N is denoted by $\text{Hom}_R(M, N)$.

Example 1: Let M be an R-module. Then the mapping $I_M: M \to M$ defined by

$$I_M(a) = a \text{ for all } a \in M$$

is an R-homomorphism of M onto M.

Solution: For all $a,b \in M$ and all $r \in R$, we have

$$I_M(a+b) = a+b = I_M(a) + I_M(b)$$

and $I_M(ra) = ra = rI_M(a)$

Further, $I_M : M \to M$ is surjective.

Hence, I_M is an R-homomorphism of M onto itself.

Remark: I_M is called the identity endomorphism of M.

Example 2: Let M be an R-module. Then the mapping $\hat{0} : M \to M$ defined by $\hat{0}(a) = 0_M$ for all $a \in M$ is an R-homomorphism of M into M.

Solution: For all $a, b \in M$ and all $r \in R$, we have

$$\hat{0}(a+b) = 0_M = 0_M + 0_M = \hat{0}(a) + \hat{0}(b)$$

$$\hat{0}(ra) = 0_M = r(0_M) = r(\hat{0}(a)).$$

Hence, $\hat{0} : M \to M$ is an R-homomorphism.

This mapping $\hat{0} : M \to M$ is called the **zero endomorphism** of M.

Example 3: Let M be an R-module and r be some fixed element of R which is a commutative ring. Then the mapping $f : M \to M$ given by

$$f(a) = ra \text{ for all } a \in M$$

is an R-homomorphism of M into itself.

Solution: Let a, b be any two elements of M. Then

$$f(a+b) = r(a+b) = ra + rb \qquad \text{[by axiom-2(i)]}$$

$$\Rightarrow \quad f(a+b) = f(a) + f(b)$$

Let $a \in M$ and $s \in R$. Then

$$f(sa) = r(sa) = (rs)a \qquad \text{[by axiom-2 (iii)]}$$

$$= (sr)a \qquad \text{[}\because R \text{ is commutative ring]}$$

$$= s(ra) \qquad \text{[by axiom-2(iii)]}$$

$$\Rightarrow \quad f(sa) = sf(a)$$

Hence, f is an R-homomorphism of M into itself.

Theorem 1: Let M and M' be two R-modules and $f : M \to M'$ be an R-homomorphism. Then

(i) $f(0_M) = 0_{M'}$

(ii) $f(-a) = -f(a)$ for all $a \in M$

(iii) $f(a-b) = f(a) - f(b)$ for all $a, b \in M$

Proof:

(i) We have

$$0_M + 0_M = 0_M$$

$$\Rightarrow \quad f(0_M + 0_M) = f(0_M)$$

$$\Rightarrow f(0_M) + f(0_M) = f(0_M) \qquad \text{[}\because f \text{ is an } R\text{-homomorphism]}$$

$$\Rightarrow f(0_M) + f(0_M) = f(0_M) + 0_{M'}$$

$$\text{[}\because 0_{M'} \in M' \text{ is the additive identity]}$$

$$\Rightarrow \qquad f(0_M) = 0_{M'} \qquad \text{[by cancellation laws in } M']$$

(ii) For all $a \in M$, we have

$$a + (-a) = 0_M$$
$$\Rightarrow \quad f(a + (-a)) = f(0_M)$$
$$\Rightarrow \quad f(a) + f(-a) = 0_{M'}$$
$$\Rightarrow \quad f(-a) = -f(a)$$

Thus, $\quad f(-a) = -f(a)$ for all $a \in M$.

(iii) For all $a, b \in M$, we have

$$f(a - b) = f(a + (-b))$$
$$= f(a) + f(-b)$$
$$= f(a) - f(b) \qquad \text{[from (ii)]}$$

Thus, $\quad f(a - b) = f(a) - f(b)$ for all $a, b \in M$.

Kernel of *R*-Homomorphism

Let M and M' be R-modules and $f : M \rightarrow M'$ be an R-homomorphism.

Then the set $K = \{x \in M : f(x) = 0_{M'}\}$ is called the **kernel of *f*** and is denoted by Ker (f).

By theorem 1, $f(0_M) = 0_{M'}$. Therefore, $0_M \in \mathrm{Ker}(f)$.

Obviously, $\mathrm{Ker}(f) = f^{-1}\{0_{M'}\}$.

Homomorphic Image

Let $f : M \rightarrow M'$ be an R-homomorphism of an R-module M into an R-module M'. Then the set $f(M) = \{f(x) : x \in M\}$ is called the **homomorphic image of *M*** under f and is denoted by $I_m(f)$.

Theorem 2: Let $f : M \rightarrow M'$ be an R-homomorphism of an R-module M into an R-module M'. Then

(i) $\mathrm{Ker}(f) = \{a \in M : f(a) = 0_{M'}\}$ is an R-submodule of M.

(ii) $I_m(f) = \{f(a) : a \in M\}$ is an R-submodule of M'.

Proof:

(i) Since $f(0_M) = 0_{M'}$, therefore $0_M \in \mathrm{Ker}(f)$. Consequently, Ker (f) is a non-void subset of M. Let a, b be any arbitrary elements of Ker(f). Then

$$f(a) = 0_{M'} \; f(b) = 0_{M'}$$
$$\therefore \quad f(a - b) = f(a) - f(b) = 0_{M'} - 0_{M'} = 0_{M'}$$
$$\Rightarrow a - b \in \mathrm{Ker}(f)$$

Thus, $a - b \in \mathrm{Ker}(f)$ for all $a, b \in \mathrm{Ker}(f)$.

Let $r \in R$ and $a \in \mathrm{Ker}(f)$. Then

$$f(ra) = rf(a) \qquad \text{[}\because f \text{ is an } R\text{-homomorphism]}$$
$$= r0_{M'} \qquad \text{[}\because a \in \mathrm{Ker} \Rightarrow f(a) = 0_{M'}\text{]}$$
$$\Rightarrow \quad f(ra) = 0_{M'} \Rightarrow ra \in \mathrm{Ker}(f)$$

Thus, $ra \in \text{Ker}(f)$ for all $a \in \text{Ker}(f)$ and all $r \in R$.

Hence, $\text{Ker}(f)$ is an R-module of M.

(ii) Since $0_M \in M$, therefore $f(0_M) = 0_{M'} \in I_m(f)$. Thus, $I_m(f)$ is a non-void subset of M'.

Let a', b' be any two elements in $I_m(f)$. Then there exist $a, b \in M$ such that $f(a) = a'$ and $f(b) = b'$.

Now,

$$a' - b' = f(a) - f(b)$$
$$\Rightarrow \qquad a' - b' = f(a - b) \qquad\qquad [\because f \text{ is an } R\text{-homomorphism}]$$
$$\Rightarrow \qquad a' - b' \in I_m(f) \qquad\qquad\qquad [\because a - b \in M]$$

Thus, $a' - b' \in I_m(f)$ for all $a', b' \in I_m(f)$.

Let $r \in R$ and $a' \in I_m(f)$. Then there exists $a \in M$ such that $f(a) = a'$.

Now $\qquad\qquad ra' = rf(a) = f(ra) \qquad [\because f \text{ is an } R\text{-homomorphism}]$
$$\Rightarrow \qquad\qquad ra' \in I_m(f) \qquad\qquad\qquad [\because ra \in M]$$

Thus, $ra' \in I_m(f)$ for all $a' \in I_m(f)$ and all $r \in R$

Hence, $I_m(f)$ is an R-submodule of M'.

Theorem 3: If $f : M \to M'$ is an R-homomorphism of an R-module M into an R-module M', then f is an R-monomorphism iff $\text{Ker}(f) = \{0_M\}$.

Proof: First, let f be an R-monomorphism of M into M' and a be an arbitrary element of $\text{Ker}(f)$. Then

$$f(a) = 0_{M'}$$
$$\Rightarrow \quad f(a) = f(0_M) \qquad\qquad\qquad\qquad [\because f(0_M) = 0_{M'}]$$
$$\Rightarrow \qquad a = 0_M \qquad\qquad\qquad\qquad [\because f \text{ is an injective map}]$$

Since a is an arbitrary element of $\text{Ker}(f)$,

$$a \in \text{Ker}(f) \Rightarrow a - 0_M \in \text{Ker}(f) \text{ for all } a \in \text{Ker}(f)$$

Hence $\text{Ker}(f) = \{0_M\}$

Conversely, let f be an R-homomorphism of an R-module M into an R-module M' such that $\text{Ker}(f) = \{0_M\}$. We have to prove that f is an R-monomorphism.

Let a, b be any two elements of M such that $f(a) = f(b)$. Then

$$f(a) - f(b) = 0_{M'}$$
$$\Rightarrow \qquad f(a - b) = 0_{M'} \qquad\qquad\qquad [\text{by Theorem 1 (iii)}]$$
$$\Rightarrow \quad a - b \in \text{Ker}(f)$$
$$\Rightarrow \qquad\qquad a - b = 0_M \qquad\qquad\qquad [\because \text{Ker} f = \{0_M\}]$$
$$\Rightarrow \qquad\qquad a = b$$

Thus, $\qquad f(a) = f(b) \Rightarrow a = b$ for all $a, b \in M$.

Hence f is an R-monomorphism.

Theorem 4: Let M and M' be R-modules and $f : M \to M'$, $g : M \to M'$ be R-homomorphisms. Then $f + g : M \to M'$ given by $(f + g)(a) = f(a) + g(a)$ for all $a \in M$ is also an R-homomorphism.

Proof: Let a, b be arbitrary elements of M. Then

$$(f + g)(a + b) = (f + g)(a) + (f + g)(b)$$
$$= \left[f(a) + g(a) \right] + \left[f(b) + g(b) \right]$$
$$= \left[(f(a) + f(b)) + \left[g(a) + g(b) \right] \right.$$

$$\text{[by comm. and assoc. of add. on } M']$$
$$= f(a + b) + g(a + b) \qquad \text{[by definition of } f + g]$$

Thus, $(f + g)(a + b) = f(a + b) + g(a + b)$ for all $a, b \in M$.

Let r be an arbitrary element of R and let a be an arbitrary element of M. Then

$$(f + g)(ra) = f(ra) + g(ra) \qquad \text{[by definition of } f + g]$$
$$= rf(a) + rg(a) \quad [\because f \text{ and } g \text{ are } R\text{-homomorphisms}]$$
$$= r[f(a) + g(a)] \qquad \text{[by axiom-2 (i)]}$$
$$= r(f + g)(a) \qquad \text{[by definition of } f + g]$$

Thus, $(f + g)(ra) = r(f + g)(a)$ for all $r \in R$ and all $a \in M$

Hence $f + g$ is an R-homomorphism of M into M'.

Sum of R-Homomorphisms

Let M and M' be R-modules and $f : M \to M'$, $g : M \to M'$ be R-homomorphisms. Then the R-homomorphism, $f + g : M \to M'$ is called the sum of f and g.

Remark: The sum $f + g$ of R-homomorphisms, f and g is also called the pointwise sum of R-homomorphisms f and g.

Theorem 5: Let M and M' be R-modules. Then the set $\text{Hom}_R(M, M')$ is an abelian group under pointwise sum of R-homomorphisms.

Proof: Let $f : M \to M'$, $g : M \to M'$ be any two R-homomorphisms. Then as proved in Theorem 4, $f + g$ is an R-homomorphism. Thus, the pointwise sum of an R-homomorphisms is a binary operation on $\text{Hom}_R(M, M')$

We now observe the following properties:

Associativity: Let f, g, h be any three R-homomorphisms in $\text{Hom}_R(M, M')$. Then

$$[(f + g) + h](a) = (f + g)(a) + h(a) \qquad \text{[by definition of pointwise sum]}$$
$$= \{ f(a) + g(a) \} + h(a) \text{ [by definition of pointwise sum]}$$
$$= f(a) + \{ g(a) + h(a) \} \text{ [by associativity of additon on } M']$$
$$= f(a) + (g + h)(a)$$

$$= [f + (g+h)](a) \text{ for all } a \in M.$$

Thus, $(f+g)+h = f+(g+h)$ for all $f,g,h \in \text{Hom}_R(M,M')$.

So, pointwise sum is an associative binary operation on $f,g,h \in \text{Hom}_R(M,M')$.

Commutativity: Let f, g be any two R- homomorphism in $\text{Hom}_R(M,M')$. Then for all $a \in M$, we have

$$\begin{aligned}
(f+g)(a) &= f(a)+g(a) && \text{[by definition of pointwise sum]} \\
&= g(a)+f(a) && \text{[by commutativity of additon on } M'] \\
&= (g+f)(a) && \text{[by definition of pointwise sum]}
\end{aligned}$$

$$f+g = g+f \quad \text{[using definition of equality of two functions]}$$

So, pointwise sum is a commutative binary operation on $\text{Hom}_R(M,M')$.

Existence of identity: The mapping $\hat{0} : M \to M'$ given by $\hat{0}(a) = 0_{M'}$ for all $a \in M$ is an R-homomorphism. Also, for any $f \in \text{Hom}_R(M,M')$, we have

$$\begin{aligned}
(\hat{0} + f)(a) &= \hat{0}(a) + f(a) && \text{[by definition of pointwise sum]} \\
&= 0_{M'} + f(a) \\
&= f(a) \text{ for all } a \in M \\
& && [\because 0_{M'} \in M' \text{ is the additive identity}]
\end{aligned}$$

$$\therefore \qquad \hat{0} + f = f$$

$$\Rightarrow \qquad \hat{0} + f = f = f + \hat{0} \quad \text{[by commutativity of pointwise sum]}$$

Thus, $\hat{0} \in \text{Hom}_R(M,M')$ such that $f + \hat{0} = f = \hat{0} + f$ for all $f \in \text{Hom}_R(M,M')$.

So, $\hat{0}$ is the additive identity.

Existence of inverse: Let f be an arbitrary element of $\text{Hom}_R(M,M')$. Consider the mapping $-f : M \to M'$ defined by $(-f)(a) = -f(a)$ for all $a \in M$. It can be easily seen that $-f \in \text{Hom}_R(M,M')$. Also, for all $a \in M$, we have

$$[f + (-f)](a) = f(a) + (-f)(a) = f(a) - f(a)$$

Thus, for each $f \in \text{Hom}_R(M,M')$, there exists $-f \in \text{Hom}_R(M,M')$ such that

$$f + (-f) = \overline{0} = (-f) + f$$

So, each element in $\text{Hom}_R(M,M')$ possesses its inverse in $\text{Hom}_R(M,M')$.

Hence, $\text{Hom}_R(M,M')$ is an abelian group under the pointwise sum of R-homomorphisms.

Theorem 6: Let M_1, M_2, M_3 and M_4 be modules and let $f_1 : M_1 \to M_2, f_2 : M_1 \to M_2, f_3 : M_2 \to M_3$ and $f_4 : M_4 \to M_1$ be R-homomorphisms. Then

(i) $f_3 o(f_1 + f_2) = f_3 o f_1 + f_3 o f_2$

(ii) $(f_1 + f_2) o f_4 = f_1 o f_4 + f_2 o f_4$

Proof:

(i) Since f_1, f_2, f_3 and f_4 are R-homomorphisms,

therefore $f_1 + f_2, f_3 o(f_1 + f_2)$, $(f_1 + f_2) o f_4$, $f_3 o f_1$, $f_3 o f_2$, $f_1 o f_4$, $f_2 o f_4$, $f_3 o f_1$, $f_3 o f_1 + f_3 o f_2$ and $f_1 o f_4 + f_2 o f_4$ are also R-homomorphisms.

For all $a \in M_1$, we have

$$[f_3 o(f_1 + f_2)](a) = f_3 \left[(f_1 + f_2)(a) \right]$$

[by the def. of composition of functions]

$$= f_3 \left[f_1(a) + f_2(a) \right] \quad \text{[by the def. of pointwise sum]}$$

$$= f_3 f_1(a) + f_3 f_2(a)$$

$$[\because f_3 : M_2 \to M_3 \text{ is an } R\text{-homomorphism}]$$

$$\therefore \quad f_3 o(f_1 + f_2) = f_3 o f_1 + f_3 o f_2$$

[by the equality of two functions]

(ii) For all $a \in M_4$, we have

$$\left[(f_1 + f_2) o f_4 \right](a) = (f_1 + f_2)(f_4)(a)$$

[by def. of composition of functions]

$$= f_1(f_4(a)) + f_2(f_4(a))$$

[by def. of pointwise sum]

$$= (f_1 o f_4)(a) + (f_2 o f_4)(a)$$

$$\therefore \quad (f_1 + f_2) o f_4 = f_1 o f_4 + f_2 o f_4$$

Projection Mapping

Let N be an R-submodule of an R-module M. Then the mapping $p : M \to M/N$ given by $p(a) = a + N$, for all $a \in M$ is called projection mapping (or natural mapping or canonical mapping).

Theorem 7: Let N be an R-submodule of an R-module M and let $p : M \to M/N$ be the projection mapping. Then $\text{Ker}(p) = N$.

Proof: Let a be an arbitrary element of $\text{Ker}(p)$. Then

$$a \in \text{Ker}(p) \Leftrightarrow p(a) = N \Leftrightarrow a + N = N \Leftrightarrow a \in N$$

Hence $\text{Ker}(p) = N$.

Theorem 8: (Main theorem for quotient modules). Let M and M' be R-modules and N be an R-submodule of M. Then for each R-homomorphism $f : M \to M'$ with $\text{Ker}(f) \supset N$, there exists a unique R-homomorphism $\varphi : M/N \to M'$ such that $\varphi o p = f$, where $p : M \to M/N$ is the projection mapping.

Moreover, $I_m(\varphi) = I_m(f)$ and $\text{Ker}(\varphi) = \text{Ker}(f)/N$.

Proof: Consider the mapping $\varphi : M / N \to M'$ defined by

$$\varphi(a + N) = f(a) \text{ for all } a \in M .$$

We observe that φ is well defined because

$$a + N = b + N$$
$$\Rightarrow \quad a - b \in N$$
$$\Rightarrow \quad a - b \in \text{Ker}(f) \qquad\qquad\qquad\qquad\qquad [\because \text{ Ker}(f) \supset N]$$
$$\Rightarrow \quad f(a - b) = 0_{M'}$$
$$\Rightarrow \quad f(a) - f(b) = 0_{M'} \qquad\qquad\qquad [\because f \text{ is an } R\text{-homomorphism}]$$
$$\Rightarrow \quad f(a) = f(b)$$
$$\Rightarrow \quad \varphi(a + N) = \varphi(b + N)$$

We shall now show that φ is an R-homomorphism.

Let $a + N, b + N$ be any two arbitrary elements of M/N. Then

$$\varphi\big[(a + N) + (b + N)\big] = \varphi\big[(a + b) + N\big]$$
$$\qquad\qquad\qquad\qquad [\text{by definition of addition on } M/N]$$
$$= f(a + b) \qquad\qquad [\text{by definition of } \varphi]$$
$$= f(a) + f(b) \qquad [\because f \text{ is an } R\text{-homomorphism}]$$
$$= \varphi(a + N) + \varphi(b + N)$$

Now, let $a + N$ be an arbitrary element of M/N and let r be an arbitrary element of R. Then

$$\varphi\big[r(a + N)\big] = \varphi(ra + N)$$
$$\qquad\qquad [\text{by definition of scalar multiplication on } M/N]$$
$$= f(ra) \qquad\qquad [\text{by definition of } \varphi]$$
$$= rf(a) \qquad\qquad [\because f \text{ is an } R\text{-homomorphism}]$$
$$= r\varphi(a + N)$$

Thus,

$$\varphi\big[(a + N) + (b + N)\big] = \varphi(a + N) + \varphi(b + N)$$

and $\varphi[r(a + N)] = r\varphi(a + N)$ for all $a + N$, $b + N \in M / N$ and all $r \in R$.

Hence $\varphi : M / N \to M'$ is an R-homomorphism.

Since $\varphi : M / N \to M'$ and $p : M \to M / N$, therefore $\varphi o p : M \to M'$.

Also, $(\varphi o p)(a) = \varphi[p(a)] = \varphi(a + N) = f(a)$ for all $a \in M$.

So, $\qquad\qquad \varphi o p = f \qquad\qquad$ [by the definition of equality of functions]

Uniqueness of φ: If possible, let $\psi : M / N \to M'$ be an R-homomorphism such that $\psi o p = f$.

Then,

$$\psi o p(a) = f(a) \text{ for all } a \in M$$
$$\Rightarrow \quad \psi[p(a)] = f(a) \text{ for all } a \in M$$
$$\Rightarrow \quad \psi(a + N) = f(a) \text{ for all } a \in M$$
$$\Rightarrow \quad \psi(a + N) = \varphi(a + N) \text{ for all } a \in M$$
$$\Rightarrow \quad \psi = \varphi$$

Hence for each R-homomorphism $f : M \to M'$ with $\mathrm{Ker}(f) \supset N$, there exists a unique R-homomorphism $\varphi : M / N \to M'$ such that $\varphi op = f$.

Now, let a' be an arbitrary element of $I_m(\varphi)$. Then

$$a' \in I_m(\varphi) \Leftrightarrow \text{there exists } a + N \in M / N \text{ such that } \varphi(a + N) = a'$$
$$\Leftrightarrow \text{there exists } a \in M \text{ such that } \varphi[p(a)] = a'$$
$$\qquad\qquad\qquad\qquad [\, p : (M) \to M / N \text{ is onto}]$$
$$\Leftrightarrow \varphi op(a) = a' \qquad\qquad\qquad [\because \varphi op = f\,]$$
$$\Leftrightarrow a' \in I_m(f)$$
$$\therefore \ I_m(\varphi) = I_m(f)$$

Since $\mathrm{Ker}(f)$ and N are R-submodules of M such that $\mathrm{Ker}(f) \supset N$, therefore the symbol $\mathrm{Ker}(f)/N$ is meaningful.

Now,

$$a + N \in \mathrm{Ker}(\varphi)$$
$$\Leftrightarrow \varphi(a + N) = 0_{M'}$$
$$\Leftrightarrow \varphi[p(a)] = 0_{M'}$$
$$\Leftrightarrow \varphi op(a) = 0_{M'}$$
$$\Leftrightarrow f(a) = 0_{M'} \qquad\qquad\qquad\qquad [\because \varphi op = f\,]$$
$$\Leftrightarrow a \in \mathrm{Ker}(f)$$
$$\Leftrightarrow a + N \in \mathrm{Ker}(f)/N$$
$$\therefore \ \mathrm{Ker}(\varphi) = \mathrm{Ker}(f)/N$$

Theorem 9: (Fundamental theorem of an R-homomorphism). Let f be an R-homomorphism of an R-module M into an R-module M' with kernel N. Then $M / N \cong I_m(f)$.

Every R-homomorphic image of an R-module M is isomorphic to some quotient module of M.

Proof: Let f be an R-homomorphism of an R-module M and R-module M' with kernel N. Then by theorem 2, N and $I_m(f)$ are R-submodules of M and M' respectively.

If $a \in M$, then $a + N \in M / N$ and $f(a) \in I_m(f)$.

Consider the mapping $\varphi : M / N \to I_m(f)$ given by

$$\varphi(a + N) = f(a) \text{ for all } a \in M$$

First of all, we will show that φ is well defined, i.e. if $a, b \in M$ such that $a + N = b + N$, then, $\varphi(a + N) = \varphi(b + N)$.

Now, $a + N = b + N$
$$\Rightarrow a - b \in N \qquad\qquad\qquad\qquad [\because (N, +) \text{ is a group}]$$
$$\Rightarrow f(a - b) = 0_{M'} \qquad\qquad\qquad\quad [\because N = \mathrm{Ker}(f)]$$
$$\Rightarrow f(a) - f(b) = 0_{M'}$$
$$\Rightarrow f(a) = f(b)$$
$$\Rightarrow \varphi(a + N) = \varphi(b + N)$$

So, φ is well defined,

We shall show that $\varphi : M/N \to I_m(f)$ is an isomorphism.

φ is injective: Let $a+N, b+N$ be any two arbitrary elements of M/N. Then

$\varphi(a+N) = \varphi(b+N)$

$\Rightarrow f(a) = f(b)$

$\Rightarrow f(a) - f(b) = 0_{M'}$

$\Rightarrow f(a-b) = 0_{M'}$ $[\because f(a-b) = f(a) - f(b)]$

$\Rightarrow a-b \in N$ $[\because N = \text{Ker}(f)]$

$\Rightarrow a+N = b+N$

So, φ is an injective.

φ is surjective: Let a' be an arbitrary element of $I_m(f)$. Then there exists $a \in M$ such that $f(a) = a'$. But $f(a)$ is image of $a+N$ under $\varphi : M/N \to M'$ thus for each $a' \in I_m(f)$, there exists $a+N \in M/N$ such that

$$\varphi(a+N) = f(a) = a'$$

Consequently, φ is surjective.

φ is an R-homomorphism: Let $a+N, b+N$ be any two arbitrary elements of M/N and r be an arbitrary element of R. Then

$$\varphi[(a+N) + (b+N)] = \varphi[(a+b) + N] \qquad \text{[by def. of add. on } M/N]$$
$$= f(a+b) \qquad\qquad\qquad \text{[by def. of } \varphi]$$
$$= f(a) + f(b)$$
$$= \varphi(a+N) + \varphi(b+N)$$

and $\qquad \varphi[r(a+N)] = \varphi(ra+N)$
$$\text{[by def. of scalar multiplication on } M/N]$$
$$= f(ra) \qquad\qquad\qquad \text{[by def. of } \varphi]$$
$$= rf(a) \qquad\qquad \text{[}\because f \text{ is an } R\text{-homomorphism]}$$
$$= r\varphi(a+N)$$

Therefore, φ is an R-homomorphism.

Hence, $\varphi : M/N \to I_m(f)$ is an R-isomorphism. Consequently, $M/N \cong I_m(f)$.

Theorem 10: (Another form of the fundamental theorem of an R-homomorphism). Let M and M' be R-modules and φ be an R-epimorphism of M onto M' with kernel N. Then there exists a unique R-isomorphism ψ of M/N onto M' such that $\psi o p = \varphi$ where $p : M \to M/N$ is the projection mapping.

Proof: We have $\text{Ker}(\varphi) = N$. Therefore $\varphi(a) = 0_{M'}$ for all $a \in M$.

Let a be an arbitrary element of M. Then, $a+N \in M/N$.

For any $a+x \in a+N$, we have

$$\varphi(a+x) = \varphi(a) + \varphi(x) \quad [\because \varphi : M \to M' \text{ is an } R\text{-homomorphism]}$$

$$= \varphi(a) + 0_{M'} \qquad [\because \; x \in N = \text{Ker}(\varphi) \; \therefore \; \varphi(x) = 0_{M'}]$$
$$= \varphi(a)$$

Therefore, φ associates each $a + x \in a + N$ to a unique element $\varphi(a) \in I_m(\varphi)$. Thus, $\varphi(a + N) = \varphi(a)$.

Consider a mapping $\psi : M / N \to M'$ given by
$$\psi(a + N) = \varphi(a) \text{ for all } a \in M.$$

ψ is well defined because for each $a + N \in M / N$, $\varphi(a)$ is a unique element of M'.

Now,
$$(\psi o p)(a) = \psi[p(a)] = \psi(a + N) \qquad [\because \; p(a) = a + N]$$
$$= \varphi(a) \text{ for all } a \in M$$
$$\therefore \qquad \psi o p = \varphi$$

We shall show that $\psi : M / N \to M'$ is an R-isomorphism.

ψ is an R-homomorphism: For any $a + N, b + N \in M / N$ and $r \in R$, we have

$$\psi[(a + N) + (b + N)] = \psi[(a + b) + N] \qquad \text{[by def. of add. on } M/N]$$
$$= \varphi(a + b) \qquad \text{[by def. of } \varphi]$$
$$= \varphi(a) + \varphi(b)$$
$$[\because \; \varphi : M \to M' \text{ is an } R\text{-homomorphism}]$$
$$= \psi(a + N) + \psi(b + N)$$

and $\qquad \psi[r(a + N)] = \psi(ra + N)$
$$\text{[by def. of scalar multiplication on } M/N]$$
$$= \varphi(ra)$$
$$= r\varphi(a) \, [\because \; \varphi : M \to M' \text{ is an } R\text{-homomorphism}]$$
$$= r\psi(a + N)$$

So, $\psi : M / N \to M'$ is an R-homomorphism.

ψ is an injection: In order to prove this, it is sufficient to show that $\text{Ker}(\psi) = N$.

Now,
$$a + N \in \text{Ker}(\psi) \Leftrightarrow \psi(a + N) = 0_{M'} \Leftrightarrow \varphi(a) = 0_{M'} \Leftrightarrow a \in \text{Ker}(\varphi) = N$$
So, $\text{Ker}(\psi) = \text{Ker}(\varphi) = N$

Thus, $\psi : M / N \to M'$ is an injection.

ψ is a surjection: To prove that ψ is surjective, it is sufficient to show that $I_m(\psi) = M'$.

Let a' be an arbitrary element of $I_m(\psi)$. Then

$a' \in I_m(\psi) \Leftrightarrow$ there exists $a + N \in M / N$ such that $\psi(a + N) = a'$
$$\Leftrightarrow \psi(p(a)) = a' \qquad [\because \; p : M \to M / N \text{ is an } R\text{-epimorphism}]$$
$$\Leftrightarrow (\psi o p)(a) = a'$$
$$\Leftrightarrow \varphi(a) = a'$$
$$\Leftrightarrow a' \in I_m(\varphi) = M' \qquad [\because \; \varphi : M \to M' \text{ is surjective}]$$

Thus, $I_m(\psi) = I_m(\varphi)$. So, ψ is a surjection.

Hence ψ is an R-isomorphism of M/N onto M' such that $\psi op = \varphi$.

Uniqueness of ψ: Let $\psi': M/N \to M'$ be an isomorphism such that $\psi' op = \varphi$. Then

$$(\psi' op)(a) = \varphi(a) \quad \text{for all } a \in M$$
$$\Rightarrow \quad \psi'(p(a)) = \varphi(a) \quad \text{for all } a \in M$$
$$\Rightarrow \quad \psi'(a+N) = \varphi(a) \quad \text{for all } a \in M \qquad [\text{by def. of } p: M \to M/N]$$
$$\Rightarrow \quad \psi'(a+N) = \psi(a+N) \text{ for all } a+N \in M/N$$
$$[\text{by def. of } \psi: M/N \to M']$$

Hence, for each R-epimorphism $\varphi: M \to M'$, there exists a unique isomorphism $\psi: M/N \to M'$ such that $\psi op = \varphi$.

Theorem 11: (First isomorphism theorem for R-modules). Let N_1 and N_2 be R-submodules of an R-module M. Then

(i) $N_1 \cap N_2$ is an R-submodule of M.

(ii) $N_1 + N_2$ is an R-submodule of M.

(iii) $N_1/N_1 \cap N_2 \cong N_1 + N_2/N_2$.

Proof: For proofs of (i) and (ii) refer Theorems 1 and 5 respectively.

(iii) Since $N_1/N_2, N_1 + N_2$ and N_2 are R-submodules of an R-module M such that $N_1 \cap N_2 \subset N_1$ and $N_2 \cap N_1 \subset N_2$, therefore symbols $N_1/N_1 \cap N_2$ and $N_1 + N_2/N_2$ are meaningful.

Consider a mapping $\varphi: N_1 \to N_1 + N_2/N_2$ given by

$$\varphi(a) = a + N_2 \text{ for all } a \in N_1$$

Now, $a \in N$

$$\Rightarrow a \in N_1 + N_2 \qquad\qquad\qquad [\because N = N_1 + N_2]$$
$$\Rightarrow \varphi(a) = a + N_2 \in N_1 + N_2/N_2$$

Therefore, φ is well defined.

φ is an R-homomorphism: For any $a, b \in N$ and $r \in R$, we have

$$\varphi(a+b) = (a+b) + N_2 \qquad\qquad [\text{by definition of } \varphi]$$
$$= (a + N_2) + (b + N_2)$$
$$[\text{by definition of addition on } N_1 + N_2/N_2]$$
$$= \varphi(a) + \varphi(b), \text{ and}$$
$$\phi(ra) = ra + N_2 \qquad\qquad\qquad [\text{by definition of } \varphi]$$
$$= r(a + N_2) \qquad [\text{by definition of addition on } N_1 + N_2/N_2]$$
$$= r\varphi(a).$$

Thus, φ is an R-homomorphism.

φ is surjective: Let $a + N_2$ be an arbitrary element of $N_1 + N_2/N_2$.

Then $a = a_1 + a_2$ for some $a_1 \in N_1$, $a_2 \in N_2$.

Thus, for each $a + N_2 \in N_1 + N_2/N_2$, there exists $a_1 \in N_1$ such that

$$\varphi(a_1) = a_1 + N_2 = a_1 + (a_2 + N_2) \qquad [\because a_2 \in N_2 \Rightarrow a_2 + N_2 = N_2]$$
$$\Rightarrow \varphi(a_1) = (a_1 + a_2) + N_2 = a + N_2.$$

So, φ is surjective.

Hence, by the fundamental theorem of an R-homomorphism, we have
$$N_1 \mathrm{Ker}(\varphi) \cong N_1 + N_2 / N_2$$

Now, $a \in \mathrm{Ker}(\varphi)$

$\Leftrightarrow \varphi(a) = N_2$ and $a \in N_1$ $[\because N_2$ is additive identity in $N_1 + N_2 / N_2]$

$\Leftrightarrow a + N_2 = N_2$ and $a \in N_1$

$\Leftrightarrow a \in N_2$ and $a \in N_1$

$\Leftrightarrow a \in N_1 \cap N_2 \qquad \therefore \mathrm{Ker}(\varphi) = N_1 \cap N_2$

Hence $N_1 / N_1 \cap N_2 \cong N_1 + N_2 / N_2$.

Theorem 12: (Second isomorphism theorem for R-modules). If N_1 and N_2 are R-submodules of an R-module M such that $N_1 \supset N_2$, then
$$(M / N_2)/(N_1 / N_2) \cong M / N_1$$

Proof: Since N_1 and N_2 are R-submodules of an R-module M, therefore, M/N_1 and M/N_2 are meaningful.

Consider a mapping $\varphi : M / N_2 \to M / N_1$ given by
$\varphi(a + N_2) = a + N_1$ for all $a + N_2 \in M / N_2$

Clearly, φ is well defined.

φ is an R-homomorphism: For any $a + N_2,\ b + N_2 \in M / N_2$ and any $r \in R$, we have

$$\varphi\big[(a + N_2) + (b + N_2)\big] = \varphi\big[(a+b) + N_2\big] \quad \text{[by def. of add. on } M/N_2]$$
$$= (a+b) + N_1$$
$$= (a + N_1) + (b + N_1) \text{ [by def. of add on } M/N_1]$$
$$= \varphi(a + N_2) + \varphi(b + N_2)$$

and

$$\varphi\big[r(a + N_2)\big] = \varphi(ra + N_2) \text{ [by def. of scalar mult. on } M/N_2]$$
$$= ra + N_1 \qquad\qquad \text{[by def. of } \varphi]$$
$$= r(a + N_1) \text{ [by def. of scalar mult. on } M/N_1]$$
$$= r\varphi(a + N_2)$$

So, φ is an R-homomorphism.

φ is surjective: Let $a + N_1$ be an arbitrary element of M / N_1. Then, $a \in M$.

Now, $\qquad\qquad a \in M \Rightarrow a + N_2 \in M / N_2$

Thus, for each $a + N_1 \in M / N_1$, there exists $a + N_2 \in M / N_2$ such that $\varphi(a + N_2) = a + N_1$.

So, φ is surjective.

Hence, by the fundamental theorem of an R-homomorphism, we have
$$(M / N_2)\mathrm{Ker}(\varphi) \cong M / N_1$$

Let $a + N_2$ be an arbitrary element of $\text{Ker}(\varphi)$. Then

$a + N_2 \in \text{Ker}(\varphi)$

$\Leftrightarrow \quad \varphi(a + N_2) = N_1 \qquad\qquad [\because N_1 \text{ is the additive identity in } M/N_1]$

$\Leftrightarrow \quad a + N_1 = N_1 \qquad\qquad\qquad\qquad\qquad [\text{by def. of } \varphi]$

$\Leftrightarrow \quad a \in N_1 \qquad\qquad\qquad\qquad\qquad [\because N_1 \text{ is subgroup}]$

$\Leftrightarrow \quad a + N_2 \in N_1 / N_2 \qquad\qquad [\because N_1 \supset N_2 \ \therefore \ N_1 / N_2 \text{ exists}]$

$\therefore \quad \text{Ker}(\varphi) = N_1 / N_2$

Hence $\left(M / N_2 \right) / \left(N_1 / N_2 \right) \cong M / N_1$

Theorem 13: Let A and B be R-submodules of R-modules M and N respectively. Then

$$(M \times N)/(A \times B) \cong (M/A) \times (N/B)$$

Proof: Consider a mapping $\varphi : M \times N \to (M/A) \times (N/B)$ given by

$$\varphi(m,n) = (m + A, n + B) \text{ for all } m \in M, n \in N .$$

φ is an R-homomorphism: Let (m, n), (a, b) be any two elements of $M \times N$ and $r \in R$. Then

$$\varphi[(m,n) + (a,b)] = \varphi\big[(m + a, n + b)\big]$$

$$= ((m + a) + A, (n + b) + B)$$

$$= ((m + A) + (a + A), (n + B) + (b + B))$$

$$\qquad\qquad [\text{by def. of add. on } M/A \text{ and } N/B]$$

$$= (m + A, n + B) + (a + A, b + B)$$

$$\qquad\qquad [\text{by def. of addition on } M/A \times N/B]$$

$$= \varphi(m,n) + \varphi(a,b)$$

and

$$\varphi[r(m,n)] = \varphi(rm, rn) = (rm + A, rn + B)$$

$$= (r(m + A), r(n + B))$$

$$[\text{by def. of scalar multiplication on } M/A \text{ and } N/B]$$

$$= r(m + A, n + B) = r\varphi(m,n)$$

So, φ is an R-homomorphism.

φ is surjective: Let $(m + A, n + B)$ be an arbitrary element of $M/A \times N/B$. Then $m \in M$, $n \in N$ such that

$$\varphi(m,n) = (m + A, n + B)$$

So, φ is an R-homomorphism

Hence, by the fundamental theorem of an R-homomorphism, we have

$$(M \times N)/\text{Ker}(\varphi) \cong (M/A) \times (N/B)$$

Now,

$\Leftrightarrow \quad \varphi(m,n) = (0_M + A, 0_N + B)$

$\Leftrightarrow \quad (m + A, n + B) = (0_M + A, 0_N + B)$

$\Leftrightarrow \quad (m+A, n+B) = (A, B)$

$\Leftrightarrow \quad m \in A, \ n \in B$

$\Leftrightarrow \quad (m, n) \in A \times B$

$\therefore \quad \text{Ker}(\varphi) = A \times B.$

Hence $(M \times N)/(A \times B) \cong (M/A) \times (N/B)$

Example 4: For any ring R, show that the assignment $(a_1, a_2, a_3) \to (a_1, a_2)$ is an R-epimorphism $R^3 \to R^2$ of R-modules. If $D \subset R^3$ is the set of all triples $(0, 0, a_3)$, deduce that D is an R-submodule with $(R^3/D) \cong R^2$.

Solution: Let $\varphi : R^3 \to R^2$ be the given mapping. Then

$$\varphi(a_1, a_2, a_3) = (a_1, a_2) \text{ for all } (a_1, a_2, a_3) \in R^3$$

φ is an R-homomorphism: For any $(a_1, a_2, a_3), (b_1, b_2, b_3) \in R^3$ and any $\lambda, \mu \in R$, we have

$$\varphi\big[\lambda(a_1, a_2, a_3) + \mu(b_1, b_2, b_3)\big] = \varphi\big[\lambda a_1 + \mu b_1, \lambda a_2 + \mu b_2, \lambda a_3 + \mu b_3\big]$$

$$= \big(\lambda a_1 + \mu b_1, \lambda a_2 + \mu b_2\big) \quad [\text{by def. of } \varphi]$$

$$= \lambda(a_1, a_2) + \mu(b_1, b_2)$$

$$= \lambda\varphi(a_1, a_2, a_3) + \mu\varphi(b_1, b_2, b_3).$$

$\therefore$ φ is an R-homomorphism.

φ is surjective: Obviously $\varphi : R^3 \to R^2$ is surjective because for each $(a_1, a_2) \in R^2$, there exists $(a_1, a_2, a_3) \in R^3$ such that

$$\varphi(a_1, a_2, a_3) = (a_1, a_2)$$

Hence, $\varphi : R^3 \to R^2$ is an epimorphism of R-modules.

We have $D = \{(0, 0, a_3) : a_3 \in R\}$

Let (a_1, a_2, a_3) be an arbitrary element of $\text{Ker}(\varphi)$. Then

$$\varphi(a_1, a_2, a_3) = (0, 0) \Rightarrow (a_1, a_2) = (0, 0) \Rightarrow a_1 = 0 = a_2.$$

Thus, $(a_1, a_2, a_3) \in \text{Ker}(\varphi) \Leftrightarrow a_1 = a_2 = 0 \Leftrightarrow (0, 0, a_3) \in \text{Ker}(\varphi)$

$\therefore \quad \text{Ker}(\varphi) = D$

Hence, D is an R-submodule of R^3 and by the fundamental theorem of an R-homomorphism, we have $(R^3/D) \cong R^2$.

EXERCISE

1. Let $f : R^n \to R$ be the mapping defined by $f(a_1, a_2, ..., a_n) = a_i$ where i is fixed.

   Then show that f is an R-homomorphism of the R-module R^n onto the R-module R. This is called the projection of R^n onto the ith component.

2. Let $f : M \to N$ be an R-homomorphism of an R-module. If f is a bijection, then show that $f^{-1} : N \to M$ is an R-homomorphism.

3. Prove $\text{Hom}_Z(Q,Q) \cong Q$ as rings.

4. Let M be an R-module and $x \in M$ be such that $rx = 0$, $r \in R$, implies $r = 0$. Then show that $Rx \cong R$ as R-modules.

5. Let M be an R-module and $A, B, C\,D$ be submodules of M such that $M = A \oplus B = C \oplus D$. If $A = C$ and show that $B \cong D$.

6. Let $f : R \to S$ be a ring homomorphism and M be a left S-module. Show that M can be made into a left R-module.

7. Let $N_1, N_2, ..., N_k$ be a family of R-submodules of an R-module M such that $N_i + \left(N_1 \cap N_2 \cap ... \cap N_{i-1} \cap N_{i+1} ... \cap N_k \right) = M$ for all $i = 1, 2, ..., k$. Show that $\dfrac{M}{\overset{k}{\underset{i=1}{\cap}} N_i} \cong \left(\dfrac{M}{N_1} \times \dfrac{M}{N_2} \times ... \times \dfrac{M}{N_k} \right)$

11.9 ALGEBRA

Throughtout this section, unless otherwise stated, R is a commutative ring with unity.

R-Algebra

Let S be a ring. Then S is called an R-algebra (or an algebra over R) if S is a unitary R-module such that for all $r \in R$ and all $a, b \in S$

$$r(ab) = (ra)b = a(rb)$$

Any field F can be regarded as an algebra over itself because F is a module over itself and $r(ab) = (ra)b = a(rb)$ for all $a, b \in F$.

Example 1: Let R be a commutative ring with unity. Then the set $R[x]$ of all polynomials over ring R is an R-algebra.

Solution: $R[x]$ is a unitary R-module under addition of polynomials and multiplication of a polynomial by a scalar as scalar multiplication.

For any $f(x) = \sum_i a_i x^i, g(x) = \sum_i b_i x^i \in R[x]$ and any $r \in R$, we have

$$r\big(f(x)g(x)\big) = r\left\{ \sum_{j+k=i} \left(a_j b_k \right) x^i \right\}$$

[by def. of multiplication of polynomials]

$$\Rightarrow r\big(f(x)g(x)\big) = \sum_{j+k=i} \left\{ r\left(a_j b_k \right) x^i \right\}$$

[by def. of scalar multiplication on module $R[x]$ over R]

$$\Rightarrow \quad r(f(x)g(x)) = \sum_{j+k=i} \left\{ (ra_j)b_k \right\} x^i$$

[by associativity of multiplication on R]

$$\Rightarrow \quad r(f(x)g(x)) = (rf(x))g(x)$$

$$\Rightarrow \quad r(f(x)g(x)) = \sum_{j+k=i} \left\{ (a_j r)b_k \right\} x^i$$

[by commutativity of multipliation on R]

$$\Rightarrow \quad r(f(x)g(x)) = \sum_{j+k=i} \left\{ a_j (rb_k) \right\} x^i$$

[by associativity of multiplication on R]

$$\Rightarrow \quad r(f(x)g(x)) = f(x)(rg(x))$$

Hence $R[x]$ is an R-algebra.

Example 2 : Let M be a unitary R-module. Then $\text{End}_R(M)$ is an algebra over R.

Solution: $\text{End}_R(M) = \text{Hom}_R(M,M)$ is an R-module. Also, for any $f \in \text{End}_R(M)$

$(1f)(a) = 1f(a) = f(a)$ for all $a \in M$ [$\because M$ is a unitary R-module]

$\therefore \qquad 1f = f$ for all $f \in \text{End}_R(M)$.

Thus, $\text{End}_R(M)$ is an unitary R-module.

For any $f, g \in \text{End}_R(M)$ and any $r \in R$, we have

$[r(fg)](a) = r(fg)(a)$

[by definition of scalar multiplication on $\text{End}_R(M)$]

$$\Rightarrow \quad [r(fg)](a) = r(f(a)g(a)) \qquad \text{[by multiplication of } fg\text{]}$$

$$\Rightarrow \quad [r(fg)](a) = (rf(a)g(a)) \qquad \text{[by M-2 (iii)]}$$

$$\Rightarrow \quad [r(fg)](a) = (rf)(a)g(a)$$

[by definition of scalar multiplication on $\text{End}_R(M)$]

$$\Rightarrow \quad [r(fg)](a) = [(rf)g](a) \text{ for all } a \in M$$

[by def. of the product of functions]

$\therefore \qquad r(fg) = (rf)g$

Similarly, we have $r(fg) = f(rg)$.

Thus, $r(fg) = (rf)g = f(rg)$

for all $f, g \in \text{End}_R(M)$ and all $r \in R$

Hence, $\text{End}_R(M)$ is an R-algebra.

11.10 FREE MODULES

Throughout this section, unless otherwise stated, R is a non-trivial (non-zero) ring with unity, that is, $1 \neq 0$ and an R-module is unitary R-module.

Linear combination: Let $a_1, a_2, ..., a_n$ be elements of an R-module M and $\lambda_1, \lambda_2, ..., \lambda_n$ be elements of ring R. Then

$$\lambda_1 a_1 + \lambda_2 a_2 + ... + \lambda_n a_n \left(\text{or, } \sum_{i=1}^{n} \lambda_i a_i \right)$$

is called a linear combination of $a_1, a_2, ..., a_n$. It is also called a linear combination of the set $S = \{a_1, a_2, ..., a_n\}$. Since there are finite number of elements in S, it is also called a finite linear combination of S.

If S is an inifite subset of M, then a linear combination of a finite subset of S is called a finite linear combination of S.

Trivial Linear Combination

Let $a_1, a_2, ..., a_n$ be elements of an R-module M. Then the linear combination

$$\lambda_1 a_1 + \lambda_2 a_2 + ... + \lambda_n a_n$$

is called a trivial linear combination of $a_1, a_2, ..., a_n$ if $\lambda_1 = \lambda_2 = ... = \lambda_n = 0$.

Remark: The trivial linear combination of any set of elements of an R-module is always the zero $0_M \in M$ because

$$0a_1 + 0a_2 + ... + 0a_n = 0_M + 0_M + ... + 0_M = 0_M$$

Non-trivial Linear Combination

Let $a_1, a_2, ..., a_n$ be elements of an R-module M. Then a linear combination

$$\lambda_1 a_1 + \lambda_2 a_2 + ... + \lambda_n a_n$$

is called a non-trivial linear combination of $a_1, a_2, ..., a_n$ if at least one $\lambda_i \neq 0$.

Example 3: If $a_1, a_2, ..., a_n$ are elements of an R-module M, then the linear combination $1a_1 + 0a_2 + ... + 0a_n$ is a non-trivial linear combination.

Remark : Note that a non-trivial combination of elements of a set in an R-module M may or may not be the zero element of M. For example $1(2, -1, 0) + (-2)(1, -1, 1) + 0(0, -1, 2)$ is a non-trivial linear combination of $(2, -1, 0)$, $(1, -1, 1)$ and $(0, -1, 2)$ in R^3 and is zero element $(0, 0, 0)$ of R^3 while a non-trivial linear combination $1(2, -1, 0) + 2(1, -1, 1) + (0, -1, 2)$ is a non-zero element of R^3.

Linear Independence

A list $(a_1, a_2, ..., a_n)$ of elements of an R-module M is called linearly independent if for any $\lambda_1, \lambda_2, ..., \lambda_n \in R$,

$$\lambda_1 a_1 + \lambda_2 a_2 + ... + \lambda_n a_n \in 0_M$$
$$\Rightarrow \lambda_1 = \lambda_2 = ... = \lambda_n = 0$$

Equivalently, a list $(a_1, a_2, ..., a_n)$ of elements of an R-module M is linearly independent if the only linear combination of $a_1, a_2, ..., a_n$ that equals to the zero in M is trival.

Example 4: Show that, the set $R^n = \{a_1, a_2, ..., a_n\}$ is a free module over ring R.

Solution: The set $S = \left\{e_1^{(n)}, e_2^{(n)}, ..., e_n^{(n)}\right\}$ is a linear independent set in R^n.

Let $a = (a_1, a_2, ..., a_n)$ be an arbitrary element of R^n. Then

$$a = (a_1, 0, ..., 0) + (0, a_2, ..., 0) + ... + (0, 0, ..., a_n)$$
$$a = a_1(1, 0, ..., 0) + a_2(0, 1, ..., 0) + ... + a_n(0, 0, ..., a_n)$$
$$a = a_1 e_1^{(n)} + a_2 e_2^{(n)} + ... + a_n e_n^{(n)}$$
$$a = a_1 e_1 + a_2 e_2^{(n)} + ... + a_n e_n^{(n)}$$

a is a linear combination of $e_1^{(n)}, e_2^{(n)}, ..., e_n^{(n)}$.

Thus, each element of R^n is a linear combination of elements in S, Consequently, S generates R^n. Hence, S is a basis for R^n and thus, R^n is a free R-module.

Remark: The basis $\{e_1^{(n)}, e_2^{(n)}, ..., e_n^{(n)}\}$ is known as the standard basis for R^n.

Example 5: Show that $R(x)$ is a free R-module.

Solution: Consider the set $B = \{1, x, x^2, x^3, ...\}$.

B is linearly independent: For any $\lambda_0, \lambda_1, \lambda_2, ...,$ in R

$$\lambda_0 1 + \lambda_1 x + \lambda_2 x^2 + ... + \lambda_n x^n + ... = 0 \qquad \text{(zero polynomial)}$$

$$\Rightarrow \lambda_0 1 + \lambda_1 x + \lambda_2 x^2 + ... + \lambda_n x^n + ... = 0.1 + 0x + 0x + 0x^2 + ... + 0x^n + ...$$
$$\Rightarrow \lambda_0 = 0 = \lambda_1 = \lambda_2 = ... = \lambda_n ...$$

[by the def. of equality of poly.]

$\therefore$ B is a linearly independent set.

B generates $R(x)$: For any $f(x) = a_0 + a_1 x + a^2 x^2 + ...$ in $R[x]$, we have

$$f(x) = a_0 1 + a_1 x + a_2 x^2 + ...$$
$\Rightarrow f(x)$ is a linear combination of $1, x, x^2, ...$

$\therefore$ B generates $R[x]$. Hence, $R[x]$ is a free R-module.

Remark: The set $\{1, 1 + x, x^2, ..., x^n, ...\}$ is also a basis for $R[x]$.

Theorem 1: Show that a cyclic group regarded as a Z-module has a basis if it is infinite.

OR

Show that a cyclic group regarded as a Z-module is free Z-module if it is infinite.

Proof: Let $G = [a]$ be an infinite additive cyclic group with identity element 0.

First suppose G is an infinite cyclic group generated by a. We have to prove that G as a Z-module has a basis. Since G-$[a]$ is infinite, therefore, $a \neq \underline{0}$ (identity element). Clearly the set B-$\{a\}$ generates G because each element of G is an integral multiple of a. Since G is an infinite cyclic group generated by a, therefore order of a is infinite. Thus, $na \neq \underline{0}$ for any $n \in Z$. In other words, $na = \underline{0}$ only when $n = 0$. So, B is a linearly independent set. Hence, B is a basis for G.

Conversely, let $G = [a]$ be a Z-module such that it has a basis. then we have to prove that G is an infinite cyclic group. Since each element of G is an integral multiple of a, therefore elements in the basis of G are also integral multiples of a. Let ma, $m \in Z$ be some basis element. Then $n(ma) = \underline{0}$, $n \in Z$ must imply $n = 0$. However, if G is a finite group of order k, then

$$k(ma) = m(ka) = m(\underline{0}).$$
$$k(ma) = \underline{0} \text{ on contradiction}$$
$$[\because 0(G) = k \Rightarrow 0(a) = k \Rightarrow ka = \underline{0}]$$

Hence, G must be infinite if it has a basis.

It follows from the above discussion that an R-module may or may not have a basis and even if it has, it need not be unique.

Theorem 2: Let M be a free R-module with a basis B and N be an R-module. If $f:B \to N$ is any mapping, then there exists a unique R-homomorphism $\varphi : M \to N$ which is extension of f that is, $\varphi(x) = f(x)$ for all $x \in B$.

Proof: We will prove the theorem only in the case in which B is finite, leaving the infinite. Suppose $O(B) = n$ and $B = \{a_1, a_2, ..., a_n\}$. Set $f(a_i) = b_i \in N, i = 1, 2, ..., n$. Let a be an arbitrary element of M. Since it is free R-module with basis B, therefore a can be written uniquely as a linear combination of elements in B. Let

$$a = \lambda_1 a_1 + \lambda_2 a_2 + ... + \lambda_n a_n \in R$$

Consider a mapping $\varphi : M \to N$ given by

$$\varphi(a) = \lambda_1 f(a_1) + \lambda_2 f(a_2) + ... + \lambda_n f(a_n).$$

Clearly, φ exists because each $a \in M$ is uniquely expressible as a linear combination of elements $a_1, a_2, ..., a_n$ and $f(a_1), f(a_2), ..., f(a_n)$ exist.

We shall prove that $\varphi : M \to N$ is an R-homomorphism.

Let a,b be any two elements of M. Then there exist $\lambda_1, \lambda_2, ..., \lambda_n, \mu_1, \mu_2, ..., \mu_n \in R$ such that

$$a = \lambda_1 a_1 + \lambda_2 a_2 + ... + \lambda_n a_n, \quad b = \mu_1 a_1 + \mu_2 a_2 + ... + \mu_n a_n$$

$$\therefore \varphi(a+b) = \varphi[\lambda_1 a_1 + \lambda_2 a_2 + ... + \lambda_n a_n + \mu_1 a_1 + \mu_2 a_2 + ... + \mu_n a_n]$$

$$[\because B \text{ is a basis for } M]$$

$$\Rightarrow \varphi(a+b) = \varphi[(\lambda_1 + \mu_1)a_1 + (\lambda_2 + \mu_2)a_2 + ... + (\lambda_n + \mu_n)a_n]$$

$$[\text{by comm. and assoc. of add. on } M]$$

$$\Rightarrow \varphi(a+b) = (\lambda_1 + \mu_1) f(a_1) + (\lambda_2 + \mu_2) f(a_2) + ... + (\lambda_n + \mu_n) f(a_n)$$
$$\text{[by def.of } \varphi]$$

$\therefore$ φ is an R-homomorphism.

Hence φ: $\text{Hom}_R(F, M) \to M^n$ is an isomorphism. Consequently, $\text{Hom}_R(F, M) \cong M^n$.

Theorem 3: Let M and M' be R-modules and F be a free module over ring R. If $p: M \to M'$ is an R-epimorphism, then for each R-homo-morphism $f: M \to M'$ there exists an R-homomorphism $g: f \to M$ such that, $f = pog$.

Proof: Let B be the set of free generators for R-module F. Let x be an arbitrary element of B. Then

$$f(x) \in M' \qquad\qquad [\because f: F \to M']$$

$\Rightarrow$ There exists $a_x \in M$ such that $p(a_x) = f(x)$

$$[\because p: M \to M' \text{ is surjective}]$$

Consider a mapping $\varphi: B \to M$ given by

$$\varphi:(x) = a_x \text{ for all } x \in B.$$

Since F is a free R-module with basis B, therefore there exists an R-homomorphism $g: f \to M$ such that g is extension of ϕ. That is,

$$g(x) = a_x \text{ for all } x \in B.$$

Clearly, for any $x \in B$.

$$(pog)(x) = p[g(x)] = p(a_x) = f(x)$$

$\because$
$$pog\ (x) = f(x) \text{ for all } x \in B.$$

$\Rightarrow$
$$pog = f \text{ on } B \Rightarrow pog = f \text{ on } F. \quad [\because B \text{ is a basis for } F]$$

Theorem 4: Let F be a free module over a ring R and M be an R-module such that $f: M \to F$ is an R-epimorphism. Then M is direct sum of $\text{Ker}(f)$ and a submodule F' of M are R-isomorphic to F.

Proof: Since F is a free R-module and $f: M \to F$ is an R-epimorphism, therefore, by theorem 3 corresponding to the identity R-homomorphism - I_F, there exists an R-homomorphism $\varphi: F \to M$ such that $fo\varphi = I_F$.

Let $F' = I_m(\varphi)$. Then F' is an R-submodule of M. Clearly for each $x \in M, (\varphi of)(x) \in F'$.

Let $y = x - (\varphi of)(x)$. Then

$$f(y) = f(x - (\varphi of)(x))$$

$$F \cong F'. \qquad\qquad [\because f: M \to F \text{ is an } R\text{-homomorphism}]$$

$$\Rightarrow f(y) = f(x) - fo\varphi(f(x))$$

$$\Rightarrow f(y) = f(x) - I_F(f(x)) \qquad \left[\because fo\varphi = I_F\right]$$
$$\Rightarrow f(y) = f(x) - f(x) = 0_F$$
$$\therefore y \in \text{Ker}(f)$$

Thus, for each $x \in M, \varphi of(x) \in F'$ and $x - (\varphi of)(x) \in \text{Ker}(f)$ such that

$$x = \left[x - (\varphi of)(x)\right] + (\varphi of)(x)$$

Therefore, $M = \text{Ker}(f) + F'$

Let, $x \in \text{Ker}(f) \cap F'$. Then, $x \in \text{Ker}(f)$ and $x \in F'$

Now, $x \in F'$

$$\Rightarrow \text{There exists } a \in F', \text{ such that, } \varphi(a) = x \qquad \left[\because F' = I_m(\varphi)\right]$$
$$\Rightarrow f(\varphi(a)) = f(x)$$
$$\Rightarrow fo\varphi(a) = f(x)$$
$$\Rightarrow I_F(a) = f(x) \qquad \left[\because fo\varphi = I_F\right]$$
$$\Rightarrow f(x) = a$$

and, $x \in \text{Ker}(f) \Rightarrow f(x) = 0_F$

$$\therefore a = 0_F \in F$$
$$\Rightarrow \varphi(a) = \varphi(0_F) = 0_M \in M \Rightarrow x = 0_M \qquad \left[\because x = \varphi(a)\right]$$

Thus, $x \in \text{Ker}(f) \cap F' \Rightarrow x = 0_M$

$$\text{Ker}(f) \cap F' = \{0_M\}$$

Hence, $M = \text{Ker}(f) \oplus F'$.

Since $\varphi : F \to M$ restricts to an R-isomorphism, therefore $F \cong F'$.

Hence, M is direct sum of Ker (f) and an R-submodule which is an R-isomorphic to F.

EXERCISE

1. Every finitely generated module is homomorphic image of a finitely generated free module. **[Hint:** *See* Theorem 3]

2. Show that every module is a homomorphic image of a free module.

3. Show that every principal left ideal in an integral domain R with unity is free as a left R-module.

4. Show that every ideal of Z is free as Z-module.

5. Prove that the direct product $M_1 x M_2 x ... x M_n$ of free R-modules M_i is again free.

6. Let R be a commutative ring with unity and $e \neq 0, 1$ be an inpotent. Prove that R cannot be a free R-module.

7. Let $\{a_1, a_2, ..., a_n\}$ be a basis of a free R-module M. Prove that $M = Ra_1 \oplus Ra_2 \oplus ... \oplus Ra_n$.

11.11 FREE MODULES AND MATRICES

Let R be a ring with unity. Consider a linear mapping (an R-homomorphism) $t: R^n \to R^m$ from free R-module R^n to free R-module R^m. Since R^m and R^m are free R-modules with standard bases $\left(e_1^{(n)}, e_2^{(n)}, ..., e_n^{(n)}\right)$ and $\left(e_1^{(m)}, e_2^{(m)}, ..., e_m^{(m)}\right)$ respectively therefore a linear mapping $t: R^n \to R^m$ can be described completely by simply listing the images $t\left(e_1^{(n)}\right), t\left(e_2^{(n)}\right), ..., t\left(e_n^{(n)}\right)$ of n basis elements of R^n. Each of these n images is an element of R^m, thus a column of m scalars in R. Consequently, the whole list of columns $t\left(e_1^{(n)}\right), t\left(e_2^{(n)}\right), ..., t\left(e_n^{(n)}\right)$ is an $m \times n$ matrix A over ring R which can be written as a list $t\left(e_1^{(n)}\right), t\left(e_2^{(n)}\right), ..., t\left(e_n^{(n)}\right)$ of n columns $t\left(e_1^{(n)}\right), t\left(e_2^{(n)}\right), ..., t\left(e_n^{(n)}\right)$, where each $t\left(e_j^{(n)}\right), j \in n$ is a list of m scalars in R thus, each linear mapping $t: R^n \to R^m$ determines an $m \times n$ matrix A over ring R.

Conversely, let $A = \left[a_{ij}\right]$ be an $m \times n$ matrix over ring. R. Then A can be considered as a list $\left(A^1, A^2, ..., A^n\right)$ of n columns $A^1, A^2, ..., A^n$, where each column is a list of m scalars in R, that is, an element of free R-module R^m. Thus, the matrix A is a list of n elements (vectors) in R^m. Since R^m is free R-module with $\left(e_1^{(m)}, e_2^{(m)}, ..., e_m^{(m)}\right)$ as a basis therefore it can be written as

$$A^j = \sum_{i=1}^{m} a_{ij} e_i^{(m)}, a_{ij} \in R \text{ for all } i \in m$$

Consider a mapping φ from the set $\left\{e_1^{(n)}, e_2^{(n)}, ..., e_n^{(n)}\right\}$ of free generators of R^n to R^m given by the rule

$$\lambda A = \left(\lambda a_{ij}\right) \text{ for all } j \in n$$

Since R^n is free module over ring R with basis $\left\{e_1^{(n)}, e_2^{(n)}, ..., e_n^{(n)}\right\}$, therefore it can be extended to a unique linear mapping (or an R-homomorphism) $t_A: R_n \to R_m$ given by the rule

$$t_A\left(e_j^{(n)}\right) = A^j$$

$$\Rightarrow \quad t_A\left(e_j^{(n)}\right) = \sum_{i=1}^{m} a_{ij} e_i^{(m)} \text{ for all } j \in n$$

Thus, each $m \times n$ matrix $A = \left[\, a_{ij} \,\right]$ over ring R determines a unique linear mapping $t : R^n \to R^m$ given by

$$t_A\left(e_j^{(n)}\right) = \sum_{i=1}^{m} a_{ij} e_i^{(m)} \text{ for all } j \in n$$

This linear mapping is called **linear transformation or linear mapping or R-homomorphism** corresponding to matrix A and is denoted by t_A.

It follows from above discussion that the assignment is a bijection from the set $R^{m \times n}$ of all $m \times n$ matrices over ring R to the set $\hom_R(R^n, R^m)$ of all linear mappings from R-module R^n to R-module R^m.

Note: Throughout this section, R will be a ring with unity unless stated otherwise.

Theorem 1: Let A and B be $m \times n$ matrices over a ring R. Then,

$$t_{A+B} = t_A + t_B.$$

Proof: Let $A = \left[\, a_{ij} \,\right], B = \left[\, b_{ij} \,\right]$ be two $m \times n$ matrices over ring R. Then $A + B = \left[\, a_{ij} + b_{ij} \,\right]$ is an $m \times n$ matrix such that $(A + B)_{ij} = a_{ij} + b_{ij}$ for all $i \in m, j \in n$.

For any $j \in n$, we have

$$t_{A+B}\left(e_j^{(n)}\right) = \sum_{i=1}^{m} \left(a_{ij} + b_{ij}\right) e_i^{(m)}$$

$$\Rightarrow \quad t_{A+B}\left(e_j^{(n)}\right) = \sum_{i=1}^{m} \left[a_{ij} e_i^{(m)} + b_{ij} e_i^{(m)} \right]$$

$$\Rightarrow \quad t_{A+B}\left(e_j^{(n)}\right) = \sum_{i=1}^{m} a_{ij} e_i^{(m)} + \sum_{i=1}^{m} b_{ij} e_i^{(m)}$$

$$\Rightarrow \quad t_{A+B}\left(e_j^{(n)}\right) = t_A\left(e_j^{(n)}\right) + t_B\left(e_j^{(n)}\right)$$

$$\Rightarrow \quad t_{A+B}\left(e_j^{(n)}\right) = \left(t_A + t_B\right)\left(e_j^{(n)}\right)$$

$\therefore \quad t_{A+B} = t_A + t_B$ on the basis $\left\{e_1^{(n)}, e_2^{(n)}, ..., e_n^{(n)}\right\}$ of R^n.

Hence $t_{A+B} = t_A + t_B$ on R^n.

Theorem 2: Let A be a matrix over a commutative ring R. Then $t_{(\lambda A)} = \lambda t_A$ for all $\lambda \in R$.

Proof: Let $A = \left[a_{ij}\right]$ be an $m \times n$ matrix over a commutative ring R.

Then, $\lambda A = \left(\lambda a_{ij}\right)$ for all $\lambda \in R$.

For any $j \in n$ we have

$$t_A\left(e_j^{(n)}\right) = \lambda\left\{t_A\left(e_j^{(n)}\right)\right\}$$

$$\Rightarrow \quad t_A\left(e_j^{(n)}\right) = \sum_{i=1}^{m} \lambda(a_{ij})e_i^{(m)} \qquad [\because R^m \text{ is a left } R\text{-module}]$$

$$\Rightarrow \quad t_A\left(e_j^{(n)}\right) = \lambda\left\{\sum_{i=1}^{m} a_{ij}e_i^{(m)}\right\} \qquad [\because R^m \text{ is a left } R\text{-module}]$$

$$\Rightarrow \quad t_A\left(e_j^{(n)}\right) = \lambda\left\{t_A\left(e_j^{(n)}\right)\right\}$$

Since R is a commutative ring, therefore λ_{tA} is an R-homomorphism (or a linear mapping) given by

$$\left(\lambda_{tA}\right)\left(e_j^{(n)}\right) = \lambda\left[t_A\left(e_j^{(n)}\right)\right]$$

$$\therefore \quad t_{\lambda A}\left(e_j^{(n)}\right) = \left(\lambda_{tA}\right)\left(e_j^{(n)}\right) \text{ for all } j \in \underline{n}.$$

$$\Rightarrow \quad t_{\lambda A = \lambda_{tA}} \text{ on the basis } \left\{e_1^{(n)}, e_2^{(n)}, ..., e_n^{(n)}\right\} \text{ of } R^n.$$

Hence $t_{\lambda A} = \lambda_{tA}$ on R^n.

EXERCISE

1. Let $A = \left[a_{ij}\right]_{m \times n}$ and $B = \left[b_{ij}\right]_{n \times p}$ be two matrices over a commutative ring R. Then, prove that

   (i) $t_{(AB)}T = t_B T o t_A T$

   (ii) $t_{(AB)\lambda} = t_{A(B\lambda)} = t_{(A\lambda)B}$ for some scalar λ

2. Let s_i / r_1 and $B = \left[b_{ij}\right]_{n \times p}$ and $C = \left[c_{ij}\right]_{n \times p}$ be two matrices over a commutative ring R. Then

$$t_{(AB)C} = t_{A(BC)} = t_A o t_{BC} = t_A o (t_B o t c).$$

3. Let, $B = \left[b_{ij} \right]_{n \times p}$ and $C = \left[c_{ij} \right]_{n \times p}$ be two matrices over a commutative ring R. Then prove that

$$t_{A(B+C)} = t_A o (t_B + t_c) = t_A o t_B + t_A o t_C.$$

4. Let A be an $n \times n$ matrix over a commutative ring R and I be the identity matrix. Then

$$t_A = t_A o t_I$$

11.12 CYCLIC MODULES

Cyclic Module

An R-module M is called a cyclic module if it is generated by a single element in it.

Thus, an R-module M is called a cyclic module if there exists an element $a \in M$ such that $M = [a]$.

Example: Show that a cyclic module generated by a is $\{ ra + na : r \in R, n \in Z \}$ and if R has unity, then $Ra = \{ ra : r \in R \}$ is a cyclic module generated by a. Also $R = R.1$ shows that R is a cyclic module over itself and is generated by 1 shows that

$$Ra_1 + Ra_2 + ... + Ra_n = \{ r_1 a_1 + r_2 a_2 + ... + r_n a_n : r_i \in R \}$$

is a module generated by the set $\{ a_1, a_2, ..., a_n \}$ but it is not cyclic.

Theorem 1: Let R be an Euclidean ring. Then any finitely generated R-module is the direct sum of finite number of cyclic modules.

Proof: Let M be a finitely generated R-module of rank n. We will prove the theorem by induction on n. If $n=1$, then M is generated by a single element, hence it is cyclic and theorem is proved.

Suppose that the theorem is true for all R-modules of rank $(n-1)$. In other words, assume that each module of rank $(n-1)$ is the direct sum of finite number of its cyclic submodules.

We know that an R-module may have many minimal generating sets, so if $\{ a_1, a_2, ..., a_n \}$ is a minimal generating set of M such that

$$r_1 a_1 + r_2 a_2 + ... + r_n a_n = 0_M \Rightarrow r_1 a_1 = r_2 a_2 = ... = r_n a_n = 0_M$$

Then, obviously, M is direct sum of $N_1, N_2 ..., N_n$ where each N_i is a cyclic module generated by a_i. Thus, in this case the theorem is true for M.

Now, let $\{ a_1, a_2, ..., a_n \}$ be a minimal generating set for M such that $r_1 b_1 + r_2 b_2 + ... + r_n b_n = 0_M$ but not all $r_i a_i$ are 0_M.

Among all possible such relations for all minimal generating sets, let

$s_1 \in R$ be such that $d(s_1)$ is the smallest positive integer (d is Euclidean map). Let the minimal generating set for which it occurs be $\{b_1, b_2, ..., b_n\}$. Thus,

$$s_1 b_1 + s_2 b_2 + ... + s_n b_n = 0_M \text{ for some } s_i \in R \qquad ...(i)$$

We claim that if $\qquad r_1 b_1 + r_2 b_2 + ... + r_n b_n = 0_M \qquad ...(ii)$

then s_i / r_1.

Since $s_1, r_1 \in R$ is an Euclidean ring therefore there exists $p_1, q_1 \in R$ such that $r_1 = p_1 s_1 + q_1$, where either $q_1 = 0$ or $d(q_1) < d(s_1)$.

Multiplying equation (i) by p_1 and subtracting it from (ii), we obtain

$$(r_1 - p s_1) b_1 + (r_2 - p s_2) b_2 + ... + (r_n - p s_n) b_n = 0_M$$
$$\Rightarrow \quad q_1 b_1 + (r_2 - p_1 s_2) b_2 + ... + (r_n - p_1 s_n) b_n = 0_M$$
$$[\because r_1 = p_1 s_1 + q_1] \quad ...(iii)$$

If $\{b_i, b2, ..., b_n\}$, then $d(q_1) < d(s_1)$ and therefore equation (iii) contradicts that $d(s_1)$ is the smallest positive integer. Therefore, we must have

$$q_1 = 0 \Rightarrow r_1 = p_1 s_1 \Rightarrow s_1 / r_1.$$

We further claim that s_1 / s_i for $i = 2, 3, ..., n$ and to assert we show that, s_1 / s_2.

Since $s_1, s_2 \in R$, so there exist $p_2, q_2 \in R$, such that $s_2 = p_2 s_1 + q_2$ where either $q_2 = 0$ or $d(q_2) < d(s_1)$. Clearly, the set of elements $\{b_1' = b_1 + p_2 b_2 + ... + p_n b_n, b_2, b_3, ..., b_n\}$ generates M and

$$s_1 b_1' + q_2 b_2 + ... + s_n b_n = 0_M$$
$$= s_1 (b_1 + p_2 b_2) + q_2 b_2 + s_3 b_3 + ... + s_n b_n$$
$$= s_1 b_1 + (s_1 p_2 + q_2) b_2 + ... + s_n b_n = s_1 b_1 + s_2 b_2 + ... + s_n b_n = 0_M \quad ...(iv)$$

If $q_2 \neq 0$, then $d(q_2) < d(s_1)$. Therefore,

$s_1 b_1' + q_2 b_2 + ... + s_n b_n = 0_M$ contradicts our choice of s_1.

So we must have $q_2 = 0 \Rightarrow s_2 = p_2 s_1 \Rightarrow s_1 / s_2$.

Similarly, it can be shown that $s_1 / s_i, i = 3, ..., n$ and we can write $s_i = p_i s_1, i = 3, ..., n$.

Now the set $\{b_1' = b_1 + p_2 b_2 + ... + p_n b_n, b_2, b_3, ..., b_n\}$ is a generating set for R-module M. Let N_1 be the cyclic module generated by b_1 and N_2 be the R-submodule generated by $b_2, b_3, ..., b_n$. Then $M = N_1 + N_2$ since the set $\{b_i, b_2, ..., b_n\}$ generates M.

If $b \in N_1 \cap N_2$, then $b \in N_1 \cap N_2$, and $b \in N_2$.

Now, $b \in N_1 \Rightarrow b = \lambda_1 b_i$. for some $\lambda_1 \in R$ and $b \in N_2$

$\Rightarrow \quad b = \lambda_2 b_2 + ... + \lambda_n b_n$ for some $\lambda_2, \lambda_3, ..., \lambda_n \in R$

$\therefore \quad n \in N, R^n$

$\Rightarrow \quad \lambda_1 b_i - \lambda_2 b_2 - ... - \lambda_n b_n = 0_M$

$\Rightarrow \quad \lambda_1 (b_1 + p_2 b_2 + ... + p_n b_n) - \lambda_2 b_2 ... - \lambda_n b_n = 0_M$

$\Rightarrow \quad \lambda_1 b_1 + (\lambda_1 b_2 - \lambda_2) b_2 + ... + (\lambda_1 p_n - \lambda_n) b_n = 0_M$

$\Rightarrow \quad s_1 / \lambda_1$

$\Rightarrow \quad \lambda_1 = s_1 k_1$ for some $k_1 \in R$. $\hfill$ [Using (ii)]

Now,

$$b = \lambda_1 b_i = (s_1 k_1) b_i = k_1 (s_1 b_i) \qquad [\because \ R \text{ is commutative}]$$

$$b = k_1 \left[s_1 (b_1 + p_2 b_2 + ... + p_n b_n) \right]$$

$$b = k_1 \left[s_1 b_1 + s_1 (p_2 b_2) + ... + s_1 (p_n b_n) \right]$$

$$b = k_1 \left[s_1 b_1 + s_1 (p_2 s_1) b_2 + ... + (p_n s_1) b_n \right]$$

$$b = k_1 \left[s_1 b_1 + s_2 b_2 + ... + s_n b_n \right] \qquad [\because s_i = p_1 s_1 \text{ for all } i = 2, 3, ..., n]$$

$$b = k_1 0_M = 0_M \qquad\qquad\qquad\qquad [\text{Using eq. (iv)}]$$

Thus, $b \in N_1 \cap N_2 \Rightarrow b = 0_M$

$\therefore \qquad\qquad N_1 \cap N_2 = \{0_M\}$

Hence $M = N_1 \oplus N_2$.

Since, M_2 is generated by $b_2, b_3, ..., b_n$, its rank is $(n-1)$. So by induction assumption N_2 is the direct sum of cyclic submodules. Hence M is direct sum of cyclic modules.

Corollary: A finite abelian group is the direct product (sum) of cyclic groups.

Proof: It is a simple consequence of the main theorem as a module is an abelian group.

Theorm 2: Let R be a ring with unity. An R-module M is cyclic iff $M \cong \dfrac{R}{I}$ for some left ideal I of R.

Proof: First, let M be a cyclic module generated by a. Then $M = Ra$.

Let $= \{r \in R : ra = 0_M\}$.

Let us first show that I is a left ideal of R.

Clearly, $0 \in R$ and $0a = 0_M \Rightarrow 0 \in I \Rightarrow I$ is non-void subset of R.

Let $r_1, r_2 \in I$. Then

$r_1 a = 0_M$ and $r2a = 0_M$

$\Rightarrow \quad r_1 a - r_2 a = 0_M$

$\Rightarrow \quad (r_1 - r_2) a = 0_M$

$\Rightarrow \quad r_1 - r_2 \in I \qquad [\because \text{ multiplication is distributive over addition}]$

Let $r \in R$ and $r_1 \in I$. Then

$$r_1 a = 0_M$$

$$\Rightarrow \quad r(r_1 a) = r 0_M$$

$$\Rightarrow \quad (r r_1) a = 0_M \quad [\because r 0_M = 0_M \text{ and multiplication is associative on } R]$$

$$\Rightarrow \quad r_1 r_1 \in I$$

So, I is a left ideal of R.

Consider a mapping $f : R \to M$ defined by $f(r) = ra$ for all $r \in R$. f is an R-homomorphism: Let $r, s, t \in R$. Then

$$\begin{aligned} f(r+s) &= (r+s)a \\ &= ra + sa \\ &= f(r) + f(s) \\ f(tr) &= (tr)a \\ &= t(ra) \\ &= tf(r) \end{aligned}$$

So, f is an R- homomorphism

f is onto: Let $x \in M$. Then $x = ra$ for some $r \in R$.

Thus, for each $x \in M$, there exists $r \in R$ such that $f(r) = ra = x$

So, $f : R \to M$ is onto.

Kernel of f is I Let $r \hat{I}$ Ker (f). Then

$$r \in \text{Ker}(f) \Leftrightarrow f(r) = 0_M \in M^- \Leftrightarrow ra = 0_M \Leftrightarrow r \in I$$

$$r \in \text{Ker}(f) = I.$$

Hence, by the fundamental theorem on an R-homomorphisms $\dfrac{R}{I} \cong M$.

Conversely, let R be a ring with unity and M be an R-module such that $M \cong \dfrac{R}{I}$ for some left ideal L of R. We have to prove that M is cyclic.

Let $I + a \in \dfrac{R}{I}$. Then

$$(I+1)(I+a) = I + (1a) \qquad [\because R \text{ is a ring with unity} \therefore I \in R]$$

$$\Rightarrow \quad (I+1)(I+a) = I + a$$

Thus, each element $I + a$ of $\dfrac{R}{I}$ is of the form $(I+1)(I+a)$.

So, $\dfrac{R}{I}$ is a left R-module generated by $1 + I$, i.e. $1 + R(1+I) = \dfrac{R}{I}$.

Consequently, $\dfrac{R}{I}$ is a cyclic module generated by $1 + I$

But, $M \cong \dfrac{R}{I}$. Hence M is a cyclic module.

11.13 NOETHERIAN AND ARTINIAN MODULES

Ascending Chain Condition

An R-module M is said to possess ascending (descending) chain condition on R-submodules, if for every ascending (descending) sequence of R submodules of M

$$M_1 \subset M_2 \subset M_3 ... \left(M_1 \supset M_2 \supset M_3 ...\right),$$

there exists a positive integer k, such that,

$$M_k = M_{k+1} = M_{k+2} = ...$$

Thus, ascending chain condition (abbreviated as Acc) means that every ascending sequence of R-submodules is finite. Similarly, descending chain condition (abbreviated as Dec) means that every descending sequence of R-submodules is finite.

Noetherian Module

An R-module M is called noetherian (artinian) if Acc (Dcc) for submodules holds in M.

If an R-module M is noetherian (artinian), then we also say that M has Acc (Dec) on submodule or simply that M has Acc (Dcc).

Example 1: Show that the ring Z of integers as a Z-module is noetherian but not artinian.

Solution: In fact, any ascending chain of ideals in Z starting with n can have at most n district terms. This shows that Z as a Z-module is noetherian. But Z as a Z-module has an infinite properly descending chain.

$$[n] \supset \left[n^2\right] \supset \left[n^3\right] \supset ...$$

of ideals (submodules) showing that Z is not artinian Z-module.

Example 2: Let P be the additive group of rational numbers whose denominators are powers of a fixed prime p, i.e.

$$P = \left\{\dfrac{m}{p^k} : m \in Z, k = 0, 1, 2, ...\right\}$$

Then P is an abelian group. Therefore, P is a Z-module. We have the ascending chain of submodules.

$$Z \subset \left[\frac{1}{p}\right] \subset \left[\frac{1}{p_2}\right] \subset \left[\frac{1}{p_3}\right] \subset \dots$$

It can be easily seen that the submodules of this chain are the only submodules of P containing Z. Therefore, $M = P/Z$ is artinian but not noetherian. On the other hand, since Z is a submodule of P, therefore P is a neither artinian nor noetherian.

Example 3: Every finite dimensional vector space is both noetherian and artinian.

Solution: Let V be an n-dimensional vector space over a field F. Let $S_1 \subset S_2 \subset S_3 \subset \dots \subset V \left(S_1 \supset S_2 \supset S_3 \dots \supseteq\right)$ be an ascending (or a descending) chain of subspaces of V. We know that if s is a proper subspace of V, then $\dim S < \dim V = n$. Thus, any properly ascending (or descending) chain of subspaces cannot have more than $n+1$ terms. Hence, V is both noetherian and artinian.

Before we give more examples, let us prove some theorems which provide us criteria for a module to be noetherian or artinian.

Theorem 1: An R-module M is noetherian iff every submodule of M is finitely generated.

Proof: Let M be a noetherian R-module. Then we have to show that every R- submodule of M is finitely generated. If possible, let N be an R-submodule of M which is not finitely generated. Then no finite list of its elements can generate N. Let $a_1 \in N$ and N_1 be the submodule generated by a_1. Clearly, $N_1 \subset N$. Choose $a_2 \in N$ such that $a_2 \notin N_1$. Let N_2 be the submodule generated by $\{a_1, a_2\}$. Then $N_1 \subset N_2$. Again by the same argument there exists an element $a_3 \in N$ such that $a_3 \notin N_2$. Let N_3 be the submodule generated by the set $\{a_1, a_2, a_3\}$. Then $N_1 \subset N_2 \subset N_3$. Proceeding in this manner, we obtain a properly ascending chain

$$N_1 \subset N_2 \subset N_3 \dots$$

of R-submodules of M which is not finite, this contradicts the fact that M is noetherian. Hence, every R-submodule of M is finitely generated. Conversely, let M be an R-module such that every R-submodule of M is finitely generated. Then we have to show that M is noetherian.

Let $N_1 \subset N_2 \subset N_3 \subset \dots$ be an ascending chain of R-submodules of M, and let $N = \cup N_i$. Then N is an R-submodule of M. Since each R-submodule of M is finitely generated, therefore it is N. Let $N = \{a_1, a_2, \dots, a_n\}$. Since each $a_i \in N$ and $N = \cup N_i$, therefore each a_i is in some module of the sequence, say N_{mi}. Let $m = \max\left(m_1, m_2, \dots, m_n\right)$. Then all a_i are in N_m. So $N_m = N$.

Hence $N_m = N_{m+1} = ... = N$

Consequently, M is noetherian.

Maximal Element

Let M be an R-module and S be a non-void family of R-submodules of M. Then an element M_0 of S is said to be maximal in S if for each N_0 in S

$$N_0 \supset M_0 \Rightarrow N_0 = M_0.$$

In other words, an R-submodule M_0 is maximal in S iff there exists no R-submodule N_0 in S satisfying $M_0 \subset N_0$.

Theorem 2: An R-module M is noetherian iff every non-void family S of R-submodules of M has a maximal elements.

Proof: Let M be a noetherian R-module and S be a non-void family of R-submodules of K. Let N_1 be an element of S. If N_1 is not maximal, then it is properly contained in an R-submodule $N_2 \in S$. If N_2 is maximal, then theorem is proved. If N_2 is not maximal, then it is properly contained in an R-submodule $N_3 \in S$. In case, S has no maximal element, we obtain an infinite sequence $N_1 \subset N_2 \subset N_3 \subset ...$ of R-submodules of M. This contradicts the fact that M is noetherian. Hence, S has a maximal element.

Conversely, let every non-void family of R-submodules of M has a maximal element. Then we have to prove that M is noetherian R-module. Let $N_1 \subset N_2 \subset N_3 \subset ...$, be an ascending chain of R-submodules of M. Then by hypothesis, the family S of all these submodules has a maximal element, say N_k. But then $N_k = N_{k+1} = ...$. Hence M is noetherian.

Combining Theorems 1 and 2, we obtain the following theorem.

Theorem 3: Let M be an R-module. Then the following are equivalent.
  (i) M is noetherian
 (ii) Every submodule of M is finitely generated.
(iii) Every non-void family S of submodules of M has a maximal element.
  The following theorem is dual to the above theorem.

Theorem 4: Let M be an R-module. Then the follwing are equivalent.
  (i) M is artinian.
 (ii) Every submodule of M is finitely generated.
(iii) Every non-void family S of submodules of M has a minimal element (that is, a submodule M_0 in S, such that, for any submodule N_0 in S with $N_0 \subset M_0$ we have $N_0 \subset M_0$.

Proof: Left as an exercise for the reader.

Let us now discuss some properties of noetherian modules.

Theorem 5: Any submodule of a noetherian (artinian) module is noetherian.

Proof: Let N be an R-submodule of a noetherian R-module M. Since any R-submodule of N is also an R-submodule of M, therefore any ascending chain of R-submodules of N is also of M. But M is noetherian. Therefore, N is also noetherian.

Theorem 6: Every R-homomorphic image of a noetherian (artinian) R-module is noetherian.

Proof: Let M' be an R-homomorphic image of a noetherian R-module M under an R-homomorphic f. Then by the fundamental theorem of R-homomorphism

$$M/\text{Ker}(f) \cong M'$$

We know that, each R-submodule as $M/\text{Ker}(f)$ is of the form $N/\text{Ker}(f)$, where N is an R-submodule of M contaning $\text{Ker}(f)$.

Since M is noetherian, therefore N is finitely generated. Let $\{a_1, a_2, ..., a_n\}$ be the set of generators of N.

Then the set $\{a_1 + \text{Ker}(f), a_2 + \text{Ker}(f), ..., a_n + \text{Ker}(f)\}$ would generate $N/\text{Ker}(f)$ Therefore every submodule of $N/\text{Ker}(f)$ is finitely generated. Consequently, every R-submodule $M/\text{Ker}(f)$ is finitely generated and thus $M/\text{Ker}(f)$ is noetherian. Hence M' is noetherian.

Theorem 7: Let M be an R-module and N be an R-submodule of M. Then, M is noetherian (artinian) iff both N and M/N are noetherian (artinian).

Proof: Let M be a noetherian R-module. Then by theorems 5 and 6, N and M/N are noetherian.

Conversely, let N and M/N be noetherian and let

$$N_1 \subset N_2 \subset N_3 ...$$

be an ascending chain of R-submodules of M contained in N. Since N is noetherian, therefore, there exists a positive integer n such that $N_1 \cap N = N_{n+k} \cap N$ for all k.

But for all k, $N_k + N$ is an R-submodule of M containng N. Therefore

$$(N_1 + N/N) \subset (N_2 + N/N) \subset (N_3 + N/N) \subset ...$$

is an ascending chain of R-submodules of M/N. As M/N is noetherian there exists a positive integer m such that

$$N_1 \cap N = N_{n+k} \cap N \text{ for all } k.$$

If $n_0 = \max(n, m)$, then

$$N_n \cap N = N_{n_0} \cap N \text{ and } \cap N(N_n + N/N) = (N_{n_0} + N/N) \text{ for all } n \geq n_0$$

But, then, $N_n + N = N_{n_0} + N$ for all $n \geq n_0$.

We claim that $N_n = N_{n_0}$ for all $n \geq n_0$.

To establish our claim, we proceed as follws:

For all $n \geq n_0$, we have

$$N_n = N_n \cap (N_n + /N) = N_n \cap (N_{n_0} + N)$$

$$[\because N_n + N = N_{n_0} + N \text{ for all } n \geq n_0]$$

$$'N_n = N_{n_0} + (N_n \cap N) \qquad [\because N_{n_0} \subset N_n \text{ for all } n \geq n_0]$$

$$N_n = N_{n_0} + (N_{n_0} \cap N) \qquad [\because N_n \cap N = N_{n_0} \cap N \text{ for all } n \geq n_0]$$

$$N_n = N_{n_0} \qquad\qquad [\because N_{n_0} \cap N \cap N_{n_0}]$$

Thus, $N_n = N_{n_0}$ for all $n \geq n_0$

Hence, there exists a positive integer n_0 such that $N_n = N_{n_0 + k}$ for all k.
Hence M is noetherian.

EXERCISE

1. Mark each of the following as true or false.
    (i) An R-homomorphism is a homomorphism of abelian groups.
    (ii) The trivial linear combination of any set of elements of an R-module M is not necessarily the zero in M.
    (iii) Every subset of a linearly independent set is linearly independent.
    (iv) Every superset of a linearly independent set is linearly independent.
    (v) The void set is linearly independent.
    (vi) Every R-module is a free R-module.
    (vii) $\{0_M\}$ is a free R-module.
    (viii) For each $n \in N, R^n$ is a free R-module, where R is a commutative ring with unity.
    (ix) Every R-module has a basis.
    (x) Any two bases for an R-module over a commutative ring R have the same number of elements.
    (xi) Every noetherian module is artinian.
    (xii) Every artinian module is noetherian.
    (xiii) Every finite abelian group is both noetherian and artinian.
    (xiv) Any submodule of a noetherian (artinian) module is noetherian (artinian).
    (xv) Every R-homomorphic image of a noetherian (artinian) module is noetherian (artinian).
2. If M is an irreducibel R-module such that $ra \neq 0_M$ for some $r \in R$ and $a \in M$, prove that end (M), i.e. the set of all homomorphisms from M to itself is a division ring.
3. Let M and M^1 be R-modules and $f : M \to M'$ be an R-epimorphism with kernel N. Then M is noetherian if M' and N are noetherian.
4. Prove that Q is not a noetherian Z-module.

5. If F is a field, then show that an F-module M is noetherian iff it is finite dimensional.

6. Let R be a commutative ring with unity and $e \neq 0$. 1 be an idempotent. Prove that R_e cannot be a free R-module.

7. Prove that the direct product $M_1 x M_2 x ... x M_k$ of free R-modules M_i is again a free R-module.

8. Prove that Q is not a free Z-module.

Answers

1. i. T		ii. F		iii. T		iv. F		v. T	
vi. T		viii. T		ix. F		x. T		xi. F	
xii. F		xiii. T		xiv. T		xv. T			

Index